D0627434

ICDA

VOLUME 2
Alphabetical Index

EIGHTH REVISION INTERNATIONAL CLASSIFICATION OF DISEASES,

ADAPTED

FOR USE IN THE

UNITED STATES

U.S. DEPARTMENT OF HEALTH, EDUCATION, AND WELFARE
PUBLIC HEALTH SERVICE
NATIONAL CENTER FOR HEALTH STATISTICS

For sale by the Superintendent of Documents, U.S. Government Printing Office
Washington, D.C. 20402 – Price $4.50 (cloth)

PUBLIC HEALTH SERVICE PUBLICATION NO. 1693, VOL. 2
December 1968

CONTENTS

INTRODUCTION

INTRODUCTION

This volume of the *International Classification of Diseases Adapted for Use in the United States* (ICDA) is the alphabetical index to the Tabular List of Volume 1. Although the Index reflects the provisions of the Tabular List with regard to the notes which affect the assignment of a code number to a diagnostic term when it is reported with other conditions, or under particular circumstances (e.g., certain conditions arising during pregnancy), it is not possible to express all such variations in the index terms. Hence, the Tabular List should be regarded as the primary coding tool. Reference should always be made back to the Tabular List and its notes to ensure that the code given by the Index fits the circumstances of a particular case.

The Index is, however, an essential adjunct to the Tabular List, since it contains a great number of diagnostic terms which do not appear in Volume 1. The terms included in a category of the Tabular List are not exhaustive; they serve as examples of the content of the category. The Index, on the other hand, is intended to include most diagnostic terms currently in use.

Because of its exhaustive nature, the Index inevitably includes many imprecise and undesirable terms. Since these terms are still occasionally encountered on medical records, coders need an indication of their assignment in the Classification, even if this is to a rubric for residual or ill-defined conditions. The presence of a term in this volume, therefore, should not be taken as sanction for its usage in good medical terminology. The ICDA is in no sense a medical nomenclature.

GENERAL ARRANGEMENT OF THE INDEX

Main Sections

The Alphabetic Index consists of four sections, as follows:

Section I. — Alphabetic index of diseases (categories 000–796), including causes of fetal deaths; the nature and anatomic site of injury (fracture, dislocation, open wound, burn, etc., categories 800–999), except for adverse effects of specific drugs and of other chemical substances (see Section III); and of the Supplementary Classifications (Y00–Y30), including those for special conditions and examinations without sickness, classification of liveborn infants according to type of birth, and a category for use in identifying fetal deaths occurring in hospitals so that a total count of births in the hospitals may be obtained. These types of terms are included in Section I because they constitute the kind of report of the case as it would be given by an attending physician or on a clinic or hospital record.

Section I also includes references to the numbers in the *Hospital Formulary of the American Hospital Formulary Service.*[1] In coding adverse effects of new drugs or of drugs not shown in Section III, the Hospital Formulary list number for that particular drug should be determined from the current edition of this publication. By turning to the numerical sequence of the Hospital Formulary number in the Index under "Effect, adverse," the appropriate ICDA category number can be found.

Section II. — Index to the external cause of injury (categories E800–E999) except for poisoning (see Section III). These items are not medical diagnoses. They are descriptions of the circumstances under which the accident or violence occurred, and of the means of injury. This section includes such terms as fire, explosion, fall, assault, collision, and submersion.

Section III. — Index to adverse effects of drugs and chemical substances. It includes the codes for adverse effects of chemical substances (categories 960–989) and the external cause of injury codes for accidental poisoning (E850–E877), suicide and self-inflicted injury by poisoning (E950–E952), and poisoning undetermined whether accidentally or purposely inflicted (E980–E982). The purpose of this section on poisonous agents is to provide both of the relevant codes, N and E, from a single reference to the Index. Some effects of drugs and other chemical substances (e.g., contact dermatitis) are not classified to N and E codes, but to disease codes. If there is any doubt whether the effect in a particular case is one of these, a search should be made for the term in Section I.

---

[1] Published by the American Society of Hospital Pharmacists, Washington, D.C. 20014.

Section IV. – Index to operations and nonsurgical procedures (categories 01–99, A1–A9 and R1–R9).

Structure

To avoid repetition, the Index is organized in the form of lead terms, which start at the extreme left of a column, and show various levels of indentation, progressing further and further to the right. A complete index term, therefore, may be comprised of several lines, sometimes quite widely separated. For example, in the entry

```
Atrophy, atrophic
  muscle, muscular      733.1
    progressive      348.2
      spinal      348.2
        specified as hereditary or familial      330.1
      pseudohypertrophic      330.3
      spinal      348.2
        Aran-Duchenne      348.2
        familial      330.1
```

the last line stands for "Atrophy muscular spinal familial."

Usually, the lead term is the name of a disease or pathological condition, while the terms indented beneath it refer either to varieties of this condition or to the anatomical sites affected by it. The disease condition should be looked up first as a lead term and then the anatomical site in alphabetical order below it. Thus, "tuberculosis of hip" will be found under T, not under H, and "stomach ulcer" under U, not under S. The adjectival forms of the disease name have frequently been placed on the same line as the noun form, e.g., "Paralysis, paralytic," indicating that one or the other of these terms may appear in combination with the terms indented beneath them. General adjectives such as "chronic," "diffuse," "epidemic" and "hereditary" usually appear in their alphabetical sequence in the Index with the instruction "*see* condition," which means that the disease name is to be looked up rather than the adjectival modifier. For example, to find "chronic bronchitis," look under B for "Bronchitis, chronic" and not under C for "Chronic." "Acute" and "chronic" may be omitted even as a second or later word in the disease name as listed in the Index, unless the two forms of the disease have different code numbers. Some important modifiers do, however, appear also as lead terms. Thus "typhoid fever" will be found under T as well as under F. Under the terms "Delivery," "Pregnancy," "Puerperal" and "Birth" appear fairly complete listings of conditions frequently qualified by these terms, in addition to the alphabetical listings of the conditions themselves with the qualifying terms as indents. In general, the anatomical site will follow in the Index immediately under the pathological condition, with any further descriptive adjective in the third indentation. It is not always feasible, however, to include a complete listing of the various combinations of modifiers which could apply to a given term. For example, under the lead term "Abscess" are indented a large number of anatomical sites with their appropriate codes. However, tuberculous abscesses are not classified to these codes but to the codes for tuberculosis of these sites. Instead of inserting an indent "tuberculous" under each anatomical site, the Index uses one single indent "tuberculous — *see* Tuberculosis, abscess" under the lead term "Abscess." In general, the types of modifiers which are not listed under each term to which they may apply are: in Section I, those indicating that a disease or condition was infectious or parasitic, malignant, neoplastic, psychogenic, hysterical, congenital, traumatic, or arose during pregnancy, childbirth or the puerperium; in Section II, those indicating transport accidents, complications of medical or surgical procedures, late effects, suicide and self-inflicted injury, homicide and assault, legal intervention, or war operations. The terms "Complications" (for medical and surgical procedures), "Late effect," "Suicide," "Assault," "Legal intervention," and "War operations" also appear as lead terms with complete lists of the appropriate categories indented under them.

In Section II (External Cause of Injury), the lead term is usually the description of the type of accident or violence, with the agency in the subordinate position. Thus, all collisions are indexed under C, with the type of vehicles involved indented below, and not under motor vehicle, railway train, etc.

Neoplasms. — A comprehensive list of the sites of neoplasms is found in the Index under "Neoplasm" where code numbers appear in three columns for "Malignant," "Benign," and "Unspecified," respectively. Terms such as "Carcinoma," "Sarcoma" and "Lymphoepithelioma" appear in their own alphabetical places in the Index followed by a reference to "Neoplasm, malignant," where the complete listing of anatomical sites appears with code numbers. Types of benign tumor such as "Adenoma" are indexed in a similar way except that the reference is to "Neoplasm, benign." Thus the coder is directed to the correct column of the three columns of code numbers for neoplasms according to malignancy and anatomical site. If the type of tumor listed in its own alphabetical position occurs in only one site, the code number is given with no reference to "Neoplasm," for instance Thymoma 226.1 or Seminoma 186.

A list of types of neoplasms classified as "malignant," "benign" and "unspecified" is given in the *Tabular List of Inclusions* (Vol. 1, pp. 99–102).

Eponyms. — Eponyms are listed under "Disease" followed by the name of the physician or the locality that is associated with the disease.

In most instances the name appears also in first position in the Index with code numbers. The best practice is to look under D for "Disease;" thus for "Addison's disease," look under D for "Disease, Addison's." A physician's name associated with a "syndrome" is indexed in the same manner as eponyms associated with diseases. Thus for "Korsakoff's syndrome," look under S for "Syndrome, Korsakoff's."

Code numbers

The code numbers which follow the terms in the Index are those of the three-digit categories to which the terms are classified. In general, if the three-digit category is subdivided into four-digit subcategories, the appropriate fourth digit is also given in the code number. There are, however, instances where a group of three-digit categories have a common fourth-digit subdivision based on a different axis of classification. An example is "Burn" (940–949), where the three-digit categories show burn by anatomical site, and the common fourth-digit subclassification is by severity. In these cases, the Index gives only the three-digit code numbers for the individual terms but lists the common fourth digits in a note under the appropriate lead term. Other examples are "Fracture," "Injury, superficial" and "Retardation, mental." In the latter case the note includes an alphabetical index to the fourth digits, rather than a list. Certain sections of the External Cause of Injury part of the Classification have common fourth-digit subdivisions identifying the injured person. These are not indexed but lists of the appropriate fourth digits will be found at the end of Section II.

Primary and secondary conditions

As a general rule, the Index makes no distinction between primary and secondary conditions. It simply provides a code number which can be used to represent a diagnostic statement in mechanical or electronic processing or for other purposes, whether or not these statements relate to primary or secondary conditions. There are, however, some commonly occurring combinations of conditions having a causal relationship which do appear in the Index. Where the classification provides a category specifically for late effects of certain conditions, an indented entry in the Index under the appropriate terms gives the code number of the late effects category. Otherwise the combination will be found under the secondary conditions but not under the primary. Thus, "paralysis" occurring as a late effect of cerebrovascular disease is indexed under "Paralysis" but not under Hemorrhage, cerebral, etc., and psychoses associated with a variety of physical conditions are indexed under "Psychosis" but not under the physical conditions. Nonpsychotic mental disorders associated with physical conditions are listed under the lead term "Disorder, mental."

Multiple diagnoses

The Tabular List includes a number of categories for the classification of two or more conditions jointly reported, e.g., "382 Otitis media with mastoiditis," "540.0 Acute appendicitis with peritonitis." Such combinations of conditions, which are specifically classified in the Tabular List, also appear in the Index. Provisions for certain other combinations which are for use in primary mortality coding only are not shown in the Index since they are not inherent in the Classification itself.

CONVENTIONS USED IN THE INDEX

Parentheses

In the Index, as in the Tabular List, parentheses have a special meaning. Any term which is followed by other terms in parentheses is classified to the given code number whether any of the terms in parentheses are reported or not. For example:

> Abscess (infectional) (metastatic) (multiple) (pyogenic) (septic)
>   adrenal (capsule) (gland) 255.9

Adrenal abscess is classified to 255.9 whether or not capsule or gland is mentioned and whether or not the abscess is described as infectional, metastatic, multiple, pyogenic or septic.

Cross-references

Some categories, particularly those subject to notes linking them with other categories, require rather complex indexing arrangements. To avoid repeating this arrangement for each of the inclusion terms involved, a cross-reference is used. This may take one of a number of forms, as in the following examples:

> Abscess (infectional) (metastatic) (multiple) (pyogenic) (septic)
>   mastoid (process) (subperiosteal) — *see* Mastoiditis

The above shows that the term "Abscess, mastoid" is to be coded in the same way as the term "Mastoiditis." On looking up the latter term, provisions will be found for coding the term in combination with various descriptions of otitis media.

Inflammation, inflamed, inflammatory (with exudation)
cornea (*see also* Keratitis) 363.9

This indicates that if the term "Inflammation of cornea" is the only term on the medical record, the code number is 363.9, but if any other information is present, the term "Keratitis" should be looked up. Alternative code numbers will be found there for the condition if further qualified as, for example, gonococcal, syphilitic, trachomatous or tuberculous.

Enlargement, enlarged—*see also* Hypertrophy
adenoids (and tonsils) 500
apertures of diaphragm (congenital) 756.8
etc.

If the site of the enlargement does not appear among the indents beneath "Enlargement," reference should be made to the indents beneath "Hypertrophy," where a more complete list of sites is given.

Septicemia, septicemic (generalized) (suppurative)
with
ectopic gestation—*see* categories 631.0–631.3

The coder is here referred, not to another part of the Index, but to a group of categories in Volume 1, one of which will be the appropriate code number. In this case, the categories 631.0, 631.1, 631.2 and 631.3 refer to different locations of the ectopic pregnancy.

Bladder—*see* condition
Hereditary—*see* condition

Anatomical sites and very general adjectival modifiers are not normally used as lead terms in the Index. The site or adjectival modifier will be found under the disease or injury reported on the medical record.

Abdomen, abdominal—*see also* condition
acute 785.5
convulsive equivalent 345.9

The term "acute abdomen" is coded to 785.5 and "abdominal convulsive equivalent" is coded to 345.9, but for other abdominal conditions, reference should be made to the disease or injury reported.

Abbreviation NEC

The letters NEC stand for "not elsewhere classified." They are added after terms classified to residual or unspecific categories and to terms in themselves ill-defined as a warning that specified forms of the conditions are classified differently and if the medical record includes more precise information the coding should be modified accordingly, e.g.

> Disease, diseased— *see also* Syndrome
> heart (organic) 429.9
> congenital NEC 746.9

The term "congenital heart disease" is classified to 746.9 only if no more precise description appears on the medical record. If a more precise term, e.g., inter-ventricular septal defect, is recorded, this term should be looked up for the appropriate code.

SECTION I

ALPHABETICAL INDEX TO DISEASES AND NATURE OF INJURY

Section I

ALPHABETICAL INDEX
TO DISEASES AND NATURE OF INJURY

Note—Numbers following the terms in this index are the diagnosis code numbers. The instruction "- *see* category - - -" or "- *see* categories - - -" following a term in the index means that reference should be made to the appropriate category number(s) in Volume 1. Look for the name of the disease or condition in the index and under this for the anatomical site. Words in parentheses () can be present or absent without changing the code number. NEC means "not elsewhere classified"; diagnoses so marked should be assigned the given number only when no more specific category is provided for the condition.

See "Introduction" for other important explanations about the use of the index.

A

Abasia (-astasia) 306.3
  hysterical 300 1
Abdomen, abdominal - *see also* condition
  acute 785.5
  convulsive equivalent 345.9
Abduction contracture, hip or other joint
  - *see* Contraction, joint
Aberrant (congenital) - *see also*
    Malposition, congenital
  adrenal gland 758.1
  breast 757.2
  endocrine gland NEC 758.3
  hepatic duct 751.6
  pancreas 751.7
  parathyroid gland 758.3
  pituitary gland 758.3
  sebaceous glands, mucous membrane,
    mouth 750.8
  spleen 758.0
  testis (descent) 752.1
  thymus gland 758.3
  thyroid gland 758.2
Aberration, mental (*see also* Disorder,
    mental) 300.9
Abetalipoproteinemia 272.1
Abiotrophy 796.0
Ablatio
  placentae - *see* Placenta, ablatio
  retinae 376

Ablation
  placenta - *see* Placenta, ablatio
  pregnant tube - *see* Pregnancy, tubal
  uterus 625.9
Ablepharia, ablepharon 744.8
Abnormal, abnormality, abnormalities -
    see also Anomaly
  alveolar ridge 525.9
  anatomical relationship NEC 758.9
  apertures, congenital, diaphragm 756.8
  autosomes 759.4
    21 759.3
  bony pelvis
    complicating delivery - *see*
      Deformity, pelvis, complicating
      delivery
    noted during pregnancy (undelivered)
      634.9
  chromosomal NEC 759.4
    autosome 759.4
      21 759.3
    sex 759.5
  communication - *see* Fistula
  coronary artery or vein 746.8
  course, eustachian tube 745.2
  dento-facial NEC 524.9
    functional 524.5
  development, developmental NEC
    758.9

Abnormal, etc. — *continued*
  urine (constituents) NEC   789.9
  uterine hemorrhage (*see also*
       Hemorrhage, uterus)   626.9
    climacteric   627
    postmenopausal   626.7
Abnormally formed uterus - *see* Anomaly,
    uterus
Abnormity (any organ or part) - *see*
    Anomaly
Abolition, language   781.5
Aborter, habitual (*see also* Abortion,
    spontaneous)   643.9
  undelivered   634.6
Abortion (complete) (incomplete)
    (inevitable) (with accidental
    hemorrhage of pregnancy) (with
    hemorrhage) (with laceration) (with
    placenta ablatio or abruptio) (with
    placenta previa) (with separation of
    placenta (premature)) (with retained
    secundines) (with unavoidable
    hemorrhage of pregnancy)   644.9
  with
    sepsis (conditions in categories 635,
        670, 671 or 673.9)   644.0
    and toxemia   644.2
    toxemia (conditions in categories 636-
        639)   644.1
    and sepsis   644.2
  accidental - *see* Abortion, spontaneous
  attempted - *see* Abortion, criminal
  criminal (with toxemia)   642.9
    with
      hemorrhage   642.1
        and sepsis   642.2
      laceration (any pelvic organ) (with
          hemorrhage) (with sepsis)
          642.3
      sepsis (conditions in categories 635,
          670, 671, or 673.9)   642.0
        and hemorrhage   642.2
      fetus   773
  fetus   773
  following threatened abortion - *see*
      Abortion, by type
  habitual - *see* Abortion, spontaneous
  homicidal - *see* Abortion, criminal
  induced NEC (*see also* Abortion,
      criminal)   642.9
    for
      legal indications (except medical) -
          see Abortion, legal
      medical indications - *see* Abortion,
          therapeutic
  legal (except medical)   641.9

Abortion, etc. — *continued*
  legal, etc. — *continued*
    with
      sepsis (conditions in categories 635,
          670, 671 or 673.9)   641.0
        and toxemia   641.2
      toxemia (conditions in categories
          636-639)   641.1
        and sepsis   641.2
    fetus   773
    medical - *see* Abortion, therapeutic
    mental hygiene problem - *see* Abortion,
        therapeutic
    missed (two months or more after death
        of fetus) (undelivered)   634.2
    aborted or delivered - *see* Abortion,
        by type
    operative - *see* Abortion, therapeutic
    other   645.9
      with
        sepsis (conditions in categories 635,
            670, 671 or 673.9)   645.0
          and toxemia   645.2
        toxemia (conditions in categories
            636-639)   645.1
          and sepsis   645.2
    psychiatric indication - *see* Abortion,
        therapeutic
    recurrent - *see* Abortion, spontaneous
    self-induced - *see* Abortion, criminal
    spontaneous   643.9
      with
        sepsis (conditions in categories 635,
            670, 671 or 673.9)   643.0
          and toxemia   643.2
        toxemia (conditions in categories
            636-639)   643.1
          and sepsis   643.2
    fetus   773
    surgical - *see* Abortion, therapeutic
    therapeutic   640.9
      with
        sepsis (conditions in categories 635,
            670, 671 or 673.9)   640.0
          and toxemia   640.2
        toxemia (conditions in categories
            636-639)   640.1
          and sepsis   640.2
    fetus   773
    threatened   632.3
      affecting fetus or newborn   769.9
    tubal - *see* Pregnancy, tubal
Abrami's disease   283.9
Abrasion - *see also* Injury, superficial
  tooth, teeth (dentifrice) (habitual) (hard
      tissues) (occupational) (ritual)
      521.2

Abrikossoff's tumor - *see* Neoplasm,
    connective tissue, benign
  malignant - *see* Neoplasm, connective
      tissue, malignant
Abruptio
  placentae - *see* Placenta, abruptio
Abruption
  placenta - *see* Placenta, abruptio
Abscess (infectional) (metastatic)
      (multiple) (pyogenic) (septic)   682.9
  with
    diabetes (mellitus) - *see* category 250
    lymphangitis - *code by* site under
        Abscess
  abdomen, abdominal
    cavity - *see* Abscess, peritoneum
    wall   682.1
  abdominopelvic - *see* Abscess,
      peritoneum
  accessory sinus (chronic) (*see also*
      Sinusitis)   503.9
  adrenal (capsule) (gland)   255.9
  alveolar   522.5
  amebic   006.0
    brain   006.9
      with liver abscess   006.0
    liver   006.0
    lung   006.9
      with liver abscess   006.0
    spleen   006.9
      with liver abscess   006.0
  ankle   682.4
  anorectal   566
  antecubital space   682.2
  antrum (chronic) (Highmore) (*see also*
      Sinusitis, antrum)   503.0
  anus   566
  apical (tooth)   522.5
    with sinus (alveolar)   522.7
  appendix   540.0
  areola   611.0
    puerperal, postpartum   678
  arm (any part, above wrist)   682.2
  artery (wall)   447
  auricle (ear) (staphylococcal)
      (streptococcal)   380
  axilla (region)   682.2
    lymph gland or node   683
  back (any part)   682.1
  Bartholin's gland (*see also* Vaginitis)
      622.1
  Bezold's - *see* Mastoiditis
  bile, biliary, duct or tract (*see also*
      Cholecystitis)   575
  bladder (wall) (*see also* Cystitis)   595
  bone (subperiosteal)   720.0

Abscess, etc. — *continued*
  bone, etc. — *continued*
    accessory sinus (chronic) (*see also*
        Sinusitis)   503.9
    chronic or old   720.1
    jaw (lower) (upper)   526.4
    mastoid - *see* Mastoiditis
    petrous - *see* Mastoiditis
    spinal (tuberculous) - *see also*
        Tuberculosis, abscess, spine
    nontuberculous   720.0
  bowel   569.9
  brain (any part)   322
    amebic   006.9
      with liver abscess   006.0
    cystic   322
    followed by cerebral fungus   324
    late effects   324
    hydrocephalus   324
  breast   611.0
    newborn   611.0
    puerperal, postpartum   678
  broad ligament (*see also* Disease,
      pelvis, inflammatory)   616.0
  Brodie's (localized) (chronic)   720.1
  bronchi   519.9
  buccal cavity   528.3
  bulbo-urethral gland (*see also*
      Urethritis)   597
  bursa - *see also* Bursitis
    pharyngeal   508.9
  buttock   682.1
  canthus   362
  cartilage (joint) (*see also* Disease, joint)
      729.9
  cecum   540.0
  cerebellum, cerebellar   322
    late effects   324
  cerebral (embolic)   322
    late effects   324
  cervical (meaning neck)   682.0
    lymph gland or node   683
    stump (*see also* Cervicitis)   620.9
  cervix (uteri) (*see also* Cervicitis)
      620.9
  cheek   682.0
    inner   528.3
  chest   510
    wall   682.1
  chin   682.0
  choroid   365
  ciliary body   364
  cold (tuberculous) - *see also*
      Tuberculosis, abscess
    articular - *see* Tuberculosis, joint
  colon (wall)   569.9

Abscess, etc. – *continued*
  colostomy or enterostomy   998.7
  conjunctiva   360
  connective tissue NEC   682.9
  cornea   363.9
  corpus
    cavernosum   607.5
    luteum (*see also* Salpingo-oophoritis)
      614
  Cowper's gland (*see also* Urethritis)
    597
  cranium   322
    late effects   324
  cul-de-sac (Douglas') (posterior) (*see
      also* Disease, pelvis,
      inflammatory)   616.0
  dental   522.5
    with sinus (alveolar)   522.7
  dento-alveolar   522.5
    with sinus (alveolar)   522.7
  diabetic - *see* category 250
  diaphragm, diaphragmatic - *see*
      Abscess, peritoneum
  Douglas' cul-de-sac or pouch (*see also*
      Disease, pelvis, inflammatory)
      616.0
  ductless gland   258.9
  ear (middle) - *see also* Otitis media
    acute   381.0
      with abscess, caries, empyema,
        disease or necrosis of
        mastoid, endomastoiditis,
        mastoiditis, osteitis of
        petrous bone, or petrositis -
        see Otitis media with these
        conditions
    external   380
    inner   384.0
  elbow   682.2
  endamebic - *see* Abscess, amebic
  epididymis (*see also* Epididymitis)   604
  epidural   322
    late effects   324
  epiglottis   508.3
  epiploon, epiploic - *see* Abscess,
      peritoneum
  esophagus   530.1
  ethmoid (bone) (chronic) (sinus) (*see
      also* Sinusitis)   503.9
  external auditory canal   380
  extradural   322
    late effects   324
  extraperitoneal - *see* Abscess,
      peritoneum
  eye   366
  eyelid   362

Abscess, etc. – *continued*
  face (any part, except eye)   682.0
  fallopian tube (*see also* Salpingo-
      oophoritis)   614
  fascia   732
  fauces   508.9
  fecal   569.9
  femoral (region)   682.4
  filaria, filarial (*see also* Infestation,
      filarial)   125.9
  finger (any)   681
  fistulous NEC   682.9
  Fochier's NEC   682.9
  foot (except toe)   682.5
  forearm   682.2
  forehead   682.0
  frontal (chronic) (sinus) (*see also*
      Sinusitis, frontal)   503.1
  gallbladder (*see also* Cholecystitis)
      575
  gastric   535
  genital organ or tract NEC
    female   629.4
      with
        abortion - *see* Abortion, by type,
          with sepsis
        ectopic gestation - *see* categories
          631.0-631.3
      arising during pregnancy   630
        fetus or newborn   763.1
      puerperal, postpartum, childbirth
          670
    male   607.5
  gingival   523.3
  gland, glandular (lymph) (acute) NEC
      683
  gluteal   682.1
  gonorrheal NEC (*see also* Gonococcus)
      098.9
  groin   682.1
  gum   523.3
  hand (except finger or thumb)   682.3
  head (except ear)   682.0
  heart (*see also* Disease, heart)   429.9
  heel   682.5
  hepatic   572
    amebic   006.0
    duct (*see also* Cholecystitis)   575
  hip   682.4
  ileocecal   540.0
  ileostomy (bud)   998.7
  iliac (region)   682.1
    fossa   540.0
  iliopsoas (tuberculous) - *see also*
      Tuberculosis, abscess, iliopsoas
    nontuberculous   732

Abscess, etc. — *continued*
  infraclavicular (fossa) 682.2
  inguinal (region) 682.1
    lymph gland or node 683
  intestine, intestinal 569.9
    rectal 566
  intracranial 322
    late effects 324
  intramammary - *see* Abscess, breast
  intra-orbital 366
  intraperitoneal - *see* Abscess,
      peritoneum
  intraspinal 322
    late effects 324
  intratonsillar 501
  iris 364
  ischiorectal 566
  jaw (bone) (lower) (upper) 526.4
  joint (*see also* Disease, joint) 729.9
      vertebral (tuberculous) - *see also*
          Tuberculosis, abscess, spine
      nontuberculous 729.1
  kidney 590.2
    with
      abortion - *see* Abortion, by type,
          with sepsis
      calculus 592
      ectopic gestation - *see* categories
          631.0-631.3
    arising during pregnancy 635.0
      fetus or newborn 763.0
    puerperal, postpartum 635.0
  knee 682.4
    joint 729.8
  labium (majus) (minus) (*see also*
      Vulvitis) 622.1
  lachrymal, lacrimal (apparatus)
      (caruncle) (gland) (sac) 368
  larynx 508.3
  leg (any part) 682.4

  lens 369.9
  lingual 529.0
    tonsil 501
  lip 528.5
  Littre's gland (*see also* Urethritis) 597
  liver 572
    amebic 006.0
    due to Endameba histolytica 006.0
    dysenteric 006.0
    tropical 006.0
  loin (region) 682.1
  lumbar (tuberculous) - *see also*
      Tuberculosis, abscess, lumbar
    nontuberculous 682.1
  lung (miliary) (putrid) 513

Abscess, etc. — *continued*
  lung, etc. — *continued*
    amebic 006.9
      with liver abscess 006.0
  lymph, lymphatic, gland or node (acute)
      683
    any site, except mesenteric 683
    mesentery 289.2
  malar 526.4
  mammary gland - *see* Abscess, breast
  marginal (anus) 566
  mastoid (process) (subperiosteal) - *see*
      Mastoiditis
  maxilla, maxillary 526.4
    molar 522.5
    premolar 522.5
    sinus (chronic) (*see also* Sinusitis,
        maxillary) 503.0
  mediastinum 513
  meibomian gland 362
  meninges (*see also* Meningitis) 320.9
    H. influenzae 320.0
      late effects 324
    late effects 324
    pneumococcal 320.1
      late effects 324
    specified organism NEC 320.8
      late effects 324
  mesentery, mesenteric - *see* Abscess,
      peritoneum
  mesosalpinx (*see also* Salpingo-
      oophoritis) 614
  mons pubis 682.1
  mouth (floor) 528.3
  mural 682.1
  muscle 732
  myocardium 422
  nabothian (follicle) (*see also* Cervicitis)
      620.9
  nasal (fossa) (septum) 508.9
    sinus (chronic) (*see also* Sinusitis)
        503.9
  nasopharyngeal 508.9
  nates 682.1
  navel (newborn) 682.1
  neck (region) 682.0
    lymph gland or node 683
  nephritic (*see also* Abscess, kidney)
      590.2
  nipple 611.0
    puerperal, postpartum 678
  nose (septum) 508.9
    external 682.0
  omentum - *see* Abscess, peritoneum
  operative wound 998.5
  orbit, orbital 369.0

Abscess, etc. — *continued*
  ossifluent - *see* Abscess, bone
  ovary, ovarian (corpus luteum) (*see also*
     Salpingo-oophoritis) 614
  oviduct (*see also* Salpingo-oophoritis)
     614
  palate (soft) 528.3
    hard 526.4
  palmar (space) 682.3
  pancreas (duct) 577.0
  paradontal 523.3
  parametric (*see also* Disease, pelvis,
     inflammatory) 616.0
  pararectal 566
  parasinus (*see also* Sinusitis) 503.9
  para-uterine (*see also* Disease, pelvis,
     inflammatory) 616.0
  paravaginal (*see also* Vaginitis) 622.1
  parietal region 682.0
  parotid (duct) (gland) 527.3
    region 528.3
  pectoral 682.1
  pelvis, pelvic
    female (*see also* Disease, pelvis,
      inflammatory) 616.0
    male (cellular tissue) 682.1
    peritoneal - *see* Abscess,
      peritoneum
  penis 607.5
    gonococcal (acute) 098.0
      chronic or duration of 2 months or
        over 098.1
  peri-anal 566
  periapical 522.5
    with sinus (alveolar) 522.7
  peri-appendiceal 540.0
  pericardial 420
  pericecal 540.0
  pericemental 523.3
  pericholecystic (*see also* Cholecystitis)
    575
  pericoronal 523.3
  peridental 523.3
  perigastric 535
  perimetric (*see also* Disease, pelvis,
     inflammatory) 616.0
  perinephric, perinephritic (*see also*
     Abscess, kidney) 590.2
  perineum, perineal (superficial) 682.1
    deep (*see also* Infection, urinary)
     599.0
    urethra (*see also* Infection, urinary)
     599.0
  periodontal (parietal) 523.3
  periosteum, periosteal 720.3
    with osteomyelitis 720.2

Abscess, etc. — *continued*
  periosteum, etc. — *continued*
    with osteomyelitis — *continued*
      acute or subacute 720.0
      chronic or old 720.1
  periproctic 566
  periprostatic (*see also* Prostatitis) 601
  perirectal (staphylococcal) 566
  perirenal (tissue) (*see also* Abscess,
     kidney) 590.2
  perisinus (nose) (*see also* Sinusitis)
    503.9
  peritoneum, peritoneal (perforated)
    (ruptured) 567.0
    with or following
      abortion - *see* Abortion, by type
        with sepsis
      appendicitis 540.0
      ectopic pregnancy - *see* categories
        631.0-631.3
    pelvic, female (*see also* Disease,
      pelvis, inflammatory) 616.0
    puerperal, postpartum 670
    tuberculous 014
      late effect or sequela 019.9
  peritonsillar 501
  perityphlitic 540.0
  peri-ureteral 593.5
  peri-urethral (*see also* Infection,
     urinary) 599.0
    gonococcal (acute) 098.0
      chronic or duration of 2 months or
        over 098.1
  peri-uterine (*see also* Disease, pelvis,
     inflammatory) 616.0
  perivesical (*see also* Cystitis) 595
  pernicious NEC 682.9
  petrous bone - *see* Mastoiditis
  phagedenic NEC 682.9
    chancroid 099.0
  pharynx, pharyngeal (lateral) 508.9
  phlegmonous NEC 682.9
  pilonidal 685
  pituitary (gland) 253.9
  pleura 510
  popliteal 682.4
  postcecal 540.0
  postlaryngeal 508.3
  postnasal 508.9
  postorbital 369.0
  postpharyngeal 508.4
  post-tonsillar 501
  post-typhoid 001
  premammary - *see* Abscess, breast
  prepatellar 682.4
  prostate (*see also* Prostatitis) 601

Abscess, etc. — *continued*
  prostate — *continued*
    gonococcal (acute) 098.0
      chronic or duration of 2 months or
        over 098.1
  psoas (tuberculous) - *see also*
      Tuberculosis, abscess, psoas
    nontuberculous 732
  puerperal, postpartum, childbirth 670
  pulmonary - *see* Abscess lung
  pulp, pulpal 522.0
  pyemic - *see* Septicemia
  pyloric valve 535
  rectovaginal septum 569.2
  rectovesical (*see also* Cystitis) 595
  rectum 566
  regional NEC 682.9
  renal (*see also* Abscess, kidney) 590.2
  retina 367
  retrobulbar 369.0
  retrocecal - *see* Abscess, peritoneum
  retrolaryngeal 508.3
  retromammary - *see* Abscess, breast
  retroperineal 682.1
  retroperitoneal - *see* Abscess,
      peritoneum
  retropharyngeal 508.4
  retrorectal 566
  retro-uterine (*see also* Disease, pelvis,
      inflammatory) 616.0
  retrovesical (*see also* Cystitis) 595
  round ligament (*see also* Disease,
      pelvis, inflammatory) 616.0
  rupture (spontaneous) NEC 682.9
  sacrum (tuberculous) - *see also*
      Tuberculosis, abscess, sacrum
    nontuberculous 720.0
  salivary (duct) (gland) 527.3
  scalp (any part) 682.0
  scapular 720.0
  sclera 369.9
  scrofulous - *see* Tuberculosis, abscess,
      scrofulous
  scrotum 607.5
  seminal vesicle 607.4
  septum (nasal) 508.9
  shoulder 682.2
  side 682.1
  sigmoid 569.9
  sinus - *see also* Sinusitis
    intracranial venous (any) 322
      late effects 324
  Skene's duct or gland (*see also*
      Urethritis) 597
  skin NEC 682.9
  sloughing NEC 682.9

Abscess, etc. — *continued*
  specified sites NEC 682.9
  spermatic cord 607.5
  sphenoidal (sinus) (*see also* Sinusitis)
      503.9
  spinal
    cord (any part) (staphylococcal) 322
      late effects 324
    epidural 322
      late effects 324
  spine (column) (tuberculous) - *see also*
      Tuberculosis, abscess, spine
    nontuberculous 720.0
  spleen 289.5
    amebic 006.9
      with liver abscess 006.0
  staphylococcal NEC 682.9
  stitch 998.5
  stomach (wall) 535
  subarachnoid 322
    late effects 324
  subareolar - *see* Abscess, breast
  subcecal 540.0
  subcutaneous NEC 682.9
  subdiaphragmatic - *see* Abscess,
      peritoneum
  subdorsal 682.1
  subdural 322
    late effects 324
  subgaleal 682.0
  subhepatic - *see* Abscess, peritoneum
  sublingual 528.3
    gland 527.3
  submammary - *see* Abscess, breast
  submandibular (region) (space) (triangle)
      682.0
    gland 527.3
  submaxillary (region) 682.0
    gland 527.3
  submental 682.0
    gland 527.3
  subpectoral 682.1
  subperiosteal - *see* Abscess, bone
  subphrenic - *see* Abscess, peritoneum
  suburethral (*see also* Infection, urinary)
      599.0
  sudoriparous 705.9
  suppurative NEC 682.9
  supraclavicular (fossa) 682.2
  suprapelvic (*see also* Disease, pelvis,
      inflammatory) 616.0
  suprapubic 682.1
  suprarenal (capsule) (gland) 255.9
  sweat gland 705.9
  temporal region 682.0
  temporosphenoidal 322
    late effects 324

Abscess, etc. — *continued*
  tendon (sheath) 732
  testicle (*see also* Orchitis) 604
  thecal 732
  thigh 682.4
  thorax 510
  throat 508.9
  thumb 681
  thymus (gland) 254
  thyroid (gland) 246
  toe (any) 681
  tongue (staphylococcal) 529.0
  tonsil(s) (lingual) 501
  tonsillopharyngeal 501
  tooth, teeth (root) 522.5
    with sinus (alveolar) 522.7
    supporting structures NEC 523.3
  trachea 508.9
  trunk 682.1
  tubal (*see also* Salpingo-oophoritis) 614
  tuberculous *see* Tuberculosis, abscess
  tubo-ovarian (*see also* Salpingo-oophoritis) 614
  tunica vaginalis 607.5
  umbilicus (newborn) 682.1
  upper respiratory 508.9
  urachus 682.1
  urethra (gland) (*see also* Urethritis) 597
  urinary (*see also* Infection, urinary) 599.0
  uterus, uterine (wall) (*see also* Endometritis) 622.0
    ligament (*see also* Disease, pelvis, inflammatory) 616.0
    neck (*see also* Cervicitis) 620.9
  uvula 528.3
  vagina (wall) (*see also* Vaginitis) 622.1
  vaginorectal (*see also* Vaginitis) 622.1
  vas deferens 607.5
  vermiform appendix 540.0
  vertebra (column) (tuberculous) - *see also* Tuberculosis, abscess, spine
    nontuberculous 720.0
  vesical (*see also* Cystitis) 595
  vesico-uterine pouch (*see also* Disease, pelvis, inflammatory) 616.0
  vitreous (humor) (pneumococcal) 369.9
  vocal cord 508.3
  von Bezold's - *see* Mastoiditis
  vulva (*see also* Vulvitis) 622.1
  vulvovaginal gland (*see also* Vaginitis) 622.1
  web space 682.3
  wrist 682.3

Absence (organ or part) (complete or partial)
  adrenal (gland) (congenital) 758.1
    acquired 255.9
  albumin in blood 275.2
  alimentary tract (congenital) 751.8
    lower 751.4
    upper 750.8
  anus (congenital) 751.3
  aorta (congenital) 747.2
  appendix, congenital 751.4
  arm (acquired) 738.8
    congenital 755.2
  artery (congenital) (peripheral) 747.6
    brain 747.8
    coronary 746.8
    pulmonary 747.6
  atrial septum 746.4
  auditory canal (congenital) (external) 745.0
  auricle (ear), congenital 745.0
  bile, biliary duct, congenital 751.5
  bladder (acquired) 596.9
    congenital 753.8
  bone, congenital NEC 756.9
  brain 740
    specified part 743.2
  breast(s) (acquired) 611.9
    congenital 757.2
  bronchus (congenital) 748.3
  canaliculus lacrimalis, congenital 744.8
  cerebellum (vermis) 743.2
  cervix (acquired) 621.9
    congenital 752.5
  chin, congenital 745.8
  cilia (congenital) 744.8
    acquired 704
  clitoris (congenital) 752.6
  coccyx, congenital 756.2
  cold sense (*see also* Disturbance, sensation) 781.6
  congenital
    lumen - *see* Atresia
    organ or site NEC - *see* Agenesis
    septum - *see* Imperfect closure
  corpus callosum 743.2
  diaphragm (with hernia) 756.8
  digestive organ(s) or tract, congenital 751.8
    lower 751.4
    upper 750.8
  ductus arteriosus 747.8
  ear (auricle) (external) (inner) (middle), congenital 745.0
    lobe, lobule 745.2

Absence, etc. — *continued*
 ejaculatory duct (congenital)   752.8
 endocrine gland NEC   758.3
 epididymis (congenital)   752.8
  acquired   607.9
 epiglottis, congenital   748.3
 epileptic   345.0
 esophagus (congenital)   750.3
 eustachian tube (congenital)   745.2
 extremity (acquired)   738.8
  congenital   755.4
  lower NEC   738.5
   congenital   755.3
  upper NEC   738.8
   congenital   755.2
 eye (acquired)   378.9
  congenital   744.0
  muscle (congenital)   744.8
 eyelid (fold) congenital   744.8
 fallopian tube(s) (acquired)   615.9
  congenital   752.5
 finger (acquired)   738.3
  congenital   755.2
 foot (acquired)   738.6
  congenital   755.3
 forearm (acquired)   738.2
  congenital   755.2
 gallbladder (acquired)   576.9
  congenital   751.6
 gamma globulin in blood   275.0
 genital organs, congenital
  female   752.8
   external   752.6
   internal NEC   752.5
  male   752.8
 genito-urinary organs, congenital NEC
   752.8
 hand (acquired)   738.2
  congenital   755.2
 heat sense (*see also* Disturbance,
   sensation)   781.6
 hymen (congenital)   752.6
 incus (acquired)   387.9
  congenital   745.0
 internal ear (congenital)   745.0
 intestine (acquired)   569.9
  congenital   751.4
 iris (congenital)   744.5
 joint, congenital NEC   755.9
 kidney(s) (acquired)   593.2
  congenital   753.0
 labium (congenital) (majus) (minus)
   752.6
 lachrymal, lacrimal apparatus
   (congenital)   744.8
 larynx (congenital)   748.3

Absence, etc. — *continued*
 leg (acquired)   738.5
  congenital   755.3
 lens (congenital)   744.8
  acquired   378.7
 limb (acquired) NEC   738.8
  congenital   755.4
   lower   755.3
   upper   755.2
 liver (congenital)   751.6
 lung (bilateral) (unilateral) (congenital)
   748.5
  acquired (any part)   519.2
  fissure or lobe   748.6
 menstruation   626.0
 muscle (congenital)   756.8
  ocular   744.8
 neutrophile   288
 nipple (congenital)   757.2
 nose (congenital)   748.1
  acquired   508.9
 ocular muscle (congenital)   744.8
 organ
  of Corti (congenital)   745.0
  or site, congenital NEC   758.8
 ovary (acquired)   615.9
  congenital   752.5
 oviduct (acquired)   615.9
  congenital   752.5
 pancreas (congenital)   751.7
  acquired   577.9
 parathyroid gland (congenital)   758.3
 parotid gland(s) (congenital)   750.8
 patella, congenital   755.7
 penis (congenital)   752.8
  acquired   607.9
 pericardium (congenital)   746.8
 pituitary gland (congenital)   758.3
 prostate (congenital)   752.8
  acquired   602
 punctum lacrimale (congenital)   744.8
 rectum (congenital)   751.3
  acquired   569.2
 respiratory organ (congenital) NEC
   748.9
 rib (acquired)   738.8
  congenital   756.4
 roof of orbit (congenital)   743.0
 sacrum, congenital   756.1
 salivary gland(s) (congenital)   750.8
 scrotum, congenital   752.8
 seminal tract or duct (congenital)
   752.8
  acquired   607.9
 septum
  atrial   746.4

Absence, etc. — *continued*
  septum — *continued*
    between aorta and pulmonary artery
      746.0
    ventricular 746.3
  sex chromosome 759.5
  skull bone 756.0
    with
      anencephalus 740
      encephalocele 743.0
      hydrocephalus 742
        with spina bifida 741.0
      microcephalus 743.1
  spermatic cord (congenital) 752.8
  spine, congenital 756.2
  spleen (congenital) 758.0
    acquired 289.5
  sternum, congenital 756.4
  stomach (acquired) (partial) 537.9
  submaxillary gland(s) (congenital)
    750.8
  superior vena cava (congenital) 747.4
  tendon (congenital) 756.8
  testis (congenital) 752.8
    acquired 607.9
  thigh (acquired) 738.5
  thumb (acquired) 738.3
    congenital 755.2
  thymus gland (congenital) 758.3
  thyroid (gland) (surgical) 246
    cartilage, congenital 748.3
    congenital 243
  toe (acquired) 738.7
    congenital 755.3
  tongue 750.0
  tooth, teeth (congenital) 520.0
    with abnormal spacing 524.3
    acquired 525.0
      with malocclusion 524.3
  trachea (cartilage) (congenital) 748.3
  transverse aortic arch (congenital)
    747.2
  umbilical artery (congenital) 747.5
  ureter (congenital) 753.4
    acquired 593.5
  urethra, congenital 753.8
  uterus (acquired) 625.9
    congenital 752.5
  uvula (congenital) 750.8
  vagina, congenital 752.6
  vas deferens (congenital) 752.8
    acquired 607.9
  vein (congenital) (peripheral) 747.6
    brain 747.8
    great 747.4
    portal 747.4

Absence, etc. — *continued*
  vein, etc. — *continued*
    pulmonary 747.4
  vena cava (congenital) (inferior)
    (superior) 747.4
  vertebra, congenital 756.2
  vulva, congenital 752.6
Absinthemia 303.9
Absinthism (*see also* Alcoholism) 303.9
Absorbent system disease 458.9
Absorption
  chemical NEC 989.9
    specified chemical or substance - *see*
      Table of adverse effects
    through placenta, fetus or newborn
      761.7
  drug NEC 977.9
    specified drug or substance - *see*
      Table of adverse effects
    through placenta, fetus or newborn
      761.7
  fat, disturbance 269.0
  lactose defect 271.8
  narcotic, through placenta, fetus or
    newborn 761.7
  protein, disturbance 269.0
  pus or septic, general - *see* Septicemia
  quinine, through placenta, fetus or
    newborn 761.7
  toxic substance, any, through placenta,
    fetus or newborn 761.7
  uremic - *see* Uremia
Abstinence symptoms, syndrome (drug)
    (narcotic) NEC 304.9
  specified drug - *see* listing under
    Dependence
Abulia 796.0
Abuse
  alcohol (*see also* Alcoholism) 303.9
  child NEC 996.8
  tobacco 989.9
Acalculia (developmental) 306.1
Acantho-ameloblastoma (*see also*
    Ameloblastoma) 210.4
Acanthocheilonemiasis 125.4
Acanthocytosis 272.1
Acantholysis 701.9
  bullosa 757.2
Acanthoma - *see also* Epithelioma
  adenoides cysticum (*see also*
    Trichoepithelioma) 216.1
  benign - *see also* Epithelioma, benign
    uterus 219.0
  malignant - *see* Epithelioma, malignant
Acanthosis (acquired) (nigricans) 701.1
  benign 757.2

Accident
  birth (see also Birth injury NEC)
    772.9
  cardiovascular - see Ischemia, heart
  cerebral (see also Disease,
    cerebrovascular, acute) 436.9
  cerebrovascular (see also Disease,
    cerebrovascular, acute) 436.9
  coronary (see also Infarct, myocardium)
    410.9
  craniovascular (see also Disease,
    cerebrovascular, acute) 436.9
  during pregnancy, to mother
    fetus or newborn 761.5
  heart, cardiac - see Disease, heart
  intra-uterine 778.9
  labor NEC 661.9
    fetus or newborn - see categories
      768.0-768.9
  vascular - see Disease, cerebrovascular,
    acute
Accidental - see condition
Accommodation
  disorder of 370.9
  insufficiency of 370.9
  paralysis of, hysterical 300.1
  spasm of 370.9
Accouchement - see Delivery
Accreta placenta (complicating delivery)
    (with hemorrhage) 652
Accretions
  tooth, teeth 523.6
Accumulation secretion, prostate 602
Acephalia, acephalism, acephaly 740
Acephalobrachia monster 759.2
Acephalochirus monster 759.2
Acephalogaster 759.2
Acephalostomus monster 759.2
Acephalothorax 759.2
Acephalus 740
Acetonemia 788.0
  diabetic 250.0
Acetonuria 789.6
Achalasia 530.0
  cardia 530.0
  digestive organs, congenital NEC
    751.8
  esophagus 530.0
  psychogenic 305.5
  pylorus 750.1
  sphincteral NEC 564.9
Achard-Thiers syndrome 255.0
Ache(s) - see Pain
Achillobursitis 731.7
Achillodynia 787.1
Achlorhydria, achlorhydric 536.0

Achlorhydria, etc. - continued
  anemia 280
  diarrhea 536.0
  neurogenic 536.0
  psychogenic 305.5
  secondary to vagotomy 998.9
Acholuric jaundice (familial)
    (splenomegalic) (see also
    Spherocytosis) 282.0
  acquired 283.9
Achondroplasia 756.5
Achrestic anemia 281.9
Achroacytosis, lachrymal, lacrimal gland
    378.3
  tuberculous 017.2
    late effect or sequela 019.9
Achroma, cutis 709.9
Achromate (acquired) (congenital) 377.3
Achromatopsia (acquired) (congenital)
    377.3
Achromia, congenital 270.8
Achylia gastrica 536.0
  neurogenic 536.0
  psychogenic 305.5
Acid
  burn - see also Burn
    from swallowing acid NEC 983.1
      specified acid - see Table of
        adverse effects
  deficiency
    amide nicotinic 262
    amino 270.9
    ascorbic 264
    folic 263.8
    nicotinic 262
    pantothenic 263.8
  intoxication 788.0
  stomach 536.0
    psychogenic 305.5
Acidemia 788.0
  argininosuccinic 270.8
Acidity, gastric (high) (low) 536.0
  psychogenic 305.5
Acidosis 788.0
  diabetic 250.0
  kidney tubular 273.8
  metabolic NEC 788.0
  renal ·
    hyperchloremic 273.8
    tubular 273.8
  respiratory 788.0
Aciduria
  argininosuccinic 270.8
  organic 270.8
  orotic (congenital) (hereditary)
    (pyrimidine deficiency) 281.4

Acladiosis 111.9
  skin 111.9
Aclasis diaphysial 756.5
Acne (pustular) (vulgaris) 706.1
  artificialis 706.1
  atrophica 706.0
  cachecticorum (Hebra) 706.1
  conglobata 706.1
  conjunctiva 706.1
  cystic 706.1
  decalvans 704
  eyelid 706.1
  frontalis 706.0
  indurata 706.1
  keloid 706.1
  necrotic, necrotica 706.0
    miliaris 704
  nodular 706.1
  occupational 706.1
  rosacea 695.3
  tropical 706.1
  varioliformis 706.0
Acnitis (primary) 017.0
  late effect or sequela 019.9
Acosta's disease 993.2
Acoustic - *see* condition
Acquired - *see* condition
Acrania (monster) 740
Acroasphyxia, chronic 443.8
Acrocephalosyndactyly 756.0
Acrocephaly 756.0
Acrochordon (*see also* Dermatofibroma)
  216.8
Acrocyanosis 443.8
  newborn 778.9
Acrodermatitis 686.9
  atrophicans (chronica) 701.9
  continua (Hallopeau) 686.9
  enteropathia 686.9
  Hallopeau's 686.9
  perstans 686.9
  pustulosa continua 686.9
  recalcitrant pustular 686.9
Acrodynia 985.0
Acrokeratosis verruciformis 757.2
Acromegaly, acromegalia 253.0
Acromicria, acromikria 756.7
Acropachyderma 757.2
Acroparesthesia 443.8
  simple (Schultze's type) 443.8
  vasomotor (Nothnagel's type) 443.8
Acropathy thyroid (*see also*
    Thyrotoxicosis) 242.2
Acrophobia 300.2
Acroscleriasis (*see also* Scleroderma)
  734.0

Acroscleroderma (*see also* Scleroderma)
  734.0
Acrosclerosis (*see also* Scleroderma)
  734.0
Actinic
  cheilitis 692.8
  dermatitis (due to sun) 692.8
  due to
    radiation, except from sun 692.7
  elastosis solar 692.8
Actinobacillosis, general 039.9
Actinobacillus muris 026.1
Actinomyces 113
  israelli (infection) 113
  muris-ratti (infection) 026.1
Actinomycosis, actinomycotic (any site)
  113
Actinoneuritis - *see* Effect, adverse,
  radioactivity
Action, heart
  disordered (*see also* Action, heart,
    irregular) 427.9
  irregular 427.9
    with
      hypertension (benign) (conditions in
        401) (*see also* Hypertension,
        heart) 402
        malignant (*see also*
          Hypertension, malignant
          with heart involvement)
          400.1
  psychogenic 305.3
Active - *see* condition
Activity functional, decrease 790.2
Acute - *see also* condition
  abdomen NEC 785.5
  gallbladder (*see also* Disease,
    gallbladder) 576.9
Acystia 753.8
Adair-Dighton syndrome 756.6
Adamantinoacanthoma - *see* Epithelioma,
  benign
Adamantinocarcinoma - *see*
  Ameloblastoma, malignant
Adamantinoma (*see also* Ameloblastoma)
  210.4
Adamantoblastoma (*see also*
  Ameloblastoma) 210.4
Adams-Stokes(-Morgagni) disease or
  syndrome (*see also* Block, heart)
  427.3
Addiction
  absinthe 303.2
  alcohol, alcoholic (ethyl) (methyl)
    (wood) 303.2
  drug (*see also* Dependence) 304.9

Addiction—*continued*
  ethyl alcohol 303.2
  methyl alcohol 303.2
  methylated spirit 303.2
  wine 303.2
Addison's
  anemia 281.0
  disease (bronze) 255.1
    tuberculous 017.9
      late effect or sequela 019.9
  keloid 701.0
Addisonian crisis or melanosis 255.1
Additional - *see also* Accessory
  chromosome(s) 759.4
    autosome(s) NEC 759.4
    sex 759.5
    21 759.3
Adduction contracture, hip or other joint
    - *see* Contraction, joint
Adenia leukemic 204.9
  acute 204.0
  chronic 204.1
Adenitis (*see also* Lymphadenitis) 289.3
  acute, unspecified site 683
  axillary 289.3
    acute 683
    chronic or subacute 289.1
  Bartholin's gland (*see also* Vaginitis)
    622.1
  bulbo-urethral gland (*see also*
    Urethritis) 597
  cervical 289.3
    acute 683
    chronic or subacute 289.1
  chancroid (Ducrey's bacillus) 099.0
  chronic, unspecified site 289.1
  Cowper's gland (*see also* Urethritis)
    597
  epidemic, acute 075
  gangrenous 683
  gonorrheal NEC 098.8
  groin 289.3
    acute 683
    chronic or subacute 289.1
  infectious 075
  inguinal 289.3
    acute 683
    chronic or subacute 289.1
  leukemic 204.9
    acute 204.0
    chronic 204.1
  lymph gland or node, except mesenteric
    289.3
    acute 683
    chronic or subacute 289.1
  mesenteric (acute) (chronic)
    (nonspecific) (subacute) 289.2

Adenitis —*continued*
  parotid gland (suppurative) 527.2
  salivary duct or gland (any)
    (suppurative) 527.2
  recurring 527.2
  scrofulous 017.1
    late effect or sequela 019.9
  Skene's duct or gland (*see also*
    Urethritis) 597
  strumous, tuberculous 017.1
    late effect or sequela 019.9
  subacute, unspecified site 289.1
  sublingual gland (suppurative) 527.2
  submandibular gland (suppurative)
    527.2
  submaxillary gland (suppurative) 527.2
  tuberculous - *see* Tuberculosis, lymph
    gland
  urethral gland (*see also* Urethritis) 597
  Wharton's duct (suppurative) 527.2
Adeno-acanthoma (*see also* Neoplasm,
  malignant) 199.1
Adenoameloblastoma (*see also*
  Ameloblastoma) 210.4
Adeno-angiosarcoma - *see* Neoplasm,
  connective tissue, malignant
Adenocancroid (*see also* Neoplasm,
  malignant) 199.1
Adenocarcinoma - *see also* Neoplasm,
  malignant
  sudoriferum, sudorificum, site
    unspecified 173.9
    specified site - *see* Neoplasm, skin,
      malignant
Adenochondroma - *see* Neoplasm, benign
Adenocystoma - *see also* Neoplasm,
  benign
  ovary 220.1
Adenocystosarcoma (breast) 217
  malignant 174
Adenofibroma (ovary) 220.9
  prostate 600
  specified site NEC - *see* Neoplasm,
    benign
Adenofibrosis
  breast 610
  endometroid 625.3
Adenoiditis 500
  acute 460
Adenoids (and tonsils) (congenital)
    (diseased) (growth) (hypertrophy)
    (infected) (of nasal fossa)
    (vegetations) 500
Adenoleukemia 204.9
  acute 204.0
  chronic 204.1

Adenolymphoma (salivary gland) 210.2
Adenoma (papillary) (sessile) - *see also*
   Neoplasm, benign
  adrenal (cortex) 226.0
   functionally active 255.0
  basophilic (pituitary) (gland) 258.0
  carcinomatous - *see* Neoplasm,
   malignant
  chromophobe (pituitary) (gland) 253.2
  cystic - *see* Cystadenoma
  eosinophilic (pituitary) 253.0
  fetal, thyroid (gland) 246
  malignant - *see* Neoplasm, malignant
  pancreas 211.6
   functionally active 251
   gastrin secreting 251
   insular tissue 251
  parathyroid (gland) 252.0
  pituitary (gland) 253.9
   basophilic 258.0
   chromophobe 253.2
   eosinophilic 253.0
  pleomorphic, salivary gland 210.2
  prostate (benign) 600
  sebaceous, sebaceum (gland) (senile)
   216.1
   breast 217
   external area or site NEC 216.1
   genital organ NEC - code as
    Neoplasm, benign, by site
   scrotum 216.1
  sudoriferous gland - *see* Adenoma,
   sweat gland
  sweat gland or duct (apocrine) (eccrine)
   216.2
   breast 217
   external area or site NEC 216.2
   genital organ NEC - code as
    Neoplasm, benign, by site
   scrotum 216.2
  testicular, ovary 256.0
  thyroid (gland) (colloid) (differentiated)
   (follicular) (Hurthle cell) (nodular)
   (nontoxic) (papillary) (simple)
   (solitary) (undifferentiated)
   241.9
   with
    hyperthyroidism 242.1
    thyrotoxicosis 242.1
   endemic 241.0
   fetal 246
   sporadic 241.1
   toxic 242.1
  toxic (thyroid gland) 242.1
  tubular of Pick 256.0
Adenomatosis - *see also* Adenoma

Adenomatosis — *continued*
  pluri-endocrine 258.1
  pulmonary 231.3
   malignant 162.1
Adenomatous
  cyst, thyroid (gland) (*see also* Adenoma,
   thyroid) 241.9
  goiter (nontoxic) (*see also* Adenoma,
   thyroid) 241.9
   with hyperthyroidism 242.1
   toxic 242.1
  lung 212.3
Adenomyoma - *see also* Neoplasm,
  benign
  prostate 600
Adenomyosarcoma (*see also* Neoplasm,
  kidney, malignant) 189.0
  not of kidney - *see* Neoplasm,
   malignant
Adenomyosis 625.3
Adenomyxoma - *see* Neoplasm, benign
Adenopathy (lymph gland) 782.7
  inguinal 782.7
  mediastinal 782.7
  mesentery 782.7
  tracheobronchial 782.7
  tuberculous (*see also* Tuberculosis,
   lymph gland) 017.1
   late effect or sequela 019.9
Adenophlegmon 683
Adenosarcoma (*see also* Neoplasm,
  kidney, malignant) 189.0
  not of kidney - *see* Neoplasm,
   malignant
Adenosclerosis 289.3
Adenosis (sclerosing) breast 610
Adentia (complete) (partial) (*see also*
  Absence, tooth) 520.0
Adherent
  labia (minora) 629.9
  pericardium (rheumatic) 393
   nonrheumatic 423
  placenta (complicating delivery) (with
   hemorrhage) 652
  scar (skin) 709.0
  tendon in scar 709.0
Adhesions, adhesive (postinfectional)
  568
  abdominal (wall) (*see also* Adhesions,
   peritoneum) 568
  amnion ʼ
   to fetus - *see* Placenta, abnormal
  appendix 543
  arachnoiditis - *see* Arachnoiditis
  bile duct (*see also* Disease, gallbladder)
   576.9

Adhesions, etc. — *continued*
  bladder (sphincter) 596.9
  bowel (*see also* Adhesions, peritoneum) 568
  cardiac (rheumatic) 398
    nonrheumatic (*see also* Disease, heart) 429.9
  cecum (*see also* Adhesions, peritoneum) 568
  cervicovaginal 621.9
    congenital 752.5
    postpartal 677.9
    old 621.9
  cervix 621.9
  clitoris 629.9
  colon (*see also* Adhesions, peritoneum) 568
  common duct (*see also* Disease, gallbladder) 576.9
  congenital - *see also* Anomaly, specified type NEC
    fingers 755.1
    omental, anomalous 751.1
    peritoneal 751.1
    toes 755.1
    tongue (to gum or roof of mouth) 750.0
  conjunctiva (acquired) 378.3
    congenital 744.8
  cornea - *see* Opacity, cornea
  diaphragm (*see also* Adhesions, peritoneum) 568
  duodenum (*see also* Adhesions, peritoneum) 568
  epididymis 607.9
  epidural - *see* Adhesions, meninges
  epiglottis 508.3
  eyelid 378.2
  gallbladder (*see also* Disease, gallbladder) 576.9
  globe 378.9
  heart (rheumatic) 398
    nonrheumatic (*see also* Disease, heart) 429.9
  ileocecal (coil) (*see also* Adhesions, peritoneum) 568
  ileum (*see also* Adhesions, peritoneum) 568
  intestine (*see also* Adhesions, peritoneum) 568
    with obstruction 560.4
      with hernia - *see* Hernia, by site, with obstruction
  intra-abdominal (*see also* Adhesions, peritoneum) 568
  iris 378.6

Adhesions, etc. — *continued*
  iris — *continued*
    to corneal graft 997.7
  joint (*see also* Disease, joint) 729.9
  labium (majus) (minus), congenital 752.6
  liver 573.9
  lung 511.0
  mediastinum 519.9
  meninges 347.9
    cerebral (any) 347.9
      congenital 743.2
    congenital 743.9
    spinal (any) 349.9
      congenital 743.3
    tuberculous (cerebral) (spinal) 013.0
      late effect or sequela 019.1
  mesenteric (*see also* Adhesions, peritoneum) 568
  nasal (septum) (to turbinates) 508.9
  ocular muscle 378.9
  omentum (*see also* Adhesions, peritoneum) 568
  organ or site, congenital NEC - *see* Anomaly, specified type NEC
  ovary 615.9
    congenital (to cecum, kidney or omentum) 752.5
  pachymeningitis - *see* Meningitis
  para-ovarian 615.9
  pelvic (peritoneal)
    female 616.1
    male (*see also* Adhesions, peritoneum) 568
    postpartal (old) 616.1
    tuberculous
      female 016.2
        late effect or sequela 019.2
      male 016.9
        late effect or sequela 019.2
  penis to scrotum (congenital) 752.8
  peri-appendiceal (*see also* Adhesions, peritoneum) 568
  pericardium (rheumatic) (*see also* Pericarditis, chronic) 393
    nonrheumatic 423
    tuberculous 017.9
      late effect or sequela 019.9
  pericholecystic (*see also* Disease, gallbladder) 576.9
  perigastric (*see also* Adhesions, peritoneum) 568
  peri-ovarian 615.9
  periprostatic 602
  perirectal (*see also* Adhesions, peritoneum) 568

Adhesions, etc. — *continued*
  perirenal (*see also* Lesion, kidney)
      593.2
  peritoneum, peritoneal   568
    with obstruction (intestinal)   560.4
      with hernia - *see* Hernia, by site,
          with obstruction
    congenital   751.1
    pelvic, female   616.1
    postpartal, pelvic   616.1
    to uterus   616.1
  peritubal   615.9
  peri-ureteral   593.5
  peri-uterine   625.9
  perivesical   596.9
  perivesicular (seminal vesicle)   607.9
  pleura, pleuritic   511.0
    tuberculous   012.1
      with pneumoconiosis (conditions in
          515)   010
    late effect or sequela   019.0
  pleuropericardial   511.0
  postpartal, old   629.9
  preputial, prepuce   607.9
  pulmonary   511.0
  pylorus (*see also* Adhesions,
      peritoneum)   568
  sciatic nerve   357.9
  seminal vesicle   607.9
  shoulder   717.1
  sigmoid flexure (*see also* Adhesions,
      peritoneum)   568
  spermatic cord (acquired)   607.9
    congenital   752.8
  spinal canal   349.9
  stomach (*see also* Adhesions,
      peritoneum)   568
  subscapular   733.9
  tendonitis (shoulder)   717.1
  testicle   607.9
  tongue, congenital (to gum or roof of
      mouth)   750.0
  trachea   519.9
  tubo-ovarian   615.9
  tunica vaginalis   607.9
  uterus   625.9
    to abdominal wall   625.9
      complicating delivery   657.9
        fetus or newborn - *see* categories
            764.0-764.9
      noted during pregnancy
          (undelivered)   634.9
  vagina (chronic)   629.7
  vitreous   378.9
Adie-Holmes syndrome   378.6
Adie's pupil or syndrome   378.6

Adiponecrosis neonatorum   778.9
Adiposis   277
  cerebralis   253.1
  dolorosa   279
Adiposity   277
  heart (*see also* Insufficiency,
      myocardial)   428
Adiposogenital dystrophy   253.1
Adjustment reaction
  adolescence   307
  adult   307
  childhood   308
  infancy   308
  late life   307
Admission for observation (without need
      for further medical care)   793.9
  check up only (no complaints or
      symptoms) - *see* Examination
  follow-up after previous treatment - *see*
      Follow-up
  suspected disorder   793.9
    accident   793.8
    malignant neoplasm   793.1
    mental   793.0
    other specified   793.8
    tuberculosis   793.8
Adnexitis (suppurative) (*see also* Salpingo-
      oophoritis)   614
Adrenal (gland) - *see* condition
Adrenalism, tuberculous   017.9
  late effect or sequela   019.9
Adrenalitis, adrenitis   255.9
  meningococcal, hemorrhagic   036.1
    with meningitis   036.0
Adrenocortical syndrome   255.0
Adrenogenital syndrome (acquired)
      255.0
  congenital   273.6
Adventitious bursa - *see* Bursitis
Adynamia
  episodica hereditaria   273.4
Adynamic ileus or intestine (*see also*
      Ileus)   560.1
Aeration lung imperfect (*see also*
      Asphyxia, newborn)   776.9
Aerobullosis   993.3
Aerocele - *see* Embolism, air
Aerodontalgia   993.2
Aero-embolism   993.3
Aero-otitis media   993.0
Aerophagy, aerophagia   305.5
  psychogenic   305.5
Aerosinusitis   993.1
Aerotitis   993.0
Affection - *see* Disease
Affections, old, sacro-iliac (joint)   726

Afibrinogenemia (*see also* Defect,
    coagulation) 286.9
  causing hemorrhage of pregnancy
    632.4
  following childbirth 675
After-cataract 374.1
Aftercare Y10.9
  adjustment of pace-setter or other
    cardiac device Y10.0
  chemotherapy Y10.3
  colostomy status Y10.2
  fracture Y10.4
  medical Y10.6
  orthopedic (without complications)
    Y10.4
  permanent dialysis Y10.1
  postoperative Y10.5
    fracture Y10.4
  postpartum Y07
  radiation Y10.3
  surgical Y10.5
Agalactia 678
Agammaglobulinemia 275.0
  with lymphopenia 275.0
  acquired (primary) (secondary) 275.0
  Bruton's X-linked 275.0
  congenital sex-linked 275.0
  Swiss type 275.0
Aganglionosis (bowel) (colon) 751.2
Age (old) (*see also* Senility) 794
Agenesis 758.8
  adrenal (gland) 758.1
  alimentary tract (complete) (partial)
    NEC 751.8
    lower 751.4
    upper 750.8
  anus, anal (canal) 751.3
  aorta 747.2
  appendix 751.4
  arm (complete) (partial) 755.2
  artery (peripheral) 747.6
    brain 747.8
    coronary 746.8
    pulmonary 747.6
    umbilical 747.5
  auditory (canal) (external) 745.0
  auricle (ear) 745.0
  bile duct or passage 751.5
  bladder 753.8
  bone NEC 756.9
  brain 740
    specified part 743.2
  breast 757.2
  bronchus 748.3
  canaliculus lacrimalis 744.8
  carpus 755.2

Agenesis—*continued*
  cartilage 756.9
  cecum 751.4
  cerebellum 743.2
  cervix 752.5
  chin 745.8
  cilia 744.8
  circulatory system, part NEC 747.8
  clavicle 755.5
  clitoris 752.6
  coccyx 756.2
  colon 751.4
  corpus callosum 743.2
  cricoid cartilage 748.3
  diaphragm (with hernia) 756.8
  digestive organ(s) or tract (complete)
    (partial) NEC 751.8
    lower 751.4
    upper 750.8
  ductus arteriosus 747.8
  duodenum 751.4
  ear (external) (inner) (middle) 745.0
    auricle 745.0
    lobe 745.2
  ejaculatory duct 752.8
  endocrine (gland) NEC 758.3
  epiglottis 748.3
  esophagus 750.3
  eustachian tube 745.2
  extrinsic muscle, eye 744.8
  eye 744.0
    adnexa 744.8
  eyelid (fold) 744.8
  face
    bones NEC 756.0
    specified part 745.8
  fallopian tube 752.5
  femur 755.3
  fibula 755.3
  finger (complete) (partial) 755.2
  foot (complete) (partial) 755.3
  gallbladder 751.6
  gastric 750.8
  genitalia, genital (organ(s))
    female 752.8
      external 752.6
      internal NEC 752.5
    male 752.8
  glottis 748.3
  gonadal 759.5
  hair 757.3
  hand (complete) (partial) 755.2
  heart 746.8
    valve 746.6
  hepatic 751.6
  humerus 755.2

Agenesis—*continued*
hymen 752.6
ileum 751.4
incus 745.0
intestine (large) (small) 751.4
iris (dilator fibers) 744.5
jaw 524.0
jejunum 751.4
kidney(s) (partial) (unilateral) 753.0
labium (majus) (minus) 752.6
labyrinth, membranous 745.0
lachrymal, lacrimal apparatus
    (congenital) 744.8
larynx 748.3
leg (complete) (partial) 755.3
lens 744.8
limb (complete) (partial) 755.4
    lower 755.3
    upper 755.2
lip 750.8
liver 751.6
lung (bilateral) (unilateral) 748.5
    fissures 748.6
    lobe 748.6
mandible 524.0
maxilla 524.0
metacarpus 755.2
metatarsus 755.3
muscle (any) 756.8
musculo-skeletal system NEC 756.8
nail(s) 757.4
neck, part 745.8
nerve 743.8
nervous system, part NEC 743.8
nipple 757.2
nose 748.1
organ
    of Corti 745.0
    or site not listed - *see* Anomaly,
        specified type NEC
osseous meatus (ear) 745.0
ovary 752.5
oviduct 752.5
pancreas 751.7
parathyroid (gland) 758.3
patella 755.7
pelvic girdle (complete) (partial) 755.7
penis 752.8
pericardium 746.8
pituitary (gland) 758.3
prostate 752.8
punctum lacrimale 744.8
radio-ulnar 755.2
radius 755.2
rectum 751.3
renal 753.0

Agenesis—*continued*
respiratory organ NEC 748.9
rib 756.4
roof or orbit 743.0
round ligament 752.8
sacrum 756.1
salivary gland 750.8
scapula 755.5
scrotum 752.8
seminal duct or tract 752.8
septum
    atrial 746.4
    between aorta and pulmonary artery
        746.0
    ventricular 746.3
shoulder girdle (complete) (partial)
    755.5
skull (bone) 756.0
    with
        anencephalus 740
        encephalocele 743.0
        hydrocephalus 742
            with spina bifida 741.0
        microcephalus 743.1
spermatic cord 752.8
spinal cord 743.3
spine 756.2
spleen 758.0
sternum 756.4
stomach 750.8
tarsus 755.3
tendon 756.8
thymus (gland) 758.3
thyroid (gland) 243
    cartilage 748.3
tibia 755.3
tibio-fibular 755.3
toe (complete) (partial) 755.3
tongue 750.0
trachea (cartilage) 748.3
ulna 755.2
ureter 753.4
urethra 753.8
urinary tract NEC 753.8
uterus 752.5
uvula 750.8
vagina 752.6
vas deferens 752.8
vein(s) (peripheral) 747.6
    brain 747.8
    great 747.4
    portal 747.4
    pulmonary 747.4
vena cava (inferior) (superior) 747.4
vermis of cerebellum 743.2
vertebra 756.2

Agenesis — *continued*
  vulva 752.6
Ageusia (*see also* Disturbance, sensation)
  781.6
Aggressive outburst 306.9
Aggressiveness 301.3
Agitated - *see* condition
Agitation 306.9
Aglossia (congenital) 750.0
Agnail (with lymphangitis) 681
Agnosia (body image) (tactile) 781.6
  verbal 781.5
    auditory 781.5
      developmental 306.1
      secondary to organic lesion 781.5
    developmental 306.1
    secondary to organic lesion 781.5
    visual 781.5
      developmental 306.1
      secondary to organic lesion 781.5
Agoraphobia 300.2
Agrammatism 781.5
Agranulocytopenia 288
Agranulocytosis (angina) (chronic)
  (cyclical) (genetic) (infantile)
  (periodic) (pernicious) 288
Agraphia (absolute) 781.5
  developmental 306.1
Ague 084.9
  brass-founders' 985.9
  dumb 084.9
  tertian 084.1
Agyria 743.2
Ailment heart - *see* Disease, heart
Ainhum (disease) 136
Air
  anterior mediastinum 519.9
  compressed disease 993.3
  embolism (artery) (cerebral) (any site)
    (traumatic) 995.0
    complicating delivery 673.0
    during pregnancy 634.8
    puerperal, postpartum 673.0
    sudden death, complicating delivery
      or puerperium 673.0
  rarefied, effects of - *see* Effect, adverse,
    high altitude
  sickness 994.6
Airplane sickness 994.6
Akureyri disease 065
  late effects 066
Alacrima (congenital) 744.8
Alactasia (hereditary) 271.8
Alalia 306.1
  secondary to organic lesion 781.5
Alastrim 050.1

Albers-Schonberg disease 756.7
Albert's disease 731.7
Albinism, albino (choroid) (cutaneous)
  (eye) (generalized) (isolated) (ocular)
  (oculo-cutaneous) (partial) 270.8
Albinismus 270.8
Albright-Bantam syndrome 273.4
Albright-Martin disease or syndrome
  273.4
Albright(-McCune)(-Sternberg) syndrome
  756.7
Albright's
  hereditary osteodystrophy 273.4
Albuminous - *see* condition
Albuminuria, albuminuric (acute) (chronic)
  (subacute) 789.0
  with
    abortion *see* Abortion, by type, with
      toxemia
  arising during pregnancy 636
    fetus or newborn 762.0
  Bence-Jones' NEC 203
  cardiac - *see* Failure, heart, congestive
  gravidarum 636
    fetus or newborn 762.0
  heart - *see* Failure, heart, congestive
  orthostatic (*see also* Lesion, kidney)
    593.2
  postural (*see also* Lesion, kidney)
    593.2
  pre-eclamptic
    with abortion - *see* Abortion, by type,
      with toxemia
    arising during pregnancy 637.0
      fetus or newborn 762.1
    puerperal, postpartum 637.0
  puerperal, postpartum 636
  scarlatinal 034.1
Albumosuria 279
  Bence-Jones' NEC 203
Alcaptonuria 270.6
Alcohol, alcoholic
  addiction 303.2
  apoplexy (cerebral) 303.9
  brain congestion 303.9
  cardiopathy 303.2
  cirrhosis (liver) 571.0
  coma 303.9
  complication NEC 303.9
  convulsive disorder 303.9
  delirium 291.0
    acute 291.0
    chronic 291.1
    tremens 291.0
  dementia 291.9
  edema, brain 303.9

Allergy, etc. — *continued*
 internal agent, etc. — *continued*
  food - *see* Allergy, food
  iodine 692.3
  iodoform 692.3
  kapok 507
  keratolytics 692.3
  leather 692.9
  light 692.9
  medicine - *see* Allergy, drug
  mercurials 692.3
  metals NEC 692.9
  nuts 692.5
  oils 692.1
  orris root 692.9
  pediculocides 692.3
  penicillin (internal use) 960.0
   contact 692.3
  petroleum products (substances in 981)
    692.4
  phenol 692.3
  physical agent (cold) (heat) 692.9
   light 692.9
  plant (contact with) (leaves) 692.6
   pollen 507
  plasters, medicated (any) 692.3
  poison
   ivy 692.6
   oak 692.6
   sumac 692.6
   vine 692.6
  pollen (any) 507
   asthma 493
   hay fever 507
  primrose 692.6
  Primula 692.6
  psychogenic 305.0
  ragweed (pollen) 507
   asthma 493
   hay fever 507
  Rhus
   diversiloba 692.6
   radicans 692.6
   toxicodendron 692.6
   venenata 692.6
  rose 507
  scabicides 692.3
  Senecio jacoboea 507
  serum (prophylactic) (therapeutic)
    999.5
   anaphylactic shock 999.4
  shock (anaphylactic) (from serum or
    immunization) (*see also*
    Anaphylactic shock) 999.4
  solvents (substances in 982) 692.2
  spice 692.5

Allergy, etc. — *continued*
 tea 692.5
 tobacco 692.9
 tree (any) (hay fever) (pollen) 507
  asthma 493
 upper respiratory 507
 vaccine - *see* Allergy, serum
Alligator skin disease 757.2
Allocheiria, allochiria (*see also*
   Disturbance, sensation) 781.6
Almeida's disease 116.2
Alopecia (aerata) (atrophicans) (celsi)
   (cicatrisata) (circumscripta)
   (disseminata) (febrile) (hereditaria)
   (mucinosa) (postinfectional)
   (pregnancy) (prematura)
   (seborrheica) (senilis) (totalis)
   (toxica) (universalis) 704
 adnata 757.3
 congenital, congenitalis 757.3
 specific 091.8
 syphilitic (secondary) 091.8
 x-ray - *see* Effect, adverse, x-ray
Alpine sickness 993.2
Alport's syndrome 759.8
Alternating - *see* condition
Altitude, high (effects) - *see* Effect,
   adverse, high altitude
Aluminosis (of lung) 516.0
Alvarez syndrome (*see also* Ischemia,
   cerebral, transient) 435.9
Alveolitis 526.5
Alveolus, alveolar - *see* condition
Alymphocytosis 275.0
Alzheimer's dementia, disease or sclerosis
   290.1
Amastia (*see also* Absence, breast)
   611.9
Amaurosis (acquired) (congenital) (*see
   also* Blindness) 379.1
 hysterical 300.1
 not specifically defined (economic)
    379.1
  both eyes 379.1
  one eye 379.3
  without statement as to eye(s)
     affected 379.1
 specifically defined (for pension
    purposes) 379.0
  both eyes 379.0
  one eye 379.2
  without statement as to eye(s)
     affected 379.0
 uremic - *see* Uremia
Amaurotic family idiocy (infantile)
   (juvenile) (late) 333.0

Amblyopia (congenital) (partial)   377.2
  exanopsia   377.2
  hysterical   300.1
  nocturnal   377.2
    vitamin A deficiency   260.0
  tobacco   377.2
  toxic NEC   377.2
  uremic - see Uremia
Ameba, amebic (histolytica)
  carrier or suspected carrier   Y05.3
  coli   006.9
    with liver abscess   006.0
  gingivalis   006.9
    with liver abscess   006.0
Amebiasis (any site)   006.9
  with liver abscess   006.0
Ameboma (any site)   006.9
  with liver abscess   006.0
Amelia   755.4
  lower limb   755.3
  upper limb   755.2
Ameloblastoma (benign) (jaw)   210.4
  malignant   143.9
    lower jaw   143.1
    specified site NEC - see Neoplasm,
      malignant
    upper jaw   143.0
  pituitary   226.2
  specified site NEC - see Neoplasm,
    benign
  tibia   213.9
Amelogenesis
  imperfecta   520.5
    non-hereditaria (segmentalis)   520.4
Amenorrhea (primary)   626.0
  hyperhormonal   256.0
Amentia (see also Retardation, mental)
  315.9
Ametropia   370.9
Amimia   781.5
Amino-acid deficiency   270.9
Amino-aciduria   270.8
Amnesia (retrograde)   780.7
  auditory   781.5
    developmental   306.1
    secondary to organic lesion   781.5
  hysterical   300.1
  psychogenic   300.1
Amnion, amniotic - see condition
Amnionitis
  causing complicated delivery   661.8
  complicating pregnancy (delivered)
    (undelivered)   634.9
  fetus or newborn   763.9
Amoral trends   301.7
Amotio retinae   376

Ampulla
  lower esophagus   530.9
  phrenic   530.9
Amputation
  any part of fetus, to facilitate delivery
    773
  cervix (uteri) (supravaginal)   621.9
    complicating delivery   657.9
      fetus or newborn - see categories
        764.0-764.9
    noted during pregnancy (undelivered)
      634.9
  congenital - see Deformity, reduction
  neuroma (traumatic) - see also Injury,
    nerve, by site
    surgical complication (late)   997.2
  stump (surgical)
    abnormal, painful, or with
      complication (late)   997.2
    traumatic - see Amputation,
      traumatic
    healed or old NEC (see also
      Absence, by site, acquired)
      738.9
  traumatic (complete) (partial)

Note — The following fourth-digit subdivisions are for use with categories 885–887
and 895–897:
    .0 Without mention of complication
    .1 Complicated
    .9 Late effect
"Complicated" includes traumatic amputation with delayed healing, delayed treatment, foreign body, or major infection.

Amputation — continued
  traumatic — continued
    arm(s) (and hand(s)) (one or both)
      887
    feet (both)   896
    finger(s) (one or both hands)   886
      with thumb(s)   885
    foot (one or both)   896
      with other leg   897
    genital organ(s) (any) (external) - see
      Wound, open, genital organs
    hand(s) (and arm(s)) (one or both)
      887
    head   874.0
    leg(s) (with other foot)   897
    nose - see Wound, open, nose
    penis - see Wound, open, penis
    sites other than limbs - see Wound,
      open

Amputation—*continued*
  traumatic—*continued*
    thumb(s) (with finger(s) of either hand)
      885
    toe(s) (one or both feet) 895
Amputee (*see also* Absence, by site,
    acquired) 738.9
Amusia
  developmental 306.1
  secondary to organic lesion 781.5
Amyelencephalus 740
Amyclia 743.3
Amygdalitis - *see* Tonsillitis
Amygdalolith 500
Amyloidosis (any site) (general)
    (generalized) (primary) (secondary)
    276
  familial 276
  genetic 276
Amylopectinosis (brancher enzyme
    deficiency) 271.1
Amyoplasia congenita 756.8
Amyotonia 733.9
  congenita 330.2
Amyotrophia, amyotrophy, amyotrophic
  733.1
  congenita 756.8
  lateral sclerosis 348.0
    syndrome residual of encephalitis
    324
  neuralgic 733.1
  paralysis 348.0
  sclerosis 348.0
  spinal progressive 348.0
Anacidity gastric 536.0
  psychogenic 305.5
Anaerosis of newborn (*see also* Asphyxia,
    newborn) 776.9
Analbuminemia 275.2
Analgesia (*see also* Anesthesia) 781.6
Analpha-lipoproteinemia 272.1
Anaphylactic shock or reaction (from
    serum or immunization) 999.4
  drug - *see* Table of adverse effects
  following sting(s) 989.4
Anaphylactoid shock or reaction - *see*
    Anaphylactic shock
Anaphylaxis - *see* Anaphylactic shock
Anaplasia cervix 621.9
Anaplastic polygonal celled tumor 199.1
Anarthria 781.5
Anarthritic rheumatoid disease 446.4
Anasarca 782.6
  cardiac (*see also* Failure, heart,
    congestive) 427.0

Anasarca—*continued*
  fetus or newborn (*see also* Disease,
    hemolytic) 775.9
  lung 514
  nutritional 269.9
  pulmonary 514
  renal (*see also* Nephrosis) 581
Anaspadias 752.3
Anastomosis
  aneurysmal 442
  arteriovenous, congenital 747.6
    ruptured of brain (*see also*
    Hemorrhage, subarachnoid)
    430.9
  intestinal 569.3
  retinal and choroidal vessels 744.8
Ancylostoma (infection) (infestation)
    126.9
  americanum 126.1
  braziliense 126.8
  caninum 126.8
  ceylonicum 126.8
  duodenale 126.0
  Necator americanum 126.1
Ancylostomiasis (intestinal) 126.9
  Ancylostoma
    americanum 126.1
    braziliense 126.8
    caninum 126.8
    ceylonicum 126.8
    duodenale 126.0
  Necator americanus 126.1
Andersen's glycogen storage disease
  271.1
Andes disease 993.2
Android pelvis 755.7
  complicating delivery 654.0
    fetus or newborn - *see* categories
    764.0-764.9
  noted during pregnancy (undelivered)
    634.9
Anectasis
  pulmonary (*see also* Syndrome,
    respiratory distress) 776.2
Anemia 285.9
  with
    disorder of
      anerobic glycolosis 282.3
      pentose phosphate pathway 282.3
    koilonychia 280
  achlorhydric 280
  achrestic 281.9
  Addison's 281.0
  adynamic 284
  agranulocytic 288
  aplastic 284

Anemia—*continued*
  aplastic—*continued*
    congenital 284
    idiopathic 284
    red cell 284
  aregenerative 284
  asiderotic 280
  atypical (primary) 285.9
  Bagdad Spring 283.9
  Balantidium coli 007.0
  Biermer's 281.0
  Bomford and Rhoad 284
  brickmakers' (*see also* Ancylostomiasis)
      126.9
  cerebral (*see also* Disease,
      cerebrovascular NEC) 438.9
  childhood 285.9
  chlorotic 280
  combined system disease 281.0
  congenital (*see also* Disease, hemolytic)
      775.9
    Heinz-body 282.2
  Cooley's (erythroblastic) (*see also*
      Thalassemia) 282.4

  deficiency 281.9
    amino-acid 281.4
    enzyme drug induced hemolytic
        282.2
    erythrocytic glutathione 282.3
    folic acid 281.2
    G SH 282.3
    G-6-PD 282.2
    GGS-R 282.3
    glucose-6-phosphate dehydrogenase
        282.2
    glutathione reductase 282.3
    iron 280
    nutritional 281.9
      with poor iron absorption 280
    PK 282.3
    protein 281.4
    pyridoxine 281.3
    pyruvate kinase 282.3
    triose phosphate isomerase 282.3
    vitamin B12 NEC 281.1
    vitamin B6 281.3
    2, 3 diphosphoglycurate mutase
        282.3
    2, 3 PG 282.3
    6 phosphogluconate dehydrogenase
        282.3
    6-PGD 282.3

  Diamond-Blackfan 284
  dibothriocephalus 123.4
  dimorphic 281.9
  diphasic 281.9

Anemia—*continued*
  diphtheritic 032
  drepanocytic (*see also* Disease, sickle
      cell) 282.5
  due to
    childbearing (not secondary to
        hemorrhage) 676
    loss of blood (acute) (chronic) 280
    myxedema 244
    pregnancy 633.9
      fetus or newborn 769.9
      iron deficiency (conditions in 280)
          633.1
      macrocytic (conditions in 281)
          633.0
  Dyke-Young type (secondary)
      (symptomatic) 283.9
  dyshemopoietic 285.8
  Egypt (*see also* Ancylostomiasis)
      126.9
  elliptocytosis (*see also* Elliptocytosis)
      282.1
  epidemic (*see also* Ancylostomiasis)
      126.9
  erythroblastic (*see also* Thalassemia)
      282.4
    familial (*see also* Thalassemia) 282.4
    fetus or newborn (*see also* Disease,
        hemolytic) 775.9
  essential 285.9
  familial erythroblastic (*see also*
      Thalassemia) 282.4
  Fanconi's 284
  favism 282.2
  general 285.9
  glucose-6-phosphate dehydrogenase
      deficiency 282.2
  goat's milk 281.2
  granulocytic 288
  Heinz-body, congenital 282.2
  hemoglobin deficiency 285.9
  hemolytic 282.9
    acquired 283.9
      with hemoglobinuria 283.9
      auto-immune 283.9
      infectious 283.9
      toxic 283.9
    acute 283.0
      due to enzyme deficiency NEC
          282.2
      fetus or newborn (*see also* Disease,
          hemolytic) 775.9
      Lederer's 283.0
    auto-immune 283.9
    chronic 282.9

Anemia—*continued*
hemolytic—*continued*
congenital (spherocytic) (*see also*
Spherocytosis) 282.0
enzyme deficiency, drug induced
282.2
familial 282.9
fetus or newborn (*see also* Disease,
hemolytic) 775.9
hereditary 282.9
due to enzyme deficiency NEC
282.2
nonspherocytic
congenital or hereditary NEC
282.3
glucose-6-phosphate
dehydrogenase deficiency
282.2
pyruvate kinase deficiency
282.3
type I 282.2
type II 282.3
type I 282.2
type II 282.3
resulting from insertion of shunt or
other internal prosthetic device
997.6
secondary 283.9
Stransky-Regala type (Hb E) (*see
also* Hemoglobinopathy)
282.5
symptomatic 283.9
hemorrhagic 280
Herrick's (*see also* Disease, sickle cell)
282.5
hookworm (*see also* Ancylostomiasis)
126.9
hyperchromic 281.9
of pregnancy 633.0
fetus or newborn 769.9
hypochromic 280
with iron-loading 285.0
familial sex linked 285.0
microcytic 280
normoblastic 280
pyridoxine-responsive 285.0
hypoplasia, red blood cells 284
hypoplastic (congenital) (familial)
(idiopathic) 284
idiopathic 285.9
infantile 285.9
infective 285.9
intertropical (*see also* Ancylostomiasis)
126.9
iron deficiency 280

Anemia—*continued*
iron deficiency—*continued*
of pregnancy 633.1
fetus or newborn 769.9
labyrinth 387.9
Lederer's (hemolytic) 283.0
leuko-erythroblastic 289.9
macrocytic 281.9
nutritional 281.9
of pregnancy 633.0
fetus or newborn 769.9
tropical 281.9
malarial (*see also* Malaria) 084.9
malignant 281.0
progressive 281.0
malnutrition 281.9
marsh 084.9
Mediterranean (*see also* Thalassemia)
282.4
megaloblastic 281.2
of infancy 281.2
of pregnancy 633.0
fetus or newborn 769.9
refractory 281.9
megalocytic 281.9
microcytic 280
due to blood loss 280
familial (*see also* Thalassemia) 282.4
hypochromic 280
miners' (*see also* Ancylostomiasis)
126.9
mycloblastic (*see also* Leukemia,
myeloid) 205.9
myelocytic (*see also* Leukemia,
myeloid) 205.9
myelopathic 289.9
myelophthisic 289.9
myeloplastic (*see also* Leukemia,
myeloid) 205.9
newborn (*see also* Disease, hemolytic)
775.9
posthemorrhagic 280
nonregenerative 284
nonspherocytic hemolytic - *see* Anemia,
hemolytic, nonspherocytic
normocytic (infectional) 285.9
due to blood loss 280
myelophthisic 284
nutritional (deficiency) 281.9
with poor iron absorption 280
of pregnancy NEC 633.9
fetus or newborn 769.9
of prematurity 280
osteosclerotic 209
paludal (*see also* Malaria) 084.9
pernicious 281.0

Anemia—continued
  pernicious—continued
    with
      combined system disease   281.0
      dorsolateral spinal degeneration
            281.0
      myelopathy   281.0
      neuropathy (peripheral)   281.0
      posterior sclerosis   281.0
    of pregnancy   633.0
      fetus or newborn   769.9
    progressive   281.0
  pleochromic   285.9
    of sprue   269.0
  portal   285.8
  posthemorrhagic   280
    of newborn   280
  pressure   285.9
  primary   285.9
  profound   285.9
  progressive   285.9
    malignant   281.0
    pernicious   281.0
  pseudoleukemica infantum   285.8
  puerperal (not secondary to
            hemorrhage)   676
    following hemorrhage complicating
            delivery   653
  pure red cell   284
  refractory (primary)   284
    with hemochromatosis   285.0
    sideroblastic   285.0
    sideropenic   280
  Rietti-Greppi-Micheli (see also
            Thalassemia)   282.4
  secondary   285.9
    to blood loss (acute) (chronic)   280
    to hemorrhage   280
  semiplastic   284
  septic   285.9
  sickle cell   282.5
  sidero-achrestic   285.0
  sideroblastic (refractory)   285.0
  sideropenic (refractory)   280
  simple (chronic)   285.9
  specified type NEC   285.8
  spherocytic (hereditary) (see also
            Spherocytosis)   282.0
  splenic   285.8
  splenomegalic   285.8
  syphilitic   095
  target cell (see also Thalassemia)
            282.4
  thalassemia (see also Thalassemia)
            282.4

Anemia—continued
  thrombocytopenic (see also
            Thrombocytopenia)   287.1
  toxic   284
    paralytic   284
  tropical, macrocytic   281.9
  tuberculous   017.9
    late effect or sequela   019.9
  von Jaksch's   285.8
  Witts'   280
  Zuelzer(-Ogden) (megaloblastic)   281.2
Anencephalus, anencephaly   740
Anergasia (see also Psychosis, organic)
            294.9
  senile   290.0
Anesthesia, anesthetic   781.6
  complication or reaction NEC   968.1
    specified anesthetic - see Table of
            adverse effects
  death from (see also Table of adverse
            effects)   968.1
    during delivery (normal)   662
  eye   378.9
  functional   300.1
  hyperesthetic, thalamic   347.9
  hysterical   300.1
  local skin lesion   781.6
  sexual (psychogenic)   305.6
Anetoderma (maculosum)   701.2
Aneuploidy NEC   759.4
Aneurin deficiency   261
Aneurysm (anastomotic) (artery) (cirsoid)
            (diffuse) (false) (fusiform) (multiple)
            (ruptured) (saccular) (varicose)
            442
  abdominal (aorta)   441.2
    dissecting   441.0
    syphilitic   093.0
  aorta, aortic (nonsyphilitic)   441.9
    abdominal   441.2
    arch   441.1
    arteriosclerotic NEC   441.9
    ascending   441.1
    congenital   747.2
    descending   441.9
      abdominal   441.2
      thoracic   441.1
    dissecting (any part)   441.0
    due to coarctation (aorta)   747.1
    sinus, right   747.2
    syphilitic   093.0
    thorax, thoracic (arch)   441.1
    transverse   441.1
    valve (heart) (see also Endocarditis,
            aortic)   395.9
  arteriosclerotic NEC   442

Aneurysm, etc.*continued*
  arteriosclerotic—*continued*
    cerebral (*see also* Ischemia, cerebral)
      437.9
      ruptured (*see also* Hemorrhage,
        subarachnoid) 430.9
    arteriovenous (congenital) (peripheral)
      747.6
    acquired 442
    brain 747.8
      ruptured (*see also* Hemorrhage,
        subarachnoid) 430.9
    retina 744.8
    traumatic (complication) (early)
      995.3
  basal - *see* Aneurysm, brain
  berry (congenital) (ruptured) (*see also*
      Hemorrhage, subarachnoid)
      430.9
  brain 442
    arteriosclerotic (*see also* Ischemia,
        cerebral) 437.9
      ruptured (*see also* Hemorrhage,
        subarachnoid) 430.9
    arteriovenous 747.8
      ruptured (*see also* Hemorrhage,
        subarachnoid) 430.9
    berry (congenital) (ruptured) (*see also*
        Hemorrhage, subarachnoid)
        430.9
    congenital 747.8
      ruptured (*see also* Hemorrhage,
        subarachnoid) 430.9
    meninges 442
      ruptured (*see also* Hemorrhage,
        subarachnoid) 430.9
    miliary (congenital) (ruptured) (*see
        also* Hemorrhage,
        subarachnoid) 430.9
    mycotic 421.0
      ruptured (*see also* Hemorrhage,
        brain) 431.9
    ruptured (*see also* Hemorrhage,
        subarachnoid) 430.9
    syphilitic (hemorrhage) 094.9
    traumatic 995.3
  cardiac (false) (*see also* Ischemia, heart)
      412.9
  carotid 442
    internal 442
      ruptured into brain (*see also*
        Hemorrhage, subarachnoid)
        430.9
    syphilitic 093.9
      intracranial 094.9
  cavernous sinus 442

Aneurysm, etc.—*continued*
  cavernous sinus—*continued*
    arteriovenous 747.8
      ruptured (*see also* Hemorrhage,
        subarachnoid) 430.9
    congenital 747.8
      ruptured (*see also* Hemorrhage,
        subarachnoid) 430.9
  central nervous system syphilitic
      094.9
  cerebral - *see* Aneurysm, brain
  chest - *see* Aneurysm, thorax
  circle of Willis 442
    congenital 747.8
      ruptured (*see also* Hemorrhage,
        subarachnoid) 430.9
    ruptured (*see also* Hemorrhage,
        subarachnoid) 430.9
  congenital (peripheral) 747.6
    specified site, except of peripheral
        vessel NEC 747.8
  conus arteriosus (*see also* Ischemia,
      heart) 412.9
  coronary (arteriosclerotic) (artery) (vein)
      (*see also* Ischemia, heart) 412.9
    congenital 746.8
    syphilitic 093.9
  cylindrical 441.9
    syphilitic 093.9
  dissecting 442
    aorta (any part) 441.0
    syphilitic 093.9
  ductus arteriosus 747.0
  femoral 442
  heart (infectional) (wall) (*see also*
      Ischemia, heart) 412.9
    congenital 746.8
    valve - *see* Endocarditis
  iliac (common) 442
  innominate (nonsyphilitic) 442
    syphilitic 093.9
  interauricular septum (*see also*
      Ischemia, heart) 412.9
  interventricular septum (*see also*
      Ischemia, heart) 412.9
  intrathoracic (nonsyphilitic) 441.1
    syphilitic 093.0
  jugular vein 453
  lower extremity 442
  malignant 093.9
  mediastinal (nonsyphilitic) 442
    syphilitic 093.9
  miliary (congenital) (ruptured) (*see also*
      Hemorrhage, subarachnoid)
      430.9

Aneurysm, etc. — *continued*
  mitral (heart) (valve) (*see also*
      Endocarditis, mitral)   394.9
  mycotic, any site   421.0
    ruptured, brain (*see also* Hemorrhage,
        brain)   431.9
  myocardium (*see also* Ischemia, heart)
      412.9
  patent ductus arteriosus   747.0
  peripheral NEC   442
    congenital   747.6
  popliteal   442
  pulmonary   442
    syphilitic   093.9
    valve (heart) (*see also* Endocarditis,
        pulmonary)   424.9
  racemose   442
    congenital   747.6
  Rasmussen's (*see also* Tuberculosis,
      pulmonary)   011.9
  renal   442
  retina (progressive)   377.0
    congenital   744.8
  sinus aortic, sinuses of Valsalva   747.2
  spinal (cord)   442
    congenital   747.6
    syphilitic (hemorrhage)   094.9
  splenic   442
  subclavian   442
    syphilitic   093.9
  syphilitic   093.9
    central nervous system   094.9
    congenital   090.5
    spine, spinal   094.9
  thorax, thoracic (arch) (nonsyphilitic)
      441.1
    dissecting   441.0
    syphilitic   093.0
  traumatic (complication) (early)   995.3
  tricuspid (heart) (valve) - *see*
      Endocarditis, tricuspid
  valve, valvular - *see* Endocarditis
  venous   456.9
    congenital   747.6
  ventricle (*see also* Ischemia, heart)   412.9
Angiectasis   458.9
Angiectopia   458.9
Angiitis   447
  allergic granulomatous   446.3
  hypersensitivity   446.2
  necrotizing   446.0
Angina (attack) (cardiac) (chest) (effort)
      (heart) (pectoris) (syndrome)
      (vasomotor)   413.9
  with hypertensive disease (conditions in
      400-404)   413.0

Angina, etc. — *continued*
  agranulocytic   288
  aphthous   074.0
  catarrhal   462
  croupous   464
  cruris   443.9
  decubitus (*see also* Insufficiency,
      coronary)   411.9
  diphtheritic   032
  erysipelatous   034.0
  erythematous   462
  exudative, chronic   506
  faucium   508.9
  gangrenous   462
    diphtheritic   032
  infectious   462
  ludovici   528.3
  Ludwig's   528.3
  malignant   462
    diphtheritic   032
  . membranous   502.0
    diphtheritic   032
  monocytic   075
  phlegmonous   501
    diphtheritic   032
  pre-infarctional (*see also* Insufficiency,
      coronary)   411.9
  pseudomembranous   101
  pultaceous, diphtheritic   032
  scarlatinal   034.1
  septic   034.0
  simple   462
  staphylococcal   462
  streptococcal   034.0
  stridulous, diphtheritic   032
  syphilitic   093.9
    congenital   090.5
  tonsil   501
  trachealis   464
  Vincent's   101
Angioblastoma - *see* Neoplasm,
      connective tissue, malignant
Angiocholecystitis (*see also* Cholecystitis)
      575
Angiocholitis (*see also* Cholecystitis)
      575
Angiochondroma (*see also* Neoplasm,
      connective tissue, malignant)
      171.9
Angioedema (allergic) (any site)
      (hereditary) (with urticaria)   708.0
Angioendothelioma (*see also*
      Hemangioendothelioma)   227.1
  Ewing's - *see* Neoplasm, bone,
      malignant

Angioendothelioma—*continued*
  malignant - *see* Neoplasm, connective
    tissue, malignant
Angiofibroma (juvenile) (nasopharynx)
    227.1
Angiofibrosarcoma - *see* Neoplasm,
    connective tissue, malignant
Angiohemophilia (A) (B) 286.3
Angioid streaks (retina) 377.1
Angiokeratoma 757.2
  diffusum corporis 272.2
Angioleucitis 683
Angiolipoma (*see also* Lipoma) 214.9
Angioma (benign) (cavernous) (congenital)
    (*see also* Hemangioma) 227.0
  placenta - *see* Placenta, abnormal
  senile 448
  serpiginosum 709.9
  spider 448
  stellate 448
Angiomatosis (*see also* Hemangioma)
    227.0
  encephalocutaneous 759.8
  encephalotrigeminal 759.8
  multiple sites 759.8
Angiomyolipoma (*see also* Lipoma)
    214.9
Angioneuromyoma - *see* Glomangioma
Angioneurosis 305.3
Angioneurotic edema (allergic) (any site)
    (hereditary) (with urticaria) 708.0
Angiopathia, angiopathy 458.9
  retinae syphilitica 093.9
  retinalis juvenalis 377.0
Angiosarcoma - *see* Neoplasm,
    connective tissue, malignant
Angiosclerosis - *see* Arteriosclerosis
Angiospasm 443.9
  brachial plexus 357.0
  cerebral (*see also* Ischemia, cerebral,
    transient) 435.9
  cervical plexus 357.0
  nerve
    autonomic 358.9
    axillary 357.1
    median 357.2
    peripheral NEC 357.9
    spinal NEC 357.9
    sympathetic 358.9
    ulnar 357.3
  peripheral NEC 443.9
  traumatic 443.9
    foot 443.9
    leg 443.9
  vessel 443.9
Anguillulosis 127.1

Angulation
  cecum (*see also* Obstruction, intestine)
    560.9
  coccyx (acquired) 735.9
    congenital 756.2
  femur (acquired) 738.5
    congenital 755.7
  intestine (large) (small) (*see also*
    Obstruction, intestine) 560.9
  sacrum (acquired) 735.9
    congenital 756.2
  sigmoid (flexure) (*see also* Obstruction,
    intestine) 560.9
  spine (*see also* Curvature, spine) 735.9
  tibia (acquired) 738.5
    congenital 755.7
  ureter 593.3
  wrist (acquired) 738.2
    congenital 755.5
Angulus
  infectiosus 686.9
Anhidrosis 705.0
Anhydration 788.0
Anhydremia 788.0
Anidrosis 705.0
Aniridia (congenital) 744.5
Aniselkonia 370.9
Anisocoria (pupil) 378.6
  congenital 744.8
Anisometropia (congenital) 370.9
  causing squint 373.9
Ankle - *see* condition
Ankyloblepharon (eyelid) (acquired)
    378.6
  filiforme (adnatum) (congenital) 744.8
  total 744.8
Ankyloglossia 750.0
Ankylosis (fibrous) (osseous) 727.9
  ankle 727.7
  cricoarytenoid (cartilage) (joint) (larynx)
    508.3
  dental 521.6
  elbow 727.2
  finger 727.4
  hip 727.5
  incostapedial joint (infectional) 386
  knee 727.6
  lumbosacral (joint) 727.0
  multiple sites 727.8
  postoperative (status) (*see also* Disease,
    joint) 729.9
  produced by surgical fusion (*see also*
    Disease, joint) 729.9
  sacro-iliac (joint) 726
  shoulder 727.1
  specified site NEC 727.8

Ankylosis, etc. — *continued*
  spine NEC   727.0
  surgical (*see also* Disease, joint)   729.9
  tooth, teeth (hard tissues)   521.6
  wrist   727.3
Ankylostoma - *see* Ancylostoma
Ankylostomiasis - *see* Ancylostomiasis
Ankylurethria (*see also* Stricture, urethra)
  598
Annular - *see also* condition
  organ or site, congenital NEC - *see*
    Distortion
  pancreas (congenital)   751.7
Anodontia (complete) (partial) (vera)
  520.0
  with abnormal spacing   524.3
  acquired   525.0
    with malocclusion   524.3
Anomaly, anomalous (congenital)
    (unspecified type)   758.9
  abdomen   758.9
  abdominal wall   756.9
  acoustic nerve   743.9
  adrenal (gland)   758.1
  alimentary tract   751.9
    lower   751.4
    upper   750.9
  ankle (joint)   755.7
  anus   751.4
  aorta (arch)   747.2
    coarctation   747.1
  aortic cusp or valve   746.6
  aqueduct of sylvius   742
    with spina bifida   741.0
  arm   755.5
  arteriovenous   747.6
  artery   747.6
    cerebral   747.8
    coronary   746.8
    peripheral   747.6
    pulmonary   747.6
    retina   744.9
    umbilical   747.5
  aryteno-epiglottic folds   748.3
  atrial
    bands   746.8
    folds   746.8
    septa   746.4
  atrioventricular excitation - *see*
    Tachycardia, paroxysmal
  auditory canal   745.3
  auricle
    ear   745.3
      causing impairment of hearing
        745.0
    heart   746.8

Anomaly, etc. — *continued*
  autosomes NEC   759.4
  back   758.9
  band
    atrial   746.8
    heart   746.8
    ventricular   746.8
  Bartholin's duct   750.9
  biliary duct or passage   751.6
  bladder   753.9
  bone NEC   756.9
    face   756.0
    skull   756.0
      with
        anencephalus   740
        encephalocele   743.0
        hydrocephalus   742
          with spina bifida   741.0
        microcephalus   743.1
  brain   743.9
    multiple   743.2
    vessel   747.8
  breast   757.9
  bronchus   748.3
  bursa   756.9
  canal of Nuck   752.9
  canthus   744.9
  capillary   747.6
  cardiac   746.9
    valve (any)   746.6
  cardiovascular system   746.9
  carpus   755.5
  caruncle lachrymal, lacrimal   744.9
  cecum   751.4
  cerebral - *see also* Anomaly, brain
    vessels   747.8
  cervix   752.5
    complicating delivery   657.9
      fetus or newborn - *see* categories
        764.0-764.9
      noted during pregnancy (undelivered)
        634.9
  cheek   745.9
  chest (wall)   756.4
  chin   745.9
  chordae tendineae   746.8
  choroid   744.9
    plexus   743.9
  chromosomes, chromosomal   759.4
    autosomes NEC   759.4
    sex   759.5
    21   759.3
  cilia   744.9
  circulatory system NEC   747.9
  clavicle   755.5
  clitoris   752.6

Anomaly, etc. – *continued*
coccyx 756.2
colon 751.4
concha (ear) 745.3
connection renal vessels with kidney 747.6
cornea 744.9
coronary artery or vein 746.8
cranium - *see* Anomaly, skull
cricoid cartliage 748.3
cystic duct 751.6
dental arch relationship 524.2
dentition 520.6
dento-facial NEC 524.9
  functional 524.5
diaphragm (apertures) NEC 756.9
digestive organ(s) or system NEC 751.9
  lower 751.4
  upper 750.9
distribution, coronary artery 746.8
ductus arteriosus 747.0
duodenum 751.4
dura (brain) 743.9
  spinal cord 743.3
ear NEC 745.3
  causing impairment of hearing 745.0
  middle (causing impairment of hearing) 745.0
Ebstein 746.6
  tricuspid valve 746.6
ectodermal 757.9
ejaculatory duct 752.9
elbow 755.5
endocrine gland NEC 758.3
epididymis 752.9
epiglottis 748.3
esophagus 750.9
eustachian tube 745.3
eye (any part) 744.9
eyelid 744.9
face 745.9
fallopian tube 752.5
fascia 756.9
femur 755.7
fibula 755.7
finger 755.5
fixation, intestine 751.1
flexion (joint) 755.9
  hip or thigh 755.6
foot 755.7
forearm 755.5
forehead (*see also* Anomaly, skull) 756.0
frontal bone (*see also* Anomaly, skull) 756.0

Anomaly, etc. – *continued*
gallbladder 751.6
gastrointestinal tract NEC 751.9
genitalia, genital organ(s) or system
  female 752.9
    external 752.6
    internal NEC 752.5
  male 752.9
genito-urinary NEC 752.9
globe (eye) 744.9
gum 750.9
hair 757.9
hand 755.5
head (*see also* Anomaly, skull) 756.0
heart 746.9
  auricle 746.8
  bands 746.8
  folds 746.8
  septum 746.8
    auricular 746.4
    ventricular 746.3
  valve (any) 746.6
  ventricle 746.8
heel 755.7
Hegglin's (*see also* Thrombocytopenia) 287.1
hepatic duct 751.6
hip 755.7
humerus 755.5
hymen 752.6
hypophyseal 758.3
ileocecal (coil) (valve) 751.4
ileum 751.4
ilium 755.7
intervertebral cartilage or disc 756.2
intestine (large) (small) 751.4
iris 744.9
ischium 755.7
jaw NEC 524.9
  size (major) 524.0
jaw-cranial base relationship 524.1
joint 755.9
kidney(s) (calyx) (pelvis) 753.9
  vessel 747.6
knee 755.7
labium (majus) (minus) 752.6
labyrinth, membranous 745.0
lachrymal, lacrimal apparatus or duct 744.9
larynx, laryngeal (muscle) 748.3
leg (upper) (lower) 755.7
lens 744.9
lid (fold) 744.9
ligament 756.9
  round 752.9

Anomaly, etc. — *continued*
  limb except reduction deformity   755.9
    lower   755.7
    upper   755.5
  lip   750.9
  liver (duct)   751.6
  lower extremity   755.7
  lumbosacral (joint) (region)   756.1
  lung (fissure) (lobe) NEC   748.6
  lymphatic system   758.9
  meningeal bands or folds, constriction
      of   743.9
  meninges   743.9
    brain   743.2
    spinal   743.3
  mesentery   751.9
  metacarpus   755.5
  metatarsus   755.7
  middle ear   745.0
  mitral (leaflets) (valve)   746.6
  mouth   750.9
  multiple NEC   759.9
  muscle   756.9
  musculoskeletal system, except limbs
      756.9
  nail   757.9
  neck (any part)   745.9
  nervous system NEC   743.9
  neurological   743.9
  nipple   757.9
  nose, nasal (bones) (cartilage) (septum)
      (sinus)   748.1
  ocular muscle   744.9
  opening, pulmonary veins   747.4
  optic nerve   743.9
  opticociliary vessels   744.9
  orbit (eye)   744.9
  organ
    of Corti   745.0
    or site NEC   758.9
  origin
    coronary artery   746.8
    innominate artery   747.6
    pulmonary artery   747.6
    renal vessels   747.6
    subclavian artery   747.6
  ovary   752.5
  oviduct   752.5
  palate (hard) (soft)   750.9
  pancreas   751.7
  papillary muscles   746.8
  parathyroid gland   758.3
  paraurethral ducts   753.9
  parotid (gland)   750.9
  patella   755.7
  Pelger-Huet   289.9

Anomaly, etc. — *continued*
  pelvic girdle   755.7
  pelvis (bony)   755.7
  penis (glans)   752.9
  pericardium   746.8
  pharynx   750.9
  pigmentation NEC   709.9
    congenital   757.2
  pituitary (gland)   758.3
  pleural folds   748.8
  portal vein   747.4
  position
    tooth, teeth   524.3
  prepuce   752.9
  prostate   752.9
  pulmonary   748.6
    artery   747.6
    circulation   747.6
    valve   746.6
    vein   747.4
  pupil   744.9
  pylorus   750.9
  radius   755.5
  rectum   751.4
  refraction   370.9
  renal   753.9
    vessel   747.6
  respiratory system NEC   748.9
  rib   756.4
    cervical   756.3
  rotation - *see also* Malrotation
    hip or thigh   755.6
  sacroiliac (joint)   755.7
  sacrum   756.1
  salivary duct or gland   750.9
  scapula   755.5
  scrotum   752.9
  sebaceous gland   757.9
  seminal duct or tract   752.9
  sense organs NEC   743.9
  sex chromosomes NEC   759.5
  shoulder (girdle) (joint)   755.5
  sigmoid (flexure)   751.4
  sinus of Valsalva   747.2
  skeleton generalized NEC   756.7
  skin (appendage)   757.9
  skull   756.0
    with
      anencephalus   740
      encephalocele   743.0
      hydrocephalus   742
        with spina bifida   741.0
      microcephalus   743.1
  specified type NEC
    adrenal (gland)   758.1

Anomaly, etc. — *continued*
  specified type NEC — *continued*
    alimentary tract (complete) (part)
      751.8
      lower   751.4
      upper   750.8
    ankle   755.7
    anus, anal (canal)   751.4
    aorta (arch)   747.2
    appendix   751.4
    arm   755.5
    artery (peripheral)   747.6
      brain   747.8
      coronary   746.8
      eye   744.8
      pulmonary   747.6
      retinal   744.8
      umbilical   747.5
    auditory canal   745.2
      causing impairment of hearing
        745.0
    bile duct or passage   751.6
    bladder   753.8
      neck   753.8
    bone(s)   756.9
      arm   755.5
      face   756.0
      leg   755.7
      pelvic girdle   755.7
      shoulder girdle   755.5
      skull   756.0
        with
          anencephalus   740
          encephalocele   743.0
          hydrocephalus   742
            with spina bifida   741.0
          microcephalus   743.1
    brain   743.2
    broad ligament   752.8
    bronchus   748.3
    canal of Nuck   752.8
    carpus   755.5
    cartilaginous   756.9
    cecum   751.4
    cervix   752.5
    chest (wall)   756.4
    chin   745.8
    circulatory system   747.8
    clavicle   755.5
    clitoris   752.6
    coccyx   756.2
    colon   751.4
    common duct   751.6
    cricoid cartilage   748.3
    cystic duct   751.6
    diaphragm   756.8

Anomaly, etc. — *continued*
  specified type NEC — *continued*
    digestive organ(s) or tract   751.8
      lower   751.4
      upper   750.8
    duodenum   751.4
    ear (auricle) (lobe)   745.2
      causing impairment of hearing
        745.0
      inner   745.0
      middle   745.0
    ejaculatory duct   752.8
    endocrine   758.3
    epiglottis   748.3
    esophagus   750.8
    eustachian tube   745.2
    eye (lid) (muscle)   744.8
    face   745.8
      bone(s)   756.0
    fallopian tube   752.5
    fascia   756.8
    femur   755.7
    fibula   755.7
    finger   755.5
    foot   755.7
    fovea centralis   744.8
    gallbladder   751.6
    Gartner's duct   752.8
    gastrointestinal tract   751.8
    genitalia, genital organ(s)
      female   752.8
        external   752.6
        internal NEC   752.5
      male   752.8
    genitourinary tract NEC   752.8
    glottis   748.3
    hair   757.3
    hand   755.5
    heart   746.8
      valve (any)   746.6
    hepatic duct   751.6
    hydatid of Morgagni   752.8
    hymen   752.6
    intestine (large) (small)   751.4
      fixational type   751.1
    jaw - *see* categories 524.0-524.9
    jejunum   751.4
    joint   755.9
    kidney   753.3
    knee   755.7
    labium (majus) (minus)   752.6
    labyrinth, membranous   745.0
    larynx   748.3
    leg   755.7
    limb except reduction deformity
      755.9

Anomaly, etc. — *continued*
  submaxillary gland   750.9
  superior vena cava   747.4
  tarsus   755.7
  tendon   756.9
  testicle   752.9
  thebesian valve   746.8
  thigh   755.7
  thorax (wall)   756.4
  throat   750.9
  thumb   755.5
  thymus gland   758.3
  thyroid (gland)   758.2
    cartilage   748.3
  tibia   755.7
  toe   755.7
  tongue   750.0
  tooth, teeth NEC   520.9
    position   524.3
    spacing   524.3
  tracheal cartilage   748.3
  trichromata   377.3
  trichromatopsia   377.3
  tricuspid (leaflet) (valve)   746.6
  trunk   758.9
  ulna   755.5
  umbilicus   758.9
  union trachea with larynx   748.3
  upper extremity   755.5
  urachus   753.9
  ureter   753.9
    obstructive   753.2
  urethra (valve)   753.9
  urinary tract   753.9
  uterus   752.5
    complicating delivery   657.9
      fetus or newborn -see categoriies
        764.0-764.9   764.9
      noted during pregnancy (undelivered)
        634.9
  vagina   752.6
  valleculae   748.3
  valve (heart)   746.6
  vas deferens   752.9
  vascular NEC   747.6
    ring   747.2
  vein(s) (peripheral)   747.6
    brain   747.8
    cerebral   747.8
    coronary   746.8
    great   747.4
    portal   747.4
    pulmonary   747.4
    retina   744.9
  vena cava (inferior) (superior)   747.4
  venous return   747.4

Anomaly, etc. — *continued*
  ventricular
    bands   746.8
    folds   746.8
    septa   746.3
  vertebra   756.2
  vesicourethral orifice   753.9
  vessels NEC   747.6
    optic papilla   744.9
  vitreous humor   744.9
  vulva   752.6
  wrist (joint)   755.5
Anomia   781.5
Anonychia   757.4
  acquired   703.9
Anophthalmos, anophthalmus (congenital)
    (globe)   744.0
  acquired   378.9
Anopsia (altitudinal)   373.9
Anorchia   752.8
Anorchism, anorchidism   752.8
Anorexia   784.0
  hysterical   300.1
  nervosa   306.5
Anosmia (*see also* Disturbance, sensation)
    781.6
  hysterical   300.1
  postinfectional   508.9
  traumatic - *see* Injury, nerve, olfactory
Anosognosia   781.6
Anosteoplasia   756.7
Anovulatory cycle   615.9
Anoxemia   796.0
  newborn (*see also* Asphyxia, newborn)
    776.9
Anoxia   796.0
  altitude   993.2
  cerebral   347.9
    newborn (*see also* Asphyxia,
      newborn)   776.9
  due to drowning   994.1
  fetus - *see* Anoxia, intra-uterine
  heart - *see* Insufficiency, coronary
  high altitude   993.2
  intra-uterine   776.4
    with
      abnormality of bones, organs or
        tissues of pelvis - *see*
        categories 764.0-764.4
      abnormality of forces of labor - *see*
        categories 767.0-767.4
      difficult labor NEC - *see* categories
        768.0-768.4
      disproportion, fetopelvic - *see*
        categories 765.0-765.4

Anoxia—*continued*
  intra-uterine—*continued*
    with—*continued*
      disproportion—*continued*
        with abnormality of bones,
          organs or tissues of pelvis
          - *see* categories 764.0-
          764.4
      malposition of fetus - *see* categories
        766.0-766.4
      myocardial - *see* Insufficiency, coronary
      newborn (*see also* Asphyxia, newborn)
        776.9
      pathological   796.0
Anteflexion - *see* Anteversion
Antepartum - *see* condition
Anterior - *see* condition
Anteversion
  cervix (*see also* Anteversion, uterus)
    624.1
  femur (neck), congenital   755.7
  uterus, uterine (cervix) (postinfectional)
    (postpartal, old)   624.1
  complicating
    delivery   657.9
      fetus or newborn - *see* categories
        764.0-764.9
      pregnancy (undelivered)   634.9
    congenital   752.5
    pregnant or gravid (undelivered)
      634.9
Anthracosilicosis   515.1
  with tuberculosis   010
Anthracosis (lung)   515.1
  with tuberculosis   010
Anthrax (any site)   022
Anthropoid pelvis   755.7
  complicating delivery   654.1
    fetus or newborn - *see* categories
      764.0-764.9
  noted during pregnancy (undelivered)
    634.9
Antimonial cholera   985.9
Antisocial personality   301.7
Antithrombinemia (*see also* Circulating
    anticoagulants)   286.5
Antithromboplastinemia (*see also*
    Circulating anticoagulants)   286.5
Antithromboplastinogenemia (*see also*
    Circulating anticoagulants)   286.5
Antitoxin complication or reaction - *see*
    Complications, vaccination
Antritis (*see also* Sinusitis, antrum)
    503.0
Antrum, antral - *see* condition
Anuria   786.5

Anuria—*continued*
  with abortion - *see* Abortion, by type,
    with toxemia
  calculous (impacted) (recurrent)   592
  congenital   753.3
  newborn   753.3
  puerperal, postpartum, childbirth   636
  sulfonamide   961.0
  traumatic (following crushing)   995.6
Anus, anal - *see* condition
Anusitis   569.2
Anxiety (neurosis) (reaction) (state)
    300.0
  depression   300.0
  hysteria   300.0
Aorta, aortic - *see* condition
Aortitis (nonsyphilitic)   446.9
  arteriosclerotic - *see* Arteriosclerosis,
    aorta
  calcific   446.9
  Doehle-Heller   093.9
  luetic   093.9
  rheumatic (*see also* Endocarditis, acute,
    rheumatic)   391.1
  rheumatoid - *see* Arthritis, rheumatoid
  specific   093.9
  syphilitic   093.9
    congenital   090.5
Apepsia   536.9
  achlorhydric   536.0
  psychogenic   305.5
Apert's syndrome   756.0
Aphagia   784.0
  psychogenic   306.5
Aphakia
  acquired   378.7
  congenital   744.8
  unilateral   378.7
Aphasia (amnestic) (ataxic) (auditory)
    (Broca's) (choreatic) (expressive)
    (global) (jargon) (motor) (nominal)
    (receptive) (semantic) (sensory)
    (syntactic) (verbal) (visual)
    (Wernicke's)   781.5
  developmental   306.1
  syphilis, tertiary   094.9
  uremic - *see* Uremia
Aphemia   781.5
Aphonia   783.5
  clericorum   783.5
  hysterical   300.1
  organic   783.5
  psychogenic   305.2
Aphthae, aphthous - *see also* condition
  Bednar's   528.2
  epizootic   079.4

Aphthae, etc. — *continued*
  fever 079.4
  stomatitis 528.2
  thrush 112
  ulcer (oral) (recurrent) 528.2
    genital organ(s) NEC
      female 629.9
      male 607.9
    larynx 508.3
Apical - *see* condition
Aplasia - *see also* Agenesis
  alveolar process (acquired) 525.9
    congenital 750.8
  aorta (congenital) 747.2
  aortic valve (congenital) 746.6
  axialis extracorticalis (congenita) 333.1
  bone marrow (myeloid) 284
  brain 740
    specific part 743.2
  bronchus 748.3
  cementum 520.4
  cerebellum 743.2
  corpus callosum 743.2
  eye 744.1
  fovea centralis (congenital) 744.8
  iris 744.5
  labyrinth, membranous 745.0
  limb (congenital) 755.4
    lower 755.3
    upper 755.2
  lung (bilateral) (congenital) (unilateral) 748.5
  nervous system NEC 743.8
  nuclear 743.8
  Pelizaeus-Merzbacher 333.1
  prostate 752.8
  red cell 284
  round ligament 752.8
  spinal cord 743.3
  testicle 752.8
  ventral horn cell 743.3
Apnea 783.2
  newborn (*see also* Asphyxia, newborn) 776.9
Apneumatosis newborn (*see also* Asphyxia, newborn) 776.9
Apophysitis (bone) (*see also* Osteochondrosis) 722.9
  calcaneus 722.4
Apoplectiform convulsions (*see also* Disease, cerebrovascular, acute) 436.9
Apoplexia, apoplexy, apoplectic (*see also* Disease, cerebrovascular, acute) 436.9
  abdominal 569.9

Apoplexia, etc. — *continued*
  adrenal - *see* Meningococcemia
  alcoholic (cerebral) 303.9
  basilar (*see also* Disease, cerebrovascular, acute) 436.9
  brain (*see also* Disease, cerebrovascular, acute) 436.9
  bulbar (*see also* Disease, cerebrovascular, acute) 436.9
  capillary (*see also* Disease, cerebrovascular, acute) 436.9
  cardiac - *see* Disease, heart
  cerebral (*see also* Disease, cerebrovascular, acute) 436.9
  chorea (*see also* Disease, cerebrovascular, acute) 436.9
  congestive (*see also* Disease, cerebrovascular, acute) 436.9
  cord, spinal 349.9
    fetus or newborn (*see also* Birth injury, spinal cord) 772.1
  embolic (*see also* Embolism, brain) 434.9
  fetus or newborn (*see also* Birth injury, brain) 772.0
  fit (*see also* Disease, cerebrovascular, acute) 436.9
  heart - *see* Disease, heart
  heat 992.0
  hemiplegia (*see also* Disease, cerebrovascular, acute) 436.9
  hemorrhagic (stroke) (*see also* Hemorrhage, brain) 431.9
  ingravescent (*see also* Disease, cerebrovascular, acute) 436.9
  lung - *see* Embolism, pulmonary
  meninges, hemorrhagic (*see also* Hemorrhage, subarachnoid) 430.9
  placenta, complicating delivery - *see* Placenta, separation
  progressive (*see also* Disease, cerebrovascular, acute) 436.9
  puerperal, postpartum, childbirth 674
  pulmonary (artery) (vein) - *see* Embolism, pulmonary
  sanguineous (*see also* Disease, cerebrovascular, acute) 436.9
  seizure (*see also* Disease, cerebrovascular, acute) 436.9
  serous (*see also* Disease, cerebrovascular, acute) 436.9
  spleen 289.5
  stroke (*see also* Disease, cerebrovascular, acute) 436.9

Apoplexia, etc. — *continued*
  thrombotic (*see also* Thrombosis, brain)
    433.9
  uremic - *see* Uremia
  uteroplacental (complicating delivery) -
    see Placenta, separation
Appendage
  intestine (epiploic) 751.4
  pre-auricular 745.1
  testicular (organ of Morgagni) 752.8
Appendicitis 541
  with perforation, peritonitis or rupture
    540.0
  acute (catarrhal) (fulminating)
    (gangrenous) (obstructive)
    (retrocecal) (suppurative) 540.9
    with perforation, peritonitis, or
      rupture 540.0
  amebic 006.9
    with liver abscess 006.0
  chronic (recurrent) 542
  exacerbation - *see* Appendicitis, acute
  gangrenous - *see* Appendicitis, acute
  healed (obliterative) 543
  interval 542
  neurogenic 542
  obstructive 542
  pneumococcal .541
  recurrent 542
  retrocecal 541
  subacute (adhesive) 542
  suppurative - *see* Appendicitis; acute
  tuberculous 014
    late effect or sequela 019.9
Appendicopathia 543
  oxyurica 127.3
Appendix, appendicular - *see also*
  condition
  Morgagni 752.8
Appetite
  depraved 306.5
  excessive 788.9
  lack or loss (*see also* Anorexia) 784.0
  perverted 306.5
    hysterical 300.1
Application forceps
  fetus or newborn (*see also* Birth injury
    NEC) 772.9
Apprehension state 300.0
Apprehensiveness, abnormal 300.0
Apraxia (classic) (ideational) (ideokinetic)
  (ideomotor) (motor) 781.5
  verbal 781.5
Aptyalism 527.7
Arachnidism 989.4
Arachnitis - *see* Arachnoiditis

Arachnodactyly 759.8
Arachnoiditis (acute) (adhesive) (basic)
  (brain) (cerebrospinal) (chiasmal)
  (chronic) (spinal) (*see also*
  Meningitis) 320.9
  H. influenzae 320.0
    late effects 324
  late effects 324
  meningococcal (chronic) 036.0
  pneumococcal 320.1
    late effects 324
  specified organism NEC 320.8
    late effects 324
  syphilitic 094.9
  tuberculous 013.0
    late effect or sequela 019.1
Araneism 989.4
Arbor virus, arbovirus (infection) NEC
  068.9
Arborization block (heart) (*see also* Block,
  heart) 427.3
Arches - *see* condition
Arcuatus uterus 752.5
Arcus (cornea)
  juvenilis 378.4
  senilis 378.4
Arc-welder's lung 516.0
Areola - *see* condition
Argentaffinoma - *see* Carcinoid
Argyll Robertson pupil or syndrome
  (syphilitic) 094.0
  nonsyphilitic 378.6
Argyria 961.2
Argyriasis 961.2
Ariboflavinosis 263.0
Arizona enteritis 008.1
Arm - *see* condition
Arnold-Chiari obstruction or syndrome
  741.0
Arrest
  any plane in pelvis·
    complicating delivery 655
      fetus or newborn - *see* categories
      765.0-765.9
  cardiac 427.2
    with
      hypertension (benign) (conditions in
      401) (*see also* Hypertension,
      heart) 402
      malignant (*see also*
        Hypertension, malignant
        with heart involvement)
        400.1
    complicating
      anesthesia NEC 968.1

Arrest—*continued*
  cardiac—*continued*
    complicating—*continued*
      anesthesia—*continued*
        specified anesthetic - *see* Table
          of adverse effects
        surgery (therapeutic)
          (nontherapeutic) 998.9
    fetus or newborn 778.9
  cardio-respiratory (*see also* Arrest,
    cardiac) 427.2
  heart - *see* Arrest, cardiac
  respiratory 796.0
    newborn (*see also* Asphyxia,
      newborn) 776.9
  sinus (*see also* Block, heart) 427.3
  transverse
    complicating delivery 656.8
    fetus or newborn - *see* categories
      766.0-766.9
Arrested development or growth
  bone 723.6
  fetus or newborn 778.9
  tracheal rings 748.3
Arrhenoblastoma
  female 256.0
  male 257.0
  malignant
    female 183.0
    male 186
Arrhythmia (auricle) (cardiac) (cordis)
  (nodal) (reflex) (sinus)
  (supraventricular) (transitory)
  (ventricle) (*see also* Action, heart,
  irregular) 427.9
  psychogenic 305.3
Arrillaga-Ayerza syndrome 426
Arsenical
  pigmentation 709.9
Arsenism (*see also* Table of adverse
  effects) 985.1
Arterial - *see* condition
Arteriectasis 447
Arteriofibrosis - *see* Arteriosclerosis
Arteriolar sclerosis - *see* Arteriosclerosis
Arteriolith - *see* Arteriosclerosis
Arteriolitis 447
  necrotizing, kidney 446.9
  renal - *see* Hypertension, kidney
Arterionephrosclerosis (*see also*
  Hypertension, kidney) 403
Arteriopathy 447
Arteriosclerosis, arteriosclerotic (artery)
  (diffuse) (disease) (general)
  (obliterans) (obliterative) (occlusive)
  (senile) (with calcification) 440.9

Arteriosclerosis, etc.—*continued*
  with
    gangrene (conditions in 445.9) 445.0
    insufficiency, myocardial (conditions
      in 428) (*see also* Ischemia,
      heart) 412.9
  aorta 440.0
    with
      gangrene (conditions in 445.9)
        445.0
      myocardial insufficiency (conditions
        in 428) (*see also* Ischemia,
        heart) 412.9
  arteries of extremities (*see also*
    Arteriosclerosis, peripheral)
    440.2
  basilar (artery) (*see also* Occlusion,
    precerebral artery) 432.9
  brain (*see also* Ischemia, cerebral)
    437.9
  cardiac (*see also* Ischemia, heart)
    412.9
  cardiopathy (*see also* Ischemia, heart)
    412.9
  cardiorenal - *see* Hypertension,
    cardiorenal
  cardiovascular (*see also* Ischemia,
    heart) 412.9
  carotid (artery) (common) (internal) (*see*
    also Occlusion, precerebral
    artery) 432.9
  central nervous system (*see also*
    Ischemia, cerebral) 437.9
  cerebral (*see also* Ischemia, cerebral)
    437.9
  cerebrospinal (*see also* Ischemia,
    cerebral) 437.9
  cerebrovascular (*see also* Ischemia,
    cerebral) 437.9
  coronary (artery) (*see also* Ischemia,
    heart) 412.9
  extremities (*see also* Arteriosclerosis,
    peripheral) 440.2
  heart (*see also* Ischemia, heart) 412.9
  and kidney - *see* Hypertension,
    cardiorenal
  disease (*see also* Ischemia, heart)
    412.9
  kidney (*see also* Hypertension, kidney)
    403
  medial (*see also* Arteriosclerosis,
    peripheral) 440.2
  Monckeberg's (*see also*
    Arteriosclerosis, peripheral)
    440.2
  parkinsonism 342

Arteriosclerosis, etc. — *continued*
  peripheral (of extremities)   440.2
    with
      gangrene (conditions in 445.9)
        445.0
      myocardial insufficiency (conditions
        in 428) (*see also* Ischemia,
        heart)   412.9
  pulmonary   426
  renal (*see also* Hypertension, kidney)
    403
    arterioles (*see also* Hypertension,
      kidney)   403
    artery   440.1
      with
        gangrene (conditions in 445.9)
          445.0
        myocardial insufficiency
          (conditions in 428) (*see*
          also Ischemia, heart)
          412.9
  retina (vascular) - *see* Arteriosclerosis,
    specified artery
  specified artery NEC   440.3
    with
      gangrene (conditions in 445.9)
        445.0
      myocardial insufficiency (conditions
        in 428) (*see also* Ischemia,
        heart)   412.9
  spinal (cord) (*see also* Ischemia,
    cerebral)   437.9
  vertebral (artery) (left) (right) (*see also*
    Occlusion, precerebral artery)
    432.9
Arteriospasm   443.9
Arteriovenous - *see* condition
Arteritis   447
  allergic   446.2
  aorta (nonsyphilitic)   446.9
    syphilitic   093.9
  aortic arch   446.6
  brain (*see also* Disease, cerebrovascular
    NEC)   438.9
    syphilitic   094.9
  cerebral (*see also* Disease,
    cerebrovascular NEC)   438.9
    syphilitic   094.9
  coronary (artery) (*see also* Ischemia,
    heart)   412.9
    rheumatic   391.9
      chronic   398
    syphilitic   093.9
  cranial (left) (right)   446.4
  deformans - *see* Arteriosclerosis
  giant cell   446.4

Arteritis — *continued*
  necrosing or necrotizing   446.0
  nodosa   446.0
  obliterans - *see* Arteriosclerosis
  rheumatic - *see* Fever, rheumatic
  senile - *see* Arteriosclerosis
  suppurative   447
  syphilitic (general)   093.9
    brain   094.9
    coronary   093.9
    spinal   094.9
  temporal   446.4
Artery, arterial - *see* condition
Arthralgia   787.3
  allergic   787.3
  psychogenic   305.1
Arthritis, arthritic (general) (inflammatory)
    (monarticular) (multiple) (static)
    715
  acute (due to pyogenic organism)
    (infective) (pneumococcal)
    (purulent) (pyemic) (pyogenic)
    (septic) (staphylococcal)
    (streptococcal) (suppurative)
    710.9
    due to nonpyogenic infection (e.g.,
      dysentery, enteritis,
      paratyphoid, Reiter's urethritis,
      typhoid)   711
    hip   710.2
    lower extremity, except hip   710.3
    specified site NEC   710.9
    spine   710.0
    upper extremity (including shoulder)
      710.1
  allergic   714.9
  ankylosing (crippling)   712.3
    spine   712.4
  atrophic (chronic)   712.3
    spine   712.4
  back (*see also* Arthritis, spine)   715
  blennorrhagic   098.3
  cervical (*see also* Arthritis, spine)   715
  chronic (any site) NEC   715
  climacteric (any site) NEC   714.9
  coccyx (*see also* Arthritis, spine)   715
  cricoarytenoid   508.3
  deformans   713.0
    spine   713.1
  degenerative (chronic)   713.0
    spine   713.1
  due to
    epiphyseal slip, nontraumatic (old)
      714.9
    infection (*see also* Arthritis,
      infectious)   714.9

Arthritis, etc. — *continued*
erythema epidemic 026.1
gonococcal 098.3
gouty 274
  acute 274
hypertrophic (chronic) 713.0
  spine 713.1
idiopathic blennorrheal 136
in caisson disease 993.3
infectious or infective NEC 714.9
  acute - *see* Arthritis, acute
  chronic 712.3
    spine 712.4
  nonpyogenic, any site 711
  subacute 712.3
    spine 712.4
lumbar (*see also* Arthritis, spine) 715
meningococcal 036.8
menopausal (any site) NEC 714.9
neuropathic (Charcot) (tabetic) 094.0
  diabetic - *see* category 250
  non-syphilitic NEC 714.9
  syringomyelic 349.0
nodosa 713.0
  spine 713.1
nonpyogenic, acute or subacute (any
    site) 711
ochronotic 270.6
palindromic (any site) 712.2
pneumococcal (acute) - *see* Arthritis,
  acute
primary progressive (chronic) 712.3
  spine 712.4
proliferative 712.3
  spine 712.4
psoriatic 696.0
purulent (acute) - *see also* Arthritis,
  acute
  chronic 714.9

pyemic or pyogenic (acute) - *see*
  Arthritis, acute

rheumatic 714.9
  acute or subacute - *see* Fever,
    rheumatic
  chronic 712.3
    spine 712.4

rheumatoid (acute) (atrophic) (chronic)
  712.3
  with spleno-adenomegaly and
    leukopenia 712.1
  juvenile 712.0
  spine 712.4

sacral, sacro-iliac, sacrococcygeal (*see
  also* Arthritis, spine) 715

scorbutic 264

Arthritis, etc. — *continued*
senile or senescent 713.0
  spine 713.1
septic (acute) - *see also* Arthritis, acute
  chronic 714.9
serum (nontherapeutic) (therapeutic)
  999.5
specified form NEC 714.9
spine (chronic) 715
  acute (pyogenic) 710.0
    non-pyogenic 711
  atrophic 712.4
  degenerative or other type classifiable
    to 713.0 713.1
  hypertrophic (with deformity) 713.1
  infectious or infective NEC 714.9
    acute 710.0
    chronic 712.4
  Marie-Strumpell 712.4
  rheumatoid or other type classifiable
    to 712.3 712.4
  traumatic (old) 714.0
  tuberculous 015.0
    late effect or sequela 019.3
staphylococcal (acute) - *see* Arthritis,
  acute
streptococcal (acute) - *see* Arthritis,
  acute
subacute - *see also* Arthritis, acute
  infectious or infective NEC 712.3
    spine 712.4
suppurative (acute) - *see also* Arthritis,
  acute
  chronic 714.9
syphilitic 094.0
  congenital 090.4
syphilitica deformans (Charcot) 094.0
toxic of menopause (any site) 714.9
traumatic (chronic) (old) (post) (any site)
  714.0
  current injury - *see* nature of injury
tuberculous - *see* Tuberculosis, arthritis
uratic 274
urethritica 136
urica 274
venereal 136
vertebral (*see also* Arthritis, spine)
  715
villous (chronic) (any site) 714.9

Arthrocele (*see also* Disease, joint)
  729.9

Arthrodesis status (*see also* Disease,
  joint) 729.9

Arthrodynia 787.3
  psychogenic 305.1

Arthrofibrosis, joint (*see also* Disease, joint)　729.9
Arthrogryposis (*see also* Disease, joint)　729.9
　multiplex congenita　755.8
Arthrokatadysis　713.0
Arthropathy (*see also* Disease, joint)　729.9
　Charcot's　094.0
　neurogenic, neuropathic (Charcot) (tabetic)　094.0
　　diabetic - *see* category 250
　　non-syphilitic NEC　714.9
　　syringomyelic　349.0
　psoriatic　696.0
　pulmonary　723.1
　syringomyelia　349.0
　tabes dorsalis　094.0
　tabetic　094.0
Arthrophytis (*see also* Disease, joint)　729.9
Arthropyosis (*see also* Disease, joint)　729.9
Arthrosis (deformans) (degenerative) (polyarticular)　713.0
　spine　713.1
Arthus' phenomenon　999.4
Articular - *see* condition
Artificial
　anus, malfunction　998.7
　menopause (symptoms) (syndrome)　627
Arytenoid - *see* condition
Asbestosis　515.2
　with tuberculosis　010
Ascariasis (intestinal) (lung)　127.0
Ascaris　127.0
　lumbricoides (infestation)　127.0
　pneumonia　127.0
Ascending - *see* condition
Aschoff's bodies (*see also* Myocarditis, rheumatic)　398
Ascites　785.3
　abdominal　785.3
　cancerous　197.6
　cardiac - *see* Disease, heart
　chylous (nonfilarial)　457
　　filarial (*see also* Infestation, filarial)　125.9
　congenital (*see also* Disease, hemolytic)　775.9
　heart - *see* Disease, heart
　hepatic - *see* Cirrhosis, liver
　joint (*see also* Disease, joint)　729.9
　liver - *see* Cirrhosis, liver

Ascites — *continued*
　malignant　197.6
　pseudochylous　785.3
　syphilitic　095
　tuberculous　014
　　late effect or sequela　019.9
Aseptic - *see* condition
Asocial
　personality or trends　301.7
Aspergillosis　117.3
Aspergillus (fumigatus) (infection)　117.3
Aspermatogenesis　606
Aspermia (testis)　606
Asphyxia, asphyxiation　796.0
　alcoholic　303.9
　antenatal (*see also* Distress, fetal)　776.3
　bedclothes　994.7
　birth (*see also* Asphyxia, newborn)　776.9
　bunny bag　994.7
　caul (*see also* Asphyxia, newborn)　776.9
　cave-in　994.7
　　crushing - *see* Injury, internal, intrathoracic
　constriction　994.7
　cord, umbilical, around neck - *see* Complications, umbilical cord
　crushing - *see* Injury, internal, intrathoracic
　drowning　994.1
　during parturition (*see also* Asphyxia, newborn)　776.9
　fetal (*see also* Distress, fetal)　776.3
　food or foreign body (in larynx, nasopharynx, pharynx, or throat)　933
　　bronchus or bronchioles　934
　　lung or trachea　934
　　nose, nasal passages　932
　gas, fumes, or vapor NEC　987.9
　　specified - *see* Table of adverse effects
　hanging　994.7
　inhalation, flame　949.0
　injury at birth (*see also* Asphyxia, newborn)　776.9
　intra-uterine (*see also* Distress, fetal)　776.3
　local　443.0
　mechanical　994.7
　　during birth (*see also* Asphyxia, newborn)　776.9
　mucus　933
　　bronchus, lung, or trachea　934

Asphyxia, etc. — *continued*
mucus — *continued*
larynx, pharynx, or throat 933
nasal passages 932
newborn (*see also* Aspiration, content
of birth canal) 776.0
vaginal (*see also* Aspiration, content
of birth canal) 776.0
newborn (blue) (livida) (pallida) (white)
776.9
with
abnormality of bones, organs or
tissues of pelvis - *see*
categories 764.0-764.4
abnormality of forces of labor - *see*
categories 767.0-767.4
difficult labor NEC - *see* categories
768.0-768.4
disproportion, fetopelvic - *see*
categories 765.0-765.4
with abnormality of bones,
organs or tissues of pelvis
- *see* categories 764.0-
764.4
malposition of fetus - *see* categories
766.0-766.4
pathological 796.0
postnatal (blue) (livida) (pallida) (white)
(*see also* Asphyxia, newborn)
776.9
mechanical 994.7
pressure 994.7
reticularis 782.3
strangulation 994.7
submersion 994.1
traumatic NEC - *see* Injury, internal,
intrathoracic
vomiting, vomitus - *see* Asphyxia, food
or foreign body

Aspiration
amniotic fluid (*see also* Aspiration,
content of birth canal) 776.0
content of birth canal 776.0
with
abnormality of bones, organs or
tissues of pelvis - *see*
categories 764.0-764.4
abnormality of forces of labor - *see*
categories 767.0-767.4
difficult labor NEC - *see* categories
768.0-768.4
disproportion, fetopelvic - *see*
categories 765.0-765.4
with abnormality of bones,
organs or tissues of pelvis
- *see* categories 764.0-764.4

Aspiration — *continued*
content of birth canal — *continued*
with — *continued*
malposition of fetus - *see* categories
766.0-766.4
food, foreign body, or gasoline (with
asphyxiation) - *see* Asphyxia, food
or foreign body
meconium (*see also* Aspiration, content
of birth canal) 776.0
mucus 933
into bronchus, lung, or trachea 934
newborn (*see also* Aspiration, content
of birth canal) 776.0
vaginal (*see also* Aspiration, content
of birth canal) 776.0
newborn (*see also* Aspiration, content
of birth canal) 776.0
syndrome of newborn (*see also*
Aspiration, content of birth
canal) 776.0
vernix caseosa (*see also* Aspiration,
content of birth canal) 776.0

Asplenia 758.0
Assam fever 085.0
Assimilation pelvis
complicating delivery - *see* Deformity,
pelvis, complicating delivery
noted during pregnancy (undelivered)
634.9
Assmann's focus (with symptoms) (*see*
also Tuberculosis, pulmonary)
011.9
Astasia(-abasia) 306.3
hysterical 300.1
Asteatosis 706.9
Astereognosis 781.6
Asterixis 573.9
Asthenia, asthenic 790.1
cardiac (*see also* Failure, heart) 782.4
psychogenic 305.3
cardiovascular (*see also* Failure, heart)
782.4
psychogenic 305.3
heart (*see also* Failure, heart) 782.4
psychogenic 305.3
hysterical 300.1
myocardial (*see also* Failure, heart)
782.4
psychogenic 305.3
nervous 300.5
neurocirculatory 305.3
neurotic 300.5
psychogenic 300.5
psychoneurotic 300.5
psychophysiologic 300.5

Asthenia, asthenic — *continued*
  reaction (psychophysiologic) 300.5
  senile 794
Asthenopia 370.9
  accommodative 370.9
  hysterical (muscular) 300.1
  psychogenic 305.8
Asthenospermia 607.9
Asthma, asthmatic (allergic, any cause)
        (bronchial) (catarrh) (infantile)
        (spasmodic) 493
  with
    bronchitis - *see* Bronchitis
    hay fever 493
  cardiac (*see also* Failure, ventricular,
        left) 427.1
  cardiobronchial (*see also* Failure,
        ventricular, left) 427.1
  cardiorenal - *see* Hypertension,
        cardiorenal
  colliers' 515.1
    tuberculous 010
  croup 493
  dropsy 493
  grinders' 515.0
    tuberculous 010
  hay 493
  heart (*see also* Failure, ventricular, left)
        427.1
  Kopp's 254
  Millar's 508.3
  millstone makers' 515.0
    tuberculous 010
  miners' 515.1
    tuberculous 010
  pneumoconiotic NEC 515.9
    with tuberculosis 010
  potters' 515.0
    tuberculous 010
  psychogenic 305.2
  pulmonary eosinophilic 519.2
  renal (*see also* Lesion, kidney) 593.2
  Rostan's (*see also* Failure, ventricular,
        left) 427.1
  sandblasters' 515.0
    tuberculous 010
  stonemasons' 515.0
    tuberculous 010
  thymic 254
  tuberculous (*see also* Tuberculosis,
        pulmonary) 011.9
Astigmatism (compound) (congenital) (any
        type) 370.3

Astroblastoma (*see also* Neoplasm,
        nervous system, malignant) 192.9
  nose 212.0
Astrocytoma (*see also* Neoplasm, nervous
        system, malignant) 192.9
  nose 212.0
Astroglioma (*see also* Neoplasm, nervous
        system, malignant) 192.9
  nose 212.0
Asymbolia 781.5
Asymmetry - *see also* Distortion
  face 745.8
  jaw 524.1
Asynergia 780.4
Asynergy 780.4
Asystole (heart) (*see also* Arrest, cardiac)
        427.2
Ataxia, ataxy, ataxic 780.4
  acute 780.4
  brain 347.9
    hereditary 332.1
  cerebellar 347.9
    hereditary (Marie's) 332.1
  cerebral 347.9
    hereditary 332.1
    palsy - *see* Palsy, cerebral
  family, familial 332.9
    cerebral (Marie's) 332.1
    spinal (Friedreich's) 332.0
  Friedreich's (heredofamilial) (spinal)
        332.0
  gait 787.6
    hysterical 300.1
  general 780.4
  hereditary NEC 332.9
  heredofamilial, Marie's 332.1
  hysterical 300.1
  locomotor (progressive) 094.0
  Marie's (cerebellar) (heredofamilial)
        332.1
  nonorganic origin 306.3
  partial 094.0
  progressive 094.0
  psychogenic 306.3
  Sanger-Brown's 332.1
  spastic 094.0
    syphilitic 094.0
  spinal
    hereditary 332.0
    progressive 094.0
  telangiectasia 275.0
Ataxia-telangiectasia 275.0
Ataxo-adynamia (*see also* Ataxia)
        780.4

Atelectasis (absorption collapse)
(complete) (compression) (massive)
(partial) (postinfective) (pressure
collapse) (pulmonary) (relaxation)
519.0
congenital (*see also* Asphyxia, newborn)
776.9
partial (*see also* Syndrome,
respiratory distress) 776.2
fetus, partial (*see also* Syndrome,
respiratory distress) 776.2
newborn (*see also* Asphyxia, newborn)
776.9
partial (*see also* Syndrome,
respiratory distress) 776.2
postnatal (*see also* Asphyxia, newborn)
776.9
partial (*see also* Syndrome,
respiratory distress) 776.2
tuberculous (*see also* Tuberculosis,
pulmonary) 011.9
late effect or sequela 019.0
Atelia - *see* Distortion
Ateliosis 253.1
Atelocardia 746.9
Atelomyelia 743.3
Atherocarcinoma - *see* Epithelioma,
malignant
Atheroma, atheromatous (*see also*
Arteriosclerosis) 440.9
aorta, aortic (*see also* Arteriosclerosis,
aorta) 440.0
valve (*see also* Endocarditis, aortic,
nonrheumatic) 424.1
artery - *see* Arteriosclerosis
basilar (artery) (*see also* Occlusion,
precerebral artery) 432.9
cerebral (arteries) (*see also* Ischemia,
cerebral) 437.9
coronary (*see also* Ischemia, heart)
412.9
degeneration - *see* Arteriosclerosis
heart, cardiac - *see* Ischemia, heart
mitral (valve) - *see* Endocarditis, mitral,
nonrheumatic
myocardium, myocardial - *see*
Ischemia, heart
pulmonary valve (heart) (*see also*
Endocarditis, pulmonary) 424.9
skin 706.2
tricuspid (heart) (valve) - *see*
Endocarditis, tricuspid,
nonrheumatic
valve, valvular - *see* Endocarditis
Atheromatosis - *see also* Arteriosclerosis
arterial congenital 272.0

Atherosclerosis - *see* Arteriosclerosis
Athetosis (acquired) 780.3
bilateral 331.9
congenital (bilateral) 331.9
double 331.9
unilateral 780.3
Athlete's
foot 110.1
heart - *see* Disease, heart
Athrepsia (due to malnutrition) 268
Athyrea (acquired) 244
congenital 243
Athyroidism (acquired) 244
congenital 243
Atonia, atony, atonic
abdominal wall 733.9
bladder (sphincter) (neurogenic NEC)
596.9
bleeding, complicating delivery 653
capillary 448
cecum 564.9
psychogenic 305.5
colon 564.9
psychogenic 305.5
congenital 778.9
dyspepsia 536.1
psychogenic 305.5
intestine 564.9
psychogenic 305.5
stomach 536.1
neurotic or psychogenic 305.5
uterus
complicating delivery 657.1
fetus or newborn - *see* categories
767.0-767.9
Atransferrinemia, congenital 280
Atresia, atretic (congenital) 758.8
alimentary organ or tract NEC 751.8
lower 751.4
upper 750.8
ani, anus, anal (canal) 751.3
aorta 747.2
arch 747.1
ring 747.2
aortic (valve) 746.6
arch 747.1
aqueduct of Sylvius 742
with spina bifida 741.0
artery NEC 747.6
cerebral 747.8
coronary 746.8
eye 744.8
pulmonary 747.3
umbilical 747.5
auditory canal (external) 745.0
bile duct 751.5

Atresia, etc. — *continued*
  bile duct — *continued*
    acquired (*see also* Obstruction,
        gallbladder)   576.0
  bladder (neck)   753.6
  bronchus   748.3
  cecum   751.4
  cervix (acquired)   621.5
    complicating delivery   657.2
      fetus or newborn - *see* categories
          764.0-764.9
    congenital   752.5
    noted during pregnancy (undelivered)
        634.9
  choana   748.0
  colon   751.4
  cystic duct   751.5
    acquired (*see also* Obstruction,
        gallbladder)   576.0
  digestive organs NEC   751.8
  duodenum   751.4
  ear canal   745.0
  ejaculatory duct   752.8
  epiglottis   748.3
  esophagus   750.3
  eustachian tube   745.2
  fallopian tube (acquired)   615.9
    congenital   752.5
  foramen of
      Luschka   742
        with spina bifida   741.0
      Magendie   742
        with spina bifida   741.0
  gallbladder   751.6
  genital organ
    external
      female   752.6
      male   752.8
    internal
      female   752.5
      male   752.8
  glottis   748.3
  gullet   750.3
  heart, any valve   746.6
  hymen   752.6
    acquired   629.7
    postinfective   629.7
  ileum   751.4
  intestine (large) (small)   751.4
  iris, filtration angle   744.2
  jejunum   751.4
  kidney   753.3
  lachrymal, lacrimal apparatus   744.8
    acquired   378.3
  larynx   748.3
  lung   748.6

Atresia, etc. — *continued*
  meatus urinarius   753.6
  mitral valve   746.6
  nares (anterior) (posterior)   748.0
  nasopharynx   748.8
  nose, nostril   748.0
    acquired   508.9
  organ or site not listed - *see* Anomaly,
      specified type NEC
  osseous meatus (ear)   745.0
  oviduct (acquired)   615.9
    congenital   752.5
  parotid duct   750.8
    acquired   527.9
  pulmonary (artery)   747.3
    valve   746.6
    vein   747.4
  pulmonic   746.6
  pupil   744.8
  rectum   751.3
  salivary duct or gland   750.8
    acquired   527.9
  sublingual duct   750.8
    acquired   527.9
  submaxillary duct or gland   750.8
    acquired   527.9
  trachea   748.3
  tricuspid valve   746.6
  ureter   753.2
  ureteropelvic junction   753.2
  ureterovesical orifice   753.2
  urethra (valvular)   753.6
  urinary tract NEC   753.2
  uterus   752.5
    acquired   625.9
  vagina (acquired)   629.7
    congenital   752.6
    postgonococcal (old)   098.1
    postinfectional   629.7
    senile   629.7
  vas deferens   752.8
  vascular NEC   747.6
    cerebral   747.8
  vein   747.6
    great   747.4
    portal   747.4
    pulmonary   747.4
  vena cava (inferior) (superior)   747.4
  vesicourethral orifice   753.6
  vulva   752.6
    acquired   629.7

Atrichia, atrichosis   704
  congenital (universal)   757.3

Atrophia
  cutis senilis   701.9

Atrophia—*continued*
  dermatologica, diffuse (idiopathic)
      701.9
  flava hepatis (acuta) (subacuta) (*see also*
      Necrosis, liver) 570
  gyrata of choroid and retina 744.8
  senilis 794
    dermatological 701.9
  unguium 703.9
    congenita 757.4
Atrophoderma, atrophodermia 701.9
  diffusum (idiopathic) 701.9
  maculatum 701.2
    et striatum 701.2
      due to syphilis 095
      syphilitic 091.2
  neuriticum 701.9
  pigmentosum 757.2
  reticulatum symmetricum faciei 701.9
  senile 701.9
  symmetrical 701.9
  vermiculata 701.9
Atrophy, atrophic
  adrenal (capsule) (gland) 255.9
  alveolar process or ridge (edentulous)
      525.1
  appendix 543
  arm 733.1
  arteriosclerotic - *see* Arteriosclerosis
  arthritis 712.3
    spine 712.4
  bladder 596.9
  bone (senile) 723.9
    due to
      infection 723.9
      tabes dorsalis (neurogenic) 094.0
    late effect, acute poliomyelitis 044
    post-traumatic 723.9
  brain (cortex) (diffuse) (parenchymatous)
      (progressive) 347.1
    alcoholic 303.2
    circumscribed 290.1
    congenital 743.9
    hereditary 333.9
    late effect, viral encephalitis 066
    senile 794
  breast 611.9
    puerperal, postpartum 678
  buccal cavity 528.9
  cardiac (*see also* Disease, heart) 429.9
  cartilage (infectional) (joint) (*see also*
      Disease, joint) 729.9
  cerebellar - *see* Atrophy, brain
  cerebral - *see* Atrophy, brain
  cervix (mucosa) (senile) (uteri) 621.6
    menopausal 621.6

Atrophy, atrophic—*continued*
  Charcot-Marie-Tooth 330.0
  choroid (central) (macular) (myopic)
      (retina) (senile) 378.6
  ciliary body 378.6
  cirrhosis (liver) - *see* Cirrhosis, portal
  conjunctiva (senile) 378.3
  corpus cavernosum 607.9
  cortical (*see also* Atrophy, brain)
      347.1
  Dejerine-Thomas 347.1
  Duchenne-Aran 348.2
  ear 387.9
  edentulous alveolar ridge 525.1
  emphysema, lung 492
  endometrium (postmenopausal) (senile)
      625.0
    cervix 621.6
  enteric 569.9
  epididymis 607.9
  eyeball 378.9
  eyelid (senile) 378.2
  facial (skin) 701.9
  facioscapulohumeral 330.3
  fallopian tube (senile) 615.9
  fatty, thymus (gland) 254
  gallbladder (*see also* Disease,
      gallbladder) 576.9
  gastric 537.9
  gastritis (acute) (chronic) 535
  gastro-intestinal 569.9
  glandular 289.3
  globe 378.9
  gum 523.2
  hair 704
  heart (brown) (*see also* Disease, heart)
      429.9
  hemifacial, Romberg 356
  infantile 268
    paralysis, acute 041
  intestine 569.9
  iris (postinfectional) 378.6
  kidney (senile) (*see also* Sclerosis, renal)
      584
    congenital 753.0
    hydronephrotic 591
    infantile 753.0
  lachrymal, lacrimal apparatus 378.3
  Landouzy-Dejerine 330.3
  laryngitis, infectional 506
  larynx 508.3
  lip 528.5
  liver (acute) (subacute) (*see also*
      Necrosis, liver) 570
    chronic (yellow) 573.9
    cirrhosis - *see* Cirrhosis, portal

Atrophy, atrophic — *continued*
liver, etc. — *continued*
  yellow (congenital) (*see also*
      Necrosis, liver) 570
    chronic 573.9
    from injection, inoculation or
        transfusion (onset within 8
        months after administration)
        999.2
    healed - *see* Cirrhosis, postnecrotic
    post-immunization 999.2
    post-transfusion 999.2
lung (senile) 519.2
  congenital 748.6
macular (dermatological) 701.2
  syphilitic, skin 091.2
    striated 095
muscle, muscular 733.1
  Duchenne-Aran 348.2
  extremity (lower) (upper) 733.1
  general 733.1
  hereditary spinal 330.1
  idiopathic 733.1
  late effect, acute poliomyelitis 044
  myelopathic (progressive) 348.2
  neuritic 330.0
  neuropathic (peroneal) (progressive)
      330.0
  peroneal 330.0
  primary (idiopathic) 733.1
  progressive 348.2
    spinal 348.2
      specified as hereditary or familial
          330.1
  pseudohypertrophic 330.3
  spinal 348.2
    Aran-Duchenne 348.2
    familial 330.1
    hereditary 330.1
    infantile 330.1
    progressive 348.2
  syphilitic 095
myocardium (*see also* Disease, heart)
    429.9
myometrium (senile) 625.0
  cervix 621.6
myotatic 733.1
nail 703.9
  congenital 757.4
nasopharynx 502.1
nerve
  abducens 373.9
  accessory 356
  acoustic or auditory 387.9
  cranial 356
    eighth (auditory) 387.9

Atrophy, atrophic — *continued*
nerve — *continued*
  cranial — *continued*
    eleventh (accessory) 356
    fifth (trigeminal) 356
    first (olfactory) 356
    fourth (trochlear) 373.9
    ninth (glossopharyngeal) 356
    second (optic) 377.6
    seventh (facial) 350
    sixth (abducens) 373.9
    tenth (pneumogastric) 356
    third (oculomotor) 373.9
    twelfth (hypoglossal) 356
  facial 350
  glossopharyngeal 356
  hypoglossal 356
  oculomotor 373.9
  olfactory 356
  pneumogastric 356
  trigeminal 356
  trochlear 373.9
  vagus (pneumogastric) 356
nervous system, congenital 743.9
neuritic 355.9
neurogenic, bone
  syringomyelic 349.0
  tabetic 094.0
old age 794
olivopontocerebellar 347.1
optic nerve (ascending) (descending)
    (familial) (hereditary) (infectional
    NEC) (Leber's) (nonfamilial)
    (papillomacular bundle)
    (postretinal) (primary) (secondary)
    (simple) 377.6
  syphilitic 094.9
    congenital 090.4
    tabes dorsalis 094.0
ovary (senile) 615.9
oviduct (senile) 615.9
palsy, diffuse 348.9
pancreas (duct) (senile) 577.9
parotid gland 527.0
patches skin 701.2
  senile 701.9
penis 607.9
pharynx 508.9
pluriglandular 258.1
polyarthritis 712.3
prostate 602
pseudohypertrophic 330.3
renal (*see also* Sclerosis, renal) 584
reticulata 701.9
retina, retinal (postinfectional) 377.1
rhinitis 502.1

Atrophy, atrophic — *continued*
  salivary duct or gland   527.0
  scar   709.0
  sclerosis lobar (of brain)   290.1
  scrotum   607.9
  seminal vesicle   607.9
  senile   794
  skin (senile)   701.9
  spermatic cord   607.9
  spinal (cord)   349.9
    acute   349.9
    muscular (chronic)   348.2
    paralysis   348.2
      acute   041
        late effects   044
  spine (column)   723.9
  spleen (senile)   289.5
  spots (skin)   701.2
    senile   701.9
  stomach   537.9
  striate and macular   701.2
    syphilitic   095
  subcutaneous   701.9
  sublingual gland   527.0
  submaxillary gland   527.0
  Sudeck's   723.0
  suprarenal (capsule) (gland)   255.9
  tarso-orbital fascia, congenital   744.8
  testicle   607.8
  throat   508.9
  thymus (fat)   254
  thyroid (gland)   246
    with
      cretinism   243
      myxedema   244
    congenital   243
  tongue (senile)   529.9
    papillae   529.4
  trachea   519.9
  tunica vaginalis   607.9
  turbinate   723.9
  upper respiratory tract   508.9
  uterus, uterine (senile)   625.0
    cervix   621.6
    due to radiation (intended effect)
      625.0
  vagina (senile)   629.9
  vas deferens   607.9
  vascular   458.9
  vertebra (senile)   723.9
  vulva (senile)   629.9
  yellow (acute) (congenital) (liver)
        (subacute) (*see also* Necrosis,
        liver)   570
Attack
  angina - *see* Angina

Attack — *continued*
  bilious (*see also* Vomiting)   784.1
  cataleptic   300.1
  cerebral (*see also* Disease,
        cerebrovascular, acute)   436.9
  coronary (*see also* Infarct, myocardium)
        410.9
  epilepsy   345.9
  epileptiform   780.2
  heart (*see also* Disease, heart)   429.9
  hemiplegia (*see also* Disease,
        cerebrovascular, acute)   436.9
  hysterical   300.1
  jacksonian - *see* Epilepsy, jacksonian
  myocardial (*see also* Insufficiency,
        myocardial)   428
  panic   300.0
  paralysis (*see also* Disease,
        cerebrovascular, acute)   436.9
  paroxysmal   780.2
  psychomotor   345.3
  schizophreniform   295.8
  sensory and motor   780.2
  syncope   782.5
  toxic, cerebral   780.2
  unconsciousness   782.5
    hysterical   300.1
  vasomotor   782.5
  vasovagal (paroxysmal) (idiopathic)
        782.5
Attrition
  gum   523.2
  tooth, teeth (hard tissues)   521.1
Atypical - *see also* condition
  distribution, vessel   747.6
  endometrium   625.9
  kidney (*see also* Lesion, kidney)   593.2
Atypism cervix   621.9
Auditory - *see* condition
Aujeszky's disease   079.8
Aura, jacksonian - *see* Epilepsy,
        jacksonian
Aurantiasis, cutis   278.1
Auricle, auricular - *see* condition
Australian
  Q fever   083.1
  X disease   062.4
    late effects   066
Autism, autistic (child) (infantile)   295.8
Autodigestion   796.0
Auto-erythrocyte sensitization   283.9
Autographism   709.9
Auto-immune
  cold sensitivity   283.9
  hemolytic anemia   283.9
  thyroiditis - *see* Thyroiditis

Auto-infection
  intestinal   569.9
  septic - *see* Septicemia
Auto-intoxication   796.0
  arising during pregnancy (*see also*
      Toxemia, arising during
      pregnancy)   637.9
  intestinal   569.9
Automatism   347.9
  epileptic   345.3
  paroxysmal, idiopathic   345.9
Autonomic, autonomous
  bladder (neurogenic NEC)   596.9
  hysteria seizure   300.1
  . imbalance   358.9
Autosensitivity, erythrocyte   283.9
Autotopagnosia   781.6
Autotoxemia   796.0
Autovaccination (not sick)   Y02
Autumn - *see* condition
Avellis' syndrome   344.9

Aviators'
  disease or sickness (*see also* Effects,
      adverse, high altitude)   993.2
  ear   993.0
  effort syndrome   305.3

Avitaminosis (multiple NEC) (*see also*
      Deficiency, vitamin)   266.9

Avulsion (traumatic)   907
  cartilage - *see* Dislocation, by site
  epiphysis of bone - *see* Fracture, by site
  external site other than limb - *see*
      Wound, open, by site
  eye   871
  head NEC (intracranial)   854.1
    complete   874.0
  internal organ or site - *see* Injury,
      internal, by site
  joint - *see* Dislocation, by site
  ligament - *see* Sprain, by site
  limb - *see* Amputation, traumatic, by
      site
  muscle - *see* Sprain, strain, by site
  nerve (root) - *see* Injury, nerve, by site
  tendon - *see* Sprain, by site
  tooth - *see* Wound, open, face
Ax-grinders' disease   515.0
  with tuberculosis   010
Axilla, axillary - *see also* condition
  breast   757.2
Axonotmesis - *see* Injury, nerve, by site
Ayala's disease   756.8
Ayerza's disease or syndrome   426
Azoospermia   606
Azotemia - *see* Uremia
Aztec ear   745.2
Azygos lobe, lung   748.6

B

Babinski-Nageotte syndrome 344.1
Babinski's syndrome 093.9
Bacillary - *see* condition
Bacilluria 789.1
 tuberculous 016.1
 late effect or sequela 019.2
Bacillus - *see* Infection, bacillus
Back - *see* condition
Backache (postural) 728.9
 psychogenic 305.1
 sacroiliac 728.7
Backflow (pyelovenous) (*see also* Lesion, kidney) 593.2
Backwardness - *see* Retardation mental, borderline
Bacteremia 038.9
 with
 abortion - *see* Abortion, by type, with sepsis .
 ectopic gestation - *see* categories 631.0-631.3
 pneumonia - *see* Pneumonia, bacterial
 gas gangrene 039.0
 gonococcal NEC 098.8
 gram-negative bacilli 038.9
 meningococcal - *see* Meningococcemia
 plague - *see* Plague
 pneumococcal 038.2
 with pneumonia - *see* Pneumonia, pneumococcal
 puerperal, postpartum, childbirth 670
 specified organism NEC 038.8
 staphylococcal 038.1
 streptococcal 038.0

Bacteria
 in blood - *see* Bacteremia
 in urine 789.1
Bacterial - *see* condition
Bactericholia (*see also* Cholecystitis) 575
Bacterid, bacteride (pustular) 686.9
Bacteriuria, bacteruria 789.1
Bad heart - *see* Disease, heart
Baelz's disease 528.5
Bagassosis 516.1
Bagging after onset of labor
 fetus or newborn (*see also* Birth injury NEC) 772.9

Bagratuni's syndrome 446.4

Bairnsdale's disease 031.9

Baker's
 cyst (knee) 731.6
 tuberculous 015.2
 late effect or sequela 019.5
 itch 692.9

Balanitis (circinata) (gangrenosa) (infectional) (vulgaris) 607.3
 due to Ducrey's bacillus 099.0
 erosiva circinata et gangrenosa 607.3
 gonococcal (acute) 098.0
 chronic or duration of 2 months or over 098.1
 nongonococcal 607.3
 phagedenic 607.3
 venereal 099.9
 xerotica obliterans 607.0

Balanoposthitis 607.3
 gonococcal (acute) 098.0
 chronic or duration of 2 months or over 098.1
 ulcerative 099.9

Balanorrhagia - *see* Balanitis
Balantidiasis 007.0
Balantidiosis 007.0
Balbuties, balbutio 306.0
Baldness (*see also* Alopecia) 704
Balfour's disease 202.2
Balkan grippe 083.1
Ballingall's disease 117.4
Balloon disease (*see also* Effect, adverse, high altitude) 993.2
Balo's disease 341
Bamberger-Marie disease 723.1
Bancroft's filariasis 125.0
Band(s)
 adhesive (*see also* Adhesions, peritoneum) 568
 anomalous or congenital - *see also* Anomaly, specified type NEC
 atrial 746.8
 heart 746.8
 intestine 751.1
 omentum 751.1
 ventricular 746.8
 cervix 621.9
 gallbladder (congenital) 751.6
 intestinal (adhesive) (*see also* Adhesions, peritoneum) 568
 obstructive 560.4
 peri-appendiceal (congenital) 751.1

Band(s) — *continued*
  peritoneal (adhesive) (*see also*
    Adhesions, peritoneum) 568
  uterus 625.9
  vagina 629.7
Bandl's ring (contraction)
  complicating delivery 657.9
  fetus or newborn - *see* categories
    767.0-767.9
Bang's disease 023.1
Bannister's disease - *see* Edema,
  angioneurotic
Banti's disease or syndrome (with
  cirrhosis) (with portal hypertension)
  - *see* Cirrhosis, liver
Bar, prostate 600
Baragnosis 781.6
Barcoo disease or rot (*see also* Ulcer,
  skin) 707.9
Bard-Pic's syndrome 157.0
Barensprung's disease 110.9
Barlow's disease 264
Barodontalgia 993.2
Baron Munchausen syndrome 306.9
Barosinusitis 993.1
Barotitis 993.0
Barotrauma 993.2
  odontalgia 993.2
  otitic 993.0
  sinus 993.1
Barraquer(-Simons) disease 279
Barre-Guillain syndrome 354
Barre-Lieou syndrome 728.1
Barrel chest 738.8
Bartholin's
  adenitis (*see also* Vaginitis) 622.1
  gland - *see* condition
Bartholinitis (suppurating) (*see also*
  Vaginitis) 622.1
Bartonellosis 089.0
Basal - *see* condition
Baseball finger 842.1
Basedow's disease 242.0
Basic - *see* condition
Basilar - *see* condition
Basophilia 289.9
Basophilism (cortico-adrenal) (Cushing's)
  (pituitary) (thymic) 258.0
Bassen-Kornzweig syndrome 272.1
Bat ear 745.2
Bateman's disease 079.0
Bathing cramp 994.1
Bathophobia 300.2
Batten-Mayou disease 333.0
Batten's disease, retina 333.0
Battered baby or child (syndrome) NEC
  996.8

Battey Mycobacterium infection 031.0
Battle exhaustion 307
Battledore placenta - *see* Placenta,
  abnormal
Baumgarten-Cruveilhier cirrhosis, disease
  or syndrome 571.8
Bauxite fibrosis (of lung) 516.0
Bayle's disease 094.1
Bazin's disease (primary) 017.0
  late effect or sequela 019.9
Beach ear 380
Beaded hair (congenital) 757.3
Beard's disease 300.5
Beat
  elbow 731.2
  hand 731.4
  knee 731.6
Beats
  escaped
    heart (*see also* Action, heart,
      irregular) 427.9
    premature (atrium) (ventricle) (*see also*
      Action, heart, irregular) 427.9
Beau's
  disease (*see also* Insufficiency,
    myocardial) 428
  lines 703.9
Bechterew's disease 712.4
Becker's disease 425
Bedclothes, asphyxiation or suffocation
  by 994.7
Bednar's aphthae 528.2
Bedsore 707.0
  with gangrene (*see also* Gangrene)
    445.9
Bedwetting (*see also* Enuresis) 786.2
Bee sting (with allergic or anaphylactic
  shock) 989.4
Behavior disorder, disturbance 306.9
  childhood (primary) 308
Behcet's syndrome 136
Behr's disease 377.1
Beigel's disease or morbus 111.2
Bejel 104.0
Belching (*see also* Eructation) 784.7
Bell's
  disease 296.1
  mania 296.1
  palsy, paralysis 350
    newborn (*see also* Birth injury, bone
      or nerve) 772.2
    syphilitic 094.9
Bence-Jones albuminuria or albumosuria
  NEC 203
Bends 993.3
Benedikt's paralysis or syndrome 344.9

Benign - *see also* condition
  prostate 600
Bennett's fracture - *see* Fracture,
  metacarpus
Benson's disease 369.9
Bent back (hysterical) 300.1
Berger's paresthesia 781.6
Bergeron's disease 300.1
Beriberi 261
  heart 261
  leprosy 030.1
  neuritis 261
Berlin's edema (traumatic) 921
Berloque's dermatitis 692.9
Bernard-Horner syndrome 358.0
Bernard-Soulier disease or thrombopathia
  287.3
Bernhardt-Roth disease 355.1
Bernhardt's disease 355.1
Bernheim's syndrome (*see also* Failure,
  heart, congestive) 427.0
Bertielliasis 123.9
Bertolotti's syndrome 756.1
Berylliosis (lung) 516.0
Beshenstvo 071
Besnier-Boeck disease 135
Besnier-Boeck-Schaumann disease 135
Besnier's
  lupus pernio 135
  prurigo 691
Best's disease 377.1
Bestiality 302.8
Beta-amino-isobutyricaciduria 270.5
Beurmann's disease 117.1
Bezoar 938
  intestine 936
  stomach 935
Bezold's abscess - *see* Mastoiditis
Bianchi's syndrome 781.5
Bicornate or bicornis uterus 752.5
  complicating delivery 657.9
    fetus or newborn - *see* categories
     764.0-764.9
  noted during pregnancy (undelivered)
    634.9
Bicuspid aortic valve 746.6
Biedl-Bardet syndrome 759.8
Bielschowsky(-Jansky)
  amaurotic familial idiocy 333.0
  disease 333.0
Biermer's anemia or disease 281.0
Biett's disease 695.4
Bifid (congenital) - *see also* Imperfect
  closure
  apex, heart 746.8
  clitoris 752.6
  kidney 753.3

Bifid, etc. — *continued*
  nose 748.1
  patella 755.7
  scrotum 752.8
  toe 755.7
  tongue 750.0
  ureter 753.4
  uterus 752.5
  uvula 749.0
    with cleft lip 749.2
Biforis uterus (suprasimplex) 752.5
Bifurcation (congenital) - *see also*
  Imperfect closure
  aorta - *see* condition
  gallbladder 751.6
  kidney pelvis 753.3
  renal pelvis 753.3
  rib 756.4
  tongue 750.0
  trachea 748.3
  ureter 753.4
  urethra 753.8
  uvula 749.0
    with cleft lip 749.2
  vertebra 756.2
Bigeminal pulse (*see also* Action, heart,
  irregular) 427.9
Bilateral - *see* condition
Bile duct - *see* condition
Bile pigments in urine 789.9
Bilharziasis (*see also* Schistosomiasis)
  120.9
  chyluria 120.0
  cutaneous 120.3
  galacturia 120.0
  hematochyluria 120.0
  intestinal 120.1
  lipemia 120.9
  lipuria 120.0
  oriental 120.2
  piarhemia 120.9
  pulmonary 120.2
  tropical hematuria 120.0
  vesical 120.0
Biliary - *see* condition
Bilious (attack) (*see also* Vomiting)
  784.1
Biliuria 789.9
Billroth's disease - *see* Disease, Billroth's
Bilocular
  stomach 536.1
Biparta, bipartite - *see also* Imperfect
  closure
  carpal scaphoid 755.5
  patella 755.7
  vagina 752.6
Bird face 756.0

Birth

Note — For classification of infants born alive in hospital whether full term, immature, single, or multiple born — *see* Newborn.
For classification of infants born dead in hospital — *see* Death, fetus.

Birth — *continued*
  abnormal, fetus or newborn - *see* categories 768.0-768.9
  accident, fetus or newborn - *see* Birth injury NEC
  complications in mother - *see* Delivery, complicated
  compression
    brain - *see* Birth, injury, brain
    during (*see also* Birth injury, brain) 772.0
  consequence, fetus or newborn - *see* Birth injury NEC
  defect - *see* Anomaly
  delayed, fetus or newborn - *see* categories 768.0-768.9
  difficult, fetus or newborn - *see* categories 768.0-768.9
  dry (protracted), fetus or newborn - *see* categories 768.0-768.9
  forced, fetus or newborn - *see* Birth injury NEC
  forceps, fetus or newborn - *see* Birth injury NEC
  hematoma of sternomastoid (*see also* Birth injury NEC) 772.9
  immature 777
  inattention, after or at 994.9
  induced, fetus or newborn - *see* Birth injury NEC
  injury (adrenal gland) (conjunctiva) (instrumental) (scalp) NEC 772.9
    with
      abnormality of bones, organs or tissues of pelvis (conditions in 764) (with asphyxia, anoxia or hypoxia) 764.3
      abnormality of forces of labor (conditions in 767) (with asphyxia, anoxia or hypoxia) 767.3
      difficult labor with other and unspecified complications (conditions in 768) (with asphyxia, anoxia or hypoxia) 768.3
      disproportion, fetopelvic (conditions in 765) (with asphyxia, anoxia or hypoxia) 765.3

Birth — *continued*
  injury, etc. — *continued*
    with — *continued*
      disproportion, fetopelvic — *continued*
        with abnormality of bones, organs or tissues of pelvis (conditions in 764) 764.3
      malposition of fetus (conditions in 766) (with asphyxia, anoxia or hypoxia) 766.3
  asphyxiation NEC 772.9
  basal ganglia - *see* Birth injury, brain
  bone or nerve 772.2
    with
      abnormality of bones, organs or tissues of pelvis (conditions in 764) (with asphyxia, anoxia or hypoxia) 764.2
      abnormality of forces of labor (conditions in 767) (with asphyxia, anoxia or hypoxia) 767.2
      difficult labor with other and unspecified complications (conditions in 768) (with asphyxia, anoxia or hypoxia) 768.2
      disproportion, fetopelvic (conditions in 765) (with asphyxia, anoxia or hypoxia) 765.2
      with abnormality of bones, organs or tissues of pelvis (conditions in 764) 764.2
      malposition of fetus (conditions in 766) (with asphyxia, anoxia or hypoxia) 766.2
  brachial plexus (*see also* Birth injury, bone or nerve) 772.2
  brain (compression) (pressure) 772.0
    with
      abnormality of bones, organs or tissues of pelvis (conditions in 764) (with asphyxia, anoxia or hypoxia) 764.0
      abnormality of forces of labor (conditions in 767) (with asphyxia, anoxia or hypoxia) 767.0
      difficult labor with other and unspecified complications (conditions in 768) (with asphyxia, anoxia or hypoxia) 768.0

Birth—*continued*
  injury, etc. — *continued*
    brain, etc. — *continued*
      with — *continued*
        disproportion, fetopelvic
          (conditions in 765) (with
          asphyxia, anoxia or
          hypoxia) 765.0
        with abnormality of bones,
          organs or tissues of
          pelvis (conditions in
          764) 764.0
        malposition of fetus (conditions
          in 766) (with asphyxia,
          anoxia or hypoxia) 766.0
        residual paralysis from - *see* Palsy,
          cerebral
    cerebellum - *see* Birth injury, brain
    complicating delivery - *see*
      Obstetrical trauma
    fracture, bone (*see also* Birth injury,
      bone or nerve) 772.2
    hemiplegia (*see also* Birth injury,
      brain) 772.0
    intracranial - *see* Birth injury, brain
    laceration
      dura - *see* Birth injury, brain
      peripheral nerves (*see also* Birth
        Injury, bone or nerve)
        772.2
    meninges
      brain (*see also* Birth injury, brain)
        772.0
      spinal cord (*see also* Birth injury,
        spinal cord) 772.1
    nerve (*see also* Birth injury, bone or
      nerve) 772.2
    paralysis (Erb's) (*see also* Birth
      injury, bone or nerve) 772.2
    spastic paraplegia (*see also* Birth
      injury, brain) 772.0
    spinal cord (hemorrhage) (paralysis)
      772.1
      with
        abnormality of bones, organs or
          tissues of pelvis
          (conditions in 764) (with
          asphyxia, anoxia or
          hypoxia) 764.1
        abnormality of forces of labor
          (conditions in 767) (with
          asphyxia, anoxia or
          hypoxia) 767.1
        difficult labor with other and
          unspecified complications
          (conditions in 768) (with
          asphyxia, anoxia or
          hypoxia) 768.1

Birth—*continued*
  injury, etc. — *continued*
    spinal cord, etc. — *continued*
      with — *continued*
        disproportion, fetopelvic
          (conditions in 765) (with
          asphyxia, anoxia or
          hypoxia) 765.1
        with abnormality of bones,
          organs or tissues of
          pelvis (conditions in
          764) 764.1
        malposition of fetus (conditions
          in 766) (with asphyxia,
          anoxia or hypoxia) 766.1
      residual paralysis from - *see* Palsy,
        cerebral
    instrumental, fetus or newborn - *see*
      Birth injury NEC
    lack of care, after or at 994.9
    multiple 769.4
    neglect, after or at 994.9
    palsy or paralysis, newborn (*see also*
      Birth injury, bone or nerve)
      772.2
    precipitate, fetus or newborn - *see*
      categories 767.0-767.9
    premature (infant) 777
    prolonged, fetus or newborn - *see*
      categories 768.0-768.9
    protracted, fetus or newborn - *see*
      categories 768.0-768.9
    retarded, fetus or newborn - *see*
      categories 767.0-767.9
    shock, fetus or newborn - *see* categories
      768.0-768.9
    tentorial tear (*see also* Birth injury,
      brain) 772.0
    trauma (*see also* Birth injury NEC)
      772.9
    twin 769.4
Birthmark - *see* Nevus
Bisalbuminemia 275.3
Biskra's button 085.1
Bite(s)
  animal - *see* Wound, open
  centipede 989.4
  chigger 133.9
  flea - *see* Injury, superficial
  human (open wound) - *see* Wound, open
    intact skin surface - *see* Contusion
  insect (nonvenomous) - *see* Injury,
    superficial
    venomous 989.4
  mad dog, death from 071

Bite(s) — *continued*
  poisonous 989.4
  reptile 989.4
    nonvenomous - *see* Wound, open
  snake 989.4
    nonvenomous - *see* Wound, open
  spider (venomous) 989.4
    nonvenomous - *see* Injury, superficial
  venomous 989.4
Black death 020.9
Black hairy tongue 529.3
Blackhead 706.1
Blackout 782.5
Bladder - *see* condition
Blast
  blindness 921
  concussion - *see* Blast injury
  injury 869.0
    abdomen or thorax - *see* Injury,
        internal, by site
    brain - *see* Concussion, brain
    ear (acoustic nerve trauma) - *see also*
        Injury, nerve, acoustic
      with perforation, tympanic
          membrane - *see* Wound,
          open, ear
Blastocytoma - *see* Neoplasm
Blastoma - *see* Neoplasm
Blastomycosis, blastomycotic (cerebral)
        (chronic) (cutaneous) (disseminated)
        (Jorge Lobo's) (keloidal) (lung)
        (pulmonary) (systemic) 116.9
  Brazilian 116.2
  European 116.0
  North American 116.1
  South American 116.2
Bleb(s) 709.9
  emphysematous (lung) 492
  lung (ruptured) 492
    congenital (*see also* Syndrome,
        respiratory distress) 776.2
  subpleura 511.2
Bleeder (familial) (hereditary) (*see also*
        Defect, coagulation) 286.9
  nonfamilial 286.9
Bleeding (*see also* Hemorrhage) 458.9
  atonic, complicating delivery 653
  capillary 448
  due to subinvolution 625.1
    puerperal 677.2
  familial (*see also* Defect, coagulation)
        286.9
  fibroid (uterus) 218
  hemorrhoids 455
  intermenstrual 626.6
  menopausal 627
  ovulation 626.6

Bleeding — *continued*
  postclimacteric 626.7
  postmenopausal 626.7
  postoperative 998.1
  preclimacteric 626.2
  puberty 626.2
  rectum, rectal 569.2
  tendencies (*see also* Defect,
        coagulation) 286.9
  umbilical stump 778.9
  uterus 626.9
    climacteric 627
    dysfunctional 626.6
    functional 626.6
  vagina, vaginal 629.5
    functional 626.6
  vicarious 626.9
Blennorrhagia, blennorrhagic - *see*
        Blennorrhea
Blennorrhea (acute) 098.0
  adultorum 098.2
  alveolaris 523.4
  chronic or duration of 2 months or over
        098.1
  inclusion (newborn) (neonatal) 078.0
  neonatorum 098.2
Blepharelosis 378.1
Blepharitis (angularis) (ciliaris) (eyelid)
        (marginal) (nonulcerative)
        (squamous) (ulcerative) 361
  scrofulous 017.2
  late effect or sequela 019.9
Blepharochalasis 378.2
  congenital 744.8
Blepharoclonus 378.9
Blepharoconjunctivitis (*see also*
        Conjunctivitis) 360
Blepharophimosis (eyelid) 378.2
  congenital 744.8
Blepharoptosis 378.2
  congenital 744.7
Blepharopyorrhea 098.2
Blepharospasm 378.2
Blessig's cyst 377.1
Blind
  bronchus (congenital) 748.3
  loop syndrome 269.0
  sac, fallopian tube (congenital) 752.5
  spot 378.6
  tract or tube, congenital NEC - *see*
        Atresia
Blindness (acquired) (congenital) 379.1
  blast 921
    with nerve injury - *see* Injury, nerve,
        optic
  Bright's - *see* Uremia

Blindness — *continued*
  color 377.3
  concussion - *see* Injury, nerve, optic
  day 378.9
  due to injury NEC - *see* Injury, nerve,
    optic
  eclipse (total) 377.9
  emotional 306.9
  hysterical 300.1
  mind 781.5
  night 378.9
    vitamin A deficiency 260.0
  not specifically defined (economic)
    379.1
    both eyes 379.1
    one eye 379.3
    without statement as to eyes affected
      379.1
  psychic 781.5
  snow 360
  specifically defined (for pension
    purposes) 379.0
    both eyes 379.0
    one eye 379.2
    without statement as to eyes affected
      379.0
  sun 377.9
  traumatic NEC - *see* Injury, nerve,
    optic
  word (developmental) 306.1
    acquired 781.5
    secondary to organic lesion 781.5
Blister - *see also* Injury, superficial
  beetle dermatitis 692.3
  fever 054
  multiple, skin, nontraumatic 709.9
Bloating 785.4
Bloch-Sulzberger disease or syndrome
  757.2
Block
  arborization (heart) (*see also* Block,
    heart) 427.3
  arrhythmic (*see also* Block, heart)
    427.3
  atrioventricular (any degree) (*see also*
    Block, heart) 427.3
  auriculoventricular (any degree) (*see
    also* Block, heart) 427.3
  bundle branch (complete) (false)
    (incomplete) (left) (right) (Wilson's
    type) (*see also* Block, heart)
    427.3
  cardiac (any degree) (*see also* Block,
    heart) 427.3
  conduction (complete) (*see also* Block,
    heart) 427.3

Block — *continued*
  foramen Magendie (acquired) 347.9
    congenital 742
  heart (any degree) (incomplete) (partial)
    427.3
    with
      hypertension (benign) (conditions in
        401) (*see also* Hypertension,
        heart) 402
        malignant (*see also*
          Hypertension, malignant
          with heart involvement)
          400.1
    congenital 746.8
  hepatic vein 453
  intraventricular (*see also* Block, heart)
    427.3
  kidney (*see also* Lesion, kidney) 593.2
    postcystoscopic 999.9
  myocardial (*see also* Block, heart)
    427.3
  nodal (*see also* Block, heart) 427.3
  optic nerve 377.6
  organ or site, congenital NEC - *see*
    Atresia
  portal (vein) 452
  sino-atrial (*see also* Block, heart)
    427.3
  sino-auricular (*see also* Block, heart)
    427.3
  spinal cord 349.9
  vein NEC 453
Blocq's disease 306.3
Blood
  constituents, abnormal NEC 788.9
  crisis 289.0
  disease 289.9
  donor Y09.9
  dyscrasia 289.9
    fetus or newborn (*see also* Disease,
      hemolytic due to
      incompatibility) 775.2
    puerperal, postpartum 675
  flukes NEC (*see also* Infestation,
    Schistosoma) 120.9
  in feces (*see also* Melena) 785.7
  in urine (*see also* Hematuria) 789.3
  mole (abortion) (*see also* Abortion,
    other) 645.9
    undelivered 634.9
  overabundant supply 289.0
  poisoning - *see* Septicemia
  pressure
    decreased, due to shock following
      injury 995.5
    fluctuating 458.9

Blood—*continued*
   pressure—*continued*
     high (*see also* Hypertension)   401
     low   458.0
   spitting (*see also* Hemoptysis)   783.1
   staining cornea   378.4
   transfusion, reaction or complication
       see Complication, transfusion
   tumor - *see* Hematoma
   vessel rupture - *see* Hemorrhage
   vomiting (*see also* Hematemesis)
     784.5
Blood-forming organs, disease   289.9
Bloodgood's disease   610
Blotch
   palpebral   378.2
Blount's disease   722.2
Blue
   baby   746.9
   disease   746.9
   dome cyst   610
   eye   128.8
   nevus   757.1
   sclera   378.6
     with fragility of bone and deafness
     756.6
Blueness (*see also* Cyanosis)   782.3
Blushing
   abnormal   782.3
   excessive   782.3
Boarder   Y09.9
   healthy person accompanying sick
     relative   Y08
Bockhart's impetigo   684
Body, bodies
   Aschoff's (*see also* Myocarditis,
     rheumatic)   398
   asteroid, vitreous   369.9
   choroid, colloid   378.6
   cytoid   377.1
   drusen   377.4
   foreign - *see* Foreign body
   loose
     joint - *see* Loose bodies in joint
     sheath, tendon   733.9
   Mallory's   034.1
   Mooser's   081.0
   Negri   071
   rice (joint) - *see* Loose bodies in joint
Boeck's
   disease   135
   lupoid (miliary)   135
   sarcoid   135
Boggy
   cervix   621.9
   uterus   625.9

Boil   680.9
   abdominal wall   680.2
   Aleppo   085.1
   ankle   680.6
   anus   680.5
   arm (any part, above wrist)   680.3
   axilla   680.3
   back (any part)   680.2
   Baghdad   085.1
   breast   680.2
   buttock   680.5
   chest wall   680.2
   corpus cavernosum   607.5
   Delhi   085.1
   ear (any part) (external)   680.0
   eyelid   362
   face (any part, except eye)   680.0
   finger (any)   680.4
   foot (any part)   680.6
   forearm   680.3
   Gafsa   085.1
   gluteal (region)   680.5
   groin   680.2
   hand (any part)   680.4
   head (any part, except face)   680.8
   heel   680.6
   hip   680.6
   knee   680.6
   lachrymal, lacrimal gland or sac   368
   leg (any part)   680.6
   lower extremity   680.6
   multiple sites NEC   680.8
   natal   085.1
   neck   680.1
   nose (septum)   680.0
   orbit, orbital   369.0
   partes posteriores   680.5
   penis   607.5
   scalp (any part)   680.8
   scrotum   607.5
   seminal vesicle   607.4
   shoulder   680.3
   skin NEC   680.9
   specified site NEC   680.8
   spermatic cord   607.5
   temple (region)   680.0
   testis   607.5
   thigh   680.6
   thumb   680.4
   toe (any)   680.6
   tropical   085.1
   trunk   680.2
   tunica vaginalis   607.5
   upper arm   680.3
   vas deferens   607.5
   vulva (*see also* Vulvitis)   622.1
   wrist   680.4

Bold hives (*see also* Urticaria) 708.9
Bombe, iris 378.6
Bomford and Rhoad anemia 284
Bone - *see* condition
Bonnevie-Ullrich syndrome 759.5
Bonnier's syndrome 387.9
Bony block of joint (*see also* Disease,
    joint) 729.9
Borderline
  intelligence - *see* Retardation, mental,
      borderline
  pelvis
    complicating delivery - *see*
        Deformity, pelvis complicating
        delivery
    noted during pregnancy (undelivered)
        634.9
Borna disease 065
  late effects 066
Bornholm disease 074.1
Borrelia vincenti (mouth) (pharynx)
    (tonsils) 101
Bostock's catarrh 507
Boston exanthem 046
Botulism 005.1
Bouba (*see also* Yaws) 102.9
Bouffee delirante 298.3
Bouillaud's disease or syndrome 391.9
Bourneville's disease 759.6
Boutonniere hand (intrinsic) 738.2
Bouveret's syndrome (*see also*
    Tachycardia, paroxysmal) 427.5
Bovine heart - *see* Hypertrophy, cardiac
Bowel - *see* condition
Bowen's
  dermatosis (precancerous) 702
  disease (skin) 702
    mouth 528.7
    penis 607.1
    scrotum 702
    tongue 529.7
  epithelioma - *see* Neoplasm, skin,
     malignant
Bowing
  femur 738.5
  forearm 738.2
  radius 738.2
  tibia 738.5
Bowleg(s) 738.5
  rachitic 265.1
Boyd's dysentery 004.2
Brachial - *see* condition
Brachycardia (*see also* Action, heart,
    irregular) 427.9
Bradycardia (any type) (sino-atrial) (sinus)
    (vagal) (*see also* Action, heart,
    irregular) 427.9

Bradypnea 783.2
Brailsford's disease 722.2
  radial head 722.2
  tarsal scaphoid 722.2
Brain - *see also* condition
  syndrome (acute) (chronic) (organic)
    (non-psychotic) (with neurotic
    reaction) (with behavioral
    reaction) 309.9
  with psychosis, psychotic reaction
    (*see also* Psychosis, organic)
    294.9
  congenital - *see* Retardation, mental
  due to or associated with specified
    physical condition - *see* listing
    under Disorder, mental
Branched chain amino-acid disease
    270.4
Branchial - *see* condition
Branchioma 210.6
Brash (water) 784.7
Brass-founders' ague 985.9
Bravais-jacksonian epilepsy - *see*
    Epilepsy, jacksonian
Braxton-Hicks contractures (undelivered)
    634.7
Braziers' disease 985.9
Break, cardiorenal - *see* Hypertension,
    cardiorenal
Breakdown, nervous (*see also* Disorder,
    mental) 300.9
Breast - *see* condition
Breath
  foul 788.9
  holder, child 308
  shortness 783.2
Breathing
  labored 783.2
  periodic 783.2
Breathlessness 783.2
Breda's disease (*see also* Yaws) 102.9
Breech
  extraction, fetus or newborn (*see also*
    Birth injury NEC) 772.9
  position (noted before delivery) 634.9
  presentation - *see* Presentation,
    abnormal
Breisky's disease 629.2
Brenneman's syndrome 289.2
Brenner
  neoplasm 220.9
  tumor 220.9
Bretonneau's disease 032
Breus' mole (abortion) (*see also* Abortion,
    other) 645.9
  undelivered 634.9
Brevicollis 756.2

Bricklayers' itch 692.9
Bright's
　blindness - *see* Uremia
　disease (*see also* Nephritis) 583
　　arteriosclerotic (*see also*
　　　Hypertension, kidney) 403
Brill-Symmers' disease 202.0
Brill-Zinsser disease 081.1
Brill's disease 081.1
　flea borne 081.0
　louse borne 081.1
Briquet's syndrome 300.1
Brissaud's infantilism 244
Brittle
　bones 756.6
　nails 703.9
　　congenital 757.4
Broad ligament - *see* condition
Brock's syndrome 519.0
Brocq's disease 691
Brodie's
　abscess (localized) (chronic) 720.1
　disease (knee) 731.6
　　breast 217
　tumor 217
Broken
　arches 736
　　congenital 755.7
　back - *see* Fracture, vertebra
　bone - *see* Fracture
　compensation - *see* Disease, heart
　down gland 683
　neck - *see* Fracture, vertebra, cervical
　nose - *see* Fracture, nose
　tooth, teeth - *see* Wound, open, face
Bromhidrosis 705.9
Bromidism
　acute 967.3
　chronic 304.3
Bromidrosiphobia 300.2
Bromidrosis 705.9
Bromism
　acute 967.3
　chronic 304.3
Bronchi, bronchial - *see* condition
Bronchiectasis (cylindrical) (diffuse)
　　(fusiform) (localized) (moniliform)
　　(postinfectional) (recurrent)
　　(saccular) 518
　congenital 748.6
　tuberculous (*see also* Tuberculosis,
　　pulmonary) 011.9
　　late effect or sequela 019.0
Bronchiolectasis - *see* Bronchiectasis
Bronchiolitis (acute) (infectional)
　　(obliterating) 466

Bronchiolitis — *continued*
　with
　　influenza, flu or grippe 472
　chronic 491
　influenzal 472
Bronchitis (asthmatic) (catarrhal) (diffuse)
　　(hypostatic) (infectional)
　　(inflammatory) (simple) 490
　with
　　influenza, flu or grippe 472
　　tracheitis 490
　　　acute 466
　　　chronic 491
　acute or subacute 466
　　with
　　　tracheitis 466
　allergic (acute) (chronic) 493
　arachidic 934
　capillary 466
　　chronic 491
　caseous (*see also* Tuberculosis,
　　pulmonary) 011.9
　Castellani's 104.9
　chronic 491
　　with
　　　tracheitis (chronic) 491
　croupous 466
　emphysematous 491
　exudative 466
　fetid 491
　fibrinous, acute or subacute 466
　grippal 472
　influenzal 472
　membranous, acute or subacute 466·
　moulders' 515.0
　　with tuberculosis 010
　obliterans 491
　obstructive 491
　pituitous 491
　plastic 466
　pneumococcal, acute or subacute 466
　pseudomembranous 466
　purulent (chronic) 491
　　acute or subacute 466
　putrid 491
　scrofulous (*see also* Tuberculosis,
　　pulmonary) 011.9
　senile 491
　septic, acute or subacute 466
　spirochetal 104.9
　suffocative, acute or subacute 466
　summer 493
　suppurative (chronic) 491
　　acute or subacute 466
　tuberculous (*see also* Tuberculosis,
　　pulmonary) 011.9

Bronchitis—*continued*
  ulcerative   491
    Vincent's   101
    Vincent's   101
    viral, acute or subacute   466
Broncho-alveolitis   485
Bronchoaspergillosis   117.3
Bronchocele   240.9
Bronchohemisporosis   117.8
Broncholithiasis   519.2
  tuberculous (*see also* Tuberculosis,
    pulmonary)   011.9
Bronchomoniliasis   112
Bronchomycosis   112
Bronchonocardiosis   113
Bronchopleuropneumonia - *see*
    Pneumonia, broncho
Bronchopneumonia - *see* Pneumonia,
    broncho
Bronchopneumonitis - *see* Pneumonia,
    broncho
Bronchopulmonary - *see* condition
Bronchopulmonitis - *see* Pneumonia,
    broncho
Bronchorrhagia   783.1
  newborn   778.2
  tuberculous (*see also* Tuberculosis,
    pulmonary)   011.9
Bronchorrhea (chronic) (purulent)   491
  acute   466
Bronchospasm   519.9
Bronchospirochetosis   104.9
Bronchostenosis   519.9
Bronchus - *see* condition
Brooke's disease (*see also*
    Trichoepithelioma)   216.1
Brown-Sequard paralysis (syndrome)
    349.5
Brucella (infection)   023.9
  abortus   023.1
  dermatitis, skin   023.9
  melitensis   023.0
  suis   023.2
Brucellosis   023.9
  brucella
    abortus   023.1
    melitensis   023.0
    suis   023.2
Bruck-Lange disease   759.8
Bruck's disease   723.9
Brugsch's syndrome   757.2
Bruhl's disease   285.8
Bruise (skin surface intact) - *see also*
    Contusion
  with
    fracture - *see* Fracture

Bruise, etc.—*continued*
  with—*continued*
    open wound - *see* Wound, open
    internal organ (abdomen, chest or
      pelvis) - *see* Injury, internal
Brushburn - *see* Burn
Bruton's X-linked agammaglobulinemia
    275.0
Bruxism   780.3
Bubbly lung syndrome (*see also*
    Syndrome, respiratory distress)
    776.2
Bubo   289.3
  blennorrhagic   098.8
  chancroidal   099.0
  climatic   099.1
  due to Hemophilus ducreyi   099.0
  gonococcal   098.8
  indolent   099.9
  inguinal   099.9
    chancroidal   099.0
    climatic   099.1
    due to H. ducreyi   099.0
    infective   099.9
    venereal   099.9
  phagedenic   099.9
  scrofulous   017.1
    late effect or sequela   019.9
  soft chancre   099.0
  suppurating   683
  syphilitic   091.0
    congenital   090.0
  tropical   099.1
  venereal   099.9
  virulent   099.0
Bubonocele   550
  gangrenous, incarcerated, irreducible,
    strangulated, or with obstruction
    (intestinal)   552
Buccal - *see* condition
Buchman's disease   722.2
Bucket handle fracture (semilunar
    cartilage) - *see* Dislocation, knee
Buckwar - *see* Dermatophytosis
Budd-Chiari syndrome   453
Budinger-Ludloff-Laewen disease   729.8
Buerger-Grutz disease   272.0
Buerger's disease   443.1
Buhl's disease (*see also* Septicemia)
    038.9
Bulbar - *see* condition
Bulbus
  cordis (left ventricle) (persistent)   746.8
Bulimia   788.9
Bulla(e)   709.9
  lung   492

Bullet wound - *see also* Wound, open
    fracture - code as Fracture, open
    internal organ (abdomen, chest, or
        pelvis) - *see* Injury, internal, by
        site, with open wound
    intracranial 851.1
Bundle
    branch block (false) (*see also* Block,
        heart) 427.3
    of His - *see* condition
Bungpagga 117.9
Bunion 730
Buphthalmia, buphthalmos (congenital)
    744.2
Buried roots 525.9
Burn (acid) (cathode ray) (caustic)
    (chemical) (electric heating
    appliance) (fire) (flame) (friction)
    (hot liquid or object) (irradiation)
    (lime) (radiation) (steam) (thermal)
    (x-ray) 949

Note—The following fourth-digit subdivisions are for use with categories
940–949:
    .0 *Unspecified degree, without men-
        tion of complication*
    .1 *First degree, without mention of
        complication*
    .2 *Second degree, without mention
        of complication*
    .3 *Third degree, without mention of
        complication*
    .8 *Complicated*
    .9 *Late effect*
"Complicated" includes burn, any degree,
with delayed healing, delayed treatment, or
major infection.

Burn, etc. — *continued*
    abdomen, abdominal (muscle) (wall) -
        see Burn, trunk
    ankle - *see* Burn, leg
    anus - *see* Burn, trunk
    arm(s) 943
        with
            head (and leg(s)) 946
                with trunk 948
            trunk (and leg(s)) 947
                with head 948
    auditory canal (external) - *see* Burn,
        head
    auricle (ear) - *see* Burn, head
    axilla - *see* Burn, arm
    back - *see* Burn, trunk

Burn, etc. — *continued*
    biceps
        brachii - *see* Burn, arm
        femoris - *see* Burn, leg
    breast(s) - *see* Burn, trunk
    brow - *see* Burn, head
    buttock(s) - *see* Burn, trunk
    canthus (eye) - *see* Burn, eye
    cervix (uteri) (*see also* Burn, internal
        organs) 949
    cheek (cutaneous) (internal) - *see* Burn,
        head
    chest wall - *see* Burn, trunk
    chin - *see* Burn, head
    clitoris - *see* Burn, trunk
    conjunctiva - *see* Burn, eye
    cornea - *see* Burn, eye
    costal region - *see* Burn, trunk
    ear (auricle) (external) (drum) (canal) -
        see Burn, head
    elbow - *see* Burn, arm
    electricity, electric current (any degree)
        (any site) (entire body) 994.8
    entire body 948
    epididymis - *see* Burn, trunk
    epigastric region - *see* Burn, trunk
    epiglottis - *see* Burn, head
    esophagus (*see also* Burn, internal
        organs) 949
    extremity
        lower - *see* Burn, leg
        upper - *see* Burn, arm
    eye(s) (only) 940
        with other sites - *see* Burn, head
    eyeball - *see* Burn, eye
    eyelid(s) - *see* Burn, eye
    face - *see* Burn, head
    finger(s) (nail) (subungual) 944
        with other site(s) - *see* Burn, arm
    flank - *see* Burn, trunk
    foot (phalanges) - *see* Burn, leg
    forearm(s) - *see* Burn, arm
    forehead - *see* Burn, head
    fourth degree - code as Burn, third
        degree
    from swallowing caustic or corrosive
        substance NEC 983.9
        specified substance - *see* Table of
            adverse effects
    full thickness - code as Burn, third
        degree
    genito-urinary organs
        external - *see* Burn, trunk
        internal (*see also* Burn, internal
            organs) 949
    globe (eye) - *see* Burn, eye

Burn, etc. — *continued*
  groin - *see* Burn, trunk
  gum - *see* Burn, head
  hand(s) (phalanges) (and wrist)   944
    with other site - *see* Burn, arm
  head (and face) (and neck) (and eye)
      941
    with
      arm(s) (and leg(s))   946
        with trunk   948
      leg(s) (and arm(s))   946
        with trunk   948
      trunk (and arm(s)) (and leg(s))   948
    eye(s) only   940
  heel - *see* Burn, leg
  hip - *see* Burn, trunk
  iliac region - *see* Burn, trunk
  inhalation   949
  internal organs   949
    from caustic or corrosive substance
       (swallowing) NEC   983.9
     specified substance - *see* Table of
       adverse effects
  interscapular region - *see* Burn, trunk
  iris - *see* Burn, eye
  knee - *see* Burn, leg
  labium (majus) (minus) - *see* Burn, trunk
  lacrimal apparatus, duct, gland or sac -
    see Burn, eye
  leg (upper) (lower)   945
    with
      head (and arm(s))   946
        with trunk   948
      trunk (and arm(s))   947
        with head   948
  lightning (any degree) (any site) (entire
    body)   994.0
  limb(s)
    lower (including foot or toe(s) - *see*
      Burn, leg
    upper (except wrist and hand) - *see*
      Burn, arm
  lip(s) - *see* Burn, head
  lumbar region - *see* Burn, trunk
  lung (*see also* Burn, internal organs)
     949
  malar region - *see* Burn, head
  mastoid region - *see* Burn, head
  membrane, tympanic - *see* Burn, head
  midthoracic region - *see* Burn, trunk
  mouth - *see* Burn, head
  multiple NEC   949
  muscle, abdominal - *see* Burn, trunk
  nasal (septum) - *see* Burn, head
  neck - *see* Burn, head
  nose (septum) - *see* Burn, head

Burn, etc. — *continued*
  occipital region - *see* Burn, head
  oesophagus (*see also* Burn, internal
    organs)   949
  orbit region - *see* Burn, eye
  palate - *see* Burn, head
  palm(s)   944
    with other site(s) - *see* Burn, arm
  parietal region - *see* Burn, head
  partial thickness - code as Burn,
    unspecified degree
  penis - *see* Burn, trunk
  perineum - *see* Burn, trunk
  pharynx - *see* Burn, head
  pleura (*see also* Burn, internal organs)
     949
  popliteal space - *see* Burn, leg
  prepuce - *see* Burn, trunk
  pubic region - *see* Burn, trunk
  pudenda - *see* Burn, trunk
  rectum (*see also* Burn, internal organs)
     949
  sac lacrimal - *see* Burn, eye
  sacral region - *see* Burn, trunk
  salivary (ducts) (glands) - *see* Burn,
    head
  scalp - *see* Burn, head
  scapular region - *see* Burn, arm
  sclera - *see* Burn, eye
  scrotum - *see* Burn, trunk
  septum, nasal - *see* Burn, head
  shoulder(s) - *see* Burn, arm
  skin NEC   949
  skull - *see* Burn, head
  sternal region - *see* Burn, trunk
  subconjunctival - *see* Burn, eye
  subcutaneous - code as Burn, third
    degree
  submaxillary region - *see* Burn, head
  submental region - *see* Burn, head
  supraclavicular fossa - *see* Burn, head
  supra-orbital - *see* Burn, head
  temple - *see* Burn, head
  temporal region - *see* Burn, head
  testicle - *see* Burn, trunk
  testis - *see* Burn, trunk
  thigh - *see* Burn, leg
  thorax (external) - *see* Burn, trunk
  throat - *see* Burn, head
  thumb(s) - *see* Burn, hand
  toe(nail) (subungual) - *see* Burn, leg
  tongue - *see* Burn, head
  tonsil - *see* Burn, head
  trunk   942
    with
      arm(s) (and leg(s))   947

Burn, etc. — *continued*
  trunk — *continued*
    with — *continued*
      arm(s) and leg(s) — *continued*
        with head   948
        head (and arm(s)) (and leg(s))   948
        leg(s) (and arm(s))   947
          with head   948
    tunica vaginalis - *see* Burn, trunk
    tympanic membrane - *see* Burn, head
    tympanum - *see* Burn, head
    uvula - *see* Burn, head
    vagina - *see* Burn, trunk
    vulva - *see* Burn, trunk
    wrist(s)   944
      with other site(s) - *see* Burn, arm
Burn's disease   722.2
Burnett's syndrome   999.9
Burning
  feet syndrome   261
  sensation (*see also* Disturbance,
      sensation)   781.6
  tongue   529.6
Bursa - *see also* condition
  pharynx   508.9
Bursitis (calcific) (inflammatory)
      (suppurative) (traumatic (old)) (with
      calcification)   731.9
  Achilles   731.7
  adhesive (scapulohumeral) (shoulder)
      717.1
  ankle   731.7
  buttock   731.5
  calcaneal   731.7
  Duplay's   717.1
  elbow   731.2
  finger   731.4
  foot   731.8

Bursitis, etc. — *continued*
  gonococcal   098.3
  hand   731.4
  hip   731.5
  knee   731.6
  olecranon   731.2
  pharyngeal   508.9
  popliteal   731.6
  prepatellar   731.6
  radiohumeral   731.2
  scapulohumeral   731.1
    adhesive   717.1
  shoulder   731.1
    adhesive   717.1
  subacromial   731.1
    adhesive   717.1
  subdeltoid   731.1
    adhesive   717.1
  syphilitic   095
  Thornwaldt, Tornwaldt   508.9
  toe   731.8
  trochanteric area   731.5
  wrist   731.3
Burst stitches or sutures (complication of
      surgery)   998.3
Bury's disease   695.9
Buschke's scleredema   734.0
Busse-Buschke disease   116.0
Buttock - *see* condition
Button
  Biskra   085.1
  Delhi   085.1
  oriental   085.1
Buttonhole hand (intrinsic)   738.2
Bwamba fever   068.2
Byssinosis   516.1
Bywater syndrome   995.6

C

Cachexia 268
  cancerous 199.1
  cardiac - *see* Disease, heart
  due to malnutrition 268
  exophthalmic 242.0
  Grawitz's 281.9
  heart - *see* Disease, heart
  hypophyseal 253.1
  hypopituitary 253.1
  lead 984
  malaria (*see also* Malaria) 084.9
  malignant 199.1
  marsh 084.9
  nervous 300.5
  old age 794
  pachydermic 244
  paludal (*see also* Malaria) 084.9
  pituitary 253.1
  renal (*see also* Lesion, kidney) 593.2
  saturnine 984
  senile 794
  Simmonds' 253.1
  splenica 289.5
  strumipriva (*see also* Hypothyroidism) 244
  tuberculous NEC (*see also* Tuberculosis) 011.9
Cafe au lait spots 709.9
Caffey's syndrome 756.7
Caisson disease 993.3
Cake
  kidney 753.3
Caked breast (puerperal, postpartum) 678
Calabar swelling 125.2
Calcaneo-apophysitis 722.4
Calcareous - *see* condition
Calcicosis 515.0
  with tuberculosis 010
Calcification
  adrenal (capsule) (gland) 255.9
    tuberculous 017.9
      late effect or sequela 019.9
  aorta - *see* Arteriosclerosis, aorta
  artery (annular) - *see* Arteriosclerosis
  auricle (ear) 387.9
  brain (cortex) - *see* Calcification, cerebral
  bronchus 519.9
  bursa - *see* Bursitis
  cardiac (*see also* Insufficiency, myocardial) 428

Calcification—*continued*
  cartilage (postinfectional) (*see also* Disease, joint) 729.9
  cerebral (cortex) 347.9
    artery (*see also* Ischemia, cerebral) 437.9
    due to toxoplasmosis (congenital) 130.2
  cervix (uteri) 621.9
  choroid plexus 347.9
  conjunctiva 378.3
  corpora cavernosa (penis) 607.9
  cortex (brain) - *see* Calcification, cerebral
  dental pulp (nodular) 522.2
  dentinal papilla 520.4
  falx cerebri - *see* Calcification, cerebral
  fascia 733.9
  gallbladder (*see also* Disease, gallbladder) 576.9
  general 279
  heart (*see also* Insufficiency, myocardial) 428
    valve - *see* Endocarditis
  intervertebral cartilage or disc (postinfectional) 729.1
  intracranial - *see* Calcification, cerebral
  joint (*see also* Disease, joint) 729.9
  kidney (*see also* Lesion, kidney) 593.2
    tuberculous 016.0
      late effect or sequela 019.2
  larynx (senile) 508.3
  lens 378.8
  ligament (*see also* Disease, joint) 729.9
    knee (medial collateral) 729.8
  lung
    active 519.2
    postinfectional 519.2
    tuberculous (*see also* Tuberculosis, pulmonary) 011.9
  lymph gland or node (postinfectional) 289.3
    tuberculous (*see also* Tuberculosis, lymph gland) 017.1
      late effect or sequela 019.9
  medial - *see* Arteriosclerosis, peripheral
  meninges (cerebral) 347.9
  metastatic 279
  muscle 733.9
  myocardium, myocardial (*see also* Insufficiency, myocardial) 428

Calculus, calculi, calculous—*continued*
 tooth, teeth 523.6
 tunica vaginalis 607.9
 ureter (impacted) (recurrent) 592
 urethra (impacted) 594
 urinary (duct) (impacted) (passage) 594
 vagina 629.9
 vesical (impacted) 594
 Wharton's duct 527.5
Caliectasis (*see also* Lesion, kidney)
 593.2
Caligo cornea - *see* Opacity, cornea
Callositas, callosity (infected) 700
Callus (infected) 700
 excessive, following fracture - code as
 Fracture, late effect
 current - *see* Fracture
Calve Perthes disease 722.1
Calve's disease 722.1
Calvities (*see also* Alopecia) 704
Cameroon fever 084.9
Camptocormia 300.1
Camurati-Engelmann disease 756.7
Canal - *see* condition
Canaliculitis 368
 Actinomyces 113
Cancer (*see also* Neoplasm, malignant)
 199.1
 acoustic (nerve) 192.0
 bile duct type, liver 155.1
 chimney-sweeps' 173.5
 dye workers' 188
 green 202.2
 hepatocellular 155.0
 mesonephritic - *see* Mesonephroma
 mule spinners' - *see* Neoplasm, skin,
 malignant
 pitch - *see* Neoplasm, skin, malignant
 radiation - *see* Neoplasm, skin,
 malignant
 radiologists' - *see* Neoplasm, skin,
 malignant
 rectum and lower bowel 154.0
 smokers' (*see also* Neoplasm, lip,
 malignant) 140.9
 larynx 161.9
 tar - *see* Neoplasm, skin, malignant
 x-ray - *see* Neoplasm, skin, malignant
Cancerous - *see also* Neoplasm,
 malignant
 ascites 197.6
 cachexia 199.1
 peritonitis 197.6
Cancerphobia 300.2
Cancroid - *see* Epithelioma, malignant
Cancrum
 oris 528.1

Cancrum—*continued*
 pudendi (*see also* Vulvitis) 622.1
Candidiasis 112
Canities (premature) 704
 congenital 757.3
Canker (sore) (mouth) 528.2
Canton fever 081.9
Capillary - *see* condition
Capsule - *see* condition
Capsulitis (joint) (*see also* Disease, joint)
 729.9
 adhesive 717.1
 thyroid - *see* Thyroiditis
Caput
 crepitus 756.0
 medusae 456.9
 succedaneum (*see also* Birth injury
 NEC) 772.9
Car sickness 994.6
Carapata disease 088.1
Carate - *see* Pinta
Carboxyhemoglobinemia 986
Carbuncle 680.9
 abdominal wall 680.2
 ankle 680.6
 anus 680.5
 arm (any part, above wrist) 680.3
 axilla 680.3
 back (any part) 680.2
 breast 680.2
 buttock 680.5
 chest wall 680.2
 corpus cavernosum 607.5
 ear (any part) (external) 680.0
 eyelid 362
 face (any part, except eye) 680.0
 finger (any) 680.4
 foot (any part) 680.6
 forearm 680.3
 gluteal (region) 680.5
 groin 680.2
 hand (any part) 680.4
 head (any part, except face) 680.8
 heel 680.6
 hip 680.6
 kidney (*see also* Abscess, kidney)
 590.2
 knee 680.6
 lachrymal, lacrimal gland or sac 368
 leg (any part) 680.6
 lower extremity 680.6
 malignant 022
 multiple sites NEC 680.8
 neck 680.1
 nose (septum) 680.0
 orbit, orbital 369.0
 partes posteriores 680.5

Cardiectasis - *see* Disease, heart
Cardiocele - *see* Disease, heart
Cardiochalasia   530.9
Cardiomalacia (*see also* Insufficiency,
    myocardial)   428
Cardiomegalia
  glycogenica diffusa   271.1
Cardiomegaly (*see also* Hypertrophy,
    cardiac)   429.0
  congenital   746.8
  glycogen   271.1
  idiopathic   425
Cardiomyopathy (congestive)
    (constrictive) (familial)
    (hypertrophic obstructive)
    (idiopathic) (obscure of Africa)
    (obstructive)   425
Cardionephritis - *see* Hypertension,
    cardiorenal
Cardionephropathy - *see* Hypertension,
    cardiorenal
Cardionephrosis - *see* Hypertension,
    cardiorenal
Cardiopathy (*see also* Disease, heart)
    429.9
  idiopathic   425
Cardiopericarditis (*see also* Pericarditis)
    423
Cardiophobia   300.2
Cardiorenal - *see* condition
Cardiorrhexis (*see also* Infarct,
    myocardium)   410.9
Cardiosclerosis (*see also* Ischemia, heart)
    412.9
Cardiosis - *see* Disease, heart
Cardiospasm (esophagus) (reflex)
    (stomach)   530.0
  congenital   750.8
  neurotic   305.5
  psychogenic   305.5
Cardiostenosis - *see* Disease, heart
Cardiovascular - *see* condition
  renal - *see* condition
Carditis (acute) (bacterial) (chronic)
    (subacute) (*see also* Disease, heart)
    429.9
  rheumatoid   712.3
Care
  child (routine)   Y00.5
  convalescent (*see also* Aftercare)
    Y10.9
  improper   994.9
  lack of (at or after birth) (infant)   994.9
  postpartum   Y07
  prenatal   Y06
  well baby   Y00.5

Caries (bone)   723.9
  cementum   521.0
  cerebrospinal (tuberculous)   015.0
    late effect or sequela   019.3
  dental (acute) (chronic) (incipient) (with
    pulp exposure)   521.0
  infected   521.0
  dentin (acute) (chronic)   521.0
  enamel (acute) (chronic) (incipient)
    521.0
  external meatus   380
  labyrinth   384.0
  mastoid process, chronic - *see*
    Mastoiditis, chronic
  middle ear   387.9
  nose   723.9
  orbit   723.9
  ossicle   387.9
  petrous bone   384.0
  sacrum (tuberculous)   015.0
    late effect or sequela   019.3
  spine, spinal (column) (tuberculous)
    015.0
    late effect or sequela   019.3
  syphilitic   095
    congenital   090.0
  tooth, teeth   521.0
  vertebra (column) (tuberculous)   015.0
    late effect or sequela   019.3
Carious teeth   521.0
Carneous mole (abortion) (*see also*
    Abortion, other)   645.9
  undelivered   634.9
Carotid body or sinus syndrome   358.1
Carotidynia   358.9
Carotinemia (dietary)   278.1
Carotinosis   278.1
  cutis   278.1
  skin   278.1
Carpal tunnel syndrome   357.2
Carpopedal spasm (*see also* Tetany)
    788.5
Carrier (state) (suspected)   Y05.9
  diphtheria   Y05.0
  dysentery   Y05.9
    amebic   Y05.3
  endameba (histolytica)   Y05.3
  infective organism NEC   Y05.9
  paratyphoid   Y05.9
  shigella   Y05.9
  typhoid   Y05.1
  venereal disease   Y05.2
Carrion's disease   089.0
Carter's
  disease   117.4
  relapsing fever (Asiatic)   088.0

Cartilage - *see* condition
Caruncle (inflamed)
  abscess, lachrymal, lacrimal   368
  amnion - *see* Placenta, abnormal
  conjunctiva   360
  eyelid   361
  labium (majus) (minus)   629.9
  urethra (benign)   599.2
  vagina (wall)   629.9
Cascado - *see* Dermatophytosis
Caseation lymphatic gland   017.1
  late effect or sequela   019.9
Castellani's bronchitis   104.9
Castration, traumatic - *see* Wound, open,
  genital organs
Cat-scratch - *see also* Injury, superficial
  disease or fever   079.3
Cat's ear   745.2
Catalepsy   300.1
  catatonic (acute)   295.2
  hysterical   300.1
Cataplexy (idiopathic)   347.0
Cataract (anterior cortical) (anterior polar)
  (atopic) (black) (capsular) (central)
  (cortical) (hypermature) (immature)
  (incipient) (mature) (nuclear) (senile)
  (toxic)   374.9
  anterior and posterior axial embryonal
    744.3
  anterior pyramidal   744.3
  blue dot   744.3
  cerulean   744.3
  complicated   374.1
  congenital   744.3
  coronary   744.3
  diabetic - *see* category 250
  due to
    infection   374.8
    radiation   374.8
  electric   374.8
  glass blowers'   374.8
  heat ray   374.8
  heterochromic   374.1
  irradiational   374.8
  lamellar   744.3
  morgagnian   374.8
  myxedema   244
  posterior, polar (capsular)   744.3
  punctate   744.3
  secondary (membrane)   374.1
  sunflower   374.0
  traumatic   374.0
  zonular (perinuclear)   744.3
Cataracta   374.9
  brunescens   374.9
  cerulea   744.3

Cataracta—*continued*
  complicata   374.1
  congenita   744.3
  coralliformis   744.3
  coronaria   744.3
  floriformis   374.0
  membranacea
    accreta   374.1
    congenita   744.3
Catarrh, catarrhal (inflammation) (*see also*
    condition)   460
  acute   460
  asthma, asthmatic   493
    with bronchitis - *see* Bronchitis
  bile duct (*see also* Cholecystitis)   575
  bilious   535
  bladder (*see also* Cystitis)   595
  Bostock's   507
  bowel - *see* Catarrh, intestinal
  bronchial   490
    acute   466
    chronic   491
    subacute   466
  cervix, cervical (canal) (uteri) (*see also*
    Cervicitis)   620.9
  chest   490
  chronic   502.1
  congestion   502.1
  due to syphilis   095
  enteric - *see* Catarrh, intestinal
  epidemic   470
  eustachian   384.0
  eye (acute) (vernal)   360
  fauces   462
  febrile   460
  fibrinous, acute   466
  gastric   535
  gastroduodenal   535
  gastro-enteric - *see* Catarrh, intestinal
  gastrohepatic   535
  gastro-intestinal - *see* Catarrh, intestinal
  hay   507
  infectious   460
  intestinal   009.9
    allergic   561
    bacterial NEC   008.3
    chronic   563.9
      ulcerative   563.1
    dietetic   561
    due to
      achylia gastrica   536.0
      Aerobacter aerogenes   008.2
      Bacillus coli   008.0
      Clostrida perfringens (C) (F)
        008.2
      enterococci   008.2

Catarrh, etc. — *continued*
  intestinal — *continued*
    due to — *continued*
      Escherichia coli 008.0
      irritating foods 561
      Paracolobactrum Arizona 008.1
      Paracolon bacillus NEC 008.2
        Arizona 008.1
      Proteus (bacillus) 008.2
      Pseudomonas aeruginosa 008.2
      specified
        bacteria NEC 008.2
        organism, nonbacterial NEC
          008.9
        virus 008.8
      Staphylococcus 008.2
      Streptococcus (anaerobic) 008.2
    lienteric 009.9
    neurogenic 564.1
    noninfectious 561
    toxic 561
    ulcerative (chronic) 563.1
    viral (*see also* Enteritis, viral) 008.9
  kidney (*see also* Lesion, kidney) 593.2
  larynx 506
  liver 070
  lung 490
    acute 466
    chronic 491
  middle ear, chronic - *see* Otitis, media,
    chronic
  mouth 528.0
  nasal (chronic) 502.1
    acute 460
  nasobronchial 502.1
  nasopharyngeal (chronic) 502.1
    acute 460
  nose - *see* Catarrh, nasal
  pituitous 502.1
  pneumococcal, acute 466
  pulmonary 490
    acute 466
    chronic 491
  renal (*see also* Lesion, kidney) 593.2
  spring (eye) 360
  stomach 535
  stomatitis 528.0
  suffocating 493
    with bronchitis - *see* Bronchitis
  summer (hay) 507
  throat 502.0
  urethra (*see also* Urethritis) 597
  uterus (*see also* Endometritis) 622.0
  vagina (*see also* Vaginitis) 622.1
  vasomotor 507
  vesical (*see also* Cystitis) 595
Catarrhus aestivus 507

Catastrophe
  abdominal 785.5
  cerebral (*see also* Disease,
    cerebrovascular, acute) 436.9
  intrauterine, fetus or newborn 778.9
Catatonia, catatonic (acute) 295.2
  dementia (praecox) 295.2
  schizophrenia 295.2
Cauda equina - *see* condition
Caul over face (*see also* Asphyxia,
  newborn) 776.9
Cauliflower ear 872.9
Causalgia 355.9
Cause
  external, general effects NEC 994.9
  not stated 796.9
  unknown 796.9
Caustic burn - *see also* Burn
  from swallowing caustic or corrosive
    substance 983.9
    specified substance - *see* Table of
      adverse effects
Cavare's disease 273.4
Cave-in, injury
  crushing (severe) (*see also* Crush, by
    site) 869.1
  suffocation 994.7
Cavernitis (penis) 607.5
Cavernoma (*see also* Hemangioma)
  227.0
  lymph vessel - *see* Lymphangioma
Cavernositis 607.5
Cavernous - *see* condition
Cavitation of lung (*see also* Tuberculosis,
  pulmonary) 011.9
  nontuberculous 519.2
Cavity
  lung - *see* Cavitation of lung
  optic papilla 744.8
  pulmonary - *see* Cavitation of lung
Cavus foot (congenital) 754.0
  acquired 738.6
Cazenave's
  disease NEC 694
  lupus 695.4
Cecitis (*see also* Appendicitis) 541
  with perforation, peritonitis, or rupture
    540.0
  acute 540.9
    with perforation, peritonitis or
      rupture 540.0
Cecum - *see* condition
Celiac
  disease (adult) 269.0
  infantilism 269.0
  rickets 269.0

Celioma - *see* Mesothelioma

Cell, cellular - *see also* condition

anterior chamber (eye) (positive
aqueous ray) 378.6

Cellulitis (diffuse) (with lymphangitis) (*see
also* Abscess) 682.9

abdominal wall 682.1

anaerobic (*see also* Gas gangrene)
039.0

ankle 682.4

anus 566

arm (any part, above wrist) 682.2

axilla 682.2

back (any part) 682.1

broad ligament (*see also* Disease,
pelvis, inflammatory) 616.0

buttock 682.1

cervical 682.0

cervix (uteri) (*see also* Cervicitis)
620.9

chest wall 682.1

chronic NEC 682.9

corpus cavernosum 607.5

drainage site (following operation)
998.5

ear (external) 380

erysipelar (*see also* Erysipelas) 035

eyelid 362

face (any part, except eye) 682.0

finger (intrathecal) (periosteal)
(subcutaneous) (subcuticular)
681

foot (except toe) 682.5

gangrenous (*see also* Gangrene) 445.9

genital organ NEC

female - *see* Abscess, genital organ,
female

male 607.5

gluteal 682.1

gonococcal NEC 098.9

groin 682.1

hand (except finger or thumb) 682.3

head (except ear) 682.0

heel 682.5

hip 682.4

jaw (region) 682.0

knee 682.4

labium (majus) (minus) (*see also*
Vulvitis) 622.1

leg (any part) 682.4

lip 528.5

mouth (floor) 528.3

multiple sites NEC 682.9

navel (newborn) 682.1

neck (region) 682.0

Cellulitis — *continued*

nose 508.9

external 682.0

orbit, orbital 369.0

palate (soft) 528.3

pectoral 682.1

pelvis, pelvic (chronic)

female (*see also* Disease, pelvis,
inflammatory) 616.0

male 682.1

penis 607.5

perineal, perineum 682.1

perirectal 566

peritonsillar 501

peri-urethral (*see also* Infection,
urinary) 599.0

peri-uterine (*see also* Disease, pelvis,
inflammatory) 616.0

pharynx 508.9

phlegmonous NEC 682.9

puerperal, postpartum, childbirth 670

rectum 566

retroperineal 682.1

retroperitoneal (*see also* Peritonitis)
567.9

round ligament (*see also* Disease,
pelvis, inflammatory) 616.0

scalp (any part) 682.0

scrotum 607.5

seminal vesicle 607.4

septic NEC 682.9

shoulder 682.2

specified sites NEC 682.9

spermatic cord 607.5

suppurative NEC 682.9

testis 607.5

thigh 682.4

thumb (intrathecal) (periosteal)
(subcutaneous) (subcuticular)
681

toe (intrathecal) (periosteal)
(subcutaneous) (subcuticular)
681

tonsil 501

trunk 682.1

tuberculous (primary) 017.0

late effect or sequela 019.9

tunica vaginalis 607.5

umbilicus (newborn) 682.1

urachus 682.1

vaccinal 999.3

vas deferens 607.5

vulva (*see also* Vulvitis) 622.1

wrist 682.3

Celothelioma - *see* Mesothelioma

Cementoma 210.4

Cementoperiostitis 523.4
Cephalematocele, cephalhematocele
due to
  birth injury (*see also* Birth injury
    NEC) 772.9
  fetus or newborn (*see also* Birth injury
    NEC) 772.9
  traumatic (*see also* Contusion, head)
    920
Cephalematoma, cephalhematoma
  (calcified)
due to
  birth injury (*see also* Birth injury
    NEC) 772.9
  fetus or newborn (*see also* Birth injury
    NEC) 772.9
  traumatic (*see also* Contusion, head)
    920
Cephalgia, cephalalgia (*see also*
    Headache) 791
  nonorganic origin 306.8
Cephalic - *see* condition
Cephalitis - *see* Encephalitis
Cephalocele 743.0
Cephaloma - *see* Neoplasm, malignant
Cephalomenia 626.9
Cephalopelvic - *see* condition
Cercomoniasis 007.9
Cerebellitis - *see* Encephalitis
Cerebellum, cerebellar - *see* condition
Cerebral - *see* condition
Cerebritis - *see* Encephalitis
Cerebromacular degeneration 333.0
Cerebromalacia (*see also* Softening, brain)
    438.9
Cerebrosidosis 272.2
Cerebrospasticity 343.1
Cerebrospinal - *see* condition
Cerebrum - *see* condition
Cerumen (accumulation) (impacted)
    387.1
Cervical - *see also* condition
  auricle 745.4
  rib 756.3

Cervicalgia 728.0

Cervicitis (acute) (nonvenereal) (subacute)
    620.9
with
  abortion - *see* Abortion, by type, with
    sepsis
  ectopic gestation - *see* categories
    631.0-631.3
  arising during pregnancy 630
    fetus or newborn 763.1
  chronic 620.0
    with ulceration 621.3

Cervicitis, etc. - *continued*
  gonococcal 098.0
    chronic or duration of 2 months or
      over 098.1
  puerperal, postpartum, childbirth 670
  senile (atrophic) 620.0
  syphilitic 095
  trichomonal 131
  tuberculous 016.2
    late effect or sequela 019.2
Cervicocolpitis (emphysematosa) (*see also*
    Cervicitis) 620.9
Cervix - *see* condition
Cesarean operation or section
  fetus or newborn (*see also* Birth injury
    NEC) 772.9
  postmortem fetus or newborn (*see also*
    Birth injury NEC) 772.9
Cestan syndrome 344.1
Cestan-Chenais paralysis 344.1
Cestode infestation NEC 123.9
Cestodiasis 123.9
Chabert's disease 022
Chafing 709.9
Chagas' disease (*see also*
    Trypanosomiasis, American)
    086.9
Chagres fever 084.0
Chalasia (cardiac sphincter) 530.9
Chalazion 378.0
Chalazoderma 757.2
Chalcosis 985.9
  cornea 378.4
  crystalline lens 378.8
  retina 377.4
Chalicosis (pulmonum) 515.0
  with tuberculosis 010
Chancre (any genital site) (hard)
    (indurated) (infecting) (primary)
    (recurrent) 091.0
  congenital 090.0
  conjunctiva 091.1
  Ducrey's 099.0
  extragenital 091.1
  eyelid 091.1
  hunterian 091.0
  lip (syphilis) 091.1
  mixed 099.9
  nipple 091.1
  Nisbet's 099.0
of
  carate 103.0
  pinta 103.0
  yaws 102.0
  palate soft 091.1
  phagedenic 099.0
  Ricord's 091.0

Chancre—*continued*
 Rollet's (syphilitic)   091.0
  gonococcal   099.9
 seronegative   091.0
 seropositive   091.0
 simple   099.0
 soft   099.0
  bubo   099.0
 urethra   091.0
 yaws   102.0
Chancroid   099.0
 anus   099.0
 penis (Ducrey's bacillus)   099.0
 perineum   099.0
 rectum   099.0
 scrotum   099.0
 urethra   099.0
 vulva   099.0
Change(s)
 arteriosclerotic - *see* Arteriosclerosis
 bone   723.9
  diabetic - *see* category 250
  in disease, unknown cause   723.9
 cardiorenal (vascular) - *see*
    Hypertension, cardiorenal
 cardiovascular - *see* Ischemia, heart
 circulatory   458.9
 color, tooth, teeth
  during formation   520.9
  posteruptive   521.7
 coronary (*see also* Ischemia, heart)
    412.9
 degenerative, spine or vertebra   713.1
 dental pulp, regressive   522.2
 heart - *see* Disease, heart
 hip joint   729.5
 hyperplastic larynx   508.3
 hypertrophic
  nasal sinus (*see also* Sinusitis)   503.9
  upper respiratory tract   508.9
 inflammatory - *see* Inflammation
 joint (*see also* Disease, joint)   729.9
  sacro-iliac   726
 knee   729.8
 malignant - *see also* Neoplasm,
    malignant
  in uterine fibroid   182.9
 mental NEC   300.9
  due to or associated with physical
     condition - *see* listing under
     Disorder, mental
 myocardium, myocardial - *see*
    Insufficiency, myocardial
 of life (*see also* Menopause)   627
 peripheral nerve   357.9
 personality (*see also* Disorder,
    personality)   301.9

Change(s)—*continued*
 personality—*continued*
  due to or associated with physical
     condition - *see* listing
     under Disorder, mental
 retina, myopic   370.0
 sacro-iliac joint   726
 senile (*see also* Senility)   794
 sensory (*see also* Disturbance,
    sensation)   781.6
 spinal cord   349.9
 trophic   357.9
 vascular   458.9
 vasomotor   443.9
 voice   783.5
  psychogenic   305.2
Chapping skin   709.9
Charcot-Marie-Tooth disease, paralysis or
    syndrome   330.0
Charcot's
 arthropathy   094.0
 cirrhosis - *see* Cirrhosis, biliary
 disease   094.0
  spinal cord   094.0
 fever (biliary) (hepatic) (intermittent)
    (*see also* Cholelithiasis)   574.9
 joint (disease)   094.0
  nonvenereal (*see also* Disease, joint)
     729.9
 syndrome   443.9
Charley-horse (quadriceps)   843
 muscle, except quadriceps - *see* Sprain,
    strain
Chataign skin   709.9
Chauffeur's fracture - *see* Fracture, ulna,
    lower end
Cheadle's disease   264
Check up
 following treatment - *see* Follow-up
 infant (not sick)   Y00.5
 postoperative - *see* Follow-up,
    postoperative
 pregnancy (normal)   Y06
 routine - *see* Examination
Chediak-Higashi syndrome   270.8
Cheek - *see* condition
Cheese itch   133.9
Cheilitis   528.5
 actinic   692.8
 acute   528.5
 catarrhal   528.5
 chronic   528.5
 exfoliativa (glandularis)   528.5
 gangrenous   528.5
 glandularis (apostematosa)   528.5
 infectional   528.5
 membranous   528.5

Cheilitis — *continued*
  suppurative 528.5
  ulcerative 528.5
  vesicular 528.5
Cheiloschisis 749.1
  with cleft palate 749.2
Cheilosis 528.5
  with
    pellagra 262
  angular 528.5
  due to
    dietary deficiency 263.0
    vitamin deficiency 263.0
Cheiromegaly 787.2
Cheiropompholyx 705.9
Cheloid (*see also* Keloid) 701.3
Chemical burn - *see also* Burn
  from swallowing chemical NEC 983.9
    specified type - *see* Table of adverse
      effects
Chemodectoma (*see also* Paraganglioma)
    226.8
  malignant 194.8
Chemosis, conjunctiva 360
Cherubism 526.9
Chest - *see* condition
Chester's disease 272.0
Cheyne-Stokes respiration 783.2
Chiari-Frommel syndrome 678
Chiari's
  disease or syndrome 453
  network 746.8
Chicken pox 052
Chiggers 133.9
Chignon 111.2
Chilblains 443.2
  lupus 443.2
Childbed fever 670
Childbirth - *see also* Delivery
  puerperal complications - *see* Puerperal
Childhood, behavior disorders (any) 308
Chill(s) 788.9
  congestive 788.9
    in malarial regions 084.9
  septic - *see* Septicemia
  urethral 599.9
Chilomastigiasis 007.9
Chimney-sweeps' cancer 173.5
Chin - *see* condition
Chiropractic dislocation - *see* Dislocation
Chloasma 709.9
  cachecticorum 709.9
  eyelid 709.9
    congenital 757.2
    hyperthyroid 242.0
  gravidarum 634.9
  idiopathic 709.9

Chloasma — *continued*
  skin 709.9
  symptomatic 709.9
Chloroleukemia 202.2
Chlorolymphosarcoma 202.2
Chloroma 202.2
Chloromyeloma 202.2
Chlorosarcoma 202.2
Chlorosarcomyeloma 202.2
Chlorosis 280
  Egyptian (*see also* Ancylostomiasis)
    126.9
  miners' (*see also* Ancylostomiasis)
    126.9
Chocolate cyst (ovary) 625.3
Choked
  disc or disk 377.5
  on food, phlegm, or vomitus NEC (*see
    also* Asphyxia, food) 933
  while vomiting NEC (*see also*
    Asphyxia, food) 933
Chokes (resulting from bends) 993.3
Cholangiectasis (*see also* Disease,
    gallbladder) 576.9
Cholangiocarcinoma 155.1
Cholangiolitis (acute) (chronic)
    (extrahepatic) (gangrenous)
    (perforated) (*see also* Cholecystitis)
    575
  intrahepatic 573.0
  paratyphoidal (*see also* Fever,
    paratyphoid) 002.9
  typhoidal 001
Cholangioma (benign) 211.5
  extrahepatic duct or passage 211.5
    malignant 156.1
  malignant 155.1
Cholangitis (catarrhal) (infective)
    (malignant) (suppurative) (*see also*
    Cholecystitis) 575
Cholecystdocholithiasis (*see also*
    Cholelithiasis) 574.9
Cholecystitis (catarrhal) (gangrenous)
    (infective) (obstructive) (perforated)
    (suppurative) 575
  with calculus, cholelithiasis, stones
    - 574.1
  paratyphoidal, current (*see also* Fever,
    paratyphoid) 002.9
  specified as acute (any condition in 575)
    575
    with cholelithiasis (any condition in
      574.9) 574.0
  typhoidal (current) 001
Choledochitis (suppurative) (*see also*
    Cholecystitis) 575

Choledocholith (*see also* Cholelithiasis) 574.9
Choledocholithiasis (*see also* Cholelithiasis) 574.9
Cholelithiasis (impacted) (multiple) (recurrent) 574.9
  with
    cholecystitis (any condition in 575, not specified as acute) 574.1
    specified as acute 574.0
    other diseases of gallbladder and biliary ducts (conditions in 576.0-576.9) 574.9
Cholemia (*see also* Jaundice) 785.2
  familial 273.5
  fetus or newborn 778.9
  Gilbert's 273.5
Cholemic gallstone (*see also* Cholelithiasis) 574.9
Choleperitoneum, choleperitonitis (*see also* Disease, gallbladder) 576.9
Cholera (algid) (Asiatic) (asphyctic) (epidemic) (gravis) (Indian) (malignant) (morbus) (pestilential) (spasmodic) 000.9
  antimonial 985.9
  bilious (*see also* Diarrhea) 009.1
  classical 000.0
  due to
    Vibrio
      cholerae (Inaba, Ogawa, Hikojima types) 000.0
      El Tor 000.1
  El Tor 000.1
  English (*see also* Enteritis) 009.2
  infantum (*see also* Diarrhea) 009.1
  nostras (*see also* Diarrhea) 009.1
  sporadic (*see also* Diarrhea) 009.1
  summer (*see also* Enteritis) 009.2
  winter (*see also* Enteritis) 009.2
Cholerine (*see also* Cholera) 000.9
Cholestasis (*see also* Disease, gallbladder) 576.9
Cholesteatoma (ear (middle)) (mastoid) (with reaction) 387.0
  malignant 160.1
    specified site NEC - *see* Neoplasm, malignant
  ovary 220.0
  specified site NEC - *see* Neoplasm, benign
Cholesteremia 279
Cholesterin in vitreous 378.9
Cholesterol
  deposit
    retina 377.4

Cholesterol — *continued*
  deposit — *continued*
    vitreous 378.9
  imbibition of gallbladder (*see also* Disease, gallbladder) 576.9
Cholesterolemia 279
  essential 272.0
  familial 272.0
  hereditary 272.0
Cholesterolosis (gallbladder) (*see also* Disease, gallbladder) 576.9
Cholesterosis (gallbladder) (*see also* Disease, gallbladder) 576.9
Cholocolic fistula (*see also* Fistula, gallbladder) 576.1
Choluria 789.9
Chondritis (purulent) (*see also* Disease, joint) 729.9
  costal 729.9
  tuberculous 015.9
    intervertebral 015.0
    late effect or sequela 019.3
    late effect or sequela 019.6
Chondroblastoma (*see also* Neoplasm, cartilage, benign) 213.9
  malignant - *see* Neoplasm, cartilage, malignant
Chondrocarcinoma - *see* Neoplasm, cartilage, malignant
Chondrodermatitis nodularis helicis or anthelicis 387.9
Chondrodysplasia 756.5
  angiomatose 756.5
  calcificans congenita 756.7
  hereditary deforming 756.5
Chondrodystrophia (fetalis) 756.5
  calcarea 756.5
  calcificans congenita 756.7
  punctata 756.7
  tarda 273.8
Chondrodystrophy (familial) (hypoplastic) 756.5
Chondroectodermal dysplasia 756.7
Chondro-endothelioma - *see* Neoplasm, bone, malignant
Chondrofibroma (*see also* Neoplasm, cartilage, benign) 213.9
Chondroma 213.2
  arytenoid 212.1
  auricular 215
  bronchi 212.3
  cricoid 212.1
  cuneiform 212.1
  ear (external) 215
  epiglottis 212.1
  eyelid 215
  larynx, laryngeal 212.1

Chondroma — *continued*
nose, nasal 212.0
pinna 215
thyroid 212.1
trachea 212.2
Chondromalacia (*see also* Disease, joint)
729.9
epiglottis 748.3
knee 729.7
larynx 748.3
patella, patellae 729.7
systemic 729.9
Chondromatosis, synovial 215
Chondrometaplasia, tenosynovial,
periarticular 215
Chondromyxoma (*see also* Chondroma)
213.2
Chondromyxosarcoma - *see* Neoplasm,
cartilage, malignant
Chondro-osteodysplasia 273.8
Morquio-Brailsford type 273.8
Chondro-osteodystrophy 273.8
Chondro-osteoma (*see also* Exostosis)
213.0
Chondropathia tuberosa 729.9
Chondrosarcoma - *see* Neoplasm,
cartilage, malignant
Chordee (nonvenereal) 607.9
congenital 752.2
gonococcal 098.1
Chorditis (fibrinous) 508.3
nodosa 508.3
tuberosa 508.3
Chordóma (*see also* Neoplasm, malignant)
199.1
benign (*see also* Neoplasm, benign)
228
clivus 170.0
nasopharynx 147
sacrococcygeal 170.6

Chorea (acute or subacute) (chronic
rheumatic) (gravis) (minor)
(rheumatic) (spasmodic)
(Sydenham's) 392.9
with
heart involvement - *see* Chorea with
rheumatic heart disease
rheumatic heart disease (chronic,
inactive, or quiescent)
(conditions in 393-398) - *see*
Rheumatic heart condition
involved
active or acute (conditions in 391)
392.0
apoplectic (*see also* Disease,
cerebrovascular, acute) 436.9

Chorea — *continued*
chronic 331.0
electric 065
late effects 066
gravidarum - *see* Eclampsia, pregnancy
habit 306.2
hereditary 331.0
Huntington's 331.0
insaniens 296.1
paralytic 347.9
posthemiplegic 344.1
pregnancy - *see* Eclampsia, pregnancy
progressive 331.0
chronic 331.0
nonhereditary 342
hereditary 331.0
Huntington's 331.0
senile 342
Choreo-athetosis 780.3
Chorio-adenoma (destruens) (placental)
181
Chorio-amnionitis
causing complicated delivery 661.8
complicating pregnancy (delivered)
(undelivered) 634.9
fetus or newborn 763.9
Chorio-angioma, placenta - *see* Placenta,
abnormal
Choriocarcinoma (placental) (*see also*
Chorionepithelioma) 181
Chorio-encephalitis, lymphocytic (acute)
(serous) 079.2
Chorio-epithelioma (*see also*
Chorionepithelioma) 181
Choriomeningitis (acute) (benign)
(lymphocytic) (serous) 079.2
Chorionepithelioma (uterus) 181
male (testicle) 186
specified site NEC - *see* Neoplasm,
malignant
Chorionitis (*see also* Scleroderma) 734.0
Chorioretinitis 366
due to toxoplasmosis 130.9
acquired 130.0
congenital (active) 130.1
late effects 130.2
juxtapapillaris 365
progressive myopia (degeneration) 366
syphilitic (late) 095
congenital 090.0
tuberculous 017.2
late effect or sequela 019.9
Choristoma - *see* Neoplasm, benign
Choroid - *see* condition
Choroideremia, choroidermia 744.8

Choroiditis (acute) (anterior) (central)
    (disseminated) (exudative) (guttate)
    (Jensen's) (juxtapapillary) (myopic)
    (suppurative) (sympathetic) (Tay's)
    365
  leprous   030.9
  syphilitic (late)   095
    congenital   090.0
  tuberculous (circumscribed) (plastic)
    017.2
    late effect or sequela   019.9
Choroidopathy   378.6
Choroidoretinitis   366
Choroidosis, central serous   377.4
Choroidretinopathy, serous   377.4
Christian-Weber disease   686.9
Christmas disease   286.1
Chromaffinoma (see also Paraganglioma)
    226.8
  adrenal (gland)   255.2
  aortic body   226.8
  malignant   194.8
    adrenal (gland)   194.0
Chromatopsia   377.3
Chromhidrosis   705.9
Chromidrosis   705.9
Chromoblastomycosis   117.2
Chromomycosis   117.2
Chromophobe adenoma   253.2
  pituitary (gland)   253.2
Chromophytosis   111.0
Chromotrichomycosis   111.8
Chronic - see condition
Chyle cyst, mesentery   457
Chylocele (nonfilarial)   457
  filarial (see also Infestation, filarial)
    125.9
  tunica vaginalis   607.9
    filarial (see also Infestation, filarial)
      125.9
Chylothorax (nonfilarial)   457
  filarial (see also Infestation, filarial)
    125.9
Chylous
  ascites   457
  cyst of peritoneum   457
  hydrocele (see also Hydrocele)   603
  hydrothorax (nonfilarial)   457
    filarial (see also Infestation, filarial)
      125.9
Chyluria   789.2
  bilharziasis   120.0
  due to
    Brugia (malayi)   125.1
    Wuchereria (bancrofti)   125.0
      malayi   125.1

Chyluria — continued
  filarial (see also Infestation, filarial)
    125.9
  filariasis (see also Infestation, filarial)
    125.9
  nonfilarial   789.2
Cicatricial (deformity) - see Cicatrix
Cicatrix (adherent) (contracted) (painful)
    (vicious)   709.0
  adenoid   500
  alveolar process   525.9
  anus   569.2
  auricle   387.9
  bile duct (see also Disease, gallbladder)
    576.9
  bladder   596.9
  bone   723.9
  brain   347.9
  cervix (postoperative) (postpartal)
    621.4
  common duct (see also Disease,
    gallbladder)   576.9
  cornea - see also Opacity, cornea
    tuberculous   017.2
      late effect or sequela   019.9
  duodenum (bulb)   537.9
  eyelid   378.2
  hypopharynx   508.9
  knee, semilunar cartilage   724.5
  lachrymal, lacrimal apparatus   378.3
  larynx   508.3
  limbus (cystoid)   378.6
  lung   519.2
  middle ear   387.9
  mouth   528.9
  muscle   733.9
  nasopharynx   508.9
  palate (soft)   528.9
  penis   607.9
  prostate   602
  rectum   569.2
  retina   377.4
  seminal vesicle   607.9
  skin   709.0
    infected   686.9
    postinfectional   709.0
    tuberculous   017.0
      late effect or sequela   019.9
  throat   508.9
  tongue   529.9
  tonsil   500
  trachea   508.9
  tuberculous NEC   011.9
    late effect or sequela   019.0
  ureter   593.5

Cicatrix, etc. — *continued*
  urethra 599.9
  uterus 625.9
  vagina 629.6
  vocal cord 508.3
  wrist, constricting (annular) 709.0
Cinchonism 961.3
Circle of Willis - *see* condition
Circular - *see also* condition
  hymen 752.6
Circulating anticoagulants 286.5
  following childbirth 675
Circulation
  collateral (venous) 458.9
    lower extremity 458.9
  defective 458.9
    congenital 747.9
    lower extremity 458.9
  embryonic 747.9
  failure 796.0
    fetus or newborn 778.9
    peripheral 782.9
  fetal, persistence 747.9
  heart, incomplete 747.9
Circulatory system - *see* condition
Circulus senilis 378.9
Circumscribed - *see* condition
Circumvallata placenta - *see* Placenta,
    abnormal
Cirrhosis, cirrhotic 571.9
  with alcohol, alcoholism 571.0
  alcoholic (liver) 571.0
  atrophic (of liver) - *see* Cirrhosis, portal
  Baumgarten-Cruveilhier 571.8
  biliary (cholangiolitic) (cholangitic)
      (cholostatic) (extrahepatic)
      (hypertrophic) (intrahepatic)
      (nonobstructive) (obstructive)
      (posthepatitic) (pericholangiolitic)
      (primary) (xanthomatous) 571.8
    with alcohol, alcoholism 571.0
    due to
      clonorchiasis 121.1
      flukes 121.3
  brain 347.9
  capsular - *see* Cirrhosis, portal
  cardiac (of liver) 571.8
    with alcohol, alcoholism 571.0
  central (liver) - *see* Cirrhosis, cardiac
  Charcot's - *see* Cirrhosis, biliary
  cholangiolitic - *see* Cirrhosis, biliary
  cholangitic - *see* Cirrhosis, biliary
  cholostatic - *see* Cirrhosis, biliary
  clitoris (hypertrophic) 629.9
  coarsely nodular - *see* Cirrhosis,
    postnecrotic

Cirrhosis, cirrhotic — *continued*
  congestive (liver) - *see* Cirrhosis,
    cardiac
  Cruveilhier-Baumgarten 571.8
  dietary - *see* Cirrhosis, portal
  due to
    bronzed diabetes 273.2
    congestive hepatomegaly - *see*
        Cirrhosis, cardiac
    cystic fibrosis 273.0
    hemachromatosis 273.2
    hepatolenticular degeneration 273.3
    passive congestion (chronic) - *see*
        Cirrhosis, cardiac
    Wilson's disease 273.3
    xanthomatosis 272.0
  extrahepatic (obstructive) - *see*
      Cirrhosis, biliary
  fatty *see* Cirrhosis, portal
  Glisson's - *see* Cirrhosis, portal
  Hanot's (hypertropic) - *see* Cirrhosis,
      biliary
  hepatic - *see* Cirrhosis, liver
  hepatolienal - *see* Cirrhosis, liver
  hobnail - *see* Cirrhosis, portal
  hypertrophic - *see* Cirrhosis, liver
    biliary - *see* Cirrhosis, biliary
    Hanot's - *see* Cirrhosis, biliary
  infectious NEC - *see* Cirrhosis, portal
  insular - *see* Cirrhosis, portal
  intrahepatic (obstructive) (primary)
      (secondary) - *see* Cirrhosis,
      biliary
  juvenile - *see* Cirrhosis, portal
  kidney (*see also* Sclerosis, renal) 584
  Laennec's (of liver) 571.0
    nonalcoholic - *see* Cirrhosis, portal
  liver (chronic) (hepatolienal)
      (hypertrophic) (nodular)
      (splenomegalic) (unilobar) (with
      Banti's disease or syndrome)
      (with congestive splenomegaly)
      (with portal hypertension) 571.9
    with alcohol, alcoholism 571.0
    alcoholic 571.0
    biliary 571.8
    cardiac 571.8
    congenital (due to failure of
        obliteration of umbilical vein)
        571.8
    pigmentary 273.2
    portal 571.8
    postnecrotic 571.8
    syphilitic 095
  lung (chronic) (*see also* Fibrosis, lung)
      517

Cirrhosis, cirrhotic—*continued*
  malarial (*see also* Malaria) 084.9
  malnutrition NEC - *see* Cirrhosis,
      portal
  metabolic NEC - *see* Cirrhosis, liver
  monolobular - *see* Cirrhosis, portal
  multilobular - *see* Cirrhosis, portal
  nephritis (*see also* Sclerosis, renal)
      584
  nodular - *see* Cirrhosis, liver
    coarse - *see* Cirrhosis, postnecrotic
    diffuse - *see* Cirrhosis, portal
    toxic - *see* Cirrhosis, postnecrotic
  nutritional (fatty) - *see* Cirrhosis, portal
  obstructive (biliary) (extrahepatic)
      (intrahepatic) - *see* Cirrhosis,
      biliary
  ovarian 615.9
  paludal (*see also* Malaria) 084.9
  pancreas (duct) 577.9
  periportal - *see* Cirrhosis, portal
  pigment, pigmentary (of liver) 273.2
  portal (of liver) 571.8
    with alcohol, alcoholism 571.0
  posthepatitic - *see* Cirrhosis,
      postnecrotic
  biliary - *see* Cirrhosis, biliary
  postnecrotic (of liver) 571.8
    with alcohol, alcoholism 571.0
  primary (intrahepatic) - *see* Cirrhosis,
      biliary
  pulmonary (*see also* Fibrosis, lung)
      517
  renal (*see also* Sclerosis, renal) 584
  septal - *see* Cirrhosis, postnecrotic
  spleen 289.5
  splenomegalic (of liver) - *see* Cirrhosis,
      liver
  stasis (liver) - *see* Cirrhosis, cardiac
  stomach 535
  Todd's - *see* Cirrhosis, biliary
  toxic (nodular) - *see* Cirrhosis,
      postnecrotic
  trabecular - *see* Cirrhosis, postnecrotic
  unilobar - *see* Cirrhosis, liver
  vascular (of liver) - *see* Cirrhosis,
      cardiac
  xanthomatous (biliary) - *see also*
      Cirrhosis, biliary
    due to xanthomatosis (familial)
        (metabolic) (primary) 272.0
Citrullinemia 270.8
Citrullinuria 270.8
Civatte's disease or poikiloderma 709.9
Clap - *see* Gonorrhea
Clark's paralysis - *see* Palsy, cerebral

Clarke-Hadfield syndrome 577.9
Clasmocytoma 200.0
Clastothrix 704
Claude Bernard-Horner syndrome 358.0
Claude's syndrome 347.9
Claudication, intermittent 443.9
  cerebral (artery) (*see also* Ischemia,
      cerebral, transient) 435.9
  spinal cord (arteriosclerotic) (*see also*
      Ischemia, cerebral, transient)
      435.9
  syphilitic 094.9
Claustrophobia 300.2
Clavus (infected) 700
Clawfoot (congenital) 754.0
  acquired 738.6
  syringomyelic 349.0
Clawhand (acquired) 738.2
  congenital 755.5
  syringomyelic 349.0
Clawtoe (congenital) 754.0
  acquired 738.7
Cleft (congenital) - *see also* Imperfect
      closure
  alveolar process 525.9
  branchial (cyst) (persistent) 745.4
  facial 749.1
    with cleft palate 749.2
  lip 749.1
    with cleft palate 749.2
  nose 748.1
  palate (complete) (incomplete) 749.0
    with cleft lip 749.2
  penis 752.8
  scrotum 752.8
  thyroid cartilage 748.3
  uvula 749.0
    with cleft lip 749.2
Cleidocranial dysostosis 755.5
Cleidotomy 773
Cleptomania 300.3
Clergyman's sore throat 783.5
Climacteric (*see also* Menopause) 627
  arthritis (any site) NEC 714.9
  depression 296.0
  disease 627
  epilepsy 345.9
  insanity 296.0
  male 607.9
  melancholia 296.0
  paranoid state 297.1
  paraphrenia 297.1
  polyarthritis NEC 714.9
  symptoms 627
Clitoris - *see* condition
Cloaca persistent 751.4

Clonorchiasis 121.1
Clonorchiosis 121.1
Clonorchis infection, liver 121.1
Clonus 780.3
Closure
  congenital, nose 748.0
  cranial sutures, premature 756.0
  defective or imperfect NEC - see
      Imperfect closure
  fistula, delayed - see Fistula
  foramen ovale, imperfect 746.4
  hymen 629.7
  interauricular septum, defective 746.4
  interventricular septum, defective
      746.3
  lacrimal duct 368
    congenital 744.8
  vagina 629.7
  valve - see Endocarditis
  vulva 629.7
Clot (blood)
  artery (obstruction) (occlusion) (see also
      Embolism) 444.9
  bladder 596.9
  brain (intradural or extradural) (see also
      Disease, cerebrovascular NEC)
      438.9
  circulation 444.9
  heart (see also Infarct, myocardium)
      410.9
  vein (see also Thrombosis) 453
Clouded state
  epileptic 345.9
  paroxysmal (idiopathic) 345.9
Cloudy
  antrum, antra 503.0
  swelling
    adrenal (gland) 255.9
    kidney (see also Lesion, kidney)
      593.2
    liver 573.9
Clubfinger 738.3
  congenital 755.5
Clubfoot (congenital) 754.9
  acquired 738.6
  paralytic 738.6
  postpoliomyelitic 044
Clubhand (congenital) 755.5
  acquired 738.2
Clubnail 703.9
  congenital 757.4
Clump, kidney 753.3
Cluttering 306.0
Clutton's joints 090.5
Coagulopathy (see also Defect,
      coagulation) 286.9

Coagulopathy — continued
  causing hemorrhage of pregnancy
      632.4
  following childbirth 675
Coal miner's
  elbow 731.2
  lung 515.1
    with tuberculosis 010
Coalition, calcaneo-scaphoid 755.7
Coarctation
  aorta 747.1
  reverse 446.6
Coated tongue 529.3
Coats' disease 377.0
Cocainism 304.4
Coccidioidomycosis 114
  lung 114
  meninges 114
  prostate 114
Coccidioidosis 114
  lung 114
  meninges 114
Coccidiosis 007.2
Cocciuria 789.1
Coccus in urine 789.1
Coccydynia 728.9
Coccygodynia 728.9
Coccyx - see condition
Cochin China
  diarrhea 269.0
    anguilluliasis 127.1
  ulcer 085.1
Cock's peculiar tumor 706.2
Cocked up toe 738.7
Codman's tumor (see also Neoplasm,
      cartilage, benign) 213.9
Cogan's syndrome 363.9
Coiling, umbilical cord - see
      Complications, umbilical cord
Coitus, painful (female) (male) 786.7
  psychogenic 305.6
Cold 460
  with influenza, flu, or grippe 472
  allergic 507
  bronchi or chest - see Bronchitis
    with
      grippe or influenza 472
  common (head) 460
  deep 464
  effects of NEC 991.9
  excessive 991.9
  exhaustion from 991.9
  exposure to 991.9
  grippy 472
  head 460
  injury syndrome (newborn) 778.3

Cold—*continued*
  on lung - *see* Bronchitis
  rose 507
  sensitivity, auto-immune 283.9
  virus 460
Coldsore 054
Colibacillosis 039.9
Colic (recurrent) 785.5
  abdomen 785.5
    psychogenic 305.5
  appendicular 543
  appendix 543
  bile duct or biliary (*see also*
      Cholelithiasis) 574.9
  bilious 785.5
  common duct (*see also* Cholelithiasis)
    574.9
  Devonshire 984
  flatulent 785.5
  gallbladder or gallstone (*see also*
      Cholelithiasis) 574.9
  hepatic (duct) (*see also* Cholelithiasis)
    574.9
  hernial - *see* Hernia
  hysterical 300.1
  infantile 785.5
  intestinal 785.5
  kidney 786.0
  lead 984
  liver (duct) (*see also* Cholelithiasis)
    574.9
  mucous 564.1
    psychogenic 305.5
  nephritic 592
  painters' 984
  pancreas 577.9
  psychogenic 305.5
  renal 786.0
  saturnine 984
  spasmodic 785.5
  ureter 786.0
  urethral 594
  uterus 625.9
  worm NEC 128.9
Colicystitis (*see also* Cystitis) 595
Colitis (acute) (catarrhal) (croupous)
      (exudative) (gangrenous) (gravis)
      (hemorrhagic) (infectious) (necrotic)
      (phlegmonous) (septic) (*see also*
      Enteritis) 009.2
  allergic 561
  amebic 006.9
    with liver abscess 006.0
  anthrax 022
  bacillary NEC 004.9
  balantidial 007.0
  chronic 563.9

Colitis—*continued*
  coccidial 007.2
  dietetic 561
  giardial 007.1
  membranous 564.1
  mucous 564.1
    psychogenic 305.5
  noninfectious 561
  pseudomucinous 564.1
  spastic 564.1
  thrombo-ulcerative (chronic) 563.1
  toxic 561
  tuberculous (ulcerative) 014
  ulcerative (chronic) 563.1
Collagen disease NEC 734.9
  nonvascular 734.9
  vascular (allergic) 446.2
Collagenosis (*see also* Collagen disease)
    734.9
  cardiovascular 425
Collapse 782.5
  adrenal 255.9
  cardiorenal - *see* Hypertension,
    cardiorenal
  cardiorespiratory - *see also* Disease,
    heart
    fetus or newborn 778.9
  cardiovascular - *see also* Disease, heart
    fetus or newborn 778.9
  circulatory (peripheral) 782.9
    fetus or newborn 778.9
  general 782.5
  heart - *see* Disease, heart
  heat 992.1
  hysterical 300.1
  labyrinth, membranous (congenital)
    745.0
  lung (massive) (*see also* Atelectasis)
    519.0
  myocardial - *see* Disease, heart
  nervous (*see also* Disorder, mental)
    300.9
  neurocirculatory 305.3
  nose 738.0
  pulmonary (*see also* Atelectasis) 519.0
  thorax 512
  trachea 519.9
  valvular - *see* Endocarditis
  vascular (peripheral) 782.9
    cerebral (*see also* Disease,
      cerebrovascular, acute) 436.9
    fetus or newborn 778.9
  vertebra 723.9
Colles' fracture (reversed) (separation) -
    see Fracture, radius, lower end
Collet-Sicard syndrome 347.9

Collet's syndrome 347.9
Colliculitis urethralis (see also Urethritis)
    597
Colliers'
    asthma - see Collier's lung
    lung 515.1
        tuberculous 010
    phthisis 010
Colloid
    degeneration 279
    tumor - see Neoplasm, benign
Coloboma (choroid) (iris) (lens) (lids) (optic
        nerve entry) (retina) (sclerotic)
        744.4
Colo-enteritis - see Enteritis
Colon - see condition
Coloptosis 569.9
Color blindness 377.3
Colostomy, malfunctioning 998.7
Colpitis (see also Vaginitis) 622.1
Colpocele 623.3
Colpocystitis (see also Vaginitis) 622.1
Colporrhexis, complicating delivery - see
        Laceration, perineum complicating
        delivery
Column, spinal, vertebral - see condition
Coma 780.0
    alcoholic 303.9
    apoplectic (see also Disease,
            cerebrovascular, acute) 436.9
    brain 780.0
    diabetic 250.0
    eclamptic (see also Eclampsia) 780.2
    epileptic 345.9
    hepatic 573.9
    hyperglycemic 250.0
    hypoglycemic 251
        diabetic 250.9
    Kussmaul's 250.0
    pre-diabetic 250.0
    uremic - see Uremia
Combat fatigue 307
Combined - see condition
Comedo 706.1
Comedocarcinoma (breast) 174
Comedomastitis 611.0
Comedones 706.1
    lanugo 757.3
Comminuted fracture - code as Fracture,
        closed
Common
    atrioventricular canal 746.5
    truncus (arteriosus) 746.0
Commotio (current)
    cerebri (without skull fracture) 850.0
        late effect 850.9

Commotio (current) - continued
    retinae 921
    spinalis - see Injury, spinal, by region
Commotion (current)
    brain (without skull fracture) 850.0
        late effect 850.9
    spinal cord - see Injury, spinal, by
            region
Communication
    abnormal - see also Fistula
        between base of aorta and pulmonary
                artery 746.0
        congenital between uterus and
                anterior abdominal wall 752.5
            bladder 752.5
            intestine 752.5
            rectum 752.5
            pericardial sac with pleural sac
                    748.8
Compensation
    broken - see Disease, heart
    failure - see Disease, heart
    neurosis, psychoneurosis 300.1
Complaint - see also Disease
    bowel, functional 564.9
        psychogenic 305.5
    intestine, functional 564.9
        psychogenic 305.5
    kidney (see also Lesion, kidney) 593.2
    miners' 515.1
        with tuberculosis 010
    summer (bowel) (intestine) 009.9
Complete - see condition
Complex
    cardiorenal - see Hypertension,
            cardiorenal
    Costen's 524.9
    Eisenmenger 746.3
    homosexual 302.0
    hypersexual 302.8
    jumped process
        spine - see Dislocation, vertebra
    primary, tuberculosis (with symptoms)
            012.0
    Taussig-Bing 746.1

Complications
    amputation stump (surgical) (late)
            997.2
        traumatic - see Amputation, traumatic
    anesthesia, anesthetic NEC 968.1
        specified agent - see Table of adverse
                effects
    blood vessel graft 997.6
    cardiac - see Disease, heart
    cardiorenal - see Hypertension,
            cardiorenal

Complications—*continued*
  transfusion—*continued*
    sepsis 999.3
    shock or reaction NEC 999.8
  transplanted organ 997.7
  trauma NEC (early) 995.9
  umbilical cord (around neck or limbs)
      (entanglement) (long) (knot)
      (rupture) (short) (tear) (torsion)
      (varices)
    during delivery (any complication)
        661.3
    fetus or newborn NEC 771.9
      compression (due to prolapse)
          771.0
      prolapse (without mention of
          compression) 771.1
    in pregnancy (any complication)
        634.9
  urethral catheter 999.9
  vaccination 999.5
    anaphylaxis NEC 999.4
    cellulitis 999.3
    encephalitis or encephalomyelitis
        999.1
    hepatitis (serum) (within 8 months of
        administration) 999.2
    infection (general) (local) NEC
        999.3
    jaundice (serum) (within 8 months of
        administration) 999.2
    meningitis 999.1
    myelitis 999.1
    protein sickness 999.5
    reaction (allergic) (serum) 999.5
      Herxheimer's 999.4
    sepsis 999.3
    serum intoxication, sickness, rash, or
        other reaction NEC 999.5
    shock (allergic) (anaphylactic) 999.4
    subacute yellow atrophy of liver
        (within 8 months of
        administration) 999.2
    vaccinia (generalized) 999.0
      localized 999.3

Compressed air disease 993.3

Compression
  with injury - *see* nature of injury
  artery 447
  brachial plexus 357.0
  brain 347.9
    due to
      injury NEC (*see also* Hemorrhage,
          brain, traumatic) 853.0
      birth (*see also* Birth injury, brain)
          772.0

Compression—*continued*
  brain—*continued*
    due to—*continued*
      laceration or contusion, brain (*see
          also* Laceration, cerebral)
          851.0
  bronchus 519.9
  by cicatrix - *see* Cicatrix
  cauda equina 357.9
  cerebral - *see* Compression, brain
  cervical plexus 357.0
  cord (umbilical) - *see* Compression,
      umbilical cord
  cranial nerve NEC (*see also* Atrophy,
      nerve, cranial) 356
  divers' squeeze 993.3
  during birth (*see also* Birth injury,
      brain) 772.0
  esophagus 530.3
  fracture - *see* Fracture
  heart - *see* Disease, heart
  intestine (*see also* Obstruction,
      intestine) 560.9
  laryngeal nerve, recurrent 508.3
  lumbosacral plexus 357.9
  lung 519.2
  lymphatic vessel 457
  medulla - *see* Compression, brain

  nerve (peripheral) (spinal) 357.9
    axillary 357.1
    cranial NEC (*see also* Atrophy,
        nerve, cranial) 356
    due to displacement of intervertebral
        disc 725.9
      cervical, cervicodorsal,
          cervicothoracic 725.0
      lumbar, lumbosacral 725.1
      specified site NEC 725.8
    median 357.2
    optic 377.6
    root NEC 728.9
    sciatic (acute) 353
    sympathetic 358.9
    traumatic - *see* Injury, nerve
    ulnar 357.3

  peripheral
    autonomic nervous system 358.9
    nerve (*see also* Compression, nerve)
        357.9
      by scar tissue 357.9

  spinal (cord) (old or not specified as
      traumatic) 349.6
    by displacement of intervertebral disc
        - *see* Displacement,
        intervertebral disc

Compression—*continued*
  spinal, etc.—*continued*
    nerve   357.9
      root NEC   728.9
        traumatic - *see* Injury, nerve,
          spinal
        traumatic - *see* Injury, nerve, spinal
        traumatic - *see also* Injury, spinal, by
          region
        with fracture, vertebra (conditions
          in 805) - *code by* region
          under Fracture, vertebra,
          with spinal cord lesion
    spondylogenic NEC   728.9
      cervical spinal cord   728.4
      thoracic spinal cord   728.6
    sympathetic nerve   358.9
    thorax   512
    trachea   519.9
    ulnar nerve (by scar tissue)   357.3
    umbilical cord
      complicating delivery   661.3
      fetus or newborn (due to prolapse)
        771.0
    vein   458.9
    vena cava (inferior) (superior)   458.9
    vertebral NEC - *see* Compression,
      spondylogenic
Compulsion, compulsive
  neurosis (obsessive)   300.3
  personality   301.4
  states (mixed)   300.3
  swearing   300.3
  tics and spasms   300.3
Concato's disease
  peritoneal   569.9
  pleural - *see* Pleurisy
Concavity chest wall   738.8
Concealed penis   752.8
Concrescence (teeth)   520.2
Concretio cordis   393
Concretion - *see also* Calculus
  appendicular   543
  canaliculus   378.3
  clitoris   629.9
  conjunctiva   378.3
  eyelid   378.2
  intestinal (impaction) (obstruction)
    560.3
    with hernia - *see* Hernia, by site, with
      obstruction
  lachrymal, lacrimal apparatus   378.3
  prepuce (male)   605
    female   629.9
    in clitoris   629.9
  salivary gland (any)   527.5

Concretion—*continued*
  seminal vesicle   607.9
  stomach   537.9
  tonsil   500
Concussion (current)   850.0
  blast (air) (hydraulic) (immersion)
    (underwater)
    abdomen or thorax - *see* Injury,
      internal, by site
    brain - *see* Concussion, brain
    ear (acoustic nerve trauma) - *see also*
      Injury, nerve, acoustic
    with perforation, tympanic
      membrane - *see* Wound,
      open, ear
  brain or cerebral (without skull fracture)
    850.0
    late effect   850.9
    repeated   850.9
  cauda equina - *see* Injury, spinal, sacral
  conus medullaris - *see* Injury, spinal,
    sacral
  hydraulic - *see* Concussion, blast
  labyrinth (*see also* Injury, intracranial)
    854.0
  late effect   850.9
  ocular   921
  osseous
    labyrinth (*see also* Injury,
      intracranial)   854.0
  spinal (cord) - *see also* Injury, spinal, by
    region
    due to
      broken
        back - *code by* region under
          Fracture, vertebra with
          spinal cord lesion
        neck (closed)   806.0
          late effect   806.9
          open   806.1
      fracture, fracture dislocation, or
        compression fracture of
        spine or vertebra - *see*
        Fracture, vertebra, with
        spinal cord lesion
  syndrome   850.9
  underwater blast - *see* Concussion,
    blast
Condition - *see also* Disease
  prostatic   602
  psychiatric   299
Conduct disturbance, child   308
Condyloma (accuminatum)   099.9
  gonorrheal   098.9
  latum   091.2
  syphilitic   091.2
    congenital   090.0

Condyloma, etc. — *continued*
  uterine cervix   099.9
  venereal, syphilitic   091.2
Confinement - *see also* Delivery
  premature, with dead fetus (less than 28
       weeks gestation) - *see* Abortion,
       by type
Conflagration - *see also* Burn
  asphyxia (by inhalation of smoke, gases,
       fumes or vapors)   987.9
Confluent - *see* condition
Confusion, confused (mental) (state)
    298.2
  psychogenic   298.2
  reactive (from emotional stress,
      psychological trauma)   298.2
Congelation   991.9
Congenital - *see also* condition
  aortic septum   747.2
  malformation - *see* Anomaly

Congestion (chronic) (passive)   796.0
  bladder   596.9
  bowel   569.9
  brain (*see also* Disease, cerebrovascular
      NEC)   438.9
    alcoholic   303.9
    malarial (*see also* Malaria)   084.9
  breast   611.9
  bronchi   519.9
  bronchial tube   519.9
  cerebral - *see* Congestion, brain
  cerebrospinal - *see* Congestion, brain
  chest   514
  circulatory NEC   458.9
  duodenum   537.9
  eye   378.9
  general   796.0
  glottis   506
  heart (*see also* Failure, heart,
      congestive)   427.0
  hepatic   573.9
  hypostatic (lung)   514
  intestine   569.9
  intracranial - *see* Congestion, brain
  kidney (*see also* Lesion, kidney)   593.2
  labyrinth   387.9
  larynx   506
  liver   573.9
  lung   514
    active or acute (*see also* Pneumonia)
      486
    congenital (*see also* Pneumonia)
      486
    hypostatic   514
  malaria, malarial (brain) (fever) (*see also*
      Malaria)   084.9

Congestion, etc. — *continued*
  medulla - *see* Congestion, brain
  orbit, orbital   378.9
  ovary   615.9
  pancreas   577.9
  pelvic, female   616.2
  pleural   511.0
  prostate (active)   602
  pulmonary - *see* Congestion, lung
  renal (*see also* Lesion, kidney)   593.2
  retina   377.4
  seminal vesicle   607.9
  spinal cord   349.9
  spleen   289.5
  stomach   537.9
  trachea   464
  urethra   599.9
  uterus   625.9
  viscera   796.0

Congestive - *see* Congestion

Conical
  cervix   621.9
  cornea   378.4
Conjoined twins   759.1
Conjugal maladjustment   307
Conjunctiva - *see* condition
Conjunctivitis (acute) (actinic) (allergic)
      (anaphylactic) (angular) (atopic)
      (catarrhal) (chronic) (dust)
      (exposure) (eczematous) (follicular)
      (glare) (infantile) (infectious)
      (influenzal) (Koch-Weeks) (light)
      (medicamentosa) (membranous)
      (Morax-Axenfeld) (newborn)
      (nodosa) (nondiphtheritic)
      (Parinaud's) (petrificans)
      (phlyctenular) (pneumococcal)
      (pseudomembranous) (purulent)
      (pustular) (simple) (staphylococcal)
      (streptococcal) (sun lamp)
      (traumatic NEC) (vernal)   360
with hay fever   507
adenoviral   078.2
blennorrhagic (neonatorum)   098.2
diphtheritic   032
due to
  syphilis   095
  toxoplasmosis (acquired)   130.0
    congenital (active)   130.1
      late effects   130.2
epidemic   078.1
gonococcal (neonatorum)   098.2
granular (trachomatous)   076
  late effect   077
inclusion   078.0
meningococcic   036.8

Conjunctivitis, etc. — *continued*
　Newcastle's　078.8
　of Beal　078.2
　rosacea　695.3
　swimming pool　078.0
　trachomatous　076
　　late effect　077
　tuberculous　017.2
　　late effect or sequela　019.9
　tularemic　021
　tularensis　021
　viral NEC　078.9
Conn's syndrome　255.0
Connective tissue - *see* condition
Consecutive - *see* condition
Consolidation lung (base) - *see*
　　　Pneumonia, lobar
Constipation (atonic) (simple) (spastic)
　　564.0
　drug induced NEC　977.9
　　specified drug or substance - *see*
　　　Table of adverse effects
　neurogenic　564.0
　psychogenic　305.5
Constitutional - *see* condition
Constitutionally substandard　301.6
Constriction
　anomalous, meningeal bands or folds
　　743.9
　asphyxiation or suffocation by　994.7
　bronchi　519.9
　canal, ear　387.9
　duodenum　537.9
　gallbladder (*see also* Obstruction,
　　　gallbladder)　576.0
　intestine (*see also* Obstruction,
　　　intestine)　560.9
　larynx　508.3
　　congenital　748.3
　organ or site, congenital NEC - *see*
　　　Atresia
　prepuce (congenital)　605
　pylorus　537.0
　　congenital or infantile　750.1
　ring (uterus), complicating delivery
　　657.9
　　fetus or newborn - *see* categories
　　　767.0-767.9
　spastic - *see also* Spasm
　　ureter　593.3
　　urethra　599.9
　stomach　537.9
　ureter　593.3
　visual field (peripheral) (functional)
　　781.0
Constrictive - *see* condition

Consumption - *see* Tuberculosis
Contact
　with
　　infective or parasitic disease NEC
　　　Y04.9
　　poliomyelitis　Y04.1
　　rabies　Y04.2
　　tuberculosis　Y04.0
　dermatitis - *see* Dermatitis
Contamination, food (*see also* Poisoning,
　　food)　005.9
Contraceptive device causing menorrhagia
　939
Contraction, contracture, contracted
　Achilles tendon　733.4
　　congenital　754.9
　anus　564.9
　axilla　733.9
　bile duct (*see also* Disease, gallbladder)
　　576.9
　bladder (neck) (sphincter)　596.2
　bowel, cecum, colon or intestine, any
　　　part (*see also* Obstruction,
　　　intestine)　560.9
　Braxton-Hicks (undelivered)　634.7
　bronchi　519.9
　burn (old) - *see* Cicatrix
　cervix (*see also* Stricture, cervix)
　　621.5
　　congenital　752.5
　cicatricial - *see* Cicatrix
　conjunctiva trachomatous, active　076
　　late effect　077
　Dupuytren's　733.5
　eyelid　378.2
　face　733.9
　fascia (lata) (postural)　733.9
　finger(s)　738.3
　　congenital　755.5
　　flexion　729.4
　　joint (*see also* Contraction, joint)
　　　729.9
　flaccid, paralytic
　　joint (*see also* Contraction, joint)
　　　729.9
　　muscle (*see also* Contraction, muscle)
　　　733.9
　　ocular (*see also* Strabismus)　373.9
　gallbladder or gall duct (*see also*
　　　Disease, gallbladder)　576.9
　hamstring　733.9
　heart valve - *see* Endocarditis
　hip (*see also* Contraction, joint)　729.5
　hourglass
　　bladder　596.2
　　congenital　753.8

Contraction, etc. — *continued*
  hourglass — *continued*
    gallbladder (*see also* Disease,
        gallbladder)   576.9
      congenital   751.6
    stomach   536.1
      congenital   750.8
      psychogenic   305.5
    hysterical   300.1
    infantile   780.3
    internal os (*see also* Stricture, cervix)
        621.5
    joint (abduction) (acquired) (adduction)
        (extension) (flexion) (paralytic
        NEC) (postinfectional NEC)
        (rotation)   729.9
      congenital NEC   755.9
        generalized or multiple   755.8
        hip   755.6
        lower limb (including pelvic girdle)
            not involving hip   755.7
        upper limb (including shoulder
            girdle)   755.5
      finger   729.9
        flexion   729.4
      hip   729.5
      hysterical   300.1
      knee   729.8
      postpoliomyelitic   044
      shoulder   729.2
      spine   729.1
    kidney (granular) (secondary) (*see also*
        Sclerosis, renal)   584
      congenital   753.3
      hydronephritic   591
      pyelonephritic (*see also* Pyelitis,
          chronic)   590.0
      tuberculous   016.0
        late effect or sequela   019.2
    ligament   733.9
      congenital   756.8
    liver - *see* Cirrhosis, liver
    muscle (flaccid) (paralytic)
        (postinfectional) (postural) NEC
        733.9
      congenital   756.8
      eye (extrinsic) (*see also* Strabismus)
          373.9
        intrinsic   378.9
      hysterical   300.1
      ischemic (Volkmann's)   995.7
      postpoliomyelitic   044
      psychogenic   305.1
        specified as conversion reaction
            300.1
    neck (*see also* Torticollis)   717.2
      psychogenic   305.1

Contraction, etc. — *continued*
    ocular muscle (*see also* Strabismus)
        373.9
    organ or site, congenital NEC - *see*
        Atresia
    outlet (pelvis) - *see* Contraction, pelvis
    palmar fascia   733.5
    paralytic
      joint (*see also* Contraction, joint)
          729.9
      muscle (*see also* Contraction, muscle)
          733.9
        ocular (*see also* Strabismus)   373.9
    pelvis (asymmetric) (general) (inlet)
        (midplane) (oblique) (outlet)
        (paralytic) (transverse)   738.8
      complicating delivery - *see*
          Deformity, pelvis, complicating
          delivery
      noted during pregnancy (undelivered)
          634.9
    plantar fascia   733.9
    premature
      auricular (*see also* Action, heart,
          irregular)   427.9
      auriculoventricular (*see also* Action,
          heart, irregular)   427.9
      heart (atrial) (auricular)
          (auriculoventricular)
          (junctional) (nodal) (ventricular)
          (*see also* Action, heart,
          irregular)   427.9
      junctional (*see also* Action, heart,
          irregular)   427.9
      ventricular (*see also* Action, heart,
          irregular)   427.9
    prostate   602
    pylorus (*see also* Pylorospasm)   784.2
    rectum, rectal (sphincter)   564.9
      psychogenic   305.5
    ring (Bandl's), complicating delivery
        657.9
      fetus or newborn - *see* categories
          767.0-767.9
    scar - *see* Cicatrix
    socket, eye   378.9
    spine (*see also* Curvature, spine)   735.9
    stomach   537.9
      hourglass   536.1
        psychogenic   305.5
      psychogenic   305.5
    tendon (sheath) (*see also* Short, tendon)
        733.9
    toe   738.7
    ureterovesical orifice (postinfectional)
        593.3
    urethra   599.9

Contraction, etc.—*continued*
  uterus 625.9
    clonic, hourglass, inefficient or tetanic
      complicating delivery 657.9
        fetus or newborn - *see* categories
          767.0-767.9
    vagina (outlet) 629.7
    vesical (neck) (urethral orifice) 596.2
    visual field 781.0
    Volkmann's (ischemic) 995.7

Contusion (skin surface intact) 929

Note—The following fourth-digit subdivisions are for use with categories
920–929:
    .0 Current injury
    .9 Late effect

Contusion—*continued*
  with
    dislocation - *see* Dislocation
    fracture - *see* Fracture
    nerve injury - *see* Injury, nerve
    open wound - *see* Wound, open
  abdomen, abdominal (muscle) (wall)
    (and other parts of trunk) 922
    organ(s) (internal) - *see* Injury,
      internal, by site
  ankle (and hip) (and thigh) (and leg)
    927
  arm 929
    lower (and elbow) (and wrist) 924
    upper (and shoulder) 923
  auditory canal (external) (meatus) (and
    other part(s) of neck, scalp, or
    face except eye) 920
  auricle, ear (and other part(s) of neck,
    scalp, or face except eye) 920
  axilla (and shoulder) (and upper arm)
    923
  back (and other part(s) of trunk) 922
  bone NEC 929
  brain (any part) (with hemorrhage)
    (without skull fracture) 851.0
    with open intracranial wound 851.1
    late effect 851.9
  breast(s) (and other part(s) of trunk)
    922
  brow (and other part(s) of neck, scalp,
    or face except eye) 920
  buttock (and other part(s) of trunk)
    922
  canthus 921
  cerebellum (*see also* Contusion, brain)
    851.0

Contusion—*continued*
  cerebral (*see also* Contusion, brain)
    851.0
  cheek(s) (and other part(s) of neck,
    scalp, or face except eye) 920
  chest (wall) (and other part(s) of trunk)
    922
  chin (and other part(s) of neck, scalp, or
    face except eye) 920
  clitoris (and other part(s) of trunk) 922
  conjunctiva (and orbit) 921
  cornea 921
  corpus cavernosum 922
  cortex (brain) (cerebral) (*see also*
    Contusion, brain) 851.0
  costal region (and other part(s) of trunk)
    922
  elbow (and forearm) (and wrist) 924
  epididymis (and other part(s) of trunk)
    922
  epigastric region (and other part(s) of
    trunk) 922
  eye (lid) (muscle) (globe) (and orbit)
    921
  face (any part, except eye(s), and neck
    or scalp) 920
  femoral triangle (and other part(s) of
    trunk) 922
  finger(s) (nail) (subungual) 926
  flank (and other part(s) of trunk) 922
  foot (and toe(s)) 928
  forearm (and elbow) (and wrist) 924
  forehead (and other part(s) of neck,
    scalp, or face except eye) 920
  genital organs, external (and other
    part(s) of trunk) 922
  globe (eye) (and orbit) 921
  groin (and other part(s) of trunk) 922
  gum(s) (and other part(s) of neck, scalp,
    or face except eye) 920
  hand(s) (except fingers alone) 925
  head (any part, except eye) (and face)
    (and neck) 920
  heel (and toe(s)) 928
  hip (and thigh) (and leg) (and ankle)
    927
  iliac region (and other part(s) of trunk)
    922
  inguinal region (and other part(s) of
    trunk) 922
  internal organs (abdomen, chest or
    pelvis) - *see* Injury, internal, by
    site
  interscapular region (and other part(s)
    of trunk) 922
  iris (eye) (and orbit) 921

Contusion—*continued*
  knee (and ankle) (and hip) (and leg) (and thigh) 927
  labium (majus) (minus) (and other part(s) of trunk) 922
  lacrimal apparatus, gland or sac (and eye) (and orbit) 921
  larynx (and other parts of neck, scalp or face, except eye) 920
  leg (upper) (lower) (and hip) (and thigh) (and ankle) 927
  lens (and other part(s) of eye and orbit) 921
  lingual (and other parts of neck, scalp or face, except eye) 920
  lip(s) (and other part(s) of neck, scalp, or face except eye) 920
  lower extremity (except foot) 927
  lumbar region (and other part(s) of trunk) 922
  malar region (and other part(s) of neck, scalp, or face except eye) 920
  mandibular joint (and other part(s) of neck, scalp, or face except eye) 920
  mastoid region (and other part(s) of neck, scalp, or face except eye) 920
  membrane, brain (*see also* Contusion, brain) 851.0
  midthoracic region (and other part(s) of trunk) 922
  mouth (and other part(s) of neck, scalp, or face except eye) 920
  multiple sites (not classifiable to same three-digit category) 929
  muscle NEC 929
  nasal (septum) (and other part(s) of neck, scalp, or face except eye) 920
  neck (and scalp, or face any part except eye) 920
  nerve (root) (with open wound) - *see* Injury, nerve, by site
  nose (and other part(s) of neck, scalp, or face except eye) 920
  occipital region (scalp) (and neck or face, except eye) 920
    lobe (*see also* Contusion, brain) 851.0
  orbit (region) (and eye) 921
  palate (soft) (and other part(s) of neck, scalp, or face except eye) 920
  parietal region (scalp) (and neck or face, except eye) 920

Contusion—*continued*
  parietal region, etc.—*continued*
    lobe (*see also* Contusion, brain) 851.0
  penis (and other part(s) of trunk) 922
  perineum (and other part(s) of trunk) 922
  pharynx (and other part(s) of neck, scalp, or face except eye) 920
  popliteal space (with other part(s) of leg except foot) 927
  prepuce (and other part(s) of trunk) 922
  pubic region (and other part(s) of trunk) 922
  pudenda (and other part(s) of trunk) 922
  quadriceps femoris 927
  rib cage (and other part(s) of trunk) 922
  sacral region (and other part(s) of trunk) 922
  salivary ducts or glands (and other part(s) of neck, scalp, or face except eye) 920
  scalp (and neck, or face any part except eye) 920
  scapular region - *see* Contusion, shoulder
  sclera (eye) (and orbit) 921
  scrotum (and other part(s) of trunk) 922
  shoulder (and upper arm) 923
  skin NEC 929
  specified site(s) NEC 929
  spermatic cord 922
  spinal cord - *see also* Injury, spinal, by region
    cauda equina - *see* Injury, spinal, sacral
    conus medullaris - *see* Injury, spinal, sacral
  sternal region (and other part(s) of trunk) 922
  stomach - *see* Injury, internal, stomach
  subconjunctival (and eye) (and orbit) 921
  subcutaneous NEC 929
  submaxillary region (and other part(s) of neck, scalp, or face except eye) 920
  submental region (and other part(s) of neck, scalp, or face except eye) 920
  subperiosteal NEC 929

Contusion—*continued*

supra-orbital (and other part(s) of neck, scalp, or face except eye) 920

supraclavicular fossa (and other parts of neck, scalp, or face except eye) 920

temple (region) (and other part(s) of neck, scalp, or face except eye) 920

testicle, testis (and other part(s) of trunk) 922

thigh (and hip) (and leg) (and ankle) 927

thorax (and other part(s) of trunk) 922

throat (and other part(s) of neck, scalp, or face except eye) 920

thumb(s) (nail) (subungual) 926

toe(s) (nail) (subungual) (and heel) (and foot) 928

tongue (and other part(s) of neck, scalp, or face except eye) 920

trunk (any part) 922

tunica vaginalis (and other part(s) of trunk) 922

tympanum (membrane) (and other part(s) of neck, scalp, or face except eye) 920

upper extremity NEC 929

uvula (and other part(s) of neck, scalp, or face except eye) 920

vagina (and other part(s) of trunk) 922

vocal cord(s) (and other parts of neck, scalp, or face except eye) 920

vulva (and other part(s) of trunk) 922

wrist (and elbow) (and forearm) 924

Conus (congenital) (any type) 744.8

acquired 378.6

medullaris syndrome 349.9

Convalescent, convalescence - *see* Aftercare

Conversion

hysteria, hysterical, any type 300.1

neurosis, any 300.1

reaction, any 300.1

Convulsions (idiopathic) 780.2

with abortion - *see* Abortion, by type, with toxemia

apoplectiform (*see also* Disease, cerebrovascular, acute) 436.9

arising during pregnancy NEC - *see* Eclampsia, pregnancy

brain 780.2

cerebral 780.2

cerebrospinal 780.2

Convulsions, etc.—*continued*

due to

injury at birth (*see also* Birth injury, brain) 772.0

trauma NEC - *see* Injury, intracranial

eclamptic (*see also* Eclampsia) 780.2

epileptic (*see also* Epilepsy) 345.9

epileptiform (*see also* Seizure, epileptiform) 780.2

epileptoid (*see also* Seizure, epileptiform) 780.2

ether - *see* Table of adverse effects, ether

febrile 780.2

generalized 780.2

hysterical 300.1

infantile 780.2

epilepsy - *see* Epilepsy

internal 780.2

jacksonian - *see* Epilepsy, jacksonian

myoclonic 780.3

newborn 780.2

paretic 094.1

pregnancy (nephritic) (uremic) - *see* Eclampsia, pregnancy

psychomotor 345.3

puerperal, postpartum - *see* Eclampsia, puerperal

reflex 780.3

scarlatinal 034.1

spasmodic 780.2

tetanus, tetanic (*see also* Tetanus) 037

thymic 254

uncinate 780.2

uremic - *see* Uremia, convulsions

Convulsive - *see also* Convulsions

equivalent, abdominal 345.9

Cooley's anemia (*see also* Thalassemia) 282.4

Cooper's

disease 610

hernia - *see* Hernia, Cooper's

irritable breast 355.9

Copra itch 133.9

Coprolith 560.3

with hernia - *see* Hernia, by site, with obstruction

Coprostasis 560.3

with hernia - *see* Hernia, by site, with obstruction

Cor

biloculare 746.5

bovinum - *see* Hypertrophy, cardiac

bovis - *see* Hypertrophy, cardiac

pulmonale 426

triatriatum, triatrium 746.8

Cor—*continued*
  triloculare 746.8
    biatriatum 746.3
    biventriculare 746.4
Corbus' disease 607.3
Cord - *see also* condition
  around neck or limbs - *see*
      Complications, umbilical cord
  bladder NEC 596.9
    tabetic 094.0
Cordis ectopia 746.8
Corditis (spermatic) 607.5
Corectopia 744.8
Cori type glycogen storage disease - *see*
    Disease, glycogen storage
Corlett's pyosis 684
Corn (infected) 700
Cornea - *see also* condition
  guttata (dystrophy) 378.4
  plana 744.8
Cornu cutaneum 702
Cornual
  gestation or pregnancy - *see* Pregnancy,
    ectopic
Coronary (artery) - *see* condition
Corpora - *see also* condition
  amylacea
    prostate 602
  cavernosa - *see* condition
Corpulence (*see also* Obesity) 277
Corpus - *see* condition
Corrigan's disease (*see also* Endocarditis,
    aortic) 395.9 '
Corrosive burn - *see* Burn
Corsican fever 084.9
Cortical - *see* condition
Cortico-adrenal - *see* condition
Coryza (acute) 460
  with grippe or influenza 472
  syphilitic 095
    congenital (chronic) 090.0
Cosmetic surgical procedure Y11.9
  for prominent
    ear Y11.1
    nose Y11.0
Costen's syndrome or complex 524.9
Costiveness (*see also* Constipation)
    564.0
Cough 783.3
  with hemorrhage (*see also* Hemoptysis)
    783.1
  affected 783.3
  bronchial 783.3
    with grippe or influenza 472
  chronic 783.3
  epidemic 783.3

Cough—*continued*
  functional 305.2
  hysterical 300.1
  laryngeal, spasmodic 783.3
  nervous 783.3
  psychogenic 305.2
  tea tasters' 112
Coupled rhythm - *see* Action, heart,
    irregular
Couvelaire uterus (complicating delivery)
    - *see* Placenta, separation
Cowper's gland - *see* condition
Cowperitis (*see also* Urethritis) 597
Cowpox 051
  vaccinia (generalized) 999.0
Coxa
  plana 722.1
  valga or vara (acquired) 738.4
    congenital 755.7
    late effects of rickets 265.1
    postpoliomyelitic 044
Coxae malum senilis 713.0
Coxalgia (nontuberculous) 787.3
  tuberculous 015.1
    late effect or sequela 019.4
Coxalgic pelvis 738.8
Coxitis 729.5
Coxsackie (virus) (infection) 079.9
  central nervous system NEC 046
  enteritis 008.8
  meningitis (aseptic) 045.0
  myocarditis 074.2
  pericarditis 074.2
  pharyngitis 074.0
  pleurodynia 074.1
  specific disease NEC 074.9
Craft neurosis 300.8
Craigiasis 007.9
Cramp(s) 787.1
  abdominal 785.5
  bathing 994.1
  colic 785.5
    psychogenic 305.5
  extremity (lower) (upper) NEC 787.1
  fireman 992.2
  heat 992.2
  immersion 994.1
  intestinal 785.5
    psychogenic 305.5
  linotypist's 300.8
  muscle (extremity) (general) 787.1
    due to immersion 994.1
    hysterical 300.1
  occupational (hand) 300.8
  salt-depletion 788.0
  stoker 992.2

Cramp(s) — *continued*
  telegrapher's   300.8
  typist's   300.8
  uterus   625.9
  writer's   300.8
Cranial - *see* condition
Cranioclasis   773
Craniocleidodysostosis   755.5
Craniofenestria (skull)   756.0
Craniolacunia (skull)   756.0
Craniopagus   759.1
Craniopathy, metabolic   723.4
Craniopharyngeal - *see* condition
Craniopharyngioma   226.2
  malignant   194.3
Craniorachischisis (totalis)   740
Cranioschisis   756.0
Craniostenosis   756.0
Craniosynostosis   756.0
Craniotabes (cause unknown)   723.9
  rachitic   265.1
  syphilitic   090.5
Craniotomy
  fetal   773
Cranium - *see* condition
Craw-craw   125.3
Crazy (*see also* Psychosis)   299
Creaking joint (*see also* Disease, joint)
  729.9
Creeping
  palsy   348.2
  paralysis   348.2
Crenated tongue   529.9
Creotoxism - *see* Poisoning, food
Crepitus
  caput   756.0
  joint (*see also* Disease, joint)   729.9
Crescent or conus choroid, congenital
  744.8
Cretin   243
  pelvis (dwarf type) (male type)   243
    complicating delivery - *see*
        Deformity, pelvis, complicating
        delivery
    noted during pregnancy (undelivered)
      634.9
Cretinism (congenital) (endemic) (goitrous)
  (nongoitrous) (sporadic)   243
  pituitary   253.1
Cretinoid degeneration   243
Creutzfeldt-Jakob syndrome   333.9
  with dementia   290.1
Crib death   796.2
Cribriform hymen   752.6
Crigler-Najjar disease or syndrome
  273.5

Criminalism   301.7
Crisis
  abdomen   785.5
  addisonian   255.1
  adrenal (cortical)   255.1
  blood   289.0
  brain, cerebral (*see also* Disease,
      cerebrovascular, acute)   436.9
  Dietl's   593.3
  emotional   307
  gastric (tabetic)   094.0
  heart (*see also* Failure, heart)   782.4
  nitritoid   961.1
  oculogyric   781.1
    late effect viral encephalitis   066
    psychogenic   305.8
  Pel's   094.0
  rectum   094.0
  renal (*see also* Lesion, kidney)   593.2
  respiratory, late effect, viral encephalitis
    066
  stomach (tabetic)   094.0
  tabetic   094.0
  thyroid (*see also* Hyperthyroidism)
    242.2
  thyrotoxic (*see also* Thyrotoxicosis)
    242.2
  vascular - *see* Disease, cerebrovascular,
    acute
Crohn's disease   563.0
Crooked septum, nasal   504
Cross eye (*see also* Strabismus)   373.9
Crossbite, posterior   524.2
Crossed ectopia of kidney   753.3
Croup, croupous (angina) (catarrhal)
      (infectious) (inflammatory)
      (laryngeal) (membranous)
      (nondiphtheritic)
      (pseudomembranous)   464
  asthmatic   493
  with bronchitis - *see* Bronchitis
  bronchial   466
  diphtheritic   032
  false   508.3
  spasmodic   508.3
    diphtheritic   032
  stridulous   508.3
    diphtheritic   032
Crouzon's disease   756.0
Crowding
  tooth, teeth   524.3
Cruchet's disease   065
  late effects   066
Cruelty in children   308
Crush, crushed, crushing
  with
    fracture - *see* Fracture

Crush, etc. — *continued*
  with — *continued*
    open wound - *see* Wound, open
    skin surface intact - *see* Contusion
    chest - *see* Injury, internal, chest
    head (without fracture) (*see also* Injury,
      intracranial) 854.0
    internal organ, abdomen, chest, or
      pelvis - *see* Injury, internal, by
      site
    nerve - *see* Injury, nerve, by site
    severe, unspecified site 869.1
    skull or cranium - *see* Fracture, skull
    spinal cord - *see* Injury, spinal, by
      region
    syndrome (complication of trauma)
      995.6
Crusta lactea 691
Cruveilhier-Baumgarten cirrhosis, disease
  or syndrome 571.8
Cruveilhier's disease 348.2
Crying, forced 308
Cryoglobulinemia 275.4
Crypt
  anal 569.2
  rectum, rectal 569.2
Cryptitis (anal) (rectal) 569.2
Cryptococcosis 116.0
Cryptococcus
  epidermicus 116.0
  neoformans, infection by 116.0
Cryptopapillitis (anus) 569.2
Cryptophthalmos (eyelid) 744.8
Cryptorchid, cryptorchism,
  cryptorchidism 752.1
Crystalluria 594
Cuban itch 050.1
Cubitus valgus or varus (acquired) 738.2
  congenital 755.5
  late effects of rickets 265.1
Curling's ulcer - *see* Ulcer, duodenum
Curvature
  organ or site, congenital NEC - *see*
    Distortion
  penis (lateral) 752.8
  Pott's (spinal) 015.0
    late effects or sequela 019.3
  radius, idiopathic, progressive
    (congenital) 755.5
  spine (acquired) (angular) (incorrect)
    (postural) 735.9
    congenital 756.2
    kyphoscoliotic 735.2
    kyphotic 735.1
    late effects of rickets 265.1

Curvature — *continued*
  spine, etc. — *continued*
    scoliotic 735.0
    tuberculous 015.0
    late effect or sequela 019.3
Cushing's
  basophilism, disease, or syndrome
    (pituitary) 258.0
  ulcer - *see also* Ulcer, stomach
    duodenum - *see* Ulcer, duodenum
Cushingoid due to steroid therapy 962.0
Cut (external) - *see* Wound, open
Cutis - *see also* condition
  hyperelastic 757.2
    acquired 701.9
  laxa - *see* Dermatolysis
  marmorata 782.3
  osteosis 709.9
  pendula - *see* Dermatolysis
  rhomboidalis nuchae 701.9
  verticis gyrata 757.2
    acquired 701.9
Cyanosis 782.3
  congenital 778.9
  conjunctiva 378.3
  enterogenous 289.9
  fetus or newborn 778.9
  paroxysmal digital 443.0
  retina, retinal 377.0
Cycle, anovulatory 615.9
Cyclencephaly 759.2
Cyclical vomiting 305.5
Cyclitic membrane 377.4
Cyclitis 364
Cyclophoria 373.9
Cyclopia, cyclops 759.2
Cycloplegia 378.6
Cyclospasm 378.6
Cyclothymia 296.3
Cyclothymic personality 301.1
Cyclotropia 373.9
Cylindroma NEC (*see also* Neoplasm,
  malignant) 199.1
  cutaneous (*see also* Adenoma, sweat
    glands) 216.2
  dermal eccrine (*see also* Adenoma,
    sweat glands) 216.2
  external area or site (*see also* Adenoma,
    sweat glands) 216.2
Cylindruria 789.9
Cyllosoma 759.2
Cynanche
  diphtheritic 032
  tonsillaris 501
Cyphosis - *see* Kyphosis

Cyst (colloid) (mucous) (retention) (serous) (simple) (solitary)

Note — In general, cysts are not neoplastic and are classified to the appropriate category for disease of the specified anatomical site. This generalization does not apply to certain types of cysts which are neoplastic in nature, for example, dermoid and epidermoid, nor does it apply to cysts of certain structures, for example, branchial cleft, which are classified as developmental anomalies.

The following listing includes some of the most frequently reported sites of cysts as well as qualifiers which indicate the type of cyst. The latter qualifiers usually are not repeated under the anatomical sites. Since the code assignment for a given site may vary depending upon the type of cyst, the coder should refer to the listings under the specified type of cyst before consideration is given to the site.

Cyst, etc. — *continued*
  accessory, fallopian tube   752.5
  adenoid (infected)   508.9
  adrenal gland   255.9
    congenital   758.1
  air, lung   519.2
  alveolar process   526.2
  amnion, amniotic - *see* Placenta,
    abnormal
  antrum   508.9
  anus   569.2
  apical   522.8
  appendix   543
  arachnoid brain   347.9
  arytenoid   508.3
  auricle (*see also* Cyst, skin)   706.2
  Baker's (knee)   731.6
    tuberculous   015.2
      late effect or sequela   019.5
  Bartholin's gland (benign)   221.2
  bile duct (*see also* Disease, gallbladder)
    576.9
  bladder (multiple) (trigone)   596.9
  Blessig   377.1
  blue dome   610
  bone (local)   723.3
    jaw   526.2
  brain   347.9
    congenital   743.2
    hydatid   122.8
    third ventricle (colloid)   743.2
  branchial (cleft)   745.4
  branchiogenic   745.4

Cyst, etc. — *continued*
  breast   610
    benign   610
    blue dome   610
    involution   610
    pedunculated   610
    sebaceous   610
    sweat glands   217
  broad ligament (benign)   221.0
  bronchogenic (congenital) (mediastinal)
    (sequestration)   748.4
  buccal   528.4
  bulbo-urethral gland   599.9
  bursa, bursal - *see also* Bursitis
    pharyngeal   508.9
  canal of Nuck   752.8
  canthus   378.2
  carcinomatous - *see* Neoplasm,
    malignant
  cauda equina   349.9
  cavum septi pellucidi NEC   347.9
  celomic (pericardium)   746.8
  cerebellopontine (angle) - *see* Cyst,
    brain
  cerebellum - *see* Cyst, brain
  cerebral - *see* Cyst, brain
  cervical lateral   745.4
  cervix   219.1
    embryonal   752.5
    nabothian (*see also* Cervicitis,
      chronic)   620.0
  chamber anterior (eye)   378.6
  chiasmal optic NEC   377.6
  chocolate (ovary)   625.3
  choledochus   751.6
  chorion - *see* Placenta, abnormal
  choroid   378.6
    plexus   347.9
  clitoris   221.2
  coccyx   723.3
  colon   569.9
  common bile duct (*see also* Disease,
    gallbladder)   576.9
  congenital NEC   758.8
    epiglottis   748.3
    esophagus   750.8
    fallopian tube   752.5
    larynx   748.3
    liver   751.6
    mediastinum   748.8
    oviduct   752.5
    peri-urethral (tissue)   753.8
    prepuce   752.8
    sublingual   750.8
    submaxillary gland   750.8
    thymus (gland)   758.3

Cyst, etc. — *continued*
  congenital NEC — *continued*
    tongue   750.0
    ureterovesical orifice   753.4
    vulva   752.6
  conjunctiva   378.3
  cornea   378.4
  corpora quadrigemina   347.9
  corpus
    albicans   615.2
    luteum (ruptured)   615.2
  Cowper's gland (benign) (infected)
      599.9
  cranial meninges   347.9
  craniobuccal pouch   253.9
  craniopharyngeal pouch   253.9
  cysticercus   123.1
  Dandy-Walker   742
    with spina bifida   741.0
  dental   522.8
    developmental   526.0
    eruption   526.0
    primordial   526.0
    root   522.8
  dentigerous   526.0
    mandible   526.0
    maxilla   526.0
  dermoid   220.0
    external area or site (*see also*
        Dermatofibroma)   216.8
    implantation
      external area or site (skin) NEC
          709.9
      iris   378.6
      vagina or vulva   629.9
    midline (*see also* Dermatofibroma)
        216.8
    skin (*see also* Dermatofibroma)
        216.8
    specified site NEC - *see* Neoplasm,
        benign
  developmental, vessels brain   225.0
  dura (cerebral)   347.9
    spinal   349.9
  ear (external) (*see also* Cyst, skin)
      706.2
  echinococcal (*see also* Cyst, hydatid)
      122.9
  endometrial   219.1
    ectopic   625.3
  endometrium (uterus)   219.1
  enteric   751.4
  enterogenous   751.4
  epidermal (inclusion) (*see also* Cyst,
      skin)   706.2
    not of skin - *see* Neoplasm, benign

Cyst, etc. — *continued*
  epidermoid (*see also* Dermatofibroma)
      216.8
    inclusion (*see also* Cyst, skin)   706.2
      not of skin - *see* Neoplasm, benign
    not of skin - *see* Neoplasm, benign
  epididymis   607.9
  epiglottis   508.3
  epiphysis cerebri   258.9
  epithelial (inclusion) (*see also* Cyst,
      skin)   706.2
    not of skin - *see* Neoplasm, benign
  epoophoron   752.8
  esophagus   530.9
  ethmoid sinus   508.9
  eye   378.9
  eyebrow (*see also* Cyst, skin)   706.2
  eyelid (sebaceous)   378.2
    infected   362
    sweat glands or ducts   216.2
  falciform ligament (inflammatory)
      573.9
  fallopian tube   221.0
  female genital organs NEC   221.9
  fimbrial   752.5
  fissural (oral region)   526.1
  follicle (graafian)   615.2
    nabothian (*see also* Cervicitis,
        chronic)   620.0
  follicular (atretic) (ovarian)   615.2
    dentigerous   526.0
  frontal sinus   508.9
  gallbladder or duct (*see also* Disease,
        gallbladder)   576.9
  ganglion - *see* Bursitis
  Gartner's duct   752.8
  gingiva   523.9
  gland of Moll   216.2
  globulo-maxillary   526.1
  graafian follicle   615.2
  granulosal lutein   615.2
  hemangiomatous - *see* Hemangioma
  hydatid   122.9
    liver   122.0
    lung   122.1
    Morgagni   752.8
    specified site NEC   122.8
  hymen   221.1
    embryonal   752.6
  hypopharynx   508.9
  hypophysis, hypophyseal (duct)
        (recurrent)   253.9
    cerebri   253.9
  implantation (dermoid)
    external area or site (skin) NEC
        709.9

Cyst, etc. — *continued*
  pancreas, etc. — *continued*
    hemorrhagic 577.9
    true 577.9
  papillomatous (*see also* Epithelioma,
      benign) 228
    malignant - *see* Epithelioma,
      malignant
    uterus 219.0
  para-ovarian 221.0
  paraphysis, cerebri 743.2
  parasitic NEC 136
  parathyroid (gland) 252.9
  paratubal 221.0
  para-urethral duct 599.9
  paroophoron 752.8
  parotid gland 527.6
  parovarian 752.8
  pelvis, female 221.9
    complicating delivery 657.9
      fetus or newborn - *see* categories
        764.0-764.9
      noted during pregnancy (undelivered)
        634.9
  penis 607.9
    sebaceous 607.9
    sweat glands 222.1
  periapical 522.8
  pericardial (congenital) 746.8
  pericoronal 526.0
  periodontal 522.8
  peripancreatic 577.9
  peritoneum 569.9
    chylous 457
  pharynx (wall) 508.9
  pilonidal (infected) (rectum) 685
    malignant 173.6
  pituitary (duct) (gland) 253.9
  placenta (amniotic) - *see* Placenta,
    abnormal
  pleura 519.9
  porencephalic 743.2
    acquired 347.9
  postanal (infected) 685
  prepuce 607.9
    congenital 752.8
  prostate 600
  pseudomucinous 220.1
  pudendum 221.2
    sebaceous 629.9
    sweat glands 221.2
  radicular 522.8
  ranular 527.6
  Rathke's pouch 253.9
  rectum (epithelium) 569.2
  renal - *see* Cyst, kidney

Cyst, etc. — *continued*
  retina 377.4
  retroperitoneal 569.9
  salivary gland or duct 527.6
  Sampson's 625.3
  sclera 378.6
  scrotum 706.2
    sebaceous 706.2
    sweat glands 216.2
  sebaceous (duct) (gland) 706.2
    breast 610
    eyelid 378.2
    genital organ NEC
      female 629.9
      male 607.9
    scrotum 706.2
  semilunar cartilage (knee) (multiple)
    724.5
  seminal vesicle 607.9
  Skene's gland 599.9
  skin (epidermal) (epithelial) (epidermoid,
    inclusion) (inclusion) (sebaceous)
    706.2
    breast 610
    eyelid 378.2
    genital organ NEC
      female 629.9
      male 607.9
    scrotum 706.2
    sweat gland or duct (*see also*
      Adenoma, sweat glands)
      216.2
  spermatic cord 607.9
  sphenoid sinus 508.9
  spinal meninges 349.9
  spine 723.3
  spleen NEC 289.5
    due to
      hemangioma 227.1
      lymphangioma 227.2
    hydatid 122.8
  spring water (pericardium) 746.8
  subdural 347.9
    spinal cord 349.9
  sublingual gland 527.6
  submaxillary gland 527.6
  suburethral 599.9
  suprarenal gland 255.9
  suprasellar - *see* Cyst, brain
  sweat gland (*see also* Adenoma, sweat
    glands) 216.2
  sympathetic nervous system 358.9
  syncytium - *see* Placenta, abnormal
  synovial - *see* Bursitis
  tarsal 378.0
  tendon (sheath) - *see* Bursitis

Cystitis (acute) (allergic) (bacillary)
(bullous) (catarrhal) (chronic) (colli)
(cystic) (cystica) (diffuse)
(emphysematous) (encrusted)
(encysted) (exudative) (gangrenous)
(glandularis) (hemorrhagic)
(incrusted) (interstitial) (leukoplakia)
(malignant) (panmural)
(phlegmonous) (purulent) (recurrent)
(septic) (subacute) (submucous)
(suppurative) (ulcerative)   595
  with
    abortion - *see* Abortion by type, with
      sepsis
    ectopic gestation - *see* categories
      631.0-631.3
  amebic   006.9
  arising
    during pregnancy   635.1
      fetus or newborn   763.1
    following delivery   635.1
  blennorrhagic   098.0
  chronic or duration of 2 months or
    over   098.1
  calculous   594
  diphtheritic   032
  gonococcal   098.0
    chronic or duration of 2 months or
      over   098.1

Cystitis, etc. — *continued*
  irradiation - *see* Effect, adverse,
    radiotherapy
  prostatic   602
  puerperal, postpartum   635.1
  syphilitic   095
  trichomoniasis   131
  tuberculous   016.1
    late effects or sequela   019.2
Cystocele
  complicating delivery   657.9
    fetus or newborn - *see* categories
      764.0-764.9
  female   623.0
  male   596.9
  noted during pregnancy (undelivered)
    634.9
Cystoepithelioma (ovary)   183.0
Cystofibroma papillare (breast)   217
Cystolithiasis   594
Cystoma - *see* Neoplasm, benign
Cystoplegia   596.3
Cystoptosis   596.9
Cystopyelitis (*see also* Pyelitis)   590.1
Cystorrhagia   596.9
Cystosarcoma phyllodes (breast)   217
  malignant   174
Cysto-urethritis (*see also* Urethritis)   597
Cysto-urethrocele (*see also* Cystocele)
  female   623.0
  male   596.9

D

Da Costa's syndrome   305.3
Dabney's grip   074.1
Dacryoadenitis, dacryadenitis (acute)
      (chronic)   368
Dacryocystitis (acute) (chronic)
      (phlegmonous)   368
   syphilitic   095
      congenital   090.0
   trachomatous, active   076
      late effect   077
   tuberculous   017.2
      late effect or sequela   019.9
Dacryocystoblenorrhea   368
Dacryocystocele   378.3
Dacryolith   378.3
Dacryolithiasis   378.3
Dacryoma   368
Dacryops   378.3
Dacryosialadenopathy, atrophic   734.9
Dacryostenosis   368
   congenital   744.8
Dactylitis   686.9
   bone (see also Osteomyelitis)   720.2
   syphilitic   095
   tuberculous   015.8
      late effect or sequela   019.6
Dactylosis spontanea   136
Dactylosymphysis   755.1
Damage
   arteriosclerotic - see Arteriosclerosis
   brain   347.9
      anoxic, hypoxic   347.9
         newborn (see also Asphyxia,
               newborn)   776.9
      child NEC - see Palsy, cerebral
      due to birth injury (see also Birth
            injury, brain)   772.0
      newborn (see also Birth injury, brain)
            772.0
   cardiorenal (vascular) - see
         Hypertension, cardiorenal
   cerebral NEC - see Damage, brain
   coronary (see also Ischemia, heart)
         412.9
   heart - see also Disease, heart
      valve - see Endocarditis
   liver   573.9
   myocardium (see also Insufficiency,
         myocardial)   428
   renal (see also Lesion, kidney)   593.2

Damage — continued
   subendocardium, subendocardial (see
         also Insufficiency, myocardial)
         428
   traumatic - see nature of injury
   vascular   458.9
Dana-Putnam syndrome   281.0
Dandruff   690
Dandy-Walker syndrome   742
   with spina bifida   741.0
Dangle foot   738.6
Danlos' syndrome   757.2
Darier-Roussy sarcoid   135
Darier's
   disease   757.2
      meaning erythema annulare
            centrifugum   695.0
      vitamin A deficiency   260.8
Darling's
   disease   115
   histoplasmosis   115
Dartre   054
Darwin's tubercle   745.2
Dawson's encephalitis   065
   late effects   066
De Beurmann-Gougerot disease   117.1
De Lange's syndrome   759.8
De Morgan's spots   448
De Quervain's
   disease   731.4
   thyroiditis   245.0
De Toni-Fanconi(-Debre) syndrome
      270.2
Dead
   fetus
      delivered
         less than 28 weeks gestation - see
               Abortion, by type
         28 weeks or more gestation - see
               Delivery
      retained (early pregnancy) (2 months
            or more after death)   634.2
         aborted or delivered - see
               Abortion, by type
         at or near term (undelivered)
               634.2
            with delivery - see Delivery
   labyrinth   384.9
   ovum, retained   634.9
Deaf and dumb   388

Deafmutism (acquired) (congenital) 388
  endemic 243
  hysterical 300.1
  syphilitic congenital 090.0
Deafness (acquired) (congenital)
    (hereditary) (bilateral) (both ears)
    (conduction type) (conductive)
    (middle ear) (mixed) (transmission)
    389.9
  with blue sclera and fragility of bone
    756.6
  aviation 993.0
    nerve injury - see Injury, nerve,
      acoustic
  boilermaker's - see Injury, nerve,
    acoustic
  complete (nerve) (perceptive) 389.0
    one ear (with normal hearing in other)
      389.2
      with
        deafness (partial) in other 389.1
        impairment of hearing in other
          389.1
  due to anomaly of ear(s) 745.0
  emotional (complete) 300.1
  functional (complete) 300.1
  high frequency - see Deafness, partial
  hysterical (complete) 300.1
  injury - see Injury, nerve, acoustic
  low frequency - see Deafness, partial
  mental 781.5
  nerve (complete) - see Deafness,
    complete
  partial - see Deafness, partial
  one ear (with normal hearing in other)
    389.9
    with
      complete, nerve, or perceptive
        deafness in other 389.1
      impairment of hearing in other
        389.1
      partial deafness in other 389.1
    complete - see Deafness, complete,
      one ear
    partial - see Deafness, partial, one ear
  partial (nerve) (perceptive) 389.9
    one ear (with normal hearing in other)
      389.9
      with complete, nerve, or perceptive
        deafness in other 389.1
  perceptive (complete) - see Deafness,
    complete
  partial - see Deafness, partial
  psychogenic (complete) 305.8
  syphilitic 094.9
  traumatic - see Injury, nerve, acoustic

Deafness, etc. - continued
  unilateral - see Deafness, one ear
  word (secondary to organic lesion)
    781.5
  developmental 306.1
Death
  after delivery (cause not stated)
    (sudden) 677.0
  anesthetic NEC (see also Table of
    adverse effects) 968.1
    complicated delivery (see also
      Delivery, complicated) 661.9
    in normal delivery 662
  cardiac - see Disease, heart
  during delivery (uncomplicated) 677.0
    anesthetic death 662
    complicated delivery (see also
      Delivery, complicated)
      661.9
  fetus, fetal (cause not stated) (intra-
    uterine) 779.9
    complicating pregnancy 634.2
    for classification of births in hospital
      Y30.2
      early (gestation less than 20 weeks)
        Y30.0
      intermediate (gestation 20-27
        weeks) Y30.1
      late (gestation 28 weeks or more)
        Y30.2
  from pregnancy NEC 634.9
  intra-uterine - see Death, fetus
  maternal, affecting fetus or newborn
    769.5
  neonatal 778.9
  sudden (cause unknown) 795
    during delivery 677.0
    under anesthesia NEC 662
    puerperal, during puerperium 677.0
  under anesthesia NEC (see also Table
    of adverse effects) 968.1
    complicated delivery (see also
      Delivery, complicated) 661.9
    normal delivery 662
Debility (congenital) (general) (infantile)
    (postinfectional) 790.1
  nervous 300.5
  old age 794
  senile 794
Decalcification
  bone 723.9
  teeth 521.9
Decapitation 874.0
  fetal (to facilitate delivery) 773
Decapsulation, kidney (see also Lesion,
    kidney) 593.2

Decay
  dental 521.0
  senile 794
  tooth, teeth 521.0
Deciduitis (acute)
  with
    abortion - *see* Abortion, by type, with
        sepsis
    ectopic gestation - *see* categories
        631.0-631.3
    causing complicated delivery 661.8
    complicating pregnancy 634.9
    fetus or newborn 763.9
    puerperal, postpartum, childbirth 670
Deciduoma (malignum) 181
Decline (general) (*see also* Debility)
    790.1
Decompensation
  cardiac (acute) (chronic) (*see also*
        Disease, heart) 429.9
  cardiorenal - *see* Hypertension,
        cardiorenal
  cardiovascular (*see also* Disease, heart)
        429.9
  heart (*see also* Disease, heart) 429.9
  hepatic 573.9
  myocardial (acute) (chronic) (*see also*
        Disease, heart) 429.9
  respiratory 519.9
Decompression sickness 993.3
Decrease, decreased
  blood
    platelets (*see also* Thrombocytopenia)
        287.1
    pressure, due to shock following
        injury 995.5
  cardiac reserve - *see* Disease, heart
  estrogen 256.1
  fragility of erythrocytes 289.9
  function
    adrenal medulla 255.9
    ovary in hypopituitarism 253.1
    parenchyma of pancreas 577.9
    pituitary (gland) (anterior) (lobe)
        253.1
      posterior (lobe) 253.9
  functional activity 790.2
  respiration, due to shock following
        injury 995.5
  tear secretion NEC 378.3
  tolerance
    fat 269.0
    glucose 788.9
    salt and water 788.9

Decubital gangrene (*see also* Gangrene)
    445.9

Decubiti - *see* Decubitus
Decubitus (ulcer) 707.0
  with gangrene (*see also* Gangrene)
    445.9
Deepening acetabulum 723.9
Defect, defective 758.9
  aortic septal 746.0
  aorticopulmonary septum 746.0
  atrial septal 746.4
  atrioventricular
    canal 746.5
    septum 746.3
  auricular septal 746.4
  bilirubin excretion 273.5
  bulbar septum 746.0
  circulation 458.9
    congenital 747.9
    newborn 747.9
  coagulation (congenital) NEC 286.9
    causing hemorrhage of pregnancy
        632.4
      complicating delivery 651.9
      fetus or newborn 769.9
    following childbirth 675
    newborn 778.2
  conduction (*see also* Block, heart)
    427.3
  bone - *see* Deafness
  congenital, organ or site not listed - *see*
        Anomaly
  cushion
    endocardial 746.8
  Descemet's membrane (periodica fugax)
        378.4
    congenital 744.8
  developmental - *see also* Anomaly
    cauda equina 743.3
  diaphragm
    with elevation, eventration or hernia
        - *see* Hernia, diaphragm
    congenital 756.8
      with elevation, eventration or
          hernia - *see* Hernia,
          diaphragm
      gross (with elevation, eventration
          or hernia) 756.8
  ectodermal, congenital 757.9
  esophagus, congenital 750.9
  extensor retinacular 733.9
  filling stomach 537.9
  hearing (*see also* Deafness) 389.9
  high grade - *see* Retardation, mental,
        mild
  interatrial septal 746.4
  interauricular septal 746.4
  interventricular septal 746.3

Defect, defective — *continued*
  interventricular septal — *continued*
    with pulmonary stenosis or atresia,
        dextraposition of aorta, and
        hypertrophy of right ventricle
        746.2
  learning, specific (reading)
        (mathematics) (strephosymbolia)
        306.1
  mental - *see* Retardation, mental
  ostium primum or secundum 746.4
  pericardium 746.8
  placental blood supply - *see* Placenta,
        abnormal
  postural, spine - *see* Curvature, spine
  pulmonic cusps, congenital 746.6
  respiratory system, congenital 748.9
  septal, heart NEC 746.8
  speech (nonorganic origin) NEC 306.0
    developmental 306.0
    secondary to organic lesion 781.5
  vascular (local) 458.9
    congenital 747.6
  ventricular septal 746.3
    with pulmonary stenosis or atresia,
        dextraposition of aorta, and
        hypertrophy of right ventricle
        746.2
    between infundibulum and anterior
        portion 746.3
    isolated anterior 746.3
  vision NEC 370.9
  visual field 781.0
  voice 783.5
  11 hydroxylase 273.6
  21 hydroxylase 273.6
  3B hydroxysteroid dehydrogenase
        273.6
Deferentitis 607.5
  gonorrheal (acute) 098.0
    chronic or duration of 2 months or
        over 098.1
Deficiencia intelligentsia - *see*
        Retardation, mental, borderline
Deficiency, deficient
  abdominal muscle syndrome 756.8
  aldolase (hereditary) 271.3
  amino-acids 270.9
  anemia - *see* Anemia
  aneurin 261
  anti-hemophilic globulin NEC 286.0
  ascorbic acid 264
  biotin 263.8
  brancher enzyme (amylopectinosis)
        271.1
  calciferol 265.9

Deficiency, deficient — *continued*
  calciferol — *continued*
    with
        osteomalacia 265.2
        rickets (*see also* Rickets) 265.0
  calcium 788.5
    dietary 269.9
  cardiac (*see also* Insufficiency,
        myocardial) 428
  carotene 260.9
  central nervous system 796.0
  ceruloplasmin 273.3
  cevitamic acid 264
  choline 263.8
  citrin 269.9
  clotting (blood) (*see also* Defect,
        coagulation) 286.9
  coagulation factor (*see also* Defect,
        coagulation) 286.9
  craniofacial axis 756.0
  cyanocobalamine 263.8
  debrancher enzyme (limit dextrinosis)
        271.1
  diet 269.9
  disaccharidase 271.8
  disease NEC 269.9
  edema 269.9
  endocrine 258.9
  ergosterol 265.9
    with
        osteomalacia 265.2
        rickets (*see also* Rickets) 265.0
  factor
    IX 286.1
    V (*see also* Defect, coagulation)
        286.9
    VII (*see also* Defect, coagulation)
        286.9
    VIII NEC 286.0
    X (*see also* Defect, coagulation)
        286.9
    XI 286.2
    XII (*see also* Defect, coagulation)
        286.9
    XIII (*see also* Defect, coagulation)
        286.9
  fibrin stabilizing factor (*see also* Defect,
        coagulation) 286.9
  folic acid 263.8
  fructokinase 271.3
  galactose-1-phosphate uridyl transferase
        271.2
  gammaglobulin in blood 275.1
  glucose-6-phosphatase 271.0
  glucose-6-phosphate dehydrogenase
        anemia 282.2

Deformity—*continued*
  abdominal wall—*continued*
    congenital 756.9
  acquired NEC 738.9
  adrenal gland (congenital) 758.1
  alimentary tract, congenital 751.9
    lower 751.4
    upper 750.9
  ankle (joint) (acquired) 738.6
    abduction, adduction, contraction,
        extension, flexion, or rotation
        729.9
    congenital 755.7
  anus (congenital) 751.4
    acquired 569.2
  aorta (arch) (congenital) 747.2
    acquired 446.9
  aortic
    cusp or valve (congenital) 746.6
      acquired (*see also* Endocarditis,
        aortic) 395.9
    ring 747.2
  appendix 751.4
  arm (acquired) 738.8
    congenital 755.5
  arteriovenous (congenital) 747.6
  artery (congenital) (peripheral) NEC
    747.6
    acquired 447
    cerebral 747.8
    coronary (congenital) 746.8
      acquired (*see also* Ischemia, heart)
        412.9
    retinal 744.9
    umbilical 747.5
  atrial septa (heart) (congenital) 746.4
  auditory canal (external) (congenital)
    (*see also* Deformity, ear) 745.3
    acquired 387.9
  auricle
    ear (congenital) (*see also* Deformity,
      ear) 745.3
      acquired 387.9
    heart (congenital) 746.8
      acquired - *see* Disease, heart
  back (acquired) - *see* Deformity, spine
  Bartholin's duct (congenital) 750.9
  bile duct (congenital) 751.6
    acquired (*see also* Disease,
      gallbladder) 576.9
  biliary duct or passage (congenital)
    751.6
    acquired (*see also* Disease,
      gallbladder) 576.9
  bladder (neck) (trigone) (sphincter)
    (acquired) 596.2

Deformity—*continued*
  bladder, etc.—*continued*
    congenital 753.9
  bone (acquired) NEC 738.8
    congenital 756.9
  brain (congenital) 743.9
    acquired 347.9
    multiple 743.2
    vessel (congenital) 747.8
  breast (acquired) 611.9
    congenital 757.9
  bronchus (congenital) 748.3
    acquired 519.9
  bursa, congenital 756.9
  canal of Nuck 752.9
  canthus (congenital) 744.9
    acquired 378.2
  capillary (acquired) 448
    congenital 747.6
  cardiac - *see* Deformity, heart
  cardiovascular system (congenital)
    746.9
  caruncle lachrymal, lacrimal (congenital)
    744.9
    acquired 378.3
  cecum (congenital) 751.4
    acquired 569.9
  cerebral (congenital) 743.9
    acquired 347.9
  cervix (uterus) (acquired) 621.9
    congenital 752.5
  cheek (acquired) 738.1
    congenital 745.9
  chest (acquired) (wall) 738.8
    congenital 756.4
    late effects of rickets 265.1
  chin (acquired) 738.1
    congenital 745.9
  choroid (congenital) 744.9
    acquired 378.6
    plexus (congenital) 743.9
      acquired 347.9
  cicatricial - *see* Cicatrix
  cilia (congenital) 744.9
    acquired 378.6
  circulatory system (congenital) 747.9
  clavicle (acquired) 738.8
    congenital 755.5
  clitoris (congenital) 752.6
    acquired 629.9
  clubfoot - *see* Clubfoot
  coccyx (acquired) 738.8
    congenital 756.2
  colon (congenital) 751.4
    acquired 569.9

Deformity—*continued*
concha (ear) (congenital) (*see also*
      Deformity, ear)   745.3
   acquired   387.9
congenital, organ or site not listed - *see
      also* Anomaly
cornea (congenital)   744.9
   acquired   378.4
coronary artery (congenital)   746.8
   acquired (*see also* Ischemia, heart)
      412.9
cranium (acquired)   738.1
   congenital (*see also* Deformity, skull,
      congenital)   756.0
cricoid cartilage (congenital)   748.3
   acquired   508.3
cystic duct (congenital)   751.6
   acquired (*see also* Disease,
      gallbladder)   576.9
diaphragm (congenital)   756.9
   acquired   733.9
digestive organ(s) or system (congenital)
      NEC   751.9
ductus arteriosus   747.9
duodenal bulb   537.9
duodenum (congenital)   751.4
   acquired   537.9
dura (congenital)   743.9
   brain   743.9
      acquired   347.9
   spinal   743.3
      acquired   349.9
ear (auricle) (external) (lobule)
      (congenital)   745.3
   acquired   387.9
   causing impairment of hearing   745.0
   internal   745.0
   late effect of trauma NEC   872.9
   middle   745.0
ectodermal (congenital) NEC   757.9
   acquired NEC   709.9
ejaculatory duct (congenital)   752.9
   acquired   607.9
elbow (joint) (acquired)   738.2
   abduction, adduction, contraction,
      extension, flexion, or rotation
      729.3
   congenital   755.5
endocrine gland NEC   758.3
epididymis (congenital)   752.9
   acquired   607.9
epiglottis (congenital)   748.3
   acquired   508.3
esophagus (congenital)   750.9
   acquired   530.9
eustachian tube (congenital) NEC 745.3

Deformity—*continued*
extremity (acquired) NEC   738.8
   congenital, except reduction
      deformity   755.9
   lower   755.7
   upper   755.5
eye (congenital)   744.9
   muscle   744.9
   acquired   378.9
eyelid (congenital)   744.9
   acquired   378.2
face (acquired)   738.1
   congenital   745.9
fallopian tube (congenital)   752.5
   acquired   615.9
femur (acquired)   738.5
   congenital   755.7
fetal, complicating delivery   655
finger (mallet) (acquired)   738.3
   congenital   755 5
   flexion contracture   729.4
flexion (joint) (acquired) (*see also*
      Contraction, joint)   729.9
   congenital NEC   755.9
   hip or thigh (acquired)   729.5
   congenital   755.6
foot (acquired)   738.6
   congenital NEC   755.7
forearm (acquired)   738.2
   congenital   755.5
forehead (acquired)   738.1
   congenital (*see also* Deformity, skull,
      congenital)   756.0
frontal bone (acquired)   738.1
   congenital (*see also* Deformity, skull,
      congenital)   756.0
gallbladder (congenital)   751.6
   acquired (*see also* Disease,
      gallbladder)   576.9
gastro-intestinal tract (congenital) NEC
      751.9
   acquired   569.9
genitalia, genital organ(s) or system
      NEC
   female (congenital)   752.9
      acquired   629.9
      external   752.6
      internal   752.5
   male (congenital)   752.9
      acquired   607.9
globe (eye) (congenital)   744.9
   acquired   378.9
gum (congenital)   750.9
   acquired   523.9
gunstock   738.2

Deformity—*continued*
  hand (boutonniere) (buttonhole) (claw)
      (intrinsic) (minus) (pill roller)
      (plus) (swan neck) (acquired)
      738.2
    congenital 755.5
  head (acquired) 738.1
    congenital (*see also* Deformity, skull,
        congenital) 756.0
  heart (congenital) 746.9
    acquired - *see* Disease, heart
    auricle (congenital) 746.8
      acquired - *see* Disease, heart
    septum 746.8
      auricular 746.4
      ventricular 746.3
    valve (congenital) 746.6
      acquired - *see* Endocarditis
    ventricle (congenital) 746.8
  heel (acquired) 738.6
    congenital 755.7
  hepatic duct (congenital) 751.6
    acquired (*see also* Disease,
        gallbladder) 576.9
  hip (joint) (acquired) 738.4
    abduction, adduction, contraction,
        extension, flexion, or rotation
        729.5
      congenital 755.6
    congenital 755.7
  hourglass - *see* Hourglass contraction
  humerus (acquired) 738.8
    congenital 755.5
  hymen (congenital) 752.6
    acquired 629.9
  hypophyseal (congenital) 758.3
  ileocecal (coil) (valve) (congenital)
      751.4
    acquired 569.9
  ileum (congenital) 751.4
    acquired 569.9
  ilium (acquired) 738.8
    congenital 755.7
  intervertebral cartilage or disc
      (acquired) (*see also*
      Displacement, intervertebral
      disc) 725.9
    congenital 756.2
  intestine (large) (small) (congenital)
      751.4
    acquired 569.9
  iris (acquired) 378.6
    congenital 744.9
  ischium (acquired) 738.8
    congenital 755.7
  jaw (acquired) (congenital) NEC 524.9

Deformity—*continued*
  joint (acquired) NEC 738.8
    congenital 755.9
    specified as abduction, adduction,
        contraction, extension, flexion,
        or rotation (*see also*
        Contraction, joint) 729.9
  kidney(s) (calyx) (pelvis) (congenital)
      753.9
    acquired (*see also* Lesion, kidney)
        593.2
    vessel (congenital) 747.6
      acquired 458.9
  Klippel-Feil 756.2
  knee (joint) (valgus) (varus) (acquired)
      738.5
    abduction, adduction, contraction,
        extension, flexion, or rotation
        729.8
    congenital 755.7
  labium (majus) (minus) (congenital)
      752.6
    acquired 629.9
  lachrymal, lacrimal apparatus or duct
      (congenital) 744.9
    acquired 378.3
  larynx (muscle) (congenital) 748.3
    acquired 508.3
    web 748.2
  leg (upper) (lower) (acquired) 738.5
    congenital 755.7
  lens (congenital) 744.9
    acquired 378.8
  lid (fold) (congenital) 744.9
    acquired 378.2
  ligament (acquired) 733.9
    congenital 756.9
  limb (acquired) NEC 738.8
    congenital, except reduction
        deformity 755.9
      lower 755.7
      upper 755.5
  lip (congenital) NEC 750.9
    acquired 528.5
  liver (congenital) 751.6
    acquired 573.9
    duct (congenital) 751.6
      acquired (*see also* Disease,
          gallbladder) 576.9
  lumbosacral (congenital) (joint) (region)
      756.1
    acquired 738.8
  lung (congenital) 748.6
    acquired 519.2
  lymphatic system, congenital 758.9
  Madelung's (radius) 755.5

Deformity — *continued*
  maxilla (acquired)   524.9
    congenital   524.9
  meninges or membrane (congenital)
      743.9
    brain   743.9
      acquired   347.9
    spinal (cord)   743.3
      acquired   349.9
  mesentery (congenital)   751.9
    acquired   569.9
  metacarpus (acquired)   738.2
    congenital   755.5
  metatarsus (acquired)   738.6
    congenital   755.7
  middle ear (congenital)   745.0
  mitral (congenital) (leaflets) (valve)
      746.6
    acquired - *see* Endocarditis, mitral
  mouth
    acquired   528.9
    congenital NEC   750.9
  multiple, congenital NEC   759.9
  muscle (acquired)   733.9
    congenital   756.9
  musculoskeletal system, congenital
      NEC   756.9
  nail (acquired)   703.9
    congenital   757.9
  nasal - *see* Deformity, nose
  neck (acquired) NEC   738.8
    congenital   745.9
  nipple (congenital)   757.9
    acquired   611.9
  nose, nasal (acquired) (cartilage)   508.9
    bone (turbinate)   738.0
    congenital   748.1
    saddle   738.0
      syphilitic   090.5
    septum   504
      congenital   748.1
    sinus (congenital)   748.1
    syphilitic (congenital)   090.5
      late   095
  ocular muscle (congenital)   744.9
    acquired   378.9
  opticociliary vessels (congenital)   744.9
  orbit (eye) (congenital)   744.9
    acquired   378.9
  organ of Corti (congenital)   745.0
  ovary (congenital)   752.5
    acquired   615.9
  oviduct (congenital)   752.5
    acquired   615.9
  palate (congenital)   750.9
    acquired   526.9

Deformity — *continued*
  palate (congenital) — *continued*
    cleft (congenital)   749.0
      with cleft lip   749.2
    soft, acquired   528.9
  pancreas (congenital)   751.7
    acquired   577.9
  parathyroid (gland)   758.3
  parotid (gland) (congenital)   750.9
    acquired   527.9
  patella (acquired)   738.5
    congenital   755.7
  pelvis, pelvic (acquired) (bony)   738.8
    complicating delivery (acquired)
        (congenital) (rachitic)   654.9
      android   654.0
      anthropoid   654.1
      combined or mixed   654.3
      fetus or newborn - *see* categories
          764.0-764.9
      flat   654.2
      pithecoid   654.1
      platypelloid   654.2
    congenital   755.7
    noted during pregnancy (any type)
        (undelivered)   634.9
    rachitic (late effect)   265.1
  penis (glans) (congenital)   752.9
    acquired   607.9
  pericardium (congenital)   746.8
    acquired - *see* Pericarditis
  pharynx (congenital)   750.9
    acquired   508.9
  Pierre Robin (congenital)   756.0
  pituitary (congenital)   758.3
  pleural fold (congenital)   748.8
  portal vein (congenital)   747.4
  posture - *see* Deformity, spine
  prepuce (congenital)   752.9
    acquired   607.9
  prostate (congenital)   752.9
    acquired   602
  pupil (congenital)   744.9
    acquired   378.6
  pylorus (congenital)   750.9
    acquired   537.9
  rachitic (acquired), old or healed   265.1
  radius (acquired)   738.2
    congenital   755.5
  rectum (congenital)   751.4
    acquired   569.2
  reduction (extremity) (limb)   755.4
    lower   755.3
    upper   755.2
  renal - *see* Deformity, kidney
  respiratory system (congenital)   748.9

Deformity—*continued*
 rib (acquired) 738.8
  congenital 756.4
   cervical 756.3
 rotation (joint) (acquired) (*see also*
    Contraction, joint) 729.9
  congenital 755.9
  hip or thigh 729.5
   congenital 755.6
 sacro-iliac joint (congenital) 755.7
  acquired 726
 sacrum (acquired) 738.8
  congenital 756.1
 saddle
  back (*see also* Deformity, spine)
    735.9
  nose 738.0
   syphilitic 090.5
 salivary gland or duct (congenital)
    750.9
  acquired 527.9
 scapula (acquired) 738.8
  congenital 755.5
 scrotum (congenital) 752.9
  acquired 607.9
 sebaceous gland, acquired 706.9
 seminal tract or duct (congenital)
    752.9
  acquired 607.9
 shoulder (joint) (acquired) 738.8
  abduction, adduction, contraction,
     extension, flexion, or rotation
     729.2
  congenital 755.5
 sigmoid (flexure) (congenital) 751.4
  acquired 569.9
 sinus of Valsalva 747.2
 skin (congenital) 757.9
  acquired NEC 709.9
 skull (acquired) 738.1
  congenital 756.0
   with
    anencephalus 740
    encephalocele 743.0
    hydrocephalus 742
     with spina bifida 741.0
    microcephalus 743.1
 soft parts, organs or tissues (of pelvis)
  complicating delivery 657.9
   fetus or newborn - *see* categories
     746.0-746.9
  noted during pregnancy (undelivered)
    634.9
 spermatic cord (congenital) 752.9
  acquired 607.9

Deformity—*continued*
 spinal
  column (acquired) - *see* Deformity,
     spine
  cord (congenital) 743.9
   acquired 349.9
   vessel (congenital) 747.6
  nerve root (congenital) 743.9
   acquired (*see also* Neuropathy,
      radicular) 728.9
 spine (acquired) (angular) (postural)
    735.9
  congenital 756.2
  kyphoscoliotic 735.2
  kyphotic 735.1
  rachitic 265.1
  scoliotic 735.0
 spleen
  acquired 289.5
  congenital 758.0
 Sprengel's (congenital) 755.5
 sternum (acquired) 738.8
  congenital 756.4
 stomach (congenital) 750.9
  acquired 537.9
 submaxillary gland (congenital) 750.9
  acquired 527.9
 talipes - *see* Talipes
 testicle (congenital) 752.9
  acquired 607.9
 thigh (acquired) 738.5
  congenital 755.7
 thorax (acquired) (wall) 738.8
  congenital 756.4
  late effects of rickets 265.1
 thumb (acquired) 738.3
  congenital 755.5
 thymus (tissue) (congenital) 758.3
 thyroid (gland) (congenital) 758.2
  cartilage 748.3
   acquired 508.3
 tibia (acquired) 738.5
  congenital 755.7
  saber 090.5
 toe (acquired) 738.7
  congenital 755.7
 tongue (congenital) 750.0
  acquired 529.9
 tooth, teeth NEC 520.9
 trachea (rings) (congenital) 748.3
  acquired 519.9
 transverse aortic arch (congenital)
    747.2
 tricuspid (congenital) (leaflets) (valve)
    746.6
  acquired - *see* Endocarditis, tricuspid

Deformity—*continued*
  trunk (acquired) 738.8
    congenital 758.9
  ulna (acquired) 738.2
    congenital 755.5
  urachus (congenital) 753.9
  ureter (opening) (congenital) 753.9
    acquired 593.5
  urethra (congenital) 753.9
    acquired 599.9
  urinary tract (congenital) 753.9
  uterus (congenital) 752.5
    acquired 625.9
  uvula (congenital) 750.9
    acquired 528.9
  vagina (congenital) 752.6
    acquired 629.9
  valve, valvular (congenital) (heart)
      746.6
    acquired - *see* Endocarditis
  vas deferens (congenital) 752.9
    acquired 607.9
  vascular (congenital) NEC 747.6
    acquired 458.9
  vein (congenital) NEC 747.6
    brain 747.8
    coronary 746.8
    great 747.4
  vena cava (inferior) (superior)
      (congenital) 747.4
  vertebra - *see* Deformity, spine
  vesico-urethral orifice (acquired) 596.2
    congenital NEC 753.9
  vessels of optic papilla (congenital)
      744.9
  visual field (contraction) 781.0
  vitreous humor (congenital) 744.9
    acquired 378.9
  vulva (congenital) 752.6
    acquired 629.9
  wrist (joint) (acquired) 738.2
    abduction, adduction, contraction,
        extension, flexion, or rotation
        729.9
    congenital 755.5
Degeneration, degenerative
  adrenal (capsule) (gland) 255.9
    fatty 255.9
    hyaline 255.9
    infectional 255.9
    lardaceous 276
  albuminoid NEC 796.0
  amyloid (any site) (general) 276
  anterior cornua, spinal cord 349.9
  aorta, aortic - *see also* Arteriosclerosis,
      aorta
    fatty 447

Degeneration, degenerative—*continued*
  aortic valve (heart) (*see also*
      Endocarditis, aortic) 395.9
  arteriovascular - *see* Arteriosclerosis
  artery, arterial (atheromatous)
      (calcareous) - *see also*
      Arteriosclerosis
    amyloid 276
    lardaceous 276
    medial (*see also* Arteriosclerosis,
        peripheral) 440.2
  articular cartilage (joint) 724.9
    elbow 724.3
    knee 724.5
    shoulder 724.1
  atheromatous - *see* Arteriosclerosis
  bacony (any site) 276
  basal nuclei (cystic) (*see also*
      Degeneration, brain) 347.9
  bone 723.9
  brachial plexus 357.0
  brain (cortical) (fatty) (infantile)
      (parenchymatous) (progressive)
      347.9
    arteriosclerotic (*see also* Ischemia,
        cerebral) 437.9
    cystic 347.9
      congenital 743.2
    familial NEC 333.9
    heredofamilial NEC 333.9
    motor centers 794
    senile 794
  breast - *see* Disease, breast
  Bruch's membrane 378.6
  bundle His' - *see* Block, heart
  calcareous NEC 279
  capillaries 448
    amyloid 276
    fatty 448
    lardaceous 276
  cardiac (brown) (calcareous) (fatty)
      (fibrous) (hyaline) (mural)
      (muscular) (pigmentary) (senile)
      (*see also* Insufficiency,
      myocardial) 428
    valve, valvular - *see* Endocarditis
  cardiorenal - *see* Hypertension,
      cardiorenal
  cardiovascular (*see also* Ischemia,
      heart) 412.9
    renal - *see* Hypertension, cardiorenal
  cerebellum - *see* Degeneration, brain
  cerebral - *see* Degeneration, brain
  cerebromacular 333.0
  cerebrospinal NEC 347.9

Degeneration, degenerative—*continued*
  cerebrovascular (*see also* Ischemia,
      cerebral) 437.9
  cervical plexus 357.0
  cervix 621.9
    due to radiation (intended effect)
      621.6
      adverse effect or misadventure
        see Effect, adverse,
        radiotherapy
  changes, spine or vertebra 713.1
  chitinous (any site) 276
  chorioretinal 378.6
  choroid (colloid) (drusen) 378.6
  cochlear 386
  colloid NEC 279
  combined (spinal cord) (subacute)
    281.0
  cornea 378.4
    familial (reticular and macular)
      378.4
    hyaline (of old scars) - *see* Opacity,
      cornea
    senile 378.4
  cortical (infantile) (parenchymatous) (*see*
    also Degeneration, brain) 347.9
  diffuse, due to arteriopathy (*see also*
    Ischemia, cerebral) 437.9
  corticostriatal spinal 333.9
  cretinoid 243
  cutis 709.9
    amyloid 276
  dental pulp 522.2
  disc disease - *see* Displacement,
    intervertebral disc
  dorsolateral (spinal cord) 281.0
  eye, macular 377.1
  fatty (diffuse) (general) 279
    localized - *see* Degeneration by site,
      fatty
  heart (brown) (calcareous) (fatty)
    (fibrous) (hyaline) (mural)
    (muscular) (pigmentary) (senile)
    (*see also* Insufficiency,
    myocardial) 428
    amyloid 276
    atheromatous (*see also* Ischemia,
      heart) 412.9
    gouty 274
  hepatolenticular (Wilson's) 273.3
  hepatorenal 573.9
  heredofamilial 333.9
    brain 333.9
    spinal cord 333.9
  hyaline (diffuse) (generalized) 734.9

Degeneration, degenerative—*continued*
  hyaline—*continued*
    localized - *see* Degeneration, by
      site
    keratitis (*see also* Keratitis) 363.9
  internal semilunar cartilage 724.5
  intestine 569.9
    amyloid 276
    lardaceous 276
  ischemic - *see* Ischemia
  joint disease (multiple) 713.0
    spine 713.1
  kidney (*see also* Sclerosis, renal) 584
    amyloid 276
    cystic, congenital 753.1
    fatty (*see also* Lesion, kidney) 593.2
    fibrocystic (congenital) 753.1
    lardaceous 276
    polycystic (congenital) 753.1
    waxy 276
  lardaceous (any site) 276
  lens 378.8
  lenticular (familial) (progressive)
    (Wilson's) (with cirrhosis of liver)
    273.3
    striate artery (*see also* Ischemia,
      cerebral) 437.9
  liver (diffuse) 573.9
    amyloid 276
    cystic 573.9
      congenital 751.6
    fatty - *see* Cirrhosis, portal
    hypertrophic 573.9
    lardaceous 276
    parenchymatous, acute or subacute
      (*see also* Necrosis, liver) 570
    pigmentary 573.9
    toxic (acute) 573.9
    waxy 276
  lung 519.2
  lymph gland 289.3
    hyaline 289.3
    lardaceous 276
  macula, macular (congenital) (cystoid)
    (disciform) (hereditary) (infantile)
    (lutea) (presenile) (primary)
    (secondary) (senile) 377.1
  medullary (*see also* Degeneration,
    brain) 347.9
  membranous labyrinth, congenital
    (causing impairment of hearing)
    745.0
  mitral (heart) (valve) - *see* Endocarditis,
    mitral
  Monckeberg's (*see also*
    Arteriosclerosis, peripheral) 440.2

Degeneration, degenerative — *continued*
  moral 301.7
  motor centers, senile 794
  mucinoid, mucinous NEC 279
  mural
    heart, cardiac (*see also* Insufficiency,
        myocardial) 428
    myocardium, myocardial (*see also*
        Insufficiency, myocardial)
        428
  muscle 733.9
    fatty 733.9
    fibrous 733.9
    heart (*see also* Insufficiency,
        myocardial) 428
    hyaline 733.9
  muscular progressive 733.9
  myelin central nervous system NEC
      341
  myocardium, myocardial (brown)
      (calcareous) (fatty) (fibrous)
      (hyaline) (mural) (pigmentary)
      (senile) (*see also* Insufficiency,
      myocardial) 428
    gouty 274
  nerve
    accessory 356
    acoustic 387.9
    auditory 387.9
    axillary 357.1
    cranial NEC (*see also* Atrophy,
        nerve, cranial) 356
    facial 350
    glossopharyngeal 356
    hypoglossal 356
    median 357.2
    olfactory 356
    optic 377.6
    peripheral NEC 357.9
    pneumogastric 356
    spinal NEC 357.9
    sympathetic NEC 358.9
    trigeminal 356
    ulnar 357.3
    vagus 356
  nervous system 347.9
    amyloid 276
    fatty 347.9
    peripheral autonomic 358.9
  nipple 611.9
  nose 508.9
  olivopontocerebellar (*see also*
      Degeneration, brain) 347.9
    hereditary familial 332.1
  osseous labyrinth 386
  ovary 615.9

Degeneration, degenerative — *continued*
  ovary — *continued*
    cystic 615.2
    microcystic 615.2
  pallidal
    with juvenile paralysis agitans 342
    pigmentary (progressive) 331.9
  pancreas 577.9
    tuberculous 017.9
      late effect or sequela 019.9
  penis 607.9
  peritoneum 569.9
  pigmentary (diffuse) (general) 279
    localized - *see* Degeneration by site
    pallidal (progressive) 331.9
  pineal gland 258.9
  pituitary (gland) 253.9
  placenta (fatty) (fibrinoid) (fibroid) - *see*
      Placenta, abnormal
  posterolateral (spinal cord) 281.0
  pulmonary valve (heart) (*see also*
      Endocarditis, pulmonary) 424.9
  pyramidal - *see* Degeneration, brain
  renal (*see also* Sclerosis, renal) 584
    fibrocystic 753.1
    polycystic 753.1
  reticulo-endothelial system 289.9
  retina (cystoid) (lattice) (senile cystic)
      377.1
    pigmentary (primary) 744.6
  saccule, congenital (causing impairment
      of hearing) 745.0
  sclerosis 347.9
  senile 794
    brain 794
    cardiac, heart or myocardium - *see*
        Insufficiency, myocardial
    motor centers 794
    retina, cystic 377.1
    vascular - *see* Arteriosclerosis
  sinus (cystic) (*see also* Sinusitis) 503.9
    polypoid 505
  skin 709.9
    amyloid 276
    colloid 709.9
  spinal (cord) 349.9
    amyloid 276
    column 723.9
    combined (subacute) 281.0
    dorsolateral 281.0
    familial 333.9
    fatty 349.9
    funicular 281.0
    heredofamilial 333.9
    posterolateral 281.0
    subacute combined 281.0

Degeneration, degenerative — *continued*
  spinal (cord) — *continued*
    tuberculous 013.9
      late effect or sequela 019.1
    spine 723.9
    spleen 289.5
      amyloid 276
      lardaceous 276
    stomach 537.9
      lardaceous 276
    sudoriparous (cystic) 705.9
    suprarenal (capsule) (gland) 255.9
    sweat gland 705.9
    synovial membrane (pulpy) - *see*
      Synovitis
    tapetoretinal 744.8
    testis (postinfectional) 607.9
    thymus (gland) 254
      fatty 254
      lardaceous 276
    thyroid (gland) 246
    tricuspid (heart) (valve) - *see*
      Endocarditis, tricuspid
    tuberculous NEC (*see also*
      Tuberculosis) 011.9
    turbinate 723.9
    uterus 625.9
      cystic 625.9
    vascular (senile) - *see* Arteriosclerosis
      hypertensive - *see* Hypertension
    Virchow's (any site) 276
    vitreous humor (with infiltration) 378.9
    Wallerian (*see also* Compression, nerve)
      357.9
      median nerve 357.2
      spinal NEC 357.9
    waxy (any site) 276
    Wilson's hepatolenticular 273.3
Deglutition
  paralysis 781.4
    hysterical 300.1
Degos' disease 446.9
Degradation disorder branched chain
  amino-acid 270.4
Dehiscence
  episiotomy 998.3
  operation wound 998.3
  postoperative 998.3
    abdomen 998.3
Dehydration 788.0
  newborn 778.9
Dejerine-Roussy syndrome 347.9
Dejerine-Sottas neuropathy 355.9
Dejerine-Thomas atrophy 347.1
Dejerine's disease 355.9

Delay, delayed
  any plane in pelvis
    complicating delivery 655
      fetus or newborn - *see* categories
        765.0-765.9
  birth or delivery NEC 657.9
    fetus or newborn - *see* categories
      768.0-768.9
  coagulation (*see also* Defect,
    coagulation) 286.9
  conduction (auriculoventricular)
    (cardiac) (intra-auricular)
    (ventricular) (*see also* Block,
    heart) 427.3
  development speech 306.9
  menstruation (cause unknown) 626.9
  primary respiration (*see also* Asphyxia,
    newborn) 776.9
  puberty 258.9
Deleage's disease 330.4
Delhi boil or button 085.1
Delinquency (juvenile) 308
Delirium, delirious 780.1
  acute 780.1
  alcoholic 291.0
    acute 291.0
    chronic 291.1
  alcoholicum 291.0
  chronic (*see also* Psychosis) 299
  eclamptic (*see also* Eclampsia) 780.2
  exhaustion (*see also* Psychosis) 299
  hysterical 300.1
  in institution for mentally disordered
    (*see also* Psychosis) 299
  maniacal 296.1
  puerperal 677.9
  thyroid (*see also* Hyperthyroidism) 242.2
  traumatic - *see also* Injury, intracranial
    with
      lesion spinal cord - *see* Injury,
        spinal, by region
      shock spinal - *see* Injury, spinal, by
        region
  tremens 291.0
  uremic - *see* Uremia
Delivery 650
  with dead fetus
    less than 28 weeks gestation - *see*
      Abortion, by type
    28 weeks or more gestation - code as
      Delivery
  complicated 661.9
    by
      abnormal, abnormality of
        bony pelvis (acquired)
          (congenital) 654.9

Delivery—*continued*
  complicated—*continued*
    by—*continued*
      eversion cervix or uterus 660.9
      face presentation 656.3
        to pubes 656.8
      fetal deformity 655
      fever during labor 661.8
      fibroid (tumor) (uterus) 657.9
      fistula (any site in pelvis) 657.9
      flat pelvis 654.2
      funnel pelvis 654.9
      hematoma 660.9
        ischial spine 660.9
        subdural (nontraumatic) 674
        vulva 660.9
      hemorrhage (atonic) (during or after
        childbirth) (intrapartum)
        (postpartum) (puerperal)
        (uterine) 653
      antepartum (concealed) (internal)
        651.9
      cerebral 674
      due to
        placenta previa 651.0
        premature separation of
          placenta (normally
          implanted) 651.1
        retained placenta 652
      placenta NEC 651.1
      pregnancy (before onset of labor)
        (concealed) 651.9
      accidental (due to premature
        separation of placenta)
        651.1
      unavoidable (due to placenta
        previa) 651.0
      hourglass contraction, uterus
        657.9
      hydramnios 661.8
      hydrocephalic fetus 655
      hyperinvolution uterus 661.8
      incomplete dilatation (cervix)
        657.2
      incoordinate uterus 657.9
      inertia uterus 657.1
      infantile
        genitalia 657.9
        pelvis (bony) 654.9
        uterus (os) 657.9
      injury (to mother) NEC 660.9
      inversion uterus 660.9
      justo minor pelvis 654.9
      laceration 658.9
        anus (sphincter) 658.2
        bladder (urinary) 660.9

Delivery—*continued*
  complicated—*continued*
    by—*continued*
      laceration—*continued*
        cervix (uteri) 660.1
        fourchette 658.0
        hymen 658.0
        pelvic organ NEC 660.9
        perineum (without mention of
          other laceration) 658.9
        extensive NEC 658.9
        first degree (fourchette)
          (hymen) (vagina) (vulva)
          658.0
        fourth degree 658.2
        muscles 658.1
        second degree (pelvic floor)
          (perineal muscles)
          (vaginal, deep) 658.1
        slight 658.0
        sphincter 658.2
        third degree (rectovaginal)
          (sphincter ani) 658.2
        peritoneum 660.9
        rectovaginal (septum) 658.2
        sphincter ani 658.2
        urethra 660.0
        uterus 660.9
        vagina, vaginal 658.0
        deep 658.1
        muscles 658.1
        vulva 658.0
      lateroversion, uterus or cervix
        657.9
      lesion uterus NEC 660.9
      mal lic 656.9
      male type pelvis 654.0
      malposition
        fetus - *see* Delivery complicated
          by abnormal presentation
        pelvic organs or tissues 657.9
        placenta 651.0
        uterus or cervix 657.9
      marginal sinus (bleeding) (rupture)
        651.1
      metrorrhagia (myopathia) (*see also*
        Delivery complicated by
        hemorrhage) 653
      metrorrhexis 659
      multiple pregnancy NEC 657.0
      Nagele's pelvis 654.9
      obstetric trauma NEC 660.9
      obstructed labor 657.9
      obstruction, expulsion fetus 657.9
      Otto's disease or pelvis 654.9
      oversize fetus 655

Delivery—*continued*
  complicated—*continued*
    by—*continued*
      stenosis or stricture—*continued*
        pelvic organ NEC 657.9
      sudden death, unknown cause
        677.0
      tear - *see* Delivery complicated by
        laceration
      tipping pelvis 654.9
      transverse
        arrest (of fetal head) 656.8
        lie 656.1
        presentation 656.1
      trauma (obstetrical) NEC 660.9
      umbilical cord condition (any)
        661.3
      varicosities of vulva 657.9
      vasa praevia 651.0
      velamentous insertion of cord
        661.3
  delayed NEC 657.9
  difficult NEC 657.9
  missed (at or near term) 634.2
  nonviable infant - *see* Abortion, by type
    specified as liveborn - code as
      Delivery
  normal 650
    anesthetic death 662
  precipitate 661.1
  premature (live birth) NEC 650
  spontaneous - *see* Delivery, normal
  term pregnancy (live birth) (stillbirth)
    NEC 650
  threatened premature - *see* Threatened
    premature delivery
  triplets NEC 657.0
  twins NEC 657.0
  uncomplicated 650
    anesthetic death 662
Delusions (paranoid) 306.9
  systematized 297.0
Dementia (*see also* Psychosis) 299
  Alzheimer's 290.1
  catatonic (acute) 295.2
  congenital (*see also* Retardation,
    mental) 315.9
  developmental (*see also* Schizophrenia)
    295.9
  due to or associated with physical
    condition - *see* listing under
    Psychosis, organic
  hebephrenic (acute) 295.1
  old age 290.0
  paralytica, paralytic 094.1
    juvenilis 090.4

Dementia—*continued*
  paralytica, paralytic—*continued*
    syphilitic 094.1
      congenital 090.4
      tabetic form 094.1
  paranoid 295.3
  paraphrenic 295.3
  paretic 094.1
  praecox (*see also* Schizophrenia)
    295.9
  presenile 290.1
  primary (acute) 295.0
  progressive, syphilitic 094.1
  puerperal NEC 294.4
  schizophrenic (*see also* Schizophrenia)
    295.9
  senile 290.0
    exhaustion 290.0
    paranoid 290.0
  simple type (acute) 295.0
  simplex (acute) 295.0
  uremic - *see* Uremia
Demineralization, ankle 723.9
Demodex folliculorum (infestation) 133.9
Demyelination, demyelinization
  central nervous system NEC 341
  global 341
Dengue (fever) 061
  sandfly 061
Dens
  in dente 520.2
  invaginatus 520.2
Density
  increased, bone (disseminated)
    (generalized) (spotted) 723.9
  lung (nodular) 519.2
Dental - *see* condition
Dentia praecox 520.6
Denticles (pulp) 522.2
Dentigerous cyst 526.0
Dentin
  irregular (in pulp) 522.3
  secondary (in pulp) 522.3
Dentinogenesis imperfecta 520.5
Dentinoma 210.4
Dentition 520.7
  abnormal 520.6
  anomaly 520.6
  delayed 520.6
  difficult 520.7
  disorder of 520.6
  precocious 520.6
  retarded 520.6
Denture sore mouth 528.9
Dependence
  with psychosis 294.3

Dependence — *continued*
dihydrocodeinone 304.0
dihydrohydroxycodeinone 304.0
dihydroisocodeine 304.0
dihydromorphine 304.0
dihydromorphinone 304.0
dihydroxcodeinone 304.0
dilaudid 304.0
dimethylmeperidine 304.1
dimethyltriptamine 304.7
dionin 304.0
diphenoxylate 304.8
dipipanone 304.1
D-lysergic acid diethylamide 304.7
DMT 304.7
dolophine 304.1
doriden 304.3
dormiral 304.2
dormison 304.3
dromoran 304.1
drug NEC 304.9
  analgesic NEC 304.8
  due to or associated with physical
        condition - *see* listing under
        Disorder, mental
  hallucinogenic 304.7
  hypnotic NEC 304.3
  narcotic NEC 304.9
  psycho-stimulant NEC 304.6
  sedative 304.3
  soporific NEC 304.3
  specified NEC 304.8
  tranquilizing 304.3
duboisine 304.8
ectylurea 304.3
endocaine 304.8
equanil 304.3
eskabarb 304.2
ethchlorvynol 304.3
ether (ethyl) (liquid) (vapor) (vinyl)
        304.8
ethidine 304.8
ethinamate 304.3
ethoheptazine 304.8
ethyl
  alcohol 303.2
  bromide 304.8
  carbamate 304.8
  chloride 304.8
  morphine 304.0
ethylene (gas) 304.8
  dichloride 304.8
ethylidine chloride 304.8
etilfen 304.2
etorphine 304.1
etoval 304.2

Dependence — *continued*
eucodal 304.0
euneryl 304.2
evipal 304.2
evipan 304.2
fentanyl 304.1
ganja 304.5
gardenal 304.2
gardenpanyl 304.2
gelsemine 304.8
gelsemium 304.8
gemonil 304.2
glucochloral 304.3
glue (airplane) (sniffing) 304.8
glutethimide 304.3
hallucinogenics 304.7
hashish 304.5
headache powder NEC 304.8
hedonal 304.3
heptabarbital 304.2
heptalgen 304.1
heptobarbitone 304.2
heroin 304.0
  salt (any) 304.0
hexethal (sodium) 304.2
hexobarbital 304.2
hycodan 304.0
hydrocodone 304.0
hydromorphinol 304.0
hydromorphinone 304.0
hydromorphone 304.0
hydroxycodeine 304.0
hypnotic NEC 304.3
Indian hemp 304.5
intranarcon 304.2
ipral 304.2
kemithal 304.2
ketobemidone 304.1
khat 304.6
kig 304.5
lactuca (virosa) extract 304.3
lactucarium 304.3
laudanum 304.0
leritine 304.1
lettuce opium 304.3
levanil 304.3
levo-dromoran 304.1
levo-iso-methadone 304.1
levorphan(ol) 304.1
librium 304.3
lomotil 304.8
lotusate 304.2
LSD 304.7
  -25 304.7
luminal 304.2

Dependence—*continued*
placidyl 304.3
pontocaine 304.8
potassium bromide 304.3
preludin 304.6
prinadol 304.1
probarbital 304.2
procaine 304.8
propanal 304.3
propoxyphene 304.8
psilocibin 304.7
psilocin 304.7
psilocybin 304.7
psilocyline 304.7
psilocyn 304.7
psycho-stimulant NEC 304.6
pyrahexyl 304.5
pyramidon 304.8
quinalbarbitone 304.2
racemoramide 304.1
racemorphan 304.1
rela 304.8
scopolamine 304.8
secobarbital 304.2
seconal 304.2
sedative NEC 304.3
sedormid 304.3
sodium bromide 304.3
soma 304.8
somnos 304.3
somonal 304.2
soneryl 304.2
spinocaine 304.8
stovaine 304.8
stramonium 304.8
sulfonal 304.3
sulfonethylmethane 304.3
sulfonmethane 304.3
surital 304.2
talbutal 304.2
tetracaine 304.8
tetrahydrocannabinol 304.5
tetronal 304.3
thebacon 304.0
thebaine 304.0
thiamil 304.2
thiamylal 304.2
thiopental 304.2
tranquilizer NEC 304.3
tribromacetaldehyde 304.8
tribromethanol 304.8
tribromomethane 304.8
trichloroethanol 304.8
trichoroethyl phosphate 304.3
triclofos 304.3
trional 304.3

Dependence—*continued*
tuinal 304.2
urethan(e) 304.8
valium 304.3
valmid 304.3
veganin 304.0
veramon 304.2
veronal 304.2
versidyne 304.8
vinbarbital 304.2
vinbarbitone 304.2
vinyl bitone 304.2
zactane 304.8
14-hydroxy-dihydromorphinone 304.0
Dependency
passive 301.6
reactions 301.6
Depersonalization (episode in neurotic
state) (neurotic) (syndrome) 300.6
Depletion, salt or sodium 788.0
causing heat exhaustion or prostration
992.4
Deposit
bone in Boeck's sarcoid 135
calcareous, calcium - *see* Calcification
cholesterin, retina or vitreous (humor)
377.4
cholesterol, retina or vitreous (humor)
377.4
crystallin, vitreous (humor) 378.9
hemosiderin in old scars of cornea - *see*
Opacity, cornea
metallic in lens 378.8
tooth, teeth (black, green, orange,
tobacco) (soft) 523.6
urate
kidney (*see also* Lesion, kidney)
593.2
Depraved appetite 306.5
Depression 790.2
acute 296.2
agitated 296.0
anxiety 300.0
arches 736
congenital 755.7
basal metabolic rate 788.9
bone marrow 289.9
cerebral 347.9
newborn (*see also* Asphyxia,
newborn) 776.9
cerebrovascular (*see also* Disease,
cerebrovascular NEC) 438.9
newborn (*see also* Asphyxia,
newborn) 776.9
chest wall 738.8
endogenous 296.2

Depression—*continued*
  functional activity   790.2
  hysterical   300.1
  involutional, climacteric, or menopausal
     296.0
  manic (*see also* Psychosis, manic-
     depressive)   296.9
  medullary   347.9
    newborn (*see also* Asphyxia,
      newborn)   776.9
  mental   300.4
  metatarsal heads - *see* Depression,
    arches
  metatarsus - *see* Depression, arches
  nervous   300.4
  neurotic   300.4
  nose   738.0
  psychogenic   300.4
  psychoneurotic   300.4
  psychotic   296.2
  reactive   300.4
    neurotic   300.4
    psychoneurotic   300.4
    psychotic   298.0
  recurrent   296.2
  respiratory center   347.9
    newborn (*see also* Asphyxia,
      newborn)   776.9
  senile   296.2
  sternum   738.8
  visual field   781.0

Depressive reaction   300.4
  involutional   296.0
  psychoneurotic   300.4

Deprivation
  food   994.2
  particular kind of food NEC   269.9
  protein (familial)   267
  symptoms, syndrome, drug (narcotic)
    (*see also* Dependence)   304.9
  vitamins (*see also* Deficiency, vitamin)
    266.9
  water   994.3

Derangement
  elbow (internal)   724.3
    current injury (*see also* Dislocation,
      elbow)   832.0
    recurrent   724.2
  gastro-intestinal   536.9
  heart - *see* Disease, heart
  joint (internal)   724.9
    current injury - *see* Dislocation
    elbow   724.3
    knee   724.5
    recurrent   724.9
    shoulder   724.1

Dearangement—*continued*
  knee (cartilage) (internal) (semilunar)
    724.5
    current injury (*see also* Dislocation,
      knee)   836.0
    recurrent   724.4
  low back NEC   729.1
  mental (*see also* Psychosis)   299
  semilunar cartilage (knee)   724.5
    current injury (*see also* Dislocation,
      knee)   836.0
  shoulder (internal)   724.1
    current injury (*see also* Dislocation,
      shoulder)   831.0
    recurrent   724.0
Dercum's disease   279
Derealization   300.6
Dermal - *see* condition
Dermalipoma   214.0

Dermaphytid - *see* Dermatophytosis

Dermatergosis - *see* Dermatitis

Dermatitis (allergic) (contact)
    (occupational) (venenata)   692.9
  ab igne   692.7
  acneform   692.9
  actinic (due to sun)   692.8
    due to
      radiation, except from sun   692.7
  ambustionis
    due to
      burn or scald - *see* Burn
      sunburn   692.8
  amebic   006.9
    with liver abscess   006.0
  anaphylactoid NEC   692.9
  arsenical   692.4
  artefacta   698.4
    psychogenic   305.0
  atopic (due to any substance)   691
    psychogenic   305.0
  atrophicans   701.9
    diffusa   701.9
    maculosa   701.2
  berlock   692.9
  berloque   692.9
  blastomycetic   116.1
  blister beetle   692.3
  brucella NEC   023.9
  bullosa   709.9
    striata pratensis   692.6
  bullous seasonal   709.9
  calorica
    due to
      burn or scald - *see* Burn
      cold   692.9
      sunburn   692.8

Dermatitis, etc. —*continued*
 caterpillar 692.9
 cercarial 120.3
 combustionis
  due to
   burn or scald - *see* Burn
   sunburn 692.8
 congelationis 443.2
 contusiformis 695.2
 diabetic - *see* category 250
 diaper 692.9
 diphtheritica 032
 due to
  acetone 692.2
  acids 692.4
  adhesive plaster 692.3
  alcohol (substances in 980) 692.4
  alkalis 692.4
  arnica 692.3
  arsenic 692.4
  cantharides 692.3
  carbon disulphide 692.2
  caustics 692.4
  chemical(s) NEC 692.4
   internal - *see* Table of adverse
    effects
   irritant NEC 692.4
  cold weather 692.9
  cosmetics 692.9
  detergents 692.0,
  drug (*see also* Table of adverse
    effects) 977.9
   applied to skin 692.3
   arnica 692.3
   contact 692.3
   fungicides 692.3
   internal use (any) - *see* Table of
    adverse effects
   iodine 692.3
   iodoform 692.3
   keratolytics 692.3
   mercurials 692.3
   pediculocides 692.3
   phenol 692.3
   scabicides 692.3
  dyes 692.9
  epidermophytosis - *see*
    Dermatophytosis
  external irritant NEC 692.9
  food 692.5
   atopic 691
  fungicides 692.3
  furs 692.9
  greases 692.1

Dermatitis, etc. —*continued*
 due to —*continued*
  hot
   objects and materials - *see* Burn
   weather or places 692.9
  infrared rays 692.7
  ingestion of drug or chemical (any) -
    see Table of adverse effects
  internal agent (chemical) (drug) - *see
    also* Table of adverse effects
   food 692.5
    atopic 691
  iodine 692.3
  iodoform 692.3
  irradiation 692.7
  keratolytics 692.3
  low temperature 692.9
  mercurials 692.3
  oils 692.1
  paint solvent 692.2
  pediculocides 692.3
  penicillin (internal use) 960.0
   contact 692.3
  petroleum products (substances in
    981) 692.4
  phenol 692.3
  plants NEC 692.6
  plasters, medicated (any) 692.3
  poison
   ivy 692.6
   oak 692.6
   sumac 692.6
   vine 692.6
  primrose 692.6
  primula 692.6
  radiation 692.7
   sun 692.8
  radioactive substance 692.7
  radium 692.7
  ragweed 692.6
  Rhus
   diversiloba 692.6
   radicans 692.6
   toxicodendron 692.6
   venenata 692.6
  scabicides 692.3
  Senecio jacoboea 692.6
  solvents (substances in 982) 692.2
   chlorocompound group 692.2
   cyclohexane group 692.2
   ester group 692.2
   glycol group 692.2
   hydrocarbon group 692.2
   ketone group 692.2
   paint 692.2
  specified agent NEC 692.9
  sunburn 692.8

Dermatitis, etc. —*continued*
due to—*continued*
  sunshine 692.8
  tetrachlorethylene 692.2
  toluene 692.2
  turpentine 692.2
  ultraviolet rays 692.7
    sun 692.8
  x-rays 692.7
 dysmenorrheica 626.9
 eczematoid NEC 692.9
 eczematous NEC 692.9
 epidemica 695.9
 escharotica - *see* Burn
 exfoliativa, exfoliative 695.9
  generalized 695.9
 facta, factitia 698.4
  psychogenic 305.0
 ficta 698.4
  psychogenic 305.0
 flexural 691
 follicularis 704
 friction 709.9
 fungus NEC 111.9
 gangrenosa, gangrenous (*see also*
    Gangrene) 445.9
  infantum 445.9
 gestationis 693
 harvest mite 133.9
 heat 692.9
 herpetiformis (bullous) (erythematous)
    (pustular) (vesicular) 693
 hiemalis 692.9
 hypostatic, hypostatica (lower
    extremity) 454.1
  ulcerated or with ulcer 454.0
 infectiosa eczematoides 686.2
 infective eczematoid 686.2
 Jacquet's 692.9
 leptus 133.9
 lichenified NEC 692.9
 maculosa nigra 709.9
 medicamentosa - *see* Dermatitis, due to
    drug
 mite 133.9
 multiformis 693
 napkin 692.9
 nummular NEC 692.9
 papillaris capillitii 706.1
 pellagrous 262
 perstans 686.9
 pruritic NEC 692.9
 psychogenic 305.0
 purulent 686.0
 pustular contagious 057.8
 pyococcal 686.0

Dermatitis, etc. —*continued*
 pyocyaneus 686.0
 pyogenica 686.0
 repens 686.9
 rodent - *see* Neoplasm, skin, malignant
 Schamberg's 709.9
 schistosome 120.3
 seasonal bullous 709.9
 seborrheic 690
  infantile 691
 sensitization NEC 692.9
 septic 686.0
 solare 692.8
 stasis (lower extremity) 454.1
  ulcerated or with ulcer 454.0
 suppurative 686.0
 traumatic NEC 709.9
 ultraviolet 692.7
  due to sun 692.8
 varicose (lower extremity) 454.1
  ulcerated or with ulcer 454.0
 vegetans 686.9
 verrucosa 117.2
Dermato-arthritis, lipoid 279
Dermatofibroma 216.8
 breast 217
 external area or site NEC 216.8
 genital organ NEC - code as Neoplasm,
    benign, by site
 scrotum 216.8
Dermatofibrosarcoma (protuberans) - *see*
    Neoplasm, skin, malignant
Dermatographia 709.9
Dermatolysis (exfoliativa) (congenital)
    757.2
 acquired 701.9
 eyelids 378.2
 palpebrarum 378.2
 senile 701.9
Dermatomegaly NEC 701.9
Dermatomucosomyositis 716.0
Dermatomycosis 111.9
 furfuracea 111.0
Dermatomyositis (acute) (chronic) 716.0
Dermatoneuritis of children 985.0
Dermatophiliasis 134.2
Dermatophytide - *see* Dermatophytosis
Dermatophytosis 110.9
 beard 110.0
 fingernails 110.9
 foot 110.1
 groin 110.9
 hand 110.9
 scalp 110.0
 scrotal 110.9
 specified site NEC 110.9

Dermatophytosis—*continued*
  tinea NEC 110.9
  toenails 110.1
  vulva 110.9
Dermatopolyneuritis 985.0
Dermatorrhexis 757.2
  acquired 701.9
Dermatosclerosis (*see also* Scleroderma) 734.0
Dermatosis 709.9
  Bowen's 702
  exfoliativa 695.9
  factitial 698.4
  gonococcal 098.8
  herpetiformis 693
  hysterical 300.1
  menstrual NEC 709.9
  occupational (*see also* Dermatitis) 692.9
  papulosa nigra 709.9
  pigmentary NEC 709.9
    progressive 709.9
    Schamberg's 709.9
  precancerous 702
  psychogenic 305.0
  pustular
    subcorneal 693
  senile NEC 709.9
Dermographia 709.9
Dermographism 709.9
Dermoid (cyst) (tumor) (ovary) (*see also* Cyst, dermoid) 220.0
Dermopathy, senile NEC 709.9
Dermophytosis - *see* Dermatophytosis
Descemet's membrane - *see* condition
Descemetocele 378.4
Descending - *see* condition
Descensus uteri (incomplete) (partial) 623.4
Desert sore (*see also* Ulcer, skin) 707.9
Desertion (newborn) 994.9
Desmoid (tumor) (*see also* Neoplasm, connective tissue, benign) 215
Despondency 300.4
Destruction
  articular facet (vertebra) 729.1
  bone 723.9
    syphilitic 095
  joint (*see also* Disease, joint) 729.9
    sacro-iliac 726
  kidney (*see also* Lesion, kidney) 593.2
  live fetus to facilitate birth NEC 773
  rectal sphincter 569.2
  septum (nasal) 508.9
  tuberculous NEC (*see also* Tuberculosis) 011.9

Destruction—*continued*
  tympanic membrane 387.9
  tympanum 387.9
  vertebral disc - *see* Displacement, intervertebral disc
Destructiveness, childhood 308
Detachment
  cartilage - *see* Sprain, strain
  cervix annular 621.9
    complicating delivery - *see* Obstetrical trauma
  choroid (old) (postinfectional) (simple) (spontaneous) 378.6
  knee, medial meniscus (old) 724.5
    current - *see* Dislocation, knee
  ligament - *see* Sprain, strain
  placenta (premature) - *see* Placenta, separation
  retina (old) (secondary) (simple) 376
  vitreous humor 378.9
Deterioration
  epileptic 293.2
  heart, cardiac (*see also* Insufficiency, myocardial) 428
  mental (*see also* Psychosis) 299
  myocardium, myocardial (*see also* Insufficiency, myocardial) 428
  senile (simple) 794
Deuteranopia (anomalous trichromat) (complete) (incomplete) 377.3
Deutschlander's disease - *see* Fracture, foot
Development
  abnormal, bone 756.9
  arrested 796.0
    bone 723.6
    fetus or newborn 778.9
    tracheal rings (congenital) 748.3
  defective, congenital - *see also* Anomaly
    cauda equina 743.3
  delayed, speech 306.9
  imperfect, congenital - *see also* Anomaly
    heart 746.9
    lungs 748.6
  improper (fetus or newborn) 778.9
  incomplete (fetus or newborn) 778.9
    bronchial tree 748.3
    organ or site not listed - *see* Hypoplasia
    respiratory system 748.9
  tardy, mental (*see also* Retardation, mental) 315.9
Developmental - *see* condition
Devergie's disease 696.4

Deviation
  conjugate (eye) (spastic) (*see also*
      Strabismus) 373.9
  esophagus 530.9
  eye, skew (*see also* Strabismus) 373.9
  organ or site, congenital NEC - *see*
      Malposition, congenital
  septum (nasal) 504
    congenital 748.1
  sexual 302.9
    bestiality 302.8
    due to or associated with physical
        condition - *see* Disorder,
        mental
    erotomania 302.8
    exhibitionism 302.4
    fetishism 302.1
    homosexuality 302.0
    lesbianism 302.0
    masochism 302.7
    narcissism 302.8
    necrophilia 302.8
    nymphomania 302.8
    pederosis 302.2
    pedophilia 302.2
    sadism 302.6
    satyriasis 302.8
    sodomy 302.0
    specified type NEC 302.8
    transvestism 302.3
    voyeurism 302.5
  trachea 519.9
  ureter (congenital) 753.4
Devic's disease 341
Devitalized tooth 522.9
Devonshire colic 984
Dextraposition, aorta 747.2
  with ventricular septal defect,
      pulmonary stenosis or atresia and
      hypertrophy of right ventricle
      746.2
Dextrinosis, limit (debrancher enzyme
      deficiency) 271.1
Dextrocardia (true) 746.8
  with
    complete transposition of viscera
      759.0
    situs inversus 759.0
Dhobie itch 110.9
Di Guglielmo's disease 207.2
Diabetes, diabetic (mellitus) (congenital)
      (controlled) (familial) (severe)
      (slight) (without acidosis or coma)
      250.9
  with
    acetonemia 250.0

Diabetes, etc. —*continued*
  with —*continued*
    acidosis 250.0
    coma (hyperglycemic) 250.0
    keto-acidosis 250.0
    ketosis 250.0
    abscess 250.9
    bone change 250.9
    bronze, bronzed 273.2
    cataract 250.9
    complication NEC 250.9
    dorsal sclerosis 250.9
    encephalomyelopathy 250.9
    gangrene 250.9
    hemochromatosis 273.2
    hepatogenous 250.9
    hypoglycemia (with coma) 250.9
    infection 250.9
    insipidus 253.9
      nephrogenic 273.8
      pituitary 253.9
      vasopressin resistant 273.8
    intercapillary glomerulosclerosis 250.9
    iritis 250.9
    irrefraction 250.9
    Lancereaux's 250.9
    lipoidosis 250.9
    maternal
      with manifest disease in the infant
        250.9
      affecting fetus or newborn 761.1
    melanosis, cornea 250.9
    nephropathy 250.9
    nephrosis 250.9
    neuralgia 250.9
    neuritis 250.9
    neurogenic 250.9
    neuropathy 250.9
    pancreatic 250.9
    phosphate 273.4
    pruritus 250.9
    renal 273.8
      true 273.8
    retinal hemorrhage 250.9
    retinitis 250.9
    retinopathy 250.9
    saccharine 250.9
    sclerosis
      dorsal 250.9
      islands of Langerhans 250.9
    steroid induced 962.0
    sugar 250.9
    ulcer 250.9
    vulvitis 250.9
    xanthoma 250.9

Diacyclothrombopathia 287.3

Diagnosis deferred 796.9

Diagonal conjugate, small
  complicating delivery - see Deformity,
    pelvis, complicating delivery
  noted during pregnancy (undelivered)
    634.9

Dialysis, anterior retinal 376

Diaphragm - see condition

Diaphragmitis 519.9

Diaphysial aclasis 756.5

Diaphysitis 723.9

Diarrhea, diarrheal (autumn) (bilious)
    (bloody) (catarrhal) (choleraic)
    (endemic) (epidemic) (gravis) (green)
    (infantile) (infectious) (lienteric)
    (parenteral) (putrefactive) (sporadic)
    (summer) (thermic) (zymotic)
    009.1
  achlorhydric 536.0
  allergic 561
  ameba coli 006.9
    with liver abscess 006.0
  amebic 006.9
    with liver abscess 006.0
  bacillary - see Dysentery, bacillary
  bacterial NEC 008.3
  balantidial 007.0
  cachectic NEC 561
  Chilomastix 007.9
  choleriformis 000.1
  chronic 563.9
    ulcerative 563.1
  coccidial 007.2
  Cochin-China 269.0
    anguilluliasis 127.1
    psilosis 269.0
  Dientameba 006.9
    with liver abscess 006.0
  dietetic 561
  due to
    achylia gastrica 536.0
    Aerobacter aerogenes 008.2
    Bacillus coli 008.0
    Clostridium perfringens (C) (F)
      008.2
    enterococci 008.2
    Escherichia coli 008.0
    irritating foods 561
    Paracolobactrum Arizona 008.1
    Paracolon bacillus NEC 008.2
      Arizona 008.1
    Proteus (bacillus) 008.2
    Pseudomonas aeruginosa 008.2
    virus NEC (see also Enteritis, viral)
      008.9
  dysenteric 009.0

Diarrhea, etc.—continued
  dyspeptic 561
  Endameba coli 006.9
    with liver abscess 006.0
  fermentative 561
  flagellate 007.9
  Flexner's (ulcerative) 004.1
  functional 564.9
    psychogenic 305.5
  Giardia lamblia 007.1
  giardial 007.1
  hill 269.0
  hyperperistalsis (nervous) 305.5
  inflammatory (see also Enteritis) 009.2
  malarial (see also Malaria) 084.9
  mite 133.9
  mycotic 117.9
  nervous 305.5
  neurogenic 564.9
  noninfectious 561
  psychogenic 305.5
  septic (see also Enteritis) 009.2
  specified
    bacteria NEC 008.2
    organism, nonbacterial NEC 008.9
  Staphylococcus 008.2
  Streptococcus (anaerobic) 008.2
  toxic 561
  tropical 269.0
  tuberculous 014
    late effect or sequela 019.9
  ulcerative (chronic) 563.1
  viral (see also Enteritis, viral) 008.9

Diastasis
  cranial bones 723.9
    congenital 756.0
  joint (traumatic) - see Dislocation
  muscle 733.9
    congenital 756.8
  recti (abdomen) 733.9
    complicating delivery 661.8
    congenital 756.8

Diastematomyelia 743.3

Diataxia, cerebral, infantile 343.9

Diathesis
  cystine (familial) 270.3
  gouty 274
  hemorrhagic (familial) 287.9
    newborn 778.2
  scrofulous 017.1
    late effect or sequela 019.9
  spasmophilic (see also Tetany) 788.5
  uric acid 274

Dibothriocephaliasis 123.4
  larval 123.5

Dibothriocephalus (latus) (infection)
    (infestation)   123.4
  larval   123.5
Dicephalus   759.1
Dichotomy teeth   520.2
Dichromat (congenital)   377.3
Dichromatopsia (congenital)   377.3
Dichuchwa   104.0
Dicroceliasis   121.9
Didelphys, didelphic (see also Double
    uterus)   752.5
Didymitis (see also Epididymitis)   604
Died - see also Death
  without
    medical attention (cause unknown)
        796.9
    sign of disease   796.3
Dietary inadequacy or deficiency   269.9
Dietl's crisis   593.3
Dieulafoy's ulcer - see Ulcer, stomach
Difficult
  birth
    fetus or newborn - see categories
        768.0-768.9
Difficulty
  mechanical, gastroduodenal stoma
        537.9
  swallowing (see also Dysphagia)   784.4
  walking   787.5
Diffuse - see condition
Diffused ganglion (see also Bursitis)
        731.9
Digestive - see condition
Diktyoma iris   190
Dilaceration, tooth   520.4
Dilatation
  anus   564.9
    venule   455
  aorta (focal) (general) (see also
        Aneurysm, aorta)   441.9
    congenital   747.2
    infectional   093.0
    syphilitic   093.0
  artery   447
  bile duct, common, cystic   751.6
    acquired (any bile duct) (see also
        Disease, gallbladder)   576.9
  bladder (sphincter)   596.9
    complicating delivery   657.9
      fetus or newborn - see categories
        764.0-764.9
    congenital   753.8
  blood vessel   458.9
  bronchi   518
  calyx (due to obstruction) (see also
        Lesion, kidney)   593.2

Dilatation—continued
  capillaries   448
  cardiac (acute) (chronic) (see also
        Disease, heart)   429.9
    congenital   746.8
    valve (any)   746.6
  cavum septi pellucidi   743.3
  cecum   564.9
    psychogenic   305.5
  cervix (uteri)
    incomplete, poor, slow
      complicating delivery   657.2
        fetus or newborn - see categories
            767.0-767.9
  colon   564.9
    congenital   751.2
    psychogenic   305.5
  duodenum   564.9
  esophagus   530.9
    congenital   750.8
    due to achalasia or cardiospasm
            530.0
  eustachian tube, congenital   745.2
  fontanel   756.0
  gallbladder (see also Disease,
        gallbladder)   576.9
  gastric   536.1
    psychogenic   305.5
  heart (acute) (chronic) (see also Disease,
        heart)   429.9
    congenital   746.8
    valve - see Endocarditis
      congenital   746.6
  ileum   564.9
    psychogenic   305.5
  inguinal rings   569.9
  jejunum   564.9
    psychogenic   305.5
  kidney (calyx) (collecting structures)
        (cystic) (parenchyma) (pelvis) (see
        also Lesion, kidney)   593.2
  lachrymal, lacrimal apparatus or duct
        378.3
  lymphatic vessel   457
  mammary duct   611.9
  Meckel's diverticulum (congenital)
        751.0
  meningeal vessels, congenital   743.9
  myocardium (acute) (chronic) (see also
        Disease, heart)   429.9
  organ or site, congenital NEC - see
        Distortion
  pancreatic duct   577.9
  pericardium - see Pericarditis
  pharynx   508.9
  prostate   602

Dilalation—*continued*
pulmonary
 artery (idiopathic) 426
 valve, congenital 746.6
pupil 378.6
rectum 564.9
saccule, congenital 745.0
sphincter ani 564.9
stomach (acute) (reflex) 536.1
 psychogenic 305.5
submaxillary duct 527.9
trachea, congenital 748.3
ureter (idiopathic) 593.5
 congenital 753.2
urethra (acquired) 599.9
vasomotor 443.9
vein 458.9
ventricular, ventricle (acute) (chronic)
  (*see also* Disease, heart) 429.9
 cerebral, congenital 743.2
 venule 458.9
 vesical orifice 596.9
Dilated, dilation - *see* Dilatation
Diminished hearing (acuity) (*see also*
  Deafness) 389.9
Diminution, sense or sensation (cold)
  (heat) (tactile) (vibratory) (*see also*
  Disturbance, sensation) 781.6
Dimitri-Sturge-Weber disease 759.8
Dimple
 parasacral 685
 pilonidal 685
 postanal 685
Dioctophyma renale (infection)
  (infestation) 128.8
Dipetalonemiasis 125.4
Diphallus 752.8
Diphtheria, diphtheritic (any site)
  (gangrenous) (hemorrhagic)
  (membranous) 032
 carrier (bacillus) Y05.0
 heart disease, old - *see* Disease, heart
 infection of wound 032
 myocarditis, old (*see also* Myocarditis)
  428
Diphyllobothriasis (intestine) 123.4
 larval 123.5
Diplacusis 387.9
Diplegia (*see also* Paralysis) 344.9
 brain or cerebral (*see also* Disease,
  cerebrovascular NEC) 438.9
 congenital (cerebral) (spastic) (spinal) -
  see Diplegia, infantile
 infantile (cerebral) (spastic) (spinal)
  343.1

Diplegia—*continued*
 infantile, etc.—*continued*
  with other types of motor disturbance
   (e.g., ataxic, athetoid, atonic,
   rigidity, or tremor) 343.9
  athetoid 343.2
   with other types of motor
    disturbance (e.g., ataxic,
    atonic, rigidity, spastic, or
    tremor) 343.9
  specified type NEC 343.9
 late effect of birth injury - *see* Diplegia,
  infantile
Diplococcus, diplococcal - *see* condition
Diplopia 781.1
Dipsomania 303.2
 with psychosis (*see also* Psychosis,
  alcoholic) 291.9
Dipylidiasis 123.9
 intestine 123.9
Direction, teeth abnormal 524.3
Dirt-eating child 308
Disability
 heart - *see* Disease, heart
 special spelling 306.1
Disarticulation (*see also* Dislocation,
  pathological) 729.9
 meaning
  dislocation, traumatic or congenital -
   see Dislocation
  traumatic amputation - *see*
   Amputation, traumatic
Disaster
 cerebrovascular (*see also* Disease,
  cerebrovascular, acute) 436.9
Disc (intervertebral) - *see* Displacement,
  intervertebral disc
Discharge
 breast (female) (male) 611.9
 continued local motor idiopathic 345.4
 diencephalic autonomic idiopathic
  345.9
 ear 381.9
 excessive urine 786.4
 nipple 611.9
 patterned motor idiopathic 345.4
 postnasal - *see* Sinusitis
 sinus from mediastinum 510
 vaginal 629.3
Discoid semilunar cartilage 724.5
Discoloration
 nails 703.9
Discomycosis 113
Discopathy (traumatic) - *see*
  Displacement, intervertebral disc

Discrepancy leg length (acquired) 738.5
  congenital 755.3

Disease, diseased - *see also* Syndrome
  Abrami's 283.9
  absorbent system 458.9
  Acosta's 993.2
  Adams-Stokes(-Morgagni) (*see also*
      Block, heart) 427.3
  Addison's (bronze) 255.1
    tuberculous 017.9
      late effect or sequela 019.9
  adenoids (and tonsils) 500
  adrenal (capsule) (gland) 255.9
    cortex 255.9
  ainhum 136
  Akureyri 065
    late effects 066
  Albers-Schonberg 756.7
  Albert's 731.7
  Albright-Martin 273.4
  Alibert-Bazin 696.0
  Alibert's 202.1
  alimentary canal 569.9
  alligator-skin 757.2
    acquired 701.1
  Almeida's 116.2
  alveoli, teeth 525.9
  Alzheimer's 290.1
  amyloid (any site) 276
  anarthritic rheumatoid 446.4
  Andes 993.2
  angiospastic 443.9
    cerebral (*see also* Ischemia, cerebral,
        transient) 435.9
    vein 458.9
  anterior chamber 378.6
  anus NEC 569.2
  aorta (nonsyphilitic) 446.9
    syphilitic 093.9
  aortic (heart) (valve) (*see also*
      Endocarditis, aortic) 395.9
  aponeuroses 733.9
  appendix 543
  aqueous (chamber) 378.6
  Arnold-Chiari 741.0
  arterial 447
    occlusive 447
  arteriocardiorenal - *see* Hypertension,
      cardiorenal
  arteriolar (obliterative) (generalized)
      447
  arteriorenal - *see* Hypertension, kidney
  arteriosclerotic - *see also*
        Arteriosclerosis
    coronary (*see also* Ischemia, heart)
        412.9

Disease, diseased—*continued*
  arteriosclerotic—*continued*
    heart (*see also* Ischemia, heart)
        412.9
    vascular - *see* Arteriosclerosis
  artery 447
    cerebral (*see also* Disease,
        cerebrovascular NEC) 438.9
  arthropod-borne NEC 089.9
  auditory canal, ear 387.9
  Aujeszky's 079.8
  auricle, ear NEC 387.9
  Australian X 062.4
    late effects 066
  auto-immune hemolytic 283.9
  aviators' (*see also* Effect, adverse, high
      altitude) 993.2
  axe-grinders' 515.0
    with tuberculosis 010
  Ayala's 756.8
  Ayerza's 426
  back bone NEC 723.9
  bacterial NEC 039.9
    zoonotic NEC 027.9
  Bairnsdale's 031.9
  Balfour's 202.2
  Ballingall's 117.4
  balloon (*see also* Effect, adverse, high
      altitude) 993.2
  Balo's 341
  Bamberger-Marie 723.1
  Bang's 023.1
  Bannister's - *see* Edema, angioneurotic
  Banti's (with cirrhosis) (with portal
        hypertension) - *see* Cirrhosis,
        liver
  Barcoo (*see also* Ulcer, skin) 707.9
  Barensprung's 110.9
  Barlow's 264
  Barraquer(-Simons) 279
  Basedow's 242.0
  Bateman's 079.0
  Batten-Mayou (retina) 333.0
  Baumgarten-Cruveilhier 571.8
  Bayle's 094.1
  Bazin's (primary) 017.0
    late effect or sequela 019.9
  Beard's 300.5
    psychogenic 300.5
  Beau's (*see also* Insufficiency,
      myocardial) 428
  Bechterew's 712.4
  Becker's 425
  Behr's 377.1
  Beigel's 111.2
  Bell's 296.1

Disease, diseased—*continued*
Benson's 369.9
Bergeron's 300.1
Berlin's 921
Bernard-Soulier's 287.3
Bernhardt(-Roth) 355.1
Besnier-Boeck(-Schaumann) 135
Best's 377.1
Beurmann's 117.1
bicuspid valve - *see* Endocarditis, mitral
Bielschowsky(-Jansky) 333.0
Biermer's 281.0
Biett's 695.4
bile duct (*see also* Disease, gallbladder)
    576.9
biliary tract (*see also* Disease,
        gallbladder) 576.9
Billroth's, meaning
    meningocele 741.9
        with hydrocephalus 741.0
    neoplasm 201
bladder 596.9
Bloch-Sulzberger 757.2
Blocq's 306.3
blood 289.9
    forming organs 289.9
    vessel 458.9
Bloodgood's 610
Blount's 722.2
blue 746.9
Boeck's 135
bone 723.9
    fibrocystic NEC 723.9
        jaw 526.2
    Paget's 721
bone-marrow 289.9
Borna 065
    late effects 066
Bornholm 074.1
Bouillaud's 391.9
Bourneville's 759.6
bowel 569.9
    functional 564.9
        psychogenic 305.5
Bowen's (skin) 702
    benign 702
    malignant - *see* Neoplasm, skin,
            malignant
    of mouth 528.7
    penis 607.1
    scrotum 7(
    tongue 529
Brailsford's 722.2
    radius, head 722.2
    tarsal, scaphoid 722.2
brain 347.9

Disease, diseased—*continued*
    brain—*continued*
        arterial, artery (*see also* Disease,
                cerebrovascular NEC) 438.9
        arteriosclerotic (*see also* Ischemia,
                cerebral) 437.9
        congenital 743.9
        degenerative - *see* Degeneration,
                brain
        infantile 347.9
        inflammatory 323
            late effects 324
        organic 347.9
            arteriosclerotic (*see also* Ischemia,
                    cerebral) 437.9
        parasitic NEC 123.9
        Pick's 290.1
        senile 794
        Brazier's 985.9
    breast 611.9
        Brodie's 217
        cystic (chronic) 610
        fibrocystic 610
        Paget's 174
        puerperal, postpartum 678
    Breda's (*see also* Yaws) 102.9
    Breisky's 629.2
    Bretonneau's 032
    Bright's (*see also* Nephritis) 583
        arteriosclerotic (*see also*
                Hypertension, kidney) 403
    Brill-Symmers' 202.0
    Brill-Zinsser 081.1
    Brill's 081.1
        flea borne 081.0
        louse borne 081.1
    Brocq's 691
        meaning
            dermatitis, herpetiformis 693
            lichen corneus obtusus 697.9
            parapsoriasis 696.2
            prurigo 698.2
    Brodie's (knee) 731.6
        breast 217
    bronchi 519.9
    bronchopulmonary 519.9
    bronze (Addison's) 255.1
        tuberculous 017.9
    Brooke's (*see also* Trichoepithelioma)
            216.1
    Brown-Sequard 349.5
    Bruck-Lange 759.8
    Bruck's 723.9
    Bruhl's 285.8
    buccal cavity 528.9
    Buchman's 722.2

Disease, diseased—*continued*
  combined system   281.0
  compressed air   993.3
  Concato's
    peritoneal   569.9
    pleural - *see* Pleurisy
  congenital NEC   796.0
  conjunctiva   378.3
    viral NEC   078.9
  connective tissue, diffuse - *see* Disease,
    collagen
  Cooper's   610
  Corbus'   607.3
  cornea   378.4
  coronary (artery) (heart) (obstructive)
    (occlusive) (vascular) (*see also*
    Ischemia, heart)   412.9
    congenital   746.8
  Corrigan's (*see also* Endocarditis,
    aortic)   395.9
  cranial nerve (*see also* Atrophy, nerve,
    cranial)   356
  Crigler-Najjer   273.5
  Crohn's   563.0
  Crouzon's   756.0
  Cruchet's   065
    late effects   066
  Cruveilhier's   348.2
  Cushing's   258.0
  cystine storage (with renal sclerosis)
    270.3
  cytomegalic inclusion (generalized)
    079.5
  Darier's   757.2
    meaning erythema annulare
      centrifugum   695.0
    vitamin A deficiency   260.8
  Darling's   115
  de Beurmann-Gougerot   117.1
  de Quervain's   731.4
  deficiency   269.9
  Degos'   446.9
  Dejerine's   355.9
  Deleage's   330.4
  demyelinating, demyelinizating   341
    brain stem   341
    central nervous system   341
  Dercum's   279
  Deutschlander's - *see* Fracture, foot
  Devergie's   696.4
  Devic's   341
  di Guglielmo's   207.2
  diaphorase deficiency   289.9
  digestive system   569.9
  Dimitri-Sturge-Weber   759.8
  disc, degenerative - *see* Displacement,
    intervertebral disc

Disease, diseased—*continued*
  discogenetic - *see* Displacement,
    intervertebral disc
  diverticular - *see* Diverticula
  Drierzynsky's   723.9
  Dubini's   065
    late effects   066
  Dubois' (thymus gland)   090.5
  Duchenne-Griesinger   330.3
  Duchenne's   094.0
    locomotor ataxia   094.0
    paralysis   348.1
    pseudohypertrophy, muscles   330.3
  ductless glands   258.9
  Duhring's   693
  Dukes(-Filatow)   057.8
  Duplay's   717.1
  Dupuytren's   733.5
  Durand-Nicolas-Favre   099.1
  Duroziez's   746.6
  Dutton's   087.9
  Eales'   377.0
  ear (chronic) (inner) NEC   387.9
  Eberth's   001
  Ebstein's
    heart   746.6
    meaning diabetes - *see* category 250
  echinococcus (*see also* Cyst, hydatid)
    122.9
  Economo's   065
    late effects   066
  Eddowes'   756.6
  Edsall's   992.2
  Eichstedt's   111.0
  endocrine glands or system NEC
    258.9
  Engelmann's   756.7
  English (*see also* Rickets)   265.0
  Engman's   686.9
  enterovirus, central nervous system
    NEC   046
  epidemic NEC   136
  epididymis   607.9
  epigastric, functional   536.9
    psychogenic   305.5
  Erb-Goldflam   733.0
  Erb's   330.3
  Erichsen's   300.1
  esophagus   530.9
    functional   530.0
    psychogenic   305.5
  Eulenburg's   330.9
  eustachian tube   387.9
  external auditory canal   387.9
  extrapyramidal   347.9
  eye (anterior chamber)   378.9

Disease, diseased—*continued*
eye (anterior chamber)—*continued*
  inflammatory NEC 369.9
  muscle 378.9
eyeball 378.9
eyelid 378.2
Fabry's 272.2
facial nerve (seventh) 350
  newborn (*see also* Birth injury, bone
    or nerve) 772.2
Fahr-Volhard (*see also* Hypertension,
    malignant with renal
    involvement) 400.3
fallopian tube 615.9
familial periodic 276
fascia 733.9
  inflammatory 732
Feer's 985.0
Felix's 722.2
fibrocaseous of lung (*see also*
    Tuberculosis, pulmonary) 011.9
fibrocystic - *see* Fibrocystic disease
Fiedler's 100.0
fifth 057.0
Filatov's 075
file-cutters' 984
fish-skin 757.2
  acquired 701.1
Flajani's 242.0
Flatau-Schilder 341
flax-dressers' 516.1
Fleischner's 722.2
fluke - *see* Infestation, fluke
Folling's 270.0
foot and mouth 079.4
Fordyce-Fox 705.9
Fordyce's (mouth) 750.8
Fothergill's 351
  meaning scarlatina anginosa 034.1
Fournier's 607.9
fourth 057.8
Fox(-Fordyce) 705.9
Francis' 021
Franklin's 275.9
Frei's 099.1
Freiberg's 722.2
Friedreich's 347.9
  combined systemic 332.0
Frommel's 678
fungous NEC 117.9
Gaisbock's 289.0
gallbladder 576.9
  with calculus, cholelithiasis, stones
    574.9
  congenital 751.6
Gamna's 289.5

Disease, diseased—*continued*
Gandy-Nanta 289.5
gannister 515.0
  with tuberculosis 010
Garre's 720.1
gastric (*see also* Disease, stomach)
    537.9
gastro-intestinal (tract) 569.9
  amyloid 276
  functional 536.9
    psychogenic 305.5
Gaucher's (adult) (infantile) 272.2
Gee(-Herter)(-Thaysen) 269.0
generalized neoplastic 199.0
genital organs NEC
  female 629.9
  male 607.9
genito-urinary system, chronic,
    maternal, affecting fetus or
    newborn 760.5
Gerlier's 079.8
Gibert's 696.3
Gierke's 271.0
Gilchrist's 116.1
Gilford-Hutchinson 258.9
Gilles de la Tourette's 347.9
Giovannini's 117.9
gland (lymph) 289.9
Glanzmann's 287.3
glass-blowers' 527.1
Glenard's 569.9
Glisson's (*see also* Rickets) 265.0
glycogen storage (Andersen's) (Cori
    types 2-7) (Forbe's) (heart)
    (McArdle-Schmid-Pearson)
    (Pompe's) 271.1
  Cori type 1 271.0
  generalized 271.1
  glucose-6-phosphatase deficiency
    271.0
  hepatorenal 271.0
  liver and kidney 271.0
  myocardium 271.1
  von Gierke's 271.0
Goldflam-Erb 733.0
Goldscheider's 757.2
Goldstein's 448
gonococcal NEC 098.9
Graves' 242.0
Greenfield's 333.1
Greesley 078.2
Griesinger's (*see also* Ancylostomiasis)
    126.9
Gruby's 110.0
Guillain-Barre 354

Disease, diseased—*continued*
  Gull and Sutton's - *see* Hypertension,
      kidney
  Gull's 244
  gum NEC 523.9
  gynecological NEC 629.9
  H 270.2
  Haff 988.9
  Hailey-Hailey 757.2
  hair (follicles) NEC 704
  Hallopeau's 701.0
  Hand-Schuller-Christian 279
  hand, foot and mouth 074.9
  Hanot's - *see* Cirrhosis, biliary
  Hansen's 030.9
    benign form 030.1
    malignant form 030.0
  Harley's 283.9
  Hartnup 270.2
  Hashimoto's 245.1
  Hass' 722.2
  heart (organic) 429.9
    with
        acute pulmonary edema (*see also*
            Failure, ventricular, left)
            427.1
        hypertension (benign) (conditions in
            401) (*see also* Hypertension,
            heart) 402
        malignant (*see also*
            Hypertension, malignant
            with heart involvement)
            400.1
        rheumatic fever (conditions in 390)
            active 391.9
            inactive or quiescent (with
                chorea) 398
    amyloid 276
    and kidney - *see* Hypertension,
        cardiorenal
    aortic (valve) (*see also* Endocarditis,
        aortic) 395.9
    artery, arterial - *see* Ischemia, heart
    black 426
    congenital NEC 746.9
        maternal, affecting fetus or
            newborn 760.1
    congestive (*see also* Failure, heart,
        congestive) 427.0
    coronary (*see also* Ischemia, heart)
        412.9
    cryptogenic 425
    fetal 746.9
        inflammatory 746.8
    fibroid (*see also* Insufficiency,
        myocardial) 428

Disease, diseased—*continued*
  heart (organic)—*continued*
    functional (*see also* Action, heart,
        irregular) 427.9
    psychogenic 305.3
    glycogen storage 271.1
    gonococcal 098.8
    hypertensive (*see also* Hypertension,
        heart) 402
    malignant (*see also* Hypertension,
        malignant with heart
        involvement) 400.1
    hyperthyroid (*see also*
        Hyperthyroidism) 242.2
    incompletely diagnosed 429.9
    ischemic (*see also* Ischemia, heart)
        412.9
        asymptomatic 414.9
            with hypertensive disease
                (conditions in 400-404)
                414.0
        diagnosed on ECG but presenting
            no symptoms 414.9
            with hypertensive disease
                (conditions in 400-404)
                414.0
    kyphoscoliotic 426
    mitral (*see also* Endocarditis, mitral)
        394.9
    muscular (*see also* Insufficiency,
        myocardial) 428
    psychogenic (functional) 305.3
    pulmonary 426
    renal - *see* Hypertension, cardiorenal
    rheumatic (chronic) (inactive) (old)
        (quiescent) (with chorea) 398
        active or acute 391.9
            with chorea (acute) (rheumatic)
                (Sydenham's) 392.0
        maternal, affecting fetus or
            newborn 760.0
    rheumatoid - *see* Arthritis,
        rheumatoid
    senile (*see also* Insufficiency,
        myocardial) 428
    syphilitic 093.9
        aortic 093.9
        asymptomatic 093.9
        congenital 090.5
    thyroid (gland) (*see also*
        Hyperthyroidism) 242.2
    thyrotoxic (*see also* Thyrotoxicosis)
        242.2
    tuberculous 017.9
        late effects or sequela 019.9

Disease, diseased—*continued*
  heart (organic)—*continued*
    valve, valvular (obstructive)
        (regurgitant) - *see also*
        Endocarditis
      congenital 746.6
    vascular - *see* Ischemia, heart
  heart arteriosclerotic or sclerotic (senile)
      (*see also* Ischemia, heart) 412.9
  heavy chain 275.9
  Heberden's 713.0
  Hebra-Jadassohn 695.0
  Hebra's 695.9
    meaning
      erythema multiforme exudativum
          695.1
      prurigo 698.2
  Heerfordt's 135
  Heidenhain's 290.1
    with dementia 290.1
  Heine-Medin 043
    late effects 044
  Heller's 295.8
  hematopoietic organs 289.9
  hemoglobin or Hb
    abnormal (mixed) NEC 282.5
      with thalassemia 282.4
    C (Hb D) (Hb G) (Hb S) (high fetal
        gene) 282.5
      with other abnormal hemoglobin
          NEC 282.5
      elliptocytosis 282.5
      sickle cell 282.5
      thalassemia 282.4
    D 282.5
      with other abnormal hemoglobin
          NEC 282.5
      Hb S 282.5
      sickle cell 282.5
      thalassemia 282.4
    E 282.5
      with other abnormal hemoglobin
          NEC 282.5
      Hb S 282.5
      sickle cell 282.5
      thalassemia 282.4
    elliptocytosis 282.5
    H 282.4
      with other abnormal hemoglobin
          NEC 282.4
      thalassemia 282.4
    I thalassemia 282.4
    M 289.9
    S - *see* Disease, sickle cell
    spherocytosis 282.5

Disease, diseased—*continued*
  hemolytic (fetus) (newborn) 775.9
    with kernicterus or nervous affection
        774.9
    due to or with
      blood dyscrasia NEC 775.2
        with kernicterus or nervous
            affection 774.2
      congenital abnormal erythrocytes
          775.2
        with kernicterus or nervous
            affection 774.2
      incompatibility
        ABO (blood group) 775.1
          with kernicterus or nervous
              affection 774.1
        blood (group) (M, N, P) NEC
            775.2
          with kernicterus or nervous
              affection 774.2
        Rh (blood group) (factor) 775.0
          with kernicterus or nervous
              affection 774.0
      Rh negative mother 775.0
        with kernicterus or nervous
            affection 774.0
  hemorrhagic 287.9
    newborn 778.2
  Henoch's 287.0
  hepatic - *see* Disease, liver
  heredodegenerative NEC 333.9
    brain 333.9
    spinal cord 333.9
  Hers' 271.1
  Heubner's 094.9
  high fetal gene or hemoglobin
        thalassemia 282.4
  Hildenbrand's 081.9
  hip (joint) NEC 729.5
    congenital 755.7
    suppurative 729.5
    tuberculous 015.1
    late effect or sequela 019.4
  Hippel's 224
  Hirschsprung's 751.2
  His-Werner 083.2
  Hodgkin's 201
  Hodgson's 441.9
  Holla (*see also* Spherocytosis) 282.0
  hoof and mouth 079.4
  hookworm (*see also* Ancylostomiasis)
        126.9
  Horton's 446.4
  Huebner-Herter 269.0
  Huguier's 218
  Hunt's 347.9

Disease, diseased—*continued*
  Huntington's 331.0
  Huppert's 203
  Hurler's 273.8
  Hutchinson-Boeck 135
  Hutchinson-Gilford 258.9
  Hutchinson's 709.9
  hyaline (diffuse) (generalized) 734.9
    membrane (lung) (*see also* Hyaline
      membrane) 776.1
  hydatid (*see also* Cyst, hydatid) 122.9
  Hyde's 697.9
  hyperkinetic heart - *see* Disease, heart
  hypertensive (*see also* Hypertension)
    401
  hypophysis 253.9
  Iceland 065
    late effects 066
  ill-defined 796.0
  inclusion 079.5
    salivary gland 079.5
  infancy, early NEC 778.9
  infective NEC 136
  inguinal gland 289.9
  internal semilunar cartilage, cystic
    724.5
  intervertebral disc - *see* Displacement,
    intervertebral disc
  intestine 569.9
    functional 564.9
      psychogenic 305.5
    lardaceous 276
    organic 569.9
    protozoal NEC 007.9
  iris 378.6
  iron
    metabolism 279
    storage 273.2
  Jadassohn's 695.0
  Jakob-Creutzfeldt 333.9
    with dementia 290.1
  Jaksch-Luzet 285.8
  Janet's 300.8
  jaw NEC 526.9
    fibrocystic 526.2
  Jensen's 365
  jigger 134.2
  joint NEC 729.9
    ankle 729.9
    Charcot's 094.0
    degenerative (multiple) 713.0
      spine 713.1
    elbow 729.3
    finger 729.9
      flexion contracture 729.4
    hip 729.5

Disease, diseased—*continued*
  joint NEC—*continued*
    hypertrophic (chronic) (degenerative)
      713.0
      spine 713.1
    knee 729.8
      chondromalacia 729.7
      loose body or cartilage 729.6
    sacro-iliac 726
    shoulder 729.2
    spine 729.1
      degenerative or hypertrophic
        (chronic) 713.1
      pseudarthrosis following fusion
        729.0
      sacro-iliac 726
    toe 729.9
    wrist 729.9
  Jungling's 135
  Kahler's 203
  Kaposi's 757.2
    lichen ruber moniliformis 697.9
    xeroderma pigmentosum 757.2
  Katayama 120.2
  kidney (functional) (pelvis) (*see also*
    Disease, renal) 593.2
    cystic (multiple) congenital 753.1
    fibrocystic (congenital) 753.1
    in gout 274
    polycystic (congenital) 753.1
  Kienbock's 722.2
  Kimmelstiel(-Wilson) - *see* category 250
  kissing 075
  Klebs' (*see also* Nephritis) 583
  Klippel's 715
  Koebner's 757.2
  Kohler's 722.2
  Korsakoff's (alcoholic) 291.1
    nonalcoholic 299
  Krabbe's 333.1
  Kraepelin-Morel (*see also*
    Schizophrenia) 295.9
  Kraft-Weber-Dimitri 759.8
  Kuf's 333.0
  Kummell's 713.2
  Kundrat's 200.1
  kuru 347.9
  Kussmaul's 446.0
  Kyasanur Forest 067.2
  Kyrle's 704
  labyrinth, ear 387.9
  lachrymal, lacrimal (apparatus) (gland)
    (organs) 378.3
  Lafora's 331.2
  Lagleyze-von Hippel 224
  Landry's 354

Disease, diseased—*continued*
  mouth 528.9
  Munchmeyer's 733.2
  Murri's 283.9
  muscle 733.9
    inflammatory 732
    ocular 378.9
  musculoskeletal system 733.9
  mycotic 117.9
  myeloproliferative 209
  myocardium, myocardial (*see also*
      Insufficiency, myocardial) 428
    primary (idiopathic) 425
    uncommon 425
  Naegeli's 287.3
  nails 703.9
  nasal 508.9
  navel (newborn) 778.9
  neoplastic, generalized 199.0
  nervous system (central) 347.9
    congenital 743.9
    inflammatory 323
      late effects 324
    sympathetic 358.9
  Nettleship's 757.2
  Neumann's 694
  neuromuscular system NEC 348.9
  Newcastle 078.8
  Nicolas(-Durand)-Favre 099.1
  Niemann-Pick 272.2
  nipple 611.9
    Paget's 174
  nose 508.9
  nucleus pulposus - *see* Displacement,
      intervertebral disc
  nutritional 269.9
  Oguchi's (retina) 378.9
  Ohara's 021
  Ollier's 756.5
  Opitz's 289.5
  Oppenheim-Urbach - *see* category 250
  Oppenheim's 330.2
  optic nerve 377.6
  orbit 378.9
  Ormond's 593.3
  Osgood-Schlatter 722.2
  Osgood's tibia 722.2
  Osler-Rendu 448
  Osler-Vaquez 208
  Osler's 208
  osteofibrocystic 252.0
  Otto's (*see also* Otto's disease or pelvis)
      713.0
  outer ear 387.9
  ovary 615.9
    cystic 615.2

Disease, diseased—*continued*
  ovary—*continued*
    polycystic 256.9
  Owren's (*see also* Defect, coagulation)
      286.9
  Paget's 721
    bone 721
    breast 174
    malignant 174
    nipple 174
    scrotum 173.5
    skin - *see* Neoplasm, skin, malignant
  palate (soft) 528.9
  Paltauf-Sternberg 201
  pancreas 577.9
    cystic 577.9
      congenital 751.7
    fibrocystic 273.0
  Panner's 722.2
  panvalvular - *see* Endocarditis, mitral
  parametrium 616.9
  parasitic NEC 136
    cerebral NEC 123.9
    intestinal NEC 129
    mouth 112
    other specified site or type - *see*
        Infestation
    skin NEC 134.9
    tongue 112
  parathyroid (gland) 252.9
  Parkinson's 342
    late effects of viral encephalitis 066
    postencephalitic 066
  parodontal 523.9
  Parrot's 090.0
  Parry's 242.0
  Parson's 242.0
  Pavy's (*see also* Lesion, kidney) 593.2
  Paxton's 111.2
  pearl-workers' 720.1
  Pel-Ebstein 201
  Pelizaeus-Merzbacher 333.1
  Pellegrini-Stieda 729.8
  pelvis, pelvic
    female NEC 629.9
    gonococcal (acute) 098.0
      chronic or duration of 2 months or
          over 098.1
    inflammatory 616.0
      with
        abortion - *see* Abortion, by type,
            with sepsis
        ectopic gestation - *see* categories
            631.0-631.3
      arising during pregnancy 630
      fetus or newborn 763.1

Disease, diseased—*continued*
  pelvis, pelvic—*continued*
    inflammatory—*continued*
      puerperal, postpartum, childbirth
        670
      organ, female NEC 629.9
      peritoneum, female NEC 616.9
  penis 607.9
    inflammatory 607.5
  peptic NEC 796.0
  periapical tissues NEC 522.9
  periodic (familial) (Reimann's) NEC
    276
  periodontal NEC 523.9
  periosteum 723.9
  peripheral
    arterial 443.9
    autonomic nervous system 358.9
    nerves (*see also* Neuropathy) 357.9
    vascular NEC 443.9
  peritoneum 569.9
    pelvic, female NEC 616.9
  Perthes' 722.1
  Petit's (*see also* Hernia, diaphragm)
    551.3
  Peutz-Jeghers 211.9
  Peyronie's 607.9
  Pfeiffer's 075
  pharynx 508.9
  Phoca's 610
  photochromogenic (acid-fast bacilli)
    (pulmonary) 031.0
    nonpulmonary 031.9
  Pick's 272.2
    brain 290.1
    liver 423
  pineal gland 258.9
  pink 985.0
  Pinkus' 697.1
  pituitary (gland) 253.9
  placenta
    causing complicated delivery 661.8
    complicating pregnancy (delivered)
      (undelivered) 634.1
    fetus or newborn 770.8
  pleura (cavity) (*see also* Pleurisy)
    511.0
  Plummer's 242.1
  pneumatic
    drill 994.9
    hammer 994.9
  policeman's 355.1
  Pollitzer's 705.9
  polycystic (congenital) 758.8
    kidney or renal 753.1
    liver or hepatic 751.6

Disease, diseased—*continued*
  polycystic (congenital)—*continued*
    lung or pulmonary 748.4
    ovary, ovaries 256.9
    spleen 758.0
  Pompe's 271.1
  Poncet's 015.9
    late effect or sequela 019.6
  Pott's 015.0
    late effect or sequela 019.3
  Poulet's 712.3
  pregnancy NEC 634.9
  Preiser's 723.0
  Pringle's (*see also* Trichoepithelioma)
    216.1
  prostate 602
  protozoal NEC 136
    intestine, intestinal NEC 007.9
  psychiatric (*see also* Psychosis) 299
  psychotic (*see also* Psychosis) 299
  Puente's 528.5
  puerperal NEC (*see also* Puerperal)
    677.9
  pulmonary - *see also* Disease, lung
    artery 426
    heart 426
    valve (*see also* Endocarditis,
      pulmonary) 424.9
  pulp (dental) NEC 522.9
  pulseless 446.6
  Putnam's 281.0
  pyramidal tract 347.9
  Quervain's 731.4
  Quincke's - *see* Edema, angioneurotic
  Quinquaud's 704
  rag-sorters' 022
  Raynaud's 443.0
  Recklinghausen's (nerves) (skin) 743.4
    bones 252.0
  Reclus' 610
    cystic 610
  rectum NEC 569.2
  Reichmann's 536.0
  Reiter's 136
  renal (functional) (pelvis) 593.2
    with
      abortion - *see* Abortion, by type,
        with toxemia
      edema (*see also* Nephrosis) 581
      hypertension (benign) (conditions in
        401) (*see also* Hypertension,
        kidney) 403
      malignant (*see also*
        Hypertension, malignant
        with renal involvement)
        400.3

Disease, diseased—*continued*
renal—*continued*
  acute - *see* Nephritis, acute
  arising during pregnancy 636
    fetus or newborn 762.0
  chronic - *see* Nephritis, chronic
  cystic, congenital 753.1
  fibrocystic (congenital) 753.1
  hypertensive (*see also* Hypertension,
    kidney) 403
  polycystic (congenital) 753.1
  puerperal, postpartum 636
  subacute - *see* Nephritis, subacute
  tubular (*see also* Nephrosis, tubular)
    593.1
Rendu-Osler-Weber 448
renovascular (arteriosclerotic) (*see also*
  Hypertension, kidney) 403
respiratory 519.9
  chronic 519.9
  upper (acute) (multiple sites) NEC
    465
    streptococcal 034.0
retina, retinal 377.4
  Batten's or Batten-Mayou 333.0
  vascular lesion 377.0
rheumatic (*see also* Rheumatism) 718
  heart - *see* Disease, heart, rheumatic
rheumatoid (heart) - *see* Arthritis,
  rheumatoid
rickettsial NEC 083.9
  other specified NEC 083.8
Riga-Fede 529.0
Riggs' 523.4
Ritter's 695.9
Robinson's (*see also* Adenoma, sweat
  glands) 216.2
Roble's 125.3
Roger's 746.3
Rokitansky's (*see also* Necrosis, liver)
  570
Romberg's 356
Rosenthal's 286.2
Rossbach's 536.0
  psychogenic 305.5
Roth's 355.1
Rowland's 272.0
Rust's 015.0
  late effect or sequela 019.3
sacro-iliac NEC 726
salivary gland or duct NEC 527.9
  inclusion 079.5
  virus 079.5
Sander's 297.0
Sanders' 078.1
sandworm 133.9

Disease, diseased—*continued*
Savill's 695.9
Schamberg's 709.9
Schaumann's 135
Schenck's 117.1
Scheuermann's 722.0
Schilder(-Flatau) 341
Schimmelbusch's 610
Schlatter-Osgood 722.2
Schlatter's tibia 722.2
Schmorl's - *see* Displacement,
  intervertebral disc
Scholz's 333.1
Schonlein's 287.0
Schuller-Christian 279
Schultz's 288
sclera 378.6
scrofulous 017.1
  late effect or sequela 019.9
scrotum 607.9
sebaceous glands NEC 706.9
semilunar cartilage, cystic 724.5
seminal vesicle 607.9
Senear-Usher 694
serum NEC 999.5
Sever's 722.2
Shaver's 516.0
Sheehan's 253.1
shipyard 078.1
sickle cell (Hb C) (Hb D) (Hb E) (Hb
  G) (Hb J) (Hb K) (Hb O) (Hb P)
  (high fetal gene) 282.5
  with other abnormal hemoglobin
    NEC 282.5
  elliptocytosis 282.5
  spherocytosis 282.5
  thalassemia 282.4
silo-fillers' 516.2
Simmonds' 253.1
Simons' 279
Sinding-Larsen 722.2
sinus - *see also* Sinusitis
  brain 347.9
Sirkari's 085.0
sixth 057.1
Skevas-Zerfus 989.4
skin NEC 709.9
  due to metabolic disorder 279
South African creeping 133.9
specific NEC - *see* Syphilis
Spielmeyer-Stock 333.0
Spielmeyer-Vogt 333.0
spinal (cord) 349.9
  congenital 743.9
spine 723.9

Disease, diseased—*continued*
　spine—*continued*
　　joint (*see also* Disease, joint, spine)
　　　729.1
　　tuberculous - *see* Tuberculosis, spine
　spleen 289.5
　　amyloid 276
　　lardaceous 276
　　organic 289.5
　　polycystic 758.0
　　postinfectional 289.5
　sponge-divers' 989.4
　Stanton's 025
　Steinert's 330.4
　Sternberg's 201
　Stevens-Johnson 695.1
　Sticker's 057.0
　Still's 712.0
　Stiller's 790.1
　Stokes-Adams (*see also* Block, heart)
　　427.3
　Stokes' 242.0
　Stokvis(-Talma) 289.9
　stomach 537.9
　　functional 536.9
　　　psychogenic 305.5
　　lardaceous 276
　　organic 537.9
　stonemasons' 515.0
　　with tuberculosis 010
　storage 279
　　glycogen (*see also* Disease, glycogen
　　　storage) 271.1
　　mucopolysaccharide 273.8
　striato-pallidal system, hereditary NEC
　　331.9
　Strumpell-Marie 712.4
　Sturge(-Weber) 759.8
　Sudeck's 723.0
　supporting structures of teeth NEC
　　525.9
　suprarenal (gland) (capsule) 255.9
　Sutton and Gull's - *see* Hypertension,
　　kidney
　Sutton's 709.9
　sweat glands NEC 705.9
　sweating 136
　Swift(-Feer) 985.0
　swimming-pool (bacillus) 031.9
　sympathetic nervous system 358.9
　syphilitic - *see* Syphilis
　Taenzer's 757.2
　Takayasu's (pulseless) 446.6
　Talma's 733.9
　Tangier 272.1
　Tay-Sachs 333.0

Disease, diseased—*continued*
　Taylor's 701.9
　tear duct 378.3
　tendon 733.9
　　inflammatory NEC 732
　testicle 607.9
　Thomsen's 330.9
　Thomson's 757.2
　Thornwaldt's 508.9
　throat 508.9
　　septic 034.0
　thrombo-embolic (*see also* Embolism)
　　444.9
　thymus (gland) 254
　thyroid (gland) NEC 246
　　heart (*see also* Hyperthyroidism)
　　　242.2
　　lardaceous 276
　Tietze's 729.9
　Tommaselli's 961.3
　tongue 529.9
　tonsils, tonsillar (and adenoids) 500
　tooth, teeth 525.9
　　hard tissues NEC 521.9
　　pulp NEC 522.9
　trachea 464
　tricuspid - *see* Endocarditis, tricuspid
　trophoblastic (*see also* Hydatidiform
　　mole) 634.0
　tsutsugamushi 081.2
　tube (fallopian) 615.9
　tuberculous NEC (*see also*
　　Tuberculosis) 011.9
　tubo-ovarian 615.9
　　inflammatory (*see also* Salpingo-
　　　oophoritis) 614
　tympanum 387.9
　umbilicus (newborn) 778.9
　Underwood's 778.9
　Unna's 690
　Unverricht(-Lundborg) 331.2
　Urbach-Oppenheim - *see* category 250
　Urbach-Wiethe 279
　ureter 593.5
　urethra 599.9
　urinary 599.9
　　bladder 596.9
　　tract 599.9
　Usher-Senear 694
　uterus (organic) 625.9
　　infective (*see also* Endometritis)
　　　622.0
　uveal tract 378.6
　vagabonds' 132
　vagina, vaginal 629.9

Disease, diseased—*continued*
Valsuani's
of pregnancy 633.0
fetus or newborn 769.9
puerperal, postpartum, childbirth
676
valve, valvular - *see* Endocarditis
Van . !eck's 722.2
Vaquez-Osler 208
Vaquez's 208
vas deferens 607.9
vascular 458.9
arteriosclerotic - *see* Arteriosclerosis
hypertensive - *see* Hypertension
obliterative 447
peripheral 443.9
occlusive 458.9
peripheral (occlusive) 443.9
vasomotor 443.9
vasospastic 443.9
vein 458.9
venereal NEC 099.9
Verneuil's 095
Verse's 279
vertebra, vertebral NEC 723.9
disc - *see* Displacement,
intervertebral disc
vibration NEC 994.9
Vidal's 698.3
Vincent's 101
Virchow's 723.4
virus (filtrable) NEC 079.9
arthropod-borne NEC 068.9
vitreous 378.9
vocal cords 508.3
Vogt-Spielmeyer 333.0
Vogt's (Cecile) 331.9
Volhard-Fahr (*see also* Hypertension,
malignant with renal
involvement) 400.3
von Bechterew's 712.4
von Economo 065
late effects 066
von Gierke's 271.0
von Graefe's 373.9
von Hippel-Lindau 759.8
von Hippel's 224
von Jaksch's 285.8
von Recklinghausen-Appelbaum 273.2
von Recklinghausen's (nerves) (skin)
743.4
bones 252.0
malignant 192.4
von Willebrand(-Jurgens') 286.3
Vrolik's 756.6
vulva 629.9

Disease, diseased—*continued*
Wagner's 709.9
Waldenstrom's 722.1
Wardrop's (with lymphangitis) 681
wasting NEC 796.0
Waterhouse-Friderichsen 036.1
with meningitis 036.0
waxy (any site) 276
Weber-Christian 686.9
Weil's 100.0
of lung 100.0
Werlhof's (*see also* Thrombocytopenia)
287.1
Werner's 258.9
Whipple's 039.9
white-spot 709.9
Whitmore's 025
Wilson's 273.3
Winckel's (*see also* Septicemia) 038.9
winter vomiting 079.8
woolsorters' 022
Ziehen-Oppenheimer 331.1
zoonotic, bacterial NEC 027.9
Disfigurement (facial) (head) 709.9
due to scar 709.0
Disgerminoma - *see* Dysgerminoma
Disinsertion, retina 376
Disintegration, complete, of the body
796.2
traumatic 869.1
Dislocation (articular) 839.7

Note — The following fourth-digit subdivisions are for use with categories 830–838:
.0 *Simple*
.1 *Compound*
.9 *Late effect*
"Simple" includes closed, complete, partial, uncomplicated, and unspecified dislocation.
"Compound" includes dislocation specified as infected or open and dislocation with foreign body.
"Chronic," "habitual," "old" or "recurrent" dislocations should be coded as indicated under the entry "Dislocation, recurrent"; and "pathological" as indicated under the entry "Dislocation, pathological."

---

with fracture - *see* Fracture
acromioclavicular (joint) 831
anatomical site
specified (simple) NEC 839.5
compound 839.6
late effect 839.9

Dislocation (articular) — *continued*
  anatomical site — *continued*
    unspecified or ill-defined (simple)
        839.7
      compound   839.8
      late effect   839.9
  ankle (scaphoid bone)   837
  arm (simple)   839.7
    compound   839.8
    late effect   839.9
  astragalus   837
  atlantoaxial (simple)   839.0
    compound   839.1
    late effect   839.9
  ·atlas (simple)   839.0
    compound   839.1
    late effect   839.9
  axis (simple)   839.0
    compound   839.1
    late effect   839.9
  back (simple)   839.7
    compound   839.8
    late effect   839.9
  breast bone (simple)   839.5
    compound   839.6
    late effect   839.9
  capsule, joint - *code by* site under
        Dislocation
  carpal (bone)   833
  carpometacarpal (joint)   833
  cartilage (joint) - *code by* site under
        Dislocation
  cervical, cervicodorsal, or
        cervicothoracic (spine)
        (vertebrae) (simple)   839.0
    compound   839.1
    late effect   839.9
  chiropractic - *code by* site under
        Dislocation
  chronic - *see* Dislocation, recurrent
  clavicle   831
  coccyx (simple)   839.5
    compound   839.6
    late effect   839.9
  collar bone   831
  congenital NEC   755.9
  coracoid   831
  costal cartilage (simple)   839.5
    compound   839.6
    late effect   839.9
  costochondral (simple)   839.5
    compound   839.6
    late effect   839.9
  cricoarytenoid articulation (simple)
        839.5
    compound   839.6

Dislocation (articular) — *continued*
  cricoarytenoid   articulation — *continued*
      late effect   839.9
  cricothyroid articulation (simple)   839.5
    compound   839.6
    late effect   839.9
  dorsal vertebrae (simple)   839.5
    compound   839.6
    late effect   839.9
  elbow   832
    recurrent   724.2
  eye   871
  eyeball   871
  femur
    distal end   836
    proximal end   835
  fibula
    distal end   837
    proximal end   836
  finger(s)   834
  foot   838
  forearm (simple)   839.7
    compound   839.8
    late effect   839.9
  fracture - *see* Fracture
  glenoid   831
  habitual - *see* Dislocation, recurrent
  hand (simple)   839.7
    compound   839.8
    late effect   839.9
  hip   835
    congenital   755.6
    recurrent   724.9
  humerus
    distal end   832
    proximal end   831
  infracoracoid   831
  innominate (pubic junction) (sacral
        junction) (simple)   839.5
    acetabulum   835
    compound   839.6
    late effect   839.9
  interphalangeal (joint)
    finger or hand   834
    foot or toe   838
  jaw (cartilage) (meniscus)   830
  knee (meniscus) (semilunar cartilage)
        836
    congenital   755.7
    habitual   724.4
    old   724.4
    recurrent   724.4
  lachrymal, lacrimal gland   378.3
  leg (simple)   839.7
    compound   839.8
    late effect   839.9

Dislocation (articular)—*continued*
  lens (complete) (crystalline) (partial)
    378.8
    congenital 744.8
    traumatic 921
  ligament - *code by* site under
    Dislocation
  lumbar (vertebrae) (simple) 839.5
    compound 839.6
    late effect 839.9
  lumbosacral (vertebrae) (simple) 839.5
    compound 839.6
    congenital 756.1
    late effect 839.9
  mandible 830
  maxilla (inferior) 830
  meniscus (knee) - *see* Dislocation, knee
  other sites - *code by* site under
    Dislocation
  metacarpal (bone)
    distal end 834
    proximal end 833
  metacarpophalangeal (joint) 834
  metatarsal (bone) 838
  metatarsophalangeal (joint) 838
  midcarpal (joint) 833
  midtarsal (joint) 838
  multiple locations (except fingers only
      or toes only) 839.7
    compound 839.8
    late effect 839.9
  navicular (bone) foot 837
  neck (simple) 839.0
    compound 839.1
    late effect 839.9
  nose (simple) 839.5
    compound 839.6
    late effect 839.9
  occiput from atlas (simple) 839.0
    compound 839.1
    late effect 839.9
  old - *see* Dislocation, recurrent
  paralytic (flaccid) (spastic) - *see*
      Dislocation, pathological
  patella 836
    congenital 755.7
  pathological 729.9
    ankle (sites classifiable to 837)
      729.9
    elbow (sites classifiable to 832)
      729.3
    finger (sites classifiable to 834)
      729.9
    hip (sites classifiable to 835) 729.5
    knee (sites classifiable to 836) 729.8
    lumbosacral joint 729.1

Dislocation (articular)—*continued*
  pathological—*continued*
    postpoliomyelitic 044
    sacro-iliac 726
    shoulder (sites classifiable to 831)
      729.2
    spine 729.1
    toe 729.9
    wrist (sites classifiable to 833) 729.9
  pelvis (simple) 839.5
    acetabulum 835
    compound 839.6
    late effect 839.9
  phalanx
    finger or hand 834
    foot or toe 838
  postpoliomyelitic 044
  radiocarpal (joint) 833
  radioulnar (joint)
    distal 833
    proximal 832
  radius
    distal end 833
    proximal end 832
  recurrent 724.9
    elbow (sites classifiable to 832)
      724.2
    hip (sites classifiable to 835) 724.9
    joint NEC 724.9
    knee (sites classifiable to 836) 724.4
    patella 724.4
    sacro-iliac 726
    shoulder (sites classifiable to 831)
      724.0
  rib (cartilage) (simple) 839.5
    compound 839.6
    congenital 756.4
    late effect 839.9
  sacrococcygeal (simple) 839.5
    compound 839.6
    late effect 839.9
  sacro-iliac (joint) (ligament) (simple)
      839.5
    compound 839.6
    congenital 755.7
    late effect 839.9
    recurrent 726
  sacrum (simple) 839.5
    compound 839.6
    late effect 839.9
  scaphoid (bone)
    ankle or foot 837
    wrist 833
  scapula 831
  semilunar cartilage, knee - *see*
      Dislocation, knee

Dislocation (articular)—*continued*
  septal cartilage (nose) (simple) 839.5
    compound 839.6
    late effect 839.9
  septum (nasal) (old) 504
  sesamoid bone - *code by* site under
      Dislocation
  shoulder (blade) (ligament) 831
    chronic 724.0
    recurrent 724.0
  skull (*see also* Injury, intracranial)
      854.0
  spine (*see also* Dislocation, vertebrae)
      839.5
    congenital 756.2
  sternoclavicular (joint) 831
  sternum (simple) 839.5
    compound 839.6
    late effect 839.9
  subglenoid 831
  symphysis
    jaw 830
    mandibular 830
    pubis (simple) 839.5
      compound 839.6
      late effect 839.9
  tarsal (bone) (joint) 838
  tarsometatarsal (joint) 838
  temporomandibular (joint) 830
  thigh
    distal end 836
    proximal end 835
  thoracic (vertebrae) (simple) 839.5
    compound 839.6
    late effect 839.9
  thumb 834
  thyroid cartilage (simple) 839.5
    compound 839.6
    late effect 839.9
  tibia
    distal end 837
    proximal end 836
  tibiofibular (joint)
    distal 837
    superior 836
  toe(s) 838
  trachea (simple) 839.5
    compound 839.6
    late effect 839.9
  ulna
    distal end 833
    proximal end 832
  vertebrae (articular process) (body)
      (simple) 839.5
    cervical, cervicodorsal or
        cervicothoracic (simple) 839.0
      compound 839.1

Dislocation (articular)—*continued*
  vertebrae, etc.—*continued*
    cervical, etc.—*continued*
      late effect 839.9
      compound 839.6
      congenital 756.2
      late effect 839.9
  wrist (scaphoid) (semilunar) (carpal
      bone) 833
  xiphoid cartilage (simple) 839.5
    compound 839.6
    late effect 839.9
Disobedience, child 308
Disorder - *see also* Disease
  accommodation 370.9
  affective (*see also* Psychosis, affective)
      296.9
  allergic (*see also* Allergy) 692.9
  amino-acid
    metabolism NEC 270.9
    renal transport NEC 270.2
  anerobic glycolosis with anemia 282.3
  articulation (*see also* Disease, joint)
      729.9
    psychogenic 305.1
  behavior NEC 306.9
    childhood (primary) 308
  carbohydrate metabolism, congenital
      271.9
  cardiac, functional (*see also* Action,
      heart, irregular) 427.9
  cardiovascular system, psychogenic
      305.3
  character NEC 301.9
  convulsive (secondary) (*see also*
      Convulsions) ˙780.2
  degradation
    branched chain amino-acid 270.4
  dentition 520.6
  digestive 536.9
    psychogenic 305.5
    system, psychogenic 305.5
  emotional (*see also* Disorder, mental)
      300.9
  endocrine 258.9
  esophagus 530.9
    functional 530.0
    psychogenic 305.5
  gastric (functional) 536.9
    motility 536.1
    psychogenic 305.5
    secretion 536.0
  gastro-intestinal (functional) NEC
      536.9
    psychogenic 305.5
  genito-urinary system, psychogenic
      305.6

Disorder—*continued*
  heart action (*see also* Action, heart,
      irregular) 427.9
  hematopoietic organs 289.9
  hemostasis, congenital (*see also* Defect,
      coagulation) 286.9
  intestinal, functional NEC 564.9
    psychogenic 305.5
  joint (*see also* Disease, joint) 729.9
    psychogenic 305.1
  kidney (functional) (*see also* Lesion,
      kidney) 593.2
  lactation 678
    puerperal, postpartum 678
  limb, psychogenic 305.1
  lipid
    metabolism, congenital 272.9
    storage 272.2
  lipoprotein deficiency, familial 272.1
  low back 729.1
    psychogenic 305.1
  menstrual NEC 626.9
    psychogenic 305.6
  mental (non-psychotic) 300.9
    due to or associated with
      abscess
        brain 309.0
      addiction
        alcohol 303.2
        drug - *see* listing under
            Dependence
      alcoholism - *see* category 303
      atrophy
        cerebral, senile 309.6
      bacteremia 309.1
      bronchopneumonia 309.1
      chorea
        Huntington's 309.8
      concussion 309.2
      contusion, cerebral 309.2
      degeneration
        brain 309.8
          senile 309.6
        central nervous system 309.8
        cerebral 309.8
          senile 309.6
      dependence
        alcohol 303.2
        drug - *see* listing under
            Dependence
      disease
        brain
          degenerative 309.8
          infective 309.0
          inflammatory 309.0
          neoplastic 309.7

Disorder—*continued*
  mental (non-psychotic)—*continued*
    due to, etc.—*continued*
      disease—*continued*
        brain—*continued*
          senile, presenile 309.6
          syphilitic 309.0
          tuberculous 309.0
          vascular 309.3
        circulatory (conditions in 393-
            458) 309.3
        degenerative, central nervous
            system 309.8
        endocrine (conditions in 240-258)
            309.5
        Jakob-Creutzfeldt 309.6
        metabolic (conditions in 240-258,
            270-279) 309.5
        nutritional (conditions in 260-
            269) 309.5
        Pelizaeus-Merzbacher 309.8
        Schilder's 309.8
      disorder
        circulatory (conditions in 393-
            458) 309.3
      disturbance
        circulatory (conditions in 393-
            458) 309.3
        growth 309.5
        metabolism, metabolic
            (conditions in 240-258,
            270-279) 309.5
        nutrition (conditions in 260-269)
            309.5
      electrocution trauma to brain
          309.2
      encephalitis 309.0
        specified type NEC 309.0
        traumatic 309.2
      encephalomyelitis 309.0
      epilepsy (conditions in 345) 309.4
      fever 309.1
        rheumatic, acute 309.1
        typhoid 309.1
        typhus 309.1
      fracture
        face bones 309.2
        skull (base) (vault) 309.2
      hemorrhage
        cerebral 309.3
          following injury 309.2
        extradural 309.3
          following injury 309.2
        subarachnoid 309.3
          following injury 309.2
        subdural 309.3
          following injury 309.2

Disorder—*continued*
  mental (non-psychotic)—*continued*
    due to, etc.—*continued*
      hypoxia (at birth) 309.2
      infection
        brain 309.0
        generalized 309.1
        intracranial 309.0
        systemic 309.1
      inflammation
        brain 309.0
      influenza 309.1
      injury
        brain (birth) (from electric
            current) (surgical) 309.2
        intracranial (conditions in 850-
            854) 309.2
      intoxication (alcoholic) - *see*
          category 303
        drug (acute) 309.1
          chronic - *see* listing under
              Dependence
        poison 309.1
        systemic 309.1
      Jakob-Creutzfeldt disease 309.6
      laceration, cerebral 309.2
      malaria 309.1
      meningitis 309.0
      neoplasm (benign) (malignant)
        brain 309.7
        cerebral (meninges) 309.7
        intracranial 309.7
        pineal (gland) 309.7
        pituitary (gland) 309.7
      physical condition NEC 309.9
      pneumonia 309.1
      poisoning (acute) 309.1
        blood 309.1
        chronic 309.1
          drug - *see* listing under
              Dependence
      pre-senility 309.6
      sclerosis
        brain 309.8
        multiple 309.8
      senility 309.6
      septicemia 309.1
      space-occupying lesion, brain
          309.7
      surgery, brain 309.2
      syphilis
        central nervous system 309.0
      trauma
        brain (birth) (from electric
            current) (surgical) 309.2
      tuberculosis 309.1

Disorder—*continued*
  mental (non-psychotic)—*continued*
    due to, etc.—*continued*
      tuberculosis—*continued*
        brain 309.0
        typhoid (fever) 309.1
        typhus (fever) 309.1
    neurotic (*see also* Neurosis) 300.9
    presbyophrenic type 309.6
    presenile 309.6
      psychotic NEC 290.1
    psychoneurotic (*see also* Neurosis)
        300.9
    psychotic (*see also* Psychosis) 299
    senile 309.6
      psychotic NEC 290.0
  metabolism NEC 279
    congenital 273.9
  micturition NEC - *see also* category
      786
    psychogenic 305.6
  movement (organic) 733.9
    hysterical 300.1
  muscle 733.9
    psychogenic 305.1
  musculoskeletal system, psychogenic
      305.1
  neurological NEC 796.0
  neuromuscular NEC 348.9
    hereditary NEC 330.9
  pancreatic internal secretion other than
      diabetes mellitus 251
  paroxysmal, mixed 780.2
  pentose phosphate pathway with
      anemia 282.3
  personality 301.9
    affective 301.1
    aggressive 301.3
    amoral 301.7
    anancastic 301.4
    anankastic 301.4
    antisocial 301.7
    asocial 301.7
    asthenic 301.6
    compulsive 301.4
    cyclothymic 301.1
    due to or associated with physical
        disorder - *see* listing under
        Disorder, mental
    dyssocial 301.7
    emotional instability 301.5
    explosive 301.3
    histrionic 301.5
    hyperthymic 301.1
    hypothymic 301.1
    hysterical 301.5

Disorder—*continued*
  personality—*continued*
    immature 301.8
    inadequate 301.6
    labile 301.5
    moral deficiency 301.7
    obsessional 301.4
    obsessive(-compulsive) 301.4
    paranoid 301.0
    passive-aggressive 301.8
    passive(-dependent) 301.6
    pathological NEC 301.9
    pseudosocial 301.7
    psychopathic 301.7
    schizoid 301.2
    unstable 301.8
  pigmentation, choroid (congenital)
      744.8
  pituitary, thalamic 258.1
  psychogenic NEC (*see also* conditioi)
      300.9
    allergic NEC 305.0
      respiratory 305.2
    anxiety 300.0
    appetite 306.5
    articulation
      joint 305.1
    asthenic 300.5
    blood 305.4
    cardiovascular (system) 305.3
    compulsive 300.3
    cutaneous 305.0
    depressive 300.4
    digestive (system) 305.5
    dysmennorrheic 305.6
    dyspneic 305.2
    eczematous 305.0
    endocrine (system) 305.7
    eye 305.8
    feeding 306.5
    functional NEC 305.9
    gastric 305.5
    gastro-intestinal (system) 305.5
    genito-urinary (system) 305.6
    heart (function) (rhythm) 305.3
    hemic 305.4
    hyperventilatory 305.2
    hypochondriacal 300.7
    hysterical 300.1
    intestinal 305.5
    joint 305.1
    learning 306.1
    limb 305.1
    lymphatic (system) 305.4
    menstrual 305.6
    micturition 305.6

Disorder—*continued*
  psychogenic NEC—*continued*
    motor 306.3
    muscle 305.1
    musculo-skeletal 305.1
    neurocirculatory 305.3
    obsessive 300.3
    occupational 300.8
    organ or part of body NEC 305.9
    organs of special sense 305.8
    paralytic NEC 305.1
    phobic 300.2
    physical NEC 305.9
    pruritic 305.0
    rectal 305.5
    respiratory (system) 305.2
    rheumatic 305.1
    sexual (function) 305.6
    skin (allergic) (pruritic) (eczematous)
        305.0
    sleep 306.4
    specified part of body NEC 305.9
    stomach 305.5
  psychomotor NEC 306.3
    hysterical 300.1
  psychoneurotic (*see also* Neurosis)
      300.9
    mixed NEC 300.8
  psychophysiologic (*see also* Disorder,
      psychosomatic) 305.9
  psychosexual 305.6
  psychosomatic NEC 305.9
    allergic NEC 305.0
      respiratory 305.2
    articulation, joint 305.1
    blood 305.4
    cardiovascular (system) 305.3
    cutaneous 305.0
    digestive (system) 305.5
    dysmennorrheic 305.6
    dyspneic 305.2
    eczematous 305.0
    endocrine (system) 305.7
    eye 305.8
    gastric 305.5
    gastro-intestinal (system) 305.5
    genito-urinary (system) 305.6
    heart (function) (rhythm) 305.3
    hemic 305.4
    hyperventilatory 305.2
    intestinal 305.5
    joint 305.1
    limb 305.1
    lymphatic (system) 305.4
    menstrual 305.6
    micturition 305.6

Disorder—*continued*
  psychosomatic NEC—*continued*
    monoplegic NEC 305.1
    muscle 305.1
    musculo-skeletal 305.1
    neurocirculatory 305.3
    organs of special sense 305.8
    paralytic NEC 305.1
    pruritic 305.0
    rectal 305.5
    respiratory (system) 305.2
    rheumatic 305.1
    sexual (function) 305.6
    skin (allergic) (eczematous) (pruritic)
        305.0
    specified part of body NEC 305.9
    stomach 305.5
  purine metabolism 270.5
  pyrimidine metabolism 270.5
  reflex 780.3
  respiration, psychogenic 305.2
  seizure 780.2
  sense of smell 781.4
    psychogenic 305.8
  sexual function, psychogenic 305.6
  skin NEC 709.9
    psychogenic (allergic) (eczematous)
        (pruritic) 305.0
  sleep 780.6
    non-organic origin 306.4
  speech NEC 306.9
    secondary to organic lesion 781.5
  steroid metabolism NEC 273.6
  stomach (functional) (*see also* Disorder,
        gastric) 536.9
  substitution 300.1
  tooth development NEC 520.9
Disorganized globe 378.9

Disorientation 306.9

Displacement, displaced
  acquired traumatic of bone, cartilage,
        joint, tendon NEC (without
        fracture) - *see* Dislocation
  adrenal gland (congenital) 758.1
  appendix retrocecal (congenital) 751.4
  auricle (congenital) 745.2
  bladder (acquired) 596.9
    congenital 753.8
  brachial plexus (congenital) 743.8
  brain stem, caudal 743.2
  canuliculus (lacrimalis) 744.8
  cerebellum, caudal 743.2
  cervix (*see also* Malposition, uterus)
        624.9
  colon (congenital) 751.1

Displacement, displaced—*continued*
  epithelium
    columnar of cervix 621.9
    cuboidal, beyond limits of external os
        752.5
  esophageal mucosa into cardia of
        stomach, congenital 750.8
  esophagus (acquired) 530.9
    congenital 750.8
  eyeball (acquired) (old) 378.9
    congenital 744.8
    current 871
  fallopian tube (acquired) 615.9
    congenital 752.5
    opening (congenital) 752.5
  gallbladder (congenital) 751.6
  gastric mucosa 750.8
    into
      duodenum 750.8
      esophagus 750.8
      Meckel's diverticulum 751.0
  globe (acquired) (old) 378.9
    current 871
  heart (congenital) 746.8
    acquired - *see* Disease, heart
  hymen (upward) (congenital) 752.6
  intervertebral disc (with neuritis,
        radiculitis, sciatica, or other pain)
        725.9
    cervical, cervicodorsal,
        cervicothoracic 725.0
      due to major trauma - *see*
          Dislocation, cervical
    due to major trauma - *see*
        Dislocation, vertebrae
    lumbar, lumbosacral 725.1
      due to major trauma - *see*
          Dislocation, lumbar
    specified NEC 725.8
      due to major trauma - *see*
          Dislocation, vertebrae
  kidney (acquired) (*see also* Lesion,
        kidney) 593.2
    congenital 753.3
  lachrymal, lacrimal apparatus or duct
        (congenital) 744.8
  macula (congenital) 744.8
  Meckel's diverticulum (congenital)
        751.0
  nail (congenital) 757.4
    acquired 703.9
  opening of Wharton's duct in mouth
        750.8
  organ or site, congenital NEC - *see*
        Malposition, congenital
  ovary (acquired) 615.0

Displacement, displaced—*continued*
  ovary (acquired)—*continued*
    congenital 752.5
    free in peritoneal cavity 752.5
    into hernial sac 615.0
    oviduct (acquired) 615.9
    congenital 752.5
  parotid gland (congenital) 750.8
  punctum lacrimale (congenital) 744.8
  sacro-iliac (joint) (congenital) 755.7
    current injury - *see* Dislocation,
      sacro-iliac
    old 726
  spleen, congenital 758.0
  stomach (congenital) 750.8
    acquired 537.9
    into thorax - *see* Hernia, diaphragm
  sublingual duct (congenital) 750.8
  tongue (downward) 750.0
  tooth, teeth 524.3
  trachea (congenital) 748.3
  ureter, opening (congenital) 753.4
  uterine opening of oviducts or fallopian
    tubes 752.5
  uterus, uterine (*see also* Malposition,
    uterus) 624.9
  ventricular septum 746.8
  with rudimentary ventricle 746.8
Disproportion (cephalopelvic) (fetus and
    pelvic) (shoulder and outlet)
  complicating delivery 655
    fetus or newborn - *see* categories
      765.0-765.9
  pelvis, pelvic (bony)
    complicating delivery - *see*
      Deformity, pelvis, complicating
      delivery
    noted during pregnancy (undelivered)
      634.9
Disruptio uteri, complicating delivery -
    see Rupture, uterus, complicating
    delivery
Disruption operation wound 998.3
Dissecting - *see* condition
Dissection
  aorta 441.0
  vascular 458.9
  wound - *see* Wound, open
Disseminated - *see* condition
Dissociation, auriculoventricular or
    atrioventricular (any degree) (*see*
    also Block, heart) 427.3
Dissociative reaction, state 300.1
Dissolution, vertebra 723.9
Distension
  abdomen 785.4

Distension—*continued*
  bladder 596.9
  cecum 569.9
  colon 569.9
  gallbladder (*see also* Disease,
    gallbladder) 576.9
  intestine 569.9
  kidney (*see also* Lesion, kidney) 593.2
  liver 573.9
  seminal vesicle 607.9
  stomach 536.1
    psychogenic 305.5
  ureter 593.5
  uterus 625.9
Distichia, distichiasis (eyelid) 744.8
Distoma hepaticum infestation 121.3
Distomiasis 121.9
  bile passages 121.3
    due to Clonorchis sinensis 121.1
  hemic 120.9
  hepatic 121.3
    due to Clonorchis sinensis 121.1
  intestinal 121.4
  liver 121.3
    due to Clonorchis sinensis 121.1
  lung 121.2
  pancreas 121.9
  pulmonary 121.2
Distomolar (fourth molar) 520.1
  causing crowding 524.3
Disto-occlusion 524.2
Distortion (congenital)
  adrenal (gland) 758.1
  ankle (joint) 755.7
  anus 751.4
  aorta 747.2
  appendix 751.4
  arm 755.5
  artery (peripheral) 747.6
    cerebral 747.8
    coronary 746.8
    pulmonary 747.6
    retinal 744.8
    umbilical 747.5
  auditory canal 745.2
    causing impairment of hearing 745.0
  bile duct or passage 751.6
  bladder 753.8
  brain 743.2
  bronchus 748.3
  cecum 751.4
  cervix (uteri) 752.5
  chest (wall) 756.4
  clavicle 755.5
  clitoris 752.6
  coccyx 756.2

Distortion (congenital)—*continued*
  colon   751.4
  common duct   751.6
  cornea   744.8
  cricoid cartilage   748.3
  cystic duct   751.6
  duodenum   751.4
  ear (auricle) (external)   745.2
    causing impairment of hearing   745.0
    inner   745.0
    middle   745.0
    ossicles   745.0
  endocrine (gland) NEC   758.3
  epiglottis   748.3
  eustachian tube   745.2
  eye (adnexa)   744.8
  face bone(s)   756.0
  fallopian tube   752.5
  femur   755.7
  fibula   755.7
  finger(s)   755.5
  foot   755.7
  gallbladder   751.6
  genitalia, genital organ(s)
    female   752.8
      external   752.6
      internal NEC   752.5
    male   752.8
  glottis   748.3
  gyri   743.2
  hand bone(s)   755.5
  heart (auricle) (ventricle)   746.8
    valve (cusp)   746.6
  hepatic duct   751.6
  humerus   755.5
  hymen   752.6
  ileum   751.4
  intestine (large) (small)   751.4
    with anomalous adhesions, fixation or
        malrotation   751.1
  jaw - *see* categories 524.0-524.9
  jejunum   751.4
  kidney   753.3
  knee (joint)   755.7
  labium (majus) (minus)   752.6
  larynx   748.3
  leg   755.7
  lens   744.8
  liver   751.6

  lumbar spine   756.1
    complicating delivery - *see*
        Deformity, pelvis, complicating
        delivery
    noted during pregnancy (undelivered)
        634.9
  lumbosacral (joint) (region)   756.1

Distortion (congenital)—*continued*
  lung (fissures) (lobe)   748.6
  nerve   743.8
  nose   748.1
  organ
    of Corti   745.0
    or site not listed - *see* Anomaly,
        specified type NEC
  ossicles, ear   745.0
  ovary   752.5
  oviduct   752.5
  pancreas   751.7
  parathyroid (gland)   758.3
  patella   755.7
  peripheral vascular system   747.6
  pituitary (gland)   758.3
  radius   755.5
  rectum   751.4
  rib   756.4
  sacroiliac joint   755.7
  sacrum   756.1
  scapula   755.5
  shoulder girdle   755.5
  skull bone(s)   756.0
    with
      anencephalus   740
      encephalocele   743.0
      hydrocephalus   742
        with spina bifida   741.0
      microcephalus   743.1
  spinal cord   743.3
  spine   756.2
  spleen   758.0
  sternum   756.4
  thorax (wall)   756.4
  thymus (gland)   758.3
  thyroid (gland)   758.2
    cartilage   748.3
  tibia   755.7
  toe(s)   755.7
  tongue   750.0
  trachea (cartilage)   748.3
  ulna   755.5
  ureter   753.4
    causing obstruction   753.2
  urethra   753.8
    causing obstruction   753.6
  uterus   752.5
  vagina   752.6
  vein (peripheral)   747.6
    great   747.4
    portal   747.4
    pulmonary   747.4
  vena cava (inferior) (superior)   747.4
  vertebra   756.2
  vulva   752.6

Distortion (congenital) — *continued*
  wrist (bones) (joint) 755.5
Distress
  abdomen 785.5
  epigastric 785.5
  fetal (syndrome) 776.3
    with
      abnormality of
        bones, organs or tissues of pelvis
          - *see* categories 764.0-
          764.4
        forces of labor - *see* categories
          767.0-767.4
        difficult labor NEC - *see* categories
          768.0-768.4
        disproportion, fetopelvic - *see*
          categories 765.0-765.4
          with abnormality of bones,
            organs or tissues of pelvis
            - *see* categories 764.0-
            764.4
        malposition of fetus - *see* categories
          766.0-766.4
  gastro-intestinal (functional) 536.9
    psychogenic 305.5
  intestinal (functional) NEC 564.9
    psychogenic 305.5
  leg 787.1
  respiratory 783.2
    fetus or newborn (*see also* Syndrome,
      respiratory distress) 776.2
  stomach 536.9
    psychogenic 305.5
Distribution vessel, atypical 747.6
  coronary artery 746.8
  spinal 747.6
Districhiasis 704
Disturbance - *see also* Disease
  absorption
    calcium 269.9
    carbohydrate 269.0
    fat 269.0
    protein 269.0
    vitamin (*see also* Deficiency, vitamin)
      266.9
  acid-base equilibrium 788.0
  assimilation, food 269.1
  auditory nerve, except deafness 781.3
  behavior 306.9
    child 308
  blood clotting (mechanism) (*see also*
    Defect, coagulation) 286.9
    hypoproteinemia 286.9
  cerebral nerve NEC 781.4
  circulatory 458.9
  conduct, child 308

Disturbance — *continued*
  co-ordination 780.4
  cortical sensibility 781.6
  cranial nerve NEC 781.4
  deep sensibility - *see* Disturbance,
    sensation
  digestive 536.9
    psychogenic 305.5
  emotional 306.9
  endocrine (gland) 258.9
  equilibrium 780.5
  feeding 306.5
    infant 269.9
    psychogenic, NEC 306.5
  fructose metabolism 271.3
  gait 787.6
    hysterical 300.1
  gastric (functional) 536.9
    motility 536.1
    psychogenic 305.5
    secretion 536.0
  gastro-intestinal (functional) 536.9
    psychogenic 305.5
  habit, child 308
  hearing, except deafness 781.3
  heart, functional (*see also* Action, heart,
    irregular) 427.9
  hormones 258.9
  innervation uterus, sympathetic,
    parasympathetic 625.9
  keratinization NEC
    gingiva 528.7
    lip 528.7
    oral (mucosa) (soft tissue) 528.7
    tongue 529.7
  learning, specific (mathematics)
    (reading) (strephosymbolia)
    306.1
  memory (*see also* Amnesia) 780.7
  mental (*see also* Disorder, mental)
    300.9
  metabolism 279
    cholesterol 279
    fat 279
    general 279
      carbohydrate 279
      iron 279
      nutrition 269.9
      phosphate 279
      sodium 788.0
    lipoids 279
    nitrogen 788.9
    phosphatides 279
  motor 780.3
  nervous functional 790.0

Disturbance—*continued*
  neuromuscular mechanism (eye) due to
      syphilis 094.9
  nutritional 269.9
    nail 703.9
  ocular motion 781.1
    psychogenic 305.8
  oculogyric 781.1
    psychogenic 305.8
  oculomotor 781.1
    psychogenic 305.8
  olfactory nerve 781.4
  optic nerve 781.0
  personality (pattern) (trait) (*see also*
      Disorder, personality) 301.9
    due to or associated with physical
        condition - *see* listing under
        Disorder, mental
  pilomotor 781.6
  polyglandular 258.1
  psychomotor 306.3
  pupillary 781.0
  reflex 780.3
  rhythm, heart (*see also* Action, heart,
      irregular) 427.9
  salivary secretion 527.7
  sensation (cold) (heat) (localization)
      (smell) (tactile discrimination,
      localization) (taste) (texture)
      (vibratory) NEC 781.6
    hysterical 300.1
  sensory - *see* Disturbance, sensation
  situational (transient) 307
  sleep 780.6
    nonorganic origin 306.4
  sociopathic 301.7
  speech NEC 306.9
    developmental 306.9
    secondary to organic lesion 781.5
  stomach (functional) (*see also*
      Disturbance, gastric) 536.9
  sympathetic (nerve) 358.9
  temperature sense - *see* Disturbance,
      sensation
  tooth structure, hereditary NEC 520.5
  touch - *see* Disturbance, sensation
  vascular 458.9
    arteriosclerotic - *see* Arteriosclerosis
  vasomotor 443.9
  vasospastic 443.9
  vision, visual NEC 781.0
Disuse atrophy, bone 723.9
Diuresis 786.4
Divers'
  palsy or paralysis 993.3
  squeeze 993.3

Diverticula, diverticulitis, diverticulosis,
    diverticulum (acute) (multiple)
    (perforated) (ruptured) 562.1
  appendix (noninflammatory) 543
  bladder (sphincter) 596.1
    congenital 753.8
  bronchus (congenital) 748.3
    acquired 518
  calyx, calyceal (kidney) (*see also*
      Lesion, kidney) 593.2
  cardia (stomach) 537.9
  cecum 562.1
    congenital 751.4
  colon 562.1
    congenital 751.4
  duodenum 562.0
    congenital 751.4
  epiphrenic (esophagus) 530.2
  esophagus (congenital) 750.8
    acquired 530.2
    epiphrenic 530.2
    pulsion 530.2
    traction 530.2
    Zenker's 530.2
  eustachian tube 384.9
  fallopian tube 615.9
  heart (congenital) 746.8
  ileum 562.0
  intestine (large) 562.1
    congenital 751.4
    small 562.0
      congenital 751.4
  jejunum 562.0
  kidney (pelvis) (calyces) (*see also*
      Lesion, kidney) 593.2
    with calculus 592
  Meckel's (displaced) (hypertrophic)
      751.0
  organ or site, congenital NEC - *see*
      Distortion
  pericardium (congenital) (cyst) 746.8
  pharyngo-esophageal (pulsion) 530.2
  pharynx (congenital) 750.8
  pulsion (esophagus) 530.2
  rectosigmoid 562.1
    congenital 751.4
  rectum 562.1
  seminal vesicle 607.4
  sigmoid 562.1
    congenital 751.4
  small intestine 562.0
  stomach 537.9
  trachea (congenital) 748.3
    acquired 519.9
  traction (esophagus) 530.2
  ureter (acquired) 593.5
    congenital 753.4

Diverticula, diverticulitis, etc. – *continued*
  ureterovesical orifice 593.5
  urethra (acquired) 599.9
    congenital 753.8
  vesical 596.1
    congenital 753.8
  Zenker's (esophagus) 530.2
Diverticulations Meckel's diverticulum
    (congenital) 751.0
Division
  cervix uteri 621.9
  external os into two openings by
      frenum 752.5
  hymen 752.6
  labia minora (congenital) 752.6
  ligament (partial or complete) (current)
      - *see also* Sprain, strain
    with open wound - *see* Wound, open
  muscle (partial or complete) (current) -
      see also Sprain, strain
    with open wound - *see* Wound, open
  nerve - *see* Injury, nerve, by site
  penis glans 752.8
  spinal cord - *see* Injury spinal, by
      region
  vein 458.9
Dizziness 780.5
  hysterical 300.1
  psychogenic 305.9
Doehle-Heller aortitis 093.9
Dog bite - *see* Wound, open
Dolichocolon 751.4
Dolichostenomelia 759.8
Donohue's syndrome 258.1
Donor Y09.9
  blood Y09.9
  bone Y09.9
  skin Y09.9

Donovanosis 099.2

Double
  albumin 275.3
  aortic arch 747.2
  auditory canal 745.2
  auricle (heart) 746.8
  bladder 753.8
  external os 752.5
  kidney with double pelvis (renal) 753.3
  meatus urinarius 753.8
  monster 759.1
  organ or site not listed - *see* Accessory
  orifice
    heart valve (any) 746.6
  pelvis (renal) with double ureter 753.4
  tongue 750.0
  ureter (one or both sides) 753.4
    with double pelvis (renal) 753.4

Double – *continued*
  urethra 753.8
  uterus 752.5
    complicating delivery 657.9
      fetus or newborn - *see* categories
          764.0-764.9
    noted during pregnancy (undelivered)
        634.9
  vision 781.1
  vulva 752.6
Douglas' pouch, cul-de-sac - *see* condition
Down's disease or syndrome 759.3
Dracontiasis 125.8
Dracunculiasis 125.8
Dracunculosis 125.8
Drainage
  abscess (spontaneous) - *see* Abscess
  anomalous
    pulmonary veins to hepatic veins or
        right atrium 747.4
  stump (amputation) (surgical) 997.2
    traumatic - *see* Amputation, traumatic
  suprapubic, bladder 596.9
Dream state, hysterical 300.1
Drepanocytic anemia (*see also* Disease,
    sickle cell) 282.5
Dressler's syndrome (*see also* Ischemia,
    heart) 412.9
Drierzynsky's disease 723.9
Drift, ulnar 738.2
Drinking (alcohol)
  excessive, to excess 303.9
    bouts, periodic 303.0
    continual 303.1
    episodic 303.0
    habitual 303.1
    periodic 303.0
Drop
  finger 738.3
  foot 738.6
  toe 738.7
  wrist 738.2
Dropped
  dead 795
  heart beats (*see also* Block, heart)
      427.3
Dropsy, dropsical 782.6
  abdomen 785.3
  amnion (complicating pregnancy) (*see*
      also Hydramnios) 634.3
  asthmatic 493
    with bronchitis - *see* Bronchitis
  bowel 785.3
  brain - *see* Hydrocephalus
  broad ligament 616.9
  cardiac, heart (*see also* Failure, heart,
      congestive) 427.0

Dropsy, dropsical—*continued*
  cardiorenal - *see* Hypertension,
      cardiorenal
  chest 511.2
  epidemic 269.9
  fallopian tube 615.1
  fetus or newborn (*see also* Disease,
      hemolytic) 775.9
  gallbladder (*see also* Disease,
      gallbladder) 576.9
  gangrenous (*see also* Gangrene) 445.9
  hepatic - *see* Cirrhosis, liver
  hernial sac - *see* Hernia, by site
  infantile (*see also* Disease, hemolytic)
      775.9
  intestine 785.3
  kidney (*see also* Nephrosis) 581
  liver - *see* Cirrhosis, liver
  lung 514
  malarial (*see also* Malaria) 084.9
  nephritic (*see also* Nephrosis) 581
  nutritional 269.9
  ovary 615.9
  pericardium - *see* Pericarditis
  peritoneum 785.3
  renal (acute) (*see also* Nephrosis) 581
  tube 615.1
  uremic - *see* Uremia
Drowned, drowning 994.1
Drug
  addiction (*see also* listing under
      Dependence) 304.9
  adverse effect or poisoning - *see* Table
      of adverse effects
  dependence (*see also* listing under
      Dependence) 304.9
  habit (*see also* listing under
      Dependence) 304.9
Drunkenness 303.9
Drusen
  body (eye) (hyaloid degeneration)
      377.4
  optic papilla 377.6
Drusenfieber 075
Dry - *see also* condition
  socket (teeth) 526.5
Dryness
  larynx 508.3
  mouth 527.7
  nose 508.9
  throat 508.9
Duane's syndrome 744.8

Dubin-Johnson disease or syndrome
    273.5

Dubini's disease 065
  late effects 066

Dubois' disease 090.5
Duchenne-Aran muscular atrophy 348.2
Duchenne-Griesinger disease 330.3
Duchenne's
  disease 094.0
    locomotor ataxia 094.0
    pseudohypertrophy, muscles 330.3
  paralysis 348.1
  syndorme 348.1
Ducrey's
  bacillus 099.0
  chancre 099.0
Duct, ductus - *see* condition
Duengero 061
Duhring's disease 693
Dukes(-Filatow) disease 057.8
Dullness - *see* Retardation, mental,
    borderline
Dumbness (*see also* Aphasia) 781.5
Dumdum fever 085.0
Dumping syndrome (postgastrectomy)
    997.9
Duodenitis (non-specific) (peptic) 535
Duodenocholangitis (*see also*
    Cholecystitis) 575
Duodenum, duodenal - *see* condition
Duplay's disease, periarthritis or
    syndrome 717.1
Duplex - *see also* Accessory
  kidney 753.3
  placenta - *see* Placenta, abnormal

Duplication - *see also* Accessory
  anus 751.4
  appendix 751.4
  biliary duct (any) 751.6
  bladder 753.8
  cecum 751.4
    and appendix 751.4
  cystic duct 751.6
  digestive organs 751.8
  esophagus 750.8
  frontonasal process 756.0
  gallbladder 751.6
  intestine (large) (small) 751.4
  kidney 753.3
  liver 751.6
  pancreas 751.7
  penis 752.8
  respiratory organs NEC 748.9
  salivary duct 750.8
  spinal cord (incomplete) 743.3
  stomach 750.8

Dupuytren's
  contraction 733.5
  disease 733.5
  fracture - *see* Fracture, ankle

Dupuytren's—*continued*
  muscle contracture 733.5
Durand-Nicolas-Favre disease 099.1
Duroziez's disease 746.6
Dust
  reticulation 515.9
    with tuberculosis 010
Dutton's
  disease 087.9
  relapsing fever (West African) 088.1
Dwarfism 258.9
  achondroplastic 756.5
  congenital 258.9
  constitutional 258.9
  hypophyseal 253.1
  infantile 258.9
  Lorain type 253.1
  nephrotic-glycosuric (with
        hypophosphatemic rickets)
        270.2
  ovarian 759.5
  pancreatic 577.9
  pituitary 253.1
  renal 593.0
Dyke-Young anemia (secondary)
      (symptomatic) 283.9
Dysacousis 781.3
Dysadaptation visual 378.6
Dysadrenocortism 255.9
Dysarthria 781.5
Dysautonomia, familial 743.8
Dysbarism 993.3
Dysbasia 787.5
  angiosclerotica intermittens 443.9
  hysterical 300.1
  lordotica (progressiva) 331.1
  nonorganic origin 306.3
  psychogenic 306.3
Dyschezia (*see also* Constipation) 564.0
Dyschondroplasia (with hemangiomata)
      756.5
Dyscranio-pyo-phalangy 759.8
Dyscrasia
  blood 289.9
    fetus or newborn (*see also* Disease,
        hemolytic due to
        incompatibility) 775.2
    puerperal, postpartum 675
  ovary 256.9
  pluriglandular 258.1
  polyglandular 258.1
Dysectasia, vesical neck 596.9
Dysendocrinism 258.1
Dysentery, dysenteric (bilious) (catarrhal)
      (diarrhea) (epidemic) (gangrenous)
      (hemorrhagic) (infectious) (sporadic)
      (tropical) (ulcerative) 009.0
    325–015 O–69—12

Dysentery, dysenteric—*continued*
  abscess, liver 006.0
  amebic 006.9
    with liver abscess 006.0
  arthritis 004.9
  asylum 004.9
  bacillary 004.9
    Boyd 004.2
    Flexner 004.1
    Schmitz(-Stutzer) 004.4
    Shiga 004.0
    Sonne 004.3
    specified type NEC 004.8
  bacterium 004.9
  balantidial 007.0
  Balantidium coli 007.0
  Boyd's 004.2
  Chilomastix 007.9
  Chinese 004.9
  choleriform 000.1
  coccidial 007.2
  Dientameba fragilis - *see* Dysentery,
        amebic
  Embadomonas 007.9
  Endameba, endamebic (coli) (williamsi) - *see*
        Dysentery, amebic
  Endolimax nana - *see* Dysentery,
        amebic
  Flexner-Boyd 004.2
  Flexner's 004.1
  Giardia lamblia 007.1
  giardial 007.1
  Hiss-Russell 004.1
  Lamblia 007.1
  leishmanial 085.0
  malarial (*see also* Malaria) 084.9
  metazoal 127.9
  Monilia 112
  protozoal NEC 007.9
  Russell's 004.8
  salmonella 003.9
    due to food 003.0
  schistosomal 120.1
  Schmitz(-Stutzer) 004.4
  Shiga 004.0
  Shigella NEC 004.9
  Sonne 004.3
  strongyloidiasis 127.1
  tuberculous 014
    late effect or sequela 019.9
  viral (*see also* Enteritis, viral) 008.9

Dysesthesia 781.6
  hysterical 300.1
Dysfunction
  adrenal 255.9
  bladder 596.9
  bleeding, uterus 626.6
  cerebral 781.7

Dysfunction—*continued*
    colon 564.9
        psychogenic 305.5
    colostomy or enterostomy 998.7
    endocrine NEC 258.9
    endometrium 625.9
    enteric stoma 998.7
    gallbladder (*see also* Disease,
        gallbladder) 576.9
    gastro-intestinal 536.9
    gland, glandular NEC 258.9
    heart (*see also* Action, heart, irregular)
        427.9
    hemoglobin 289.9
    hepatic 573.9
    hypophysis 253.9
    kidney (*see also* Lesion, kidney) 593.2
    liver 573.9
        constitutional 273.5
    ovary 256.9
    papillary muscle (*see also* Action, heart,
        irregular) 427.9
    pituitary (gland) 253.9
    placental - *see* Placenta, insufficiency
    polyglandular 258.1
    pylorus 537.9
    rectum 564.9
        psychogenic 305.5
    senile 794
    stomach 536.9
        psychogenic 305.5
    suprarenal 255.9
    testicular 257.9
    thyroid 246
    uterus, complicating delivery 657.9
        fetus or newborn - *see* categories
            767.0-767.9

Dysgenesis
    ovarian 759.5
    reticular 275.0
    seminiferous tubule 759.5

Dysgerminoma (malignant)
    female (ovary) 183.0
        benign 220.9
    male (testes) 186
        benign 222.0

Dysgeusia 781.4
Dysgraphia 780.4
Dyshidrosis 705.9
Dysidrosis 705.9
Dysinsulinism 251
Dyskeratosis (*see also* Keratosis) 701.1
    cervix 621.9
    congenital 757.2
    follicularis 757.2
    uterus NEC 625.9

Dyskinesia 780.4
    biliary (*see also* Disease, gallbladder)
        576.9
    hysterical 300.1
    intestinal 569.9
    nonorganic origin 306.3
    psychogenic 306.3
Dyslexia (congenital) (developmental)
        306.1
    secondary to organic lesion 781.5
Dysmaturity (*see also* Immaturity) 777
    lung (*see also* Syndrome, respiratory
        distress) 776.2
Dysmenorrhea (exfoliative) (membranous)
        (primary) 626.3
    essential 626.3
    psychogenic 305.6
Dysmetria 780.4
Dysnomia 781.5
Dysorexia 784.0
    hysterical 300.1
Dysostosis
    cleidocranial, cleidocranialis 755.5
    craniofacial 756.0
    mandibulofacial, incomplete 756.0
    multiplex 273.8
Dyspareunia (female) (male) 786.7
    psychogenic 305.6
Dyspepsia (allergic) (congenital)
        (functional) (gastro-intestinal)
        (neurogenic) (occupational) (reflex)
        536.9
    atonic 536.1
        psychogenic 305.5
    catarrhal 535
    diarrhea 561
        psychogenic 305.5
    intestinal 564.9
        psychogenic 305.5
    nervous 305.5
    neurotic 305.5
    psychogenic 305.5
Dysphagia 784.4
    functional 300.1
    hysterical 300.1
    nervous 300.1
    psychogenic 305.5
    sideropenic 280
Dysphasia 781.5
Dysphonia 783.5
    clericorum 783.5
    functional 300.1
    hysterical 300.1
    psychogenic 305.2
    spastica 508.3
Dyspituitarism 253.9

Dysplasia - *see also* Anomaly
  brain 743.9
  cervix 621.9
  chondroectodermal 756.7
  chondromatose 756.5
  diaphysial, progressive 756.7
  ectodermal (anhidrotic) (congenital)
      (hereditary) 757.9
  epiphysealis 756.9
    multiplex 756.7
    punctata 756.7
  epiphysis 756.9
    multiple 756.7
  epithelial
    uterine cervix 621.9
  eye 744.1
  fibrous
    bone NEC 723.9
    diaphysial, progressive 756.7
    jaw 526.9
    monostotic 723.9
    polyostotic 756.7
  hip, congenital 755.7
  joint 755.9
  leg 755.7
  mammary (gland) (benign) 611.9
    cystic 610
  metaphyseal 756.9
  monostotic fibrous 723.9
  muscle 756.9
  nervous system (general) 743.9
  neuro ectodermal 759.8
  oculodentodigital 759.8
  periosteum 723.9
  polyostotic fibrous 756.7
  retinal 744.9
  spinal cord 743.9

Dyspnea (nocturnal) (paroxysmal) 783.2
  asthmatic (bronchial) 493
    with bronchitis - *see* Bronchitis
  cardiac (*see also* Failure, ventricular,
      left) 427.1
  cardiac (*see also* Failure, ventricular,
      left) 427.1
  functional 300.1
  hyperventilation 783.2
  hysterical 300.1
  newborn (*see also* Syndrome,
      respiratory distress) 776.2
  psychogenic 305.2
  uremic - *see* Uremia

Dyspraxia 780.4

Dysproteinemia 275.9
  transient with copper deficiency 281.4

Dysrhythmia, cerebral or cortical 781.7

Dyssynergia
  biliary (*see also* Disease, gallbladder)
      576.9
  cerebellaris myoclonica 347.9
Dysthyroidism 246
Dystocia, complicating delivery 657.9
  affecting fetus or newborn - *see*
      categories 768.0-768.9
  cervical 657.2
    fetus or newborn - *see* categories
        764.0-764.9
  fetal - *see also* Presentation, abnormal,
      complicating delivery
    deformity or abnormal size 655
      fetus or newborn - *see* categories
          765.0-765.9
    fetus or newborn - *see* categories
        766.0-766.9
  maternal - *see* Dystocia, cervical
  pelvis, pelvic (inlet) (midplane) (outlet)
      - *see also* Deformity, pelvis,
      complicating delivery
    fetus or newborn - *see* categories
        764.0-764.9
  positional - *see also* Presentation,
      abnormal, complicating delivery
    fetus or newborn - *see* categories
        766.0-766.9
  shoulder girdle 655
    fetus or newborn *see* categories
        765.0-765.9
Dystonia
  deformans progressive 331.1
  lenticularis 331.1
  musculorum deformans 331.1
  torsion 331.1
Dystonic
  movements 780.3
  syndrome, residual of encephalitis 066
Dystrophy, dystrophia 796.0
  adiposogenital 253.1
  breviocollis 756.2
  cervical (sympathetic) 358.9
  cornea (endothelial) (epithelial) (lipid)
      (marginal) 378.4
  dermatochondrocorneal 378.4
  Erb's 330.3
  familial
    hyperplastic periosteal 756.7
    osseous 273.8
  Fuchs' 378.4
  Gower's muscular 330.3
  hair 704
  Landouzy-Dejerine 330.3
  Leyden-Moebius 330.3
  muscular 330.4

Dystrophy, dystrophia—*continued*
  muscular—*continued*
    congenital NEC   330.4
    distal   330.3
    Duchenne type   330.3
    Erb type   330.3
    facioscapulohumeral   330.3
    Gower's   330.3
    hereditary NEC   330.4
    Landouzy-Dejerine type   330.3
    limb-girdle   330.3
    progressive (hereditary)   330.3
      Charcot-Marie(-Tooth) type   330.0
      spinal   330.1
    pseudohypertrophic (infantile)   330.3
  myocardium, myocardial (*see also*
     Insufficiency, myocardial)   428
  myotonica   330.4

Dystropy, dystrophia—*continued*
  nail   703.9
    congenital   757.4
  nutritional   267
  oculocerebrorenal   270.8
  ovarian   615.9
  papillary (and pigmentary) (*see also*
     Acanthosis)   701.1
  pituitary (gland)   253.1
  polyglandular   258.1
  Salzmann's nodular   378.4
  skin NEC   709.9
  sympathetic (reflex)   358.9
  unguium   703.9
    congenital   757.4
Dysuria   786.0
  psychogenic   305.6

E

Eales' disease 377.0

Ear - *see also* condition
tropical 111.9
wax 387.1

Earache 384.9

Eberth's disease 001

Ebstein's
anomaly heart 746.6
disease, meaning diabetes - *see* category 250

Eccentro-osteochondrodysplasia 273.8

Ecchondroma (*see also* Exostosis) 213.0

Ecchondrosis (*see also* Exostosis) 213.0

Ecchordosis physaliphora 756.0

Ecchymosis (multiple) 458.9
conjunctiva 378.3
eye (traumatic) 921
eyelids (traumatic) 921
newborn 778.2
traumatic - *see* Contusion

Echinococcosis 122.9
liver 122.0
lung 122.1
mammary 122.8
specified site NEC 122.8

Echinococcus (granulosus) (infection)
(multilocularis) - *see*
Echinococcosis

Echinorhynchiasis 127.4

Echinostomiasis 121.9

Echo virus NEC 079.9

Echolalia 781.5

Eclampsia, eclamptic (coma) (convulsions)
(delirium) 780.2
with abortion - *see* Abortion, by type,
with toxemia
antepartum - *see* Eclampsia, pregnancy
arising during pregnancy 637.1
fetus or newborn 762.2
female 780.2
child-bearing age NEC - *see*
Eclampsia, pregnancy
not associated with pregnancy or
childbirth 780.2
gravidarum - *see* Eclampsia, pregnancy
male 780.2
pregnancy (nephritic) (uremic) 637.1
fetus or newborn 762.2
puerperal, postpartum 637.1
uremic 792

Eclampsia, eclamptic — *continued*
uremic — *continued*
with abortion - *see* Abortion, by type ,
with toxemia
arising during pregnancy - *see*
Eclampsia, pregnancy
puerperal, postpartum 637.1

Economo's disease 065
late effects 066

Ectasia, ectasis
aorta, (*see also* Aneurysm, aorta)
441.9
breast 611.9
capillary 448
cornea - *see* Staphyloma
mammary duct 611.9
papillary 448
scar, cornea 378.4
sclera - *see* Staphyloma

Ecthyma 686.9
contagiosum 079.8
gangrenosum 686.0
infectiosum 057.8

Ectocardia 746.8

Ectodermal dysplasia, congenital 757.2

Ectodermosis
erosiva pluriorificialis 695.1

Ectopic, ectopia (congenital) 758.8
abdominal viscera 751.8
due to defect in anterior abdominal
wall 756.8
auricular beats - *see* Action, heart,
irregular
bladder 753.5
bone and cartilage in lung 748.6
brain 743.2
breast tissue 757.2
cardiac 746.8
cerebral 743.2
cordis 746.8
endometrium (any site) 625.3
gastric mucosa 750.8
gestation - *see* Pregnancy, ectopic
heart 746.8
kidney (crossed) (pelvis) 753.3
lens 744.8
lentis 744.8
mole - *see* Pregnancy, ectopic
organ or site NEC - *see* Malposition,
congenital

Ectopic, ectopia — *continued*
  ovarian tumor - *see* Teratoma
  pancreas 751.7
  pregnancy - *see* Pregnancy, ectopic
  renal 753.3
  testis 752.1
  ureter 753.4
  ventricular beats - *see* Action, heart,
     irregular
  vesicae 753.5
Ectromelia 755.4
  lower limb 755.3
  upper limb 755.2
Ectropion 378.9
  anus 569.1
  cervix - *see* Eversion, cervix
  congenital 744.8
  eyelid 378.2
    congenital 744.8
  iris, cicatricial 378.6
  lip (congenital) 750.8
    acquired 528.5
  paralytic 378.2
  rectum 569.1
  senile 378.2
  urethra 599.9
  uvea, spastic 378.6
Eczema (acute) (allergic) (chronic)
    (erythematous) (fissum)
    (occupational) (rubrum) (squamous)
    692.9
  asthma 691
  atopic (due to any substance) 691
  contact NEC 692.9
  dermatitis NEC 692.9
  due to
    specified cause - *see* Dermatitis, due
      to
  dyshydrotic 705.9
  flexural 691
  gouty 274
  hypertrophicum 701.9
  hypostatic - *see* Varicose vein
  impetiginous 686.9
  infantile (due to any substance)
    (intertriginous) (seborrheic) 691
  intertriginous NEC 692.9
    infantile 691
  intrinsic 691
  lichenified NEC 692.9
  marginatum 110.9
  nummular NEC 692.9
  psychogenic 305.0
  pustular 686.9
  seborrheic 690
    infantile 691

Eczema — *continued*
  solare 692.7
  stasis (lower extremity) 454.1
    ulcerated or with ulcer 454.0
  vaccination, vaccinatum 999.0
  varicose - *see* Eczema, stasis
Eddowes' syndrome 756.6
Edema, edematous 782.6
  with nephritis (*see also* Nephrosis)
    581
  angioneurotic (allergic) (any site)
    (hereditary) (with urticaria)
    708.0
  angiospastic 443.9
  Berlin's (traumatic) 921
  brain (*see also* Disease, cerebrovascular
    NEC) 438.9
    alcoholic 303.9
    due to injury at birth (*see also* Birth
      injury, brain) 772.0
    fetus or newborn (*see also* Birth
      injury, brain) 772.0
  cardiac (*see also* Failure, heart,
    congestive) 427.0
  cardiovascular (*see also* Failure, heart,
    congestive) 427.0
  cerebral - *see* Edema, brain
  cerebrospinal vessel - *see* Edema, brain
  cervix (uteri) (acute) 621.9
    puerperal, postpartum 677.9
  circumscribed, acute 708.0
  conjunctiva 360
  connective tissue 782.6
  due to lymphatic obstruction 457
  epiglottis - *see* Edema, glottis
  essential, acute 708.0
  extremities, lower - *see* Edema, legs
  eyelid NEC 361
  familial, hereditary (legs) 757.0
  famine 269.9
  fetus or newborn 778.9
  glottis, glottic, glottidis (obstructive)
    (passive) 508.2
    allergic 708.0
  heart (*see also* Failure, heart,
    congestive) 427.0
  heat 992.7
  hereditary (legs) 757.0
  inanition 269.9
  infectious 782.6
  iris 364
  joint (*see also* Disease, joint) 729.9
  larynx - *see* Edema, glottis
  legs 782.6
    hereditary 757.0

Edema, edematous — *continued*
  localized, due to venous obstruction
    458.9
    lower extremity 458.9
  lower extremities - *see* Edema, legs
  lung 514
    acute 519.1
      with heart condition or failure
        (conditions in 429 or 782.4)
        (*see also* Failure, ventricular,
        left) 427.1
    chronic 514
    terminal 514
  lymphatic 457
  macula 377.0
  malignant (*see also* Gas gangrene)
    039.0
  Milroy's 757.0
  nutritional 269.9
  orbit, circulatory 458.9
  penis 607.9
  periodic 708.0
  pharynx 508.9
  pulmonary - *see* Edema, lung
  Quincke's 708.0
  renal (*see also* Nephrosis) 581
  retina (disc) 377.0
  salt 788.0
  scrotum 607.9
  starvation 269.9
  subglottic - *see* Edema, glottis
  supraglottic - *see* Edema, glottis
  toxic NEC 782.6
  traumatic NEC 782.6
  vulva (acute) 629.9
Edentulous (acquired) 525.0
  congenital (deficiency of tooth buds)
    520.0
Edsall's disease 992.2
Effect, adverse
  altitude (high) - *see* Effect, adverse, high
    altitude
  antitoxin - *see* Complications,
    vaccination
  atmospheric pressure
    high 993.3
    low - *see* Effect, adverse, high
      altitude
  blood (derivatives) (serum) (transfusion)
    - *see* Complications, transfusion
  chemical subst. NEC 989.9
    specified - *see* Table of adverse
      effects
  cobalt, radioactive - *see* Effect, adverse,
    radioactive substance
  cold (temperature) (weather) 991.9

Effect, adverse — *continued*
  cold — *continued*
    chilblains 443.2
    frostbite - *see* Frostbite
  drug (*see also* Table of adverse effects)
    977.9

Note — The coding of adverse effects of drugs is keyed to the continually revised Hospital Formulary of the American Hospital Formulary Service (AHFS) published under the direction of the American Society of Hospital Pharmacists.

The following section of this index gives the ICDA categories in 960–977 which correspond approximately to the numerical subdivisions of the AHFS list of drugs.

Effect, adverse — *Continued*
  drug — *Continued*
    AHFS List
    4:00 antihistamine drugs 963.0
    8:04 amebacides (*see also* 961.1,
      961.3) 961.9
    8:08 anthelmintics 961.9
    8:12.04 antifungal antibiotics 960.1
    8:12.08 chloramphenicol 960.2
    8:12.12 erythromycins 960.3
    8:12.16 penicillins 960.0
    8:12.20 streptomycins 960.4
    8:12.24 tetracyclines 960.5
    8:12.28 other antibiotics 960.9
    8:16 antitubercular agents 961.9
    8:20 plasmodicides 961.3
    8:24 sulfonamides 961.0
    8:26 sulfones 961.9
    8:28 treponemicides (*see also* 961.1)
      961.9
    8:32 trichomonacides (*see also* 961.1,
      961.3) 961.9
    8:36 urinary germicides 961.9
    8:40 other anti-infective agents 961.9
    10:00 antineoplastic agents 963.1
    12:04 parasympathomimetic (cholin-
      ergic) agents 972.0
    12:08 parasympatholytic (cholinergic
      blocking) agents 972.1
    12:12 sympathomimetic (adrenergic)
      agents 972.2
    12:16 sympatholytic (adrenergic
      blocking) agents 973.5
    12:20 skeletal muscle relaxants (*see
      also* 976.9) 968.0
    16:00 blood derivatives (*see also* 964.4)
      964.9
    20:04.04 iron preparations 964.0

Effect, adverse—*continued*
  drug—*continued*
    88:04 vitamin A 963.6
    88:08 vitamin B complex 963.6
    88:12 vitamin C 963.6
    88:16 vitamin D 963.6
    88:20 vitamin E 963.6
    88:24 vitamin K activity 964.3
    88:28 multivitamin preparations 963.6
    92:00 unclassified therapeutic agents 977.8
  electric current (burn) (incineration) (shock) 994.8
  electricity (burn) (incineration) (shock) 994.8
  exertion (excessive) 994.5
  exposure 994.4
  external cause NEC 994.9
  fall out (radioactive) 990.0
  fluoroscopy 990.1
  foodstuffs
    allergic reaction (*see also* Allergy, food) 692.5
    noxious NEC 988.9
      specified type - *see* Table of adverse effects
  gases, fumes, or vapors - *see* Table of adverse effects
  glue (airplane) sniffing 304.8
  heat - *see* Heat
  high altitude 993.2
    anoxia 993.2
    on ears 993.0
    on sinuses 993.1
    polycythemia 289.0
  hot weather - *see* Heat
  hunger 994.2
  immunization - *see* Complications, vaccination
  immunological agents - *see* Complications, vaccination
  implantation (removable)
    isotope or radium 990.5
    burn - *see* Burn
  infrared (radiation) (rays) 990.9
    allergy, allergic reaction (skin) 692.7
    burn - *see* Burn
    dermatitis or eczema 692.7
  infusion - *see* Complications, infusion
  ingestion or injection of isotope (therapeutic) 990.5
    diagnostic 990.2
  irradiation - *see* Effect, adverse, radiation
  isotope (radioactive) - *see* Effect, adverse, radioactive substance

Effect, adverse—*continued*
  lack of care of infants 994.9
  lightning 994.0
  lirugin - *see* Complications, vaccination
  mesothorium - *see* Effect, adverse, radioactive substance
  motion 994.6
  overheated places - *see* Heat
  polonium - *see* Effect, adverse, radioactive substance
  radiation (early reaction) (late effect) 990.9
    allergy, allergic reaction (skin) 692.7
    burn - *see* Burn
    dermatitis or eczema - *see* Dermatitis, due to, radiation
    diagnostic 990.3
      fluoroscopy 990.1
      isotope (radioactive) 990.2
      roentgenography 990.1
      tracer substance 990.2
      x-ray 990.1
    from
      fall out 990.0
      radioactive isotope or substance - *see* Effect, adverse, radioactive substance
      x-rays - *see* Effect, adverse, x-rays
    infrared - *see* Effect, adverse, infrared
    natural NEC 990.0
    therapeutic - *see* Effect, adverse, radiotherapy
    ultraviolet - *see* Effect, adverse, ultraviolet
  radioactive substance (early reaction) (late effect) 990.0
    allergy, allergic reaction (skin) 692.7
    burn - *see* Burn
    dermatitis or eczema 692.7
    diagnostic (ingested) (injected) 990.2
    industrial or occupational 990.0
    not diagnostic or therapeutic 990.0
    therapeutic 990.6
      bomb 990.4
      external 990.4
      implant (removable) 990.5
      ingested 990.5
      injected 990.5
      internal 990.5
    tracer (ingested) (injected) 990.2
  radioactivity (early reaction) (late effect) 990.0
    from
      fall out 990.0
      natural radiation 990.0

Effect, adverse—*continued*
  radioactivity, etc.—*continued*
    from—*continued*
      radioactive substance or isotope -
        see Effect, adverse,
        radioactive substance
      x-rays or roentgen rays - *see*
        Effect, adverse, x-rays
      industrial or occupational hazard
        990.0
      not diagnostic or therapeutic   990.0
  radiotherapy (early reaction) (late effect)
    990.6
    allergy, allergic reaction (skin)   692.7
    burn - *see* Burn
    dermatitis or eczema   692.7
    external (by cobalt, other isotope or
      radium used as a bomb) (by
      roentgen rays) (by x-rays)
      990.4
    internal (by implantation of isotope,
      radium or radon) (by ingestion
      or injection of isotope)   990.5
  radium - *see* Effect, adverse,
    radioactive substance
  roentgen rays - *see* Effect, adverse, x-
    rays
  roentgenography   990.1
  roentgenoscopy   990.1
  serum (prophylactic) (therapeutic) - *see*
    Complications, vaccination
  submersion   994.1
  teletherapy   990.4
  thirst   994.3
  transfusion - *see* Complications,
    transfusion
  ultraviolet (radiation) (rays)   990.9
    allergy, allergic reaction (skin)   692.7
    burn - *see also* Burn
      from sun   692.8
    dermatitis or eczema - *see*
      Dermatitis, due to, ultraviolet
      rays
  uranium - *see* Effect, adverse,
    radioactive substance
  vaccine (any) - *see* Complications,
    vaccination
  whole blood - *see* Complications,
    transfusion
  x-rays (early reaction) (late effect)
    990.0
    allergy, allergic reaction (skin)   692.7
    burn - *see* Burn
    dermatitis or eczema   692.7
    diagnostic   990.1
    industrial or occupational   990.0

Effect, adverse—*continued*
  x-rays, etc.—*continued*
    not diagnostic or therapeutic   990.0
    therapeutic   990.4
Effort syndrome (aviators') (psychogenic)
  305.3
Effusion
  amniotic fluid, complicating delivery
    661.8
  brain (serous) (*see also* Disease,
    cerebrovascular NEC)   438.9
  bronchial (*see also* Bronchitis)   490
  cerebral (*see also* Disease,
    cerebrovascular NEC)   438.9
  cerebrospinal (*see also* Meningitis)
    320.9
    vessel   438.9
  chest - *see* Effusion, pleura
  intracranial (*see also* Disease,
    cerebrovascular NEC)   438.9
  joint (*see also* Disease, joint)   729.9
  meninges (*see also* Meningitis)   320.9
  pericardium - *see* Pericarditis
  peritoneal (chronic)   569.9
  pleura, pleurisy, pleuritic,
      pleuropericardial   012.2
    with pneumoconiosis (conditions in
        515)   010
    fetus or newborn   511.2
    malignant   197.2
    nontuberculous   511.2
      bacterial   511.1
      pneumococcal   511.1
      staphylococcal   511.1
      streptococcal   511.1
    tuberculous   012.1
      with pneumoconiosis (conditions in
          515)   010
      late effect or sequela   019.0
  pulmonary - *see* Effusion, pleura
  spinal (*see also* Meningitis)   320.9
  thorax, thoracic - *see* Effusion, pleura
Egg shell nails   703.9
  congenital   757.4
Egyptian
  splenomegaly   120.1
Ehlers-Danlos syndrome   757.2
Eichstedt's disease   111.0
Eisenmenger's
  complex   746.3
  syndrome   746.3
Ejaculation semen, painful   786.7
  psychogenic   305.6
Ekbom syndrome   781.6
El Tor cholera   000.1

Elastic skin 757.2
  acquired 701.9
Elastoma 757.2
  juvenile 757.2
Elastomyofibrosis 746.7
  acquired 425
Elastosis
  atrophicans 701.9
  perforans serpiginosa 704
  senilis 701.9
Elbow - see condition
Electric current, electricity, effects (burn)
    (concussion) (incineration) (shock)
    994.8
  burn from heating appliance - see Burn
Electrocution 994.8
Electrolyte imbalance 788.0
Elephantiasis 457
  arabum (see also Infestation, filarial)
    125.9
  congenital (any site) 757.2
  due to
    Brugia (malayi) 125.1
    Wuchereria (bancrofti) 125.0
      malayi 125.1
  eyelid 457
  filarial (see also Infestation, filarial)
    125.9
  filariensis (see also Infestation, filarial)
    125.9
  glandular 457
  graecorum 030.9
  lymphangiectatic 457
    scrotum 457
  lymphatic vessel 457
  neuromatosa 743.4
  scrotum 457
  streptococcal 457
  surgical 998.9
    postmastectomy 997.3
  telangiectodes 457
  vulva (nonfilarial) 629.9
Elevation
  basal metabolic rate 788.9
  blood pressure (see also Hypertension)
    401
  body temperature (of unknown origin)
      (see also Pyrexia) 788.6
  conjugate eye 373.2
  diaphragm, congenital 756.8
  scapula, congenital 755.5
  venous pressure 458.9
Elliptocytosis (hereditary) 282.1
  Hb C (disease) (trait) 282.5
  hemoglobin disease 282.5
  sickle cell (disease) (trait) 282.5

Ellis-van Creveld syndrome 756.7
Ellison-Zollinger syndrome 251
Elongated - see Elongation
Elongation (congenital) - see also
      Distortion
  bone 756.9
  cervix (uteri) 752.5
    acquired 621.9
  colon 569.9
    congenital 751.4
  common bile duct 751.6
  cystic duct 751.6
  frenulum, penis 752.8
  labia minora, acquired 629.9
  ligamentum patellae 756.8
  petiolus (epiglottidis) 748.3
  tooth, teeth 520.2
  uvula 750.8
    acquired 528.9
Emaciation (due to malnutrition) 268
Embadomoniasis 007.9
Embarrassment heart, cardiac - see
      Disease, heart
Embedded
  tooth, teeth 520.6
    with abnormal position (same or
        adjacent tooth) 524.3
Embolic - see condition
Embolism (septic) 444.9
  with
    abortion - see Abortion, by type, with
        sepsis
    ectopic gestation - see categories
        631.0-631.3
  air (any site) (traumatic) 995.0
    complicating delivery 673.0
    fetus or newborn - see categories
        768.0-768.9
    during pregnancy 634.8
    puerperal, postpartum, childbirth
        673.0
  amniotic fluid (postpartum) (puerperal)
      (pulmonary) 673.1
    complicating delivery 673.1
  aorta, aortic 444.1
    abdominal 444.0
    bifurcation 444.0
    saddle 444.0
    thoracic 444.1
  artery 444.9
    auditory, internal (see also Occlusion,
        precerebral artery) 432.9
    basilar (see also Occlusion,
        precerebral artery) 432.9

Embolism (septic) — *continued*
  artery — *continued*
    carotid (common) (internal) (*see also*
      Occlusion, precerebral artery)
      432.9
    cerebellar (anterior inferior) (posterior
      inferior) (superior) (*see also*
      Occlusion, precerebral artery)
      432.9
    cerebral (*see also* Embolism, brain)
      434.9
    choroidal (anterior) (*see also*
      Occlusion, precerebral artery)
      432.9
    communicating posterior (*see also*
      Occlusion, precerebral artery)
      432.9
    coronary (*see also* Infarct,
      myocardium) 410.9
    extremity (lower) (upper) 444.4

    hypophyseal (*see also* Occlusion,
      precerebral artery) 432.9
    mesenteric (with gangrene) 444.2
    ophthalmic 377.0

    pontine (*see also* Occlusion,
      precerebral artery) 432.9
    pulmonary - *see* Embolism,
      pulmonary
    renal 444.3
    retinal 377.0
    vertebral (left) (right) (*see also*
      Occlusion, precerebral artery)
      432.9
  birth, mother - *see* Embolism, puerperal
  brain 434.9
    with
      hypertension (benign) (conditions in
        401) 434.0
        malignant (*see also*
          Hypertension, malignant
          with cerebrovascular
          involvement) 400.2
    puerperal, postpartum, childbirth
      674
  capillary 448

  cardiac (*see also* Infarct, myocardium)
    410.9
  carotid (artery) (common) (internal) (*see
    also* Occlusion, precerebral
    artery) 432.9
  causing sudden death after delivery -
    see Embolism, puerperal
  cavernous sinus (venous) - *see*
    Embolism, intracranial venous
    sinus

Embolism (septic) — *continued*
  cerebral (*see also* Embolism, brain)
    434.9
  coronary (artery or vein) (systemic) (*see
    also* Infarct, myocardium) 410.9
  extremities 444.4
  eye 377.0
  fat (cerebral) (pulmonary) (systemic)
    995.1
    complicating delivery - *see*
      Obstetrical trauma
  femoral 444.4
    vein 453
  heart (*see also* Infarct, myocardium)
    410.9
    fatty (*see also* Infarct, myocardium)
      410.9
  hepatic (vein) 453
  intestine (artery) (vein) (with gangrene)
    444.2
  intracranial (*see also* Embolism, brain)
    434.9
    venous sinus (any) 321
      late effects 324
      nonpyogenic (*see also* Disease,
        cerebrovascular NEC)
        438.9
  kidney (artery) 444.3
  lateral sinus (venous) - *see* Embolism,
    intracranial venous sinus
  longitudinal sinus (venous) - *see*
    Embolism, intracranial venous
    sinus
  lower extremity 444.4
  lung (massive) - *see* Embolism,
    pulmonary
  meninges (*see also* Embolism, brain)
    434.9
  mesenteric (artery) (vein) (with
    gangrene) 444.2
  multiple NEC 444.9
  ophthalmic 377.0
  paradoxical NEC 444.9
  penis 607.9
  peripheral arteries NEC 444.4
  pituitary 253.1
  portal (vein) 452
  precerebral artery (*see also* Occlusion,
    precerebral artery) 432.9
  puerperal, postpartum, childbirth
    673.9
    air 673.0
    amniotic fluid 673.1
    brain or cerebral 674
    cardiac 677.9
    heart 677.9

Embolism (septic) — *continued*
puerperal, etc. — *continued*
  intracranial (venous sinus) 674
  lung NEC 673.9
  pulmonary NEC 673.9
  pyemic (any site) 670
  septic (any site) 670
  specified site NEC 677.9
pulmonary (artery) (vein) 450
  with
    abortion - *see* Abortion, by type,
      with sepsis
    ectopic gestation - *see* categories
      631.0-631.3
    complicating pregnancy (undelivered)
      634.9
    puerperal, postpartum, childbirth
      673.9
    septic or pyemic 670
pyemic (multiple) 038.9
  with
    abortion - *see* Abortion, by type,
      with sepsis
    ectopic gestation - *see* categories
      631.0-631.3
    pneumococcal 038.2
      with pneumonia 481
    puerperal, postpartum, childbirth (any
      organism) 670
    specified organism NEC 038.8
    staphylococcal 038.1
    streptococcal 038.0
renal (artery) 444.3

retina, retinal 377.0
septicemic - *see* Embolism, pyemic
sinus - *see* Embolism, intracranial
  venous sinus
spinal cord (*see also* Disease,
    cerebrovascular NEC) 438.9
  pyogenic origin 322
  late effects 324
spleen, splenic (artery) 444.9

umbilicus (cord) - *see* Complications,
    umbilical cord
vein 453
  cerebral (*see also* Embolism, brain)
    434.9
  coronary (*see also* Infarct,
      myocardium) 410.9
  hepatic 453
  mesenteric (with gangrene) 444.2
  portal 452
  pulmonary - *see* Embolism,
      pulmonary
vessels of brain (*see also* Embolism,
    brain) 434.9

Embolus - *see* Embolism
Embryoma - *see also* Neoplasm,
    malignant
  benign - *see also* Neoplasm, benign
    ovary 220.0
  liver 155.0
Embryonic
  circulation 747.9
  heart 747.9
  rest, malignant - *see also* Neoplasm,
      malignant
    liver 155.0
  tumor, mixed - *see also* Neoplasm,
      connective tissue, malignant
    liver 155.0
  vas deferens 752.8
Embryopathia 778.9
Embryotomy 773

Embryotoxon 744.8
Emesis (*see also* Vomiting) 784.1
  gravidarum - *see* Hyperemesis,
      gravidarum
Emissions, nocturnal (semen) 607.9
Emmetropia 370.9
Emotional
  crisis 307
  disorder (*see also* Disorder, mental)
    300.9
  instability (excessive) 306.9
  upset 307
Emotionality, pathological 306.9

Emotogenic disease (*see also* Disorder,
    psychogenic) 305.9
Emphysema (atrophic) (bullous)
    (compensatory) (essential)
    (hypertrophic) (interlobular)
    (interstitial) (lung) (mediastinal)
    (obstructive) (postural) (pulmonary)
    (senile) (subpleural) (unilobular)
    (vesicular) 492
  cellular tissue 995.9
    surgical 998.9
  congenital (*see also* Syndrome,
      respiratory distress) 776.2
  conjunctiva 378.3
  connective tissue 995.9
    surgical 998.9
  eye 378.9
  eyelid 378.2
    surgical 998.9
    traumatic 995.9
  fetus or newborn (*see also* Syndrome,
      respiratory distress) 776.2
  laminated tissue 995.9
    surgical 998.9
  orbit, orbital 378.9

Emphysema — *continued*
　subcutaneous　995.9
　　due to trauma　995.9
　　surgical　998.9
　surgical　998.9
　thymus (gland) (congenital)　254
　traumatic　995.9
　tuberculous (*see also* Tuberculosis,
　　　　pulmonary)　011.9
　late effect or sequela　019.0
Empyema (chest) (diaphragmatic) (double)
　　　　(encapsulated) (general) (interlobar).
　　　　(lung) (mesial) (necessitatis)
　　　　(perforating chest wall) (pleura)
　　　　(pneumococcal) (residual)
　　　　(sacculated) (streptococcal)
　　　　(supradiaphragmatic)　510
　accessory sinus (chronic) (*see also*
　　　　Sinusitis)　503.9
　acute　510
　antrum (chronic) (*see also* Sinusitis,
　　　　antrum)　503.0
　brain (any part) (*see also* Abscess,
　　　　brain)　322
　ethmoidal (chronic) (sinus) (*see also*
　　　　Sinusitis)　503.9
　extradural (*see also* Abscess, brain)
　　　　322
　frontal (chronic) (sinus) (*see also*
　　　　Sinusitis, frontal)　503.1
　gallbladder (*see also* Cholecystitis)
　　　　575
　mastoid (process) acute - *see*
　　　　Mastoiditis, acute
　maxilla, maxillary　526.4
　　sinus (chronic) (*see also* Sinusitis,
　　　　maxillary)　503.0
　nasal sinus (chronic) (*see also* Sinusitis)
　　　　503.9
　sinus - *see* Sinusitis
　sphenoidal (sinus) (*see also* Sinusitis)
　　　　503.9
　subarachnoid (*see also* Abscess, brain)
　　　　322
　subdural (*see also* Abscess, brain)　322
　tuberculous　012.1
　　with pneumoconiosis (conditions in
　　　　515)　010
　　late effect or sequela　019.0
　ureter (*see also* Ureteritis)　593.5

Encephalitis (bacterial) (chronic)
　　　　(hemorrhagic) (idiopathic)
　　　　(nonepidemic) (postexanthematous)
　　　　(postinfectious) (posttraumatic)
　　　　(spurious) (subacute) (toxic)　323
　acute - *see also* Encephalitis, viral

Encephalitis, etc. — *continued*
　acute — *continued*
　　arthropod-borne - *see* Encephalitis,
　　　　viral, arthropod-borne
　　childhood (cerebellar)　323
　　　late effects　324
　　nonviral NEC　323
　　　late effects　324
　alcoholic　303.2
　arthropod-borne - *see* Encephalitis,
　　　　viral, arthropod-borne
　California　062.9
　　late effects　066
　Central European　063.2
　　late effects　066
　Czechoslovakian　063.2
　　late effects　066
　Dawson's　065
　　late effects　066
　due to actinomycosis　113
　endemic　065
　　late effects　066
　epidemic　065
　　late effects　066
　equine (acute) (infectious) (viral)　062.9
　　Eastern　062.2
　　　late effects　066
　　Venezuelan　068.2
　　Western　062.1
　　　late effects　066
　Far Eastern　063.0
　　late effects　066
　following vaccination or other
　　　　immunization procedure　999.1
　herpes　054
　Ilheus　062.9
　　late effects　066
　inclusional　065
　　late effects　066
　infectious (acute) (virus) NEC　065
　　late effects　066
　　　paralysis agitans syndrome　066
　　　parkinsonism　066
　influenzal　474
　　lethargic　065
　　late effects　066
　Japanese (B type)　062.0
　　late effects　066
　Langat　063.9
　　late effects　066
　late effects　324
　lead　984
　lethargic (acute) (infectious) (influenzal)
　　　　065
　　late effects　066
　louping ill　063.1

Encephalitis, etc. — *continued*
  louping ill — *continued*
    late effects 066
  lupus 734.1
  lymphatica 079.2
  Mengo 065
    late effects 066
  meningococcal 036.0
  mumps 072
  Murray Valley 062.4
    late effects 066
  myoclonic 065
    late effects 066
  narcolepsy 323
    late effects 324
  otitic (*see also* Otitis media) 381.9
  parasitic NEC 123.9
  periaxialis (concentrica) (diffuse) 341
  postchickenpox 052
  post-immunization 999.1
  postmeasles 055
  postvaccinal (smallpox) 999.1
  Powassen 063.9
    late effects 066
  Russian autumnal 062.0
    late effects 066
  Russian spring-summer type (taiga)
    063.0
    late effects 066
  saturnine 984
  serous 046
  St. Louis type 062.3
    late effects 066
  summer 062.0
    late effects 066
  suppurative 322
    late effects 324
  syphilitic 094.9
    congenital 090.4
  torula, torular 116.0
  toxoplasmic or due to toxoplasmosis
    130.9
    acquired 130.0
    congenital (active) 130.1
      late effects 130.2
  trichinosis 124
  tuberculous 013.9
    late effects or sequela 019.1
  type B 062.0
    late effects 066
  type C 062.3
    late effects 066
  Vienna type 065
    late effects 066
  viral, virus 065
    arthropod-borne 064
      late effects 066

Encephalitis, etc. — *continued*
  viral, virus — *continued*
    arthropod-borne — *continued*
      mosquito-borne 062.9
        Australian X disease 062.4
          late effects 066
        California virus 062.9
          late effects 066
        Eastern equine 062.2
          late effects 066
        Ilheus virus 062.9
          late effects 066
        Japanese 062.0
          late effects 066
        late effects 066
        Murray Valley 062.4
          late effects 066
        other 062.9
          late effects 066
        St. Louis 062.3
          late effects 066
        type
          B 062.0
            late effects 066
          C 062.3
            late effects 066
        Western equine 062.1
          late effects 066
      tick-borne 063.9
        biundulant 063.9
          late effects 066
        Central European 063.2
          late effects 066
        Czechoslovakian 063.2
          late effects 066
        diphasic meningo-encephalitis
          063.2
          late effects 066
        Far Eastern 063.0
          late effects 066
        Langat 063.9
          late effects 066
        late effects 066
        louping ill 063.1
          late effects 066
        other 063.9
          late effects 066
        Powassen 063.9
          late effects 066
        Russian spring-summer (taiga)
          063.0
          late effects 066
  late effects 066
    diabetes insipidus 066
    dystonic syndrome 066
    myasthenic syndrome 066

Encephalitis, etc. — *continued*
　viral, virus — *continued*
　　late effects — *continued*
　　　myelitic syndrome　066
　　　oculogyric crisis　066
　　　oculomotor syndrome　066
　　　pyramidopallidonigral syndrome 066
　　　respiratory crisis　066
　　　tic　066
　　Wickman's, influenzal　474
Encephalocele　743.0
Encephaloid (tumor) - *see* Neoplasm,
　　malignant
Encephaloma　238.1
Encephalomalacia (brain) (cerebellar)
　　(cerebral) (*see also* Softening, brain)
　　438.9
Encephalomeningitis - *see* Meningo-
　　encephalitis
Encephalomeningocele　743.0
Encephalomeningomyelitis - *see* Meningo-
　　encephalomyelitis
Encephalomeningopathy　781.7
Encephalomyelitis (chronic) (disseminated,
　　acute) (granulomatous)
　　(hemorrhagic necrotizing, acute)
　　(myalgic, benign)
　　(postexanthematous)
　　(postinfectious) (*see also*
　　Encephalitis)　323
　　due to or resulting from vaccination
　　　(any)　999.1
　　postvaccinal (smallpox)　999.1
Encephalomyelocele　743.0
Encephalomyelomeningitis - *see* Meningo-
　　encephalomyelitis
Encephalomyeloneuropathy　781.7
Encephalomyelopathy　781.7
Encephalomyeloradiculitis (acute)　354
Encephalomyeloradiculopathy　781.7
Encephalopathia hyperbilirubinemica,
　　newborn (*see also* Disease,
　　hemolytic, by type, with
　　kernicterus)　774.9
Encephalopathy (acute) (toxic)　781.7
　anoxic - *see* Damage, brain, anoxic
　arteriosclerotic (*see also* Ischemia,
　　cerebral)　437.9
　congenital　743.9
　demyelinating (callosal)　341
　diabetic - *see* category 250
　due to
　　alcohol (ethyl)　303.9
　　birth injury (*see also* Birth injury,
　　　brain)　772.0

Encephalopathy — *continued*
　due to — *continued*
　　birth injury — *continued*
　　　spinal cord (*see also* Birth injury,
　　　　spinal cord)　772.1
　　hyperinsulinism - *see*
　　　Hyperinsulinism
　　lack of vitamin (*see also* Deficiency,
　　　vitamin)　263.9
　　serum (nontherapeutic) (therapeutic)
　　　999.5
　　syphilis　094.9
　　trauma (late effect) (without skull
　　　fracture)　850.9
　　　current　850.0
　　vaccination　999.5
　hepatic　573.9
　hyperbilirubinemic, newborn (*see also*
　　　Disease, hemolytic, by type, with
　　　kernicterus)　774.9
　hypertensive (*see also* Disease,
　　　cerebrovascular, acute, with
　　　hypertension)　436.0
　hypoglycemic　251
　hypoxic - *see* Damage, brain, anoxic
　infantile cystic necrotizing (congenital)
　　　341
　lead　984
　leuco-polio　333.1
　metabolic NEC　279
　pellagrous　262
　saturnine　984
　subcortical progressive (Schilder)　341
　traumatic (late effect) (without skull
　　　fracture)　850.9
　　current　850.0
　vitamin B deficiency NEC　263.9
　Wernicke's　263.9
Encephalorrhagia (*see also* Hemorrhage,
　　　brain)　431.9
Enchondroma - *see also* Chondroma
　multiple, congenital　756.5
Enchondromatosis (cartilaginous)
　　　(multiple)　756.5
Enchondroses multiple (cartilaginous)
　　　756.5
Encopresis (*see also* Incontinence, feces)
　　　785.6
Encystment - *see* Cyst
Endameba
　gingivalis　006.9
　　with liver abscess　006.0
　histolytica　006.9
　　with liver abscess　006.0
　infection　006.9
　　with liver abscess　006.0

Endamebiasis   006.9

with liver abscess   006.0

Endarteritis (bacterial, subacute)
    (infective) (septic)   447

brain, cerebral or cerebrospinal (*see
    also* Ischemia, cerebral)   437.9

deformans - *see* Arteriosclerosis

embolic (*see also* Embolism)   444.9

obliterans - *see also* Arteriosclerosis

pulmonary   426

retina   377.0

senile - *see* Arteriosclerosis

syphilitic   093.9

brain or cerebral   094.9

congenital   090.5

spinal   094.9

tuberculous   017.9

late effect or sequela   019.9

Endemic - *see* condition

Endocarditis (chronic) (indeterminate)
    (interstitial) (marantic) (nonbacterial
    thrombotic) (residual) (sclerotic)
    (sclerous) (senile) (valvular)   424.9

with

rheumatic fever (conditions in 390)

active - *see* Endocarditis, acute,
    rheumatic

inactive or quiescent (with chorea)
    397.9

acute or subacute   421.9

rheumatic (aortic) (mitral) (pulmonary)
    (tricuspid)   391.1

with chorea (acute) (rheumatic)
    (Sydenham's)   392.0

aortic (chronic) (heart) (inactive) (valve)
    (with chorea)   395.9

with

mitral disease (conditions in 394.9)
    396.9

active or acute   391.1

with chorea (acute) (rheumatic)
    (Sydenham's)   392.0

specified as rheumatic
    (conditions in 394.0)
    396.0

active or acute   391.1

with chorea (acute)
    (rheumatic)
    (Sydenham's)   392.0

rheumatic fever (conditions in 390)

active - *see* Endocarditis, acute,
    rheumatic

inactive or quiescent (with
    chorea)   395.0

with mitral disease (conditions
    in 394)   396.0

Endocarditis—*continued*
aortic—*continued*

active or acute   391.1

with chorea (acute) (rheumatic)
    (Sydenham's)   392.0

arteriosclerotic   424.1

congenital   746.6

hypertensive   424.1

nonrheumatic   424.1

acute or subacute   421.9

rheumatic   395.0

with mitral disease (conditions in
    394)   396.0

active or acute   391.1

with chorea (acute) (rheumatic)
    (Sydenham's)   392.0

active or acute   391.1

with chorea (acute) (rheumatic)
    (Sydenham's)   392.0

arteriosclerotic   424.9

atypical verrucous (Libman-Sacks)
    734.1

bacterial (acute) (any valve) (chronic)
    (subacute)   421.0

congenital   746.7

fetal   746.7

gonococcal   098.8

hypertensive   424.9

infectious or infective (acute) (any
    valve) (chronic) (subacute)
    421.0

lenta (acute) (any valve) (chronic)
    (subacute)   421.0

Libman-Sacks   734.1

Loeffler's   421.0

malignant (acute) (any valve) (chronic)
    (subacute)   421.0

meningococcal   036.8

mitral (chronic) (double) (fibroid) (heart)
    (inactive) (valve) (with chorea)
    394.9

with

aortic valve disease (conditions in
    395.9)   396.9

active or acute   391.1

with chorea (acute) (rheumatic)
    (Sydenham's)   392.0

specified as rheumatic
    (conditions in 395.0)
    396.0

active or acute   391.1

with chorea (acute)
    (rheumatic)
    (Sydenham's)   392.0

Endometritis (acute) (chronic)
        (nonspecific) (purulent) (septic)
        (suppurative)   622.0
    with
        abortion - see Abortion, by type, with
            sepsis
        ectopic gestation - see categories
            631.0-631.3
    arising during pregnancy   630
        fetus or newborn   763.1
    blenorrhagic   098.0
        chronic or duration of 2 months or
            over   098.1
    cervix, cervical (see also Cervicitis)
        620.9
        hyperplastic   621.2
    decidual
        with
            abortion - see Abortion, by type,
                with sepsis
            ectopic gestation - see categories
                631.0-631.3
        complicating pregnancy   634.9
            fetus or newborn   763.9
        puerperal, postpartum, childbirth
            670
    gonorrheal   098.0
        chronic or duration of 2 months or
            over   098.1
    hyperplastic   625.2
        cervix   621.2
    polypoid - see Endometritis,
        hyperplastic
    puerperal, postpartum, childbirth   670
    senile (atrophic)   622.0
    tuberculous   016.2
        late effect or sequela   019.2
Endometrium - see condition
Endomyocarditis - see Endocarditis
Endomyofibrosis   425
Endopericarditis - see Endocarditis
Endoperineuritis - see Neuritis
Endophlebitis (see also Phlebitis)   451.9
Endophthalmitis (acute) (allergic) (globe)
        (metastatic) (subacute)   366
Endosteitis - see Osteomyelitis
Endothelioma, endotheliomatosis (blood
        vessel) (see also
        Hemangioendothelioma)   227.1
    bone (diffuse) - see Neoplasm, bone,
        malignant
    lymph gland or node   200.0
    lymph vessel   227.2
        malignant - see Neoplasm, connective
            tissue, malignant

Endotheliosarcoma - see Neoplasm,
        connective tissue, malignant
    bone - see Neoplasm, bone, malignant
Endotheliosis   287.9
    hemorrhagic infectional   287.9
    reticular   279
Endotrachelitis (see also Cervicitis)   620.9
Enema rash   692.9
Engelmann's disease   756.7
English disease (see also Rickets)   265.0
Engman's disease   686.9
Engorgement
    breast   611.9
        puerperal, postpartum   678
    liver   573.9
    lung   514
    pulmonary   514
    stomach   536.9
Enlargement, enlarged - see also
        Hypertrophy
    adenoids (and tonsils)   500
    apertures of diaphragm (congenital)   756.8
        with eventration or hernia (see also
            Hernia, diaphragm)   551.3
    gingival   523.9
    heart, cardiac (see also Hypertrophy,
        cardiac)   429.0
    liver (see also Hypertrophy, liver)   785.1
    lymph gland or node   782.7
    organ or site, congenital NEC - see
        Anomaly, specified type NEC
    parathyroid (gland)   252.0
    prostate, simple   600
    spleen - see Splenomegaly
    thymus (gland) (congenital)   254
    thyroid (gland) (see also Goiter)   240.9
    tongue   529.9
    tonsils (and adenoids)   500
Enophthalmos   781.1
Enostosis   232.0
Entamebiasis - see Amebiasis
Entamebic - see Ameba
Entanglement
    umbilical cord - see Complications,
        umbilical cord
Enteralgia   785.5
Enteric - see condition
Enteritis (acute) (catarrhal) (choleraic)
        (congestive) (croupous) (diarrheal)
        (epidemic) (exudative) (follicular)
        (gangrenous) (hemorrhagic)
        (infantile) (infectious) (lienteric)
        (necrotic) (necroticans) (perforative)
        (phlegmonous)
        (pseudomembranous) (septic)
        (zymotic)   009.2

Enterospasm 564.1
  psychogenic 305.5
Enterostenosis (*see also* Obstruction,
    intestine) 560.9
Entrance, air into vein (*see also*
    Embolism, air) 995.0
Entropion (cicatricial) (eyelid) (spastic)
    378.1
  congenital 744.8
  late effect of trachoma (healed) 077
Enucleation of eye 871

Enuresis 786.2
  habit disturbance 306.6
  nocturnal 786.2
    psychogenic 306.6
  nonorganic origin 306.6
  pregnancy 634.9
  psychogenic 306.6
Eosinophilia 289.9
  allergic 289.9
  pulmonary 519.2

Eosinophilic - *see also* condition
  granuloma (bone) 279
  infiltration lung 519.2

Ependymitis (acute) (cerebral) (chronic)
    (granular) (*see also* Meningitis)
    320.9
Ependymoblastoma (*see also* Neoplasm,
    nervous system, malignant) 192.9
Ependymoma (*see also* Neoplasm,
    nervous system, malignant) 192.9
  benign (*see also* Neoplasm, nervous
      system, benign) 225.9
Ependymopathy 347.9
  spinal cord 349.9
Ephelides, ephelis 709.9
Ephemeral fever (*see also* Pyrexia)
    788.6
Epiblepharon (congenital) 744.8
Epicanthus, epicanthic fold (eyelid)
    (congenital) 744.8
Epicondylitis (elbow) 731.2
Epicystitis (*see also* Cystitis) 595
Epidemic - *see* condition
Epidermis, epidermal - *see* condition
Epidermization
  cervix 621.9
Epidermodysplasia verruciformis 757.2
Epidermoid (cyst) (*see also*
    Dermatofibroma) 216.8
  cancer or carcinoma (*see also*
      Epithelioma, malignant) 199.1
  in situ - *see* Carcinoma, in situ
  intradermal 702
  cholesteatoma - *see* Cholesteatoma

Epidermoid (cyst) — *continued*
  inclusion (*see also* Cyst, skin) 706.2
    not of skin - *see* Neoplasm, benign
    not of skin - *see* Neoplasm, benign
Epidermolysis
  bullosa 757.2
  necroticans combustiformis 695.1
    due to drug (*see also* Table of
        adverse effects) 977.9
Epidermophytid - *see* Dermatophytosis
Epidermophytosis (infected) - *see*
    Dermatophytosis
Epididymis - *see* condition
Epididymitis (acute) (nonvenereal)
    (recurrent) (residual) 604
  blennorrhagic 098.0
    chronic or duration of 2 months or
        over 098.1
  caseous 016.2
    late effect or sequela 019.2
  gonococcal 098.0
    chronic or duration of 2 months or
        over 098.1
  syphilitic 095
  tuberculous 016.2
    late effect or sequela 019.2
Epididymo-orchitis (*see also* Epididymitis)
    604
Epidural - *see* condition
Epigastritis 535
Epigastrium, epigastric - *see* condition
Epigastrocele 551.2
  gangrenous, incarcerated, irreducible,
      strangulated or with obstruction
      (intestinal) 553.2
Epiglottiditis 508.3
Epiglottis - *see* condition
Epignathus 759.1
Epilepsia
  myoclonia 331.2
  partialis continua 345.2
  procursiva 345.3
Epilepsy, epileptic (idiopathic) 345.9
  abdominal 345.9
  absence 345.0
  akinetic 345.0
    psychomotor 345.3
  alcoholic 303.2
  automatism 345.3
  brain 345.9
  Bravais-jacksonian - *see* Epilepsy,
      jacksonian
  cerebral 345.9
  climacteric 345.9
  clonic 345.1
  clouded state 345.9

Epilepsy, epileptic — *continued*
  coma 345.9
  communicating 345.9
  congenital 345.9
    focal - *see* Epilepsy, partial
  convulsions 345.9
  cortical - *see also* Epilepsy, jacksonian
    focal - *see* Epilepsy, partial
    motor 345.4
  cysticercosis 123.1
  deterioration 293.2
  due to syphilis 094.9
  equivalent 345.9
  fit 345.9
  focal - *see* Epilepsy, partial
  functional 345.9
  generalized 345.9
    convulsive 345.1
    flexion 345.1
    non-convulsive 345.0
  grand mal 345.1
  jacksonian (focal) 345.5
    motor type 345.4
    sensory type 345.5
  Kojevnikov's 345.2
  Kojewnikoff's 345.2
  laryngeal 783.3
  major 345.1
  migraine basis 345.9
  minor 345.0
  mixed (type) 345.9
  motor partial 345.4
  musicogenic 345.9
  myoclonus, myoclonic 345.1
    progressive familial 331.2
  parasitic NEC 123.9
  parkinsonian 342
    late effect, viral encephalitis 066
  partial (focalized) 345.5
    abdominal type 345.5
    motor type 345.4
    psychomotor type 345.3
    psychosensory type 345.5
    secondarily generalized 345.5
    sensory type 345.5
    somatomotor type 345.4
    somatosensory type 345.5
    temporal lobe type 345.3
    visceral type 345.5
    visual type 345.5
  peripheral 345.5
  petit mal 345.0
  progressive familial myoclonic 331.2
  psychomotor 345.3
  psychosensory 345.5
  senile 345.9

Epilepsy, epileptic — *continued*
  somatomotor 345.4
  somatosensory 345.5
  status (any type) 345.2
  symptomatic 345.5
  temporal lobe 345.3
  tonic(-clonic) 345.1
  traumatic (injury unspecified) 854.9
    injury specified - *code to* type of
      injury
  uncinate (gyrus) 345.3
  Unverricht(-Lundborg) (familiar
      myoclonic) 331.2
  visceral 345.5
  visual 345.5
Epiloia 759.6
Epimenorrhea 626.4
Epipharyngitis (*see also* Nasopharyngitis)
    460
Epiphora 378.3
Epiphyseolysis, epiphysiolysis (*see also*
    Osteochondrosis) 722.9
Epiphysitis (*see also* Osteochondrosis)
    722.9
  syphilitic (congenital) 090.0
  vertebral 722.0
Epiplocele 551.9
  gangrenous, incarcerated, irreducible,
      strangulated or with obstruction
      (intestinal) 553.9
Epiploitis (*see also* Peritonitis) 567.9
Epiplosarcomphalocele (*see also* Hernia,
    umbilicus) 551.1
Episcleritis 369.9
  gouty 274
  periodica fugax 369.9
    angioneurotic - *see* Edema,
      angioneurotic
  staphylococcal 369.9
  suppurative 369.9
  syphilitic 095
  tuberculous 017.2
    late effect or sequela 019.9
Episode
  brain (*see also* Disease,
      cerebrovascular, acute) 436.9
  cerebral (*see also* Disease,
      cerebrovascular, acute) 436.9
  depersonalization (in neurotic state)
      300.6
  psychotic (*see also* Psychosis) 299
  schizophrenic (acute) NEC 295.4
Epispadias
  female 753.8
  male 752.3

Episplenitis 289.5

Epistaxis (multiple) 783.0
  vicarious menstruation 626.9

Epithelioma (squamous cell) (*see also*
      Neoplasm) 239.9
  adamantinum (*see also* Ameloblastoma)
      210.4
  adenoides cysticum (*see also*
        Trichoepithelioma) 216.1
    bronchus 212.3
    lacrimal sac 224
  auricular canal (external) 232.2
  basal cell - *see* Neoplasm, skin,
      malignant
  benign (*see also* Neoplasm, benign)
      228
    auricular canal (external) 216.0
    breast (intracystic) (intraductal) (skin
        of) 217
    calcifying (*see also*
        Trichoepithelioma) 216.1
    cystic (*see also* Trichoepithelioma)
        216.1
    external area or site NEC 216.0
    genital organ NEC - code as
        neoplasm, benign, by site
    jaw 210.4
      skin of 216.0
    lip 210.0
      skin of 216.0
    nose 212.0
      skin of 216.0
    scrotum 216.0
    skin NEC 216.0
    uterus 219.9
    squamous cell 219.0
  Bowen's - *see* Neoplasm, skin,
      malignant
  chorionic (*see also* Chorionepithelioma)
      181
  external area or site NEC - *see*
      Neoplasm, skin
  jaw 239.0
    skin of 232.2
  lip 239.0
    skin of 232.2
  malignant (*see also* Neoplasm,
      malignant) 199.1
    auricular canal (external) 173.2
    external area or site NEC - *see*
        Neoplasm, skin, malignant
    jaw 143.1
      skin of 173.3
    lip (*see also* Neoplasm, lip, malignant)
        140.9

Epithelioma – *continued*
  malignant – *continued*
    lip – *continued*
      skin of 173.0
    nose 160.0
      skin of 173.3
    skin NEC - *see* Neoplasm, skin,
        malignant
  melanotic - *see* Melanoma
  nose 231.0
    skin of 232.2
  radium - *see* Neoplasm, skin, malignant
  skin NEC 232.2
  x-ray - *see* Neoplasm, skin, malignant
Epithelium, epithelial - *see* condition
Epituberculosis (with symptoms) - *see*
      Tuberculosis, pulmonary
Eponychia 757.4
Epstein's nephrosis or syndrome (*see also*
      Nephrosis) 581
Epulis (gingiva) 210.4
  giant cell 523.9
  malignant 143.9
    lower 143.1
    upper 143.0
Equinia 024
Equinovarus (congenital) 754.1
  acquired 738.6
Equivalent
  convulsive (abdominal) 345.9
  epileptic (psychic) 345.9
Erb-Goldflam disease or syndrome
      733.0
Erb(-Duchenne) paralysis (birth injury)
      (newborn) (*see also* Birth injury,
      bone or nerve) 772.2
Erb's
  disease 330.3
  palsy, paralysis (brachial) (birth)
      (newborn) (*see also* Birth injury,
      bone or nerve) 772.2
  spinal (spastic) syphilitic 094.9
  pseudohypertrophic muscular dystrophy
      330.3
Erection (painful) 786.6
Ergosterol deficiency (vitamin D) 265.9
  with
    osteomalacia 265.2
    rickets (*see also* Rickets) 265.0
Ergotism (ergotized grain) 988.2
  from ergot used as drug 976.0
Erichsen's disease 300.1
Erosio interdigitalis blastomycetica 112
Erosion
  artery 447
  bone 723.9

Erosion—*continued*
  bronchus 519.9
  cartilage (joint) (*see also* Disease, joint)
      729.9
  cervix (uteri) (acquired) (chronic)
      (congenital) 621.3
  cornea (recurrent) (*see also* Keratitis)
      363.0
    traumatic - *see* Injury, superficial,
        cornea
  dental (idiopathic) (occupational) 521.3
  esophagus 530.9
  gastric - *see* Ulcer, stomach
  intestine 569.9
  lymphatic vessel 457
  sclera 378.6
  spine, aneurysmal 094.9
  spleen 289.5
  stomach - *see* Ulcer, stomach
  teeth (idiopathic) (occupational) 521.3
  urethra 599.9
  uterus 625.9
  vertebra 723.9
Erotomania 302.8
Error
  in diet 269.9
  refractive 370.9
Eructation 784.7
  nervous 305.5
  psychogenic 305.5
Eruption
  drug - *see* Dermatitis, due to drug
  Hutchinson, summer 709.9
  Kaposi varicelliform 054
  polymorphous
    light 692.7
  ringed 695.9
  skin 788.2
    creeping (meaning hookworm) 126.8
    due to chemical, drug, or poison - *see*
        also Dermatitis, due to
      internal use - *see* Table of adverse
          effects
    erysipeloid 027.1
    feigned 698.4
    Kaposi's, varicelliform 054
    lichenoid, axilla 698.3
    resulting from
      prophylactic inoculation or
          vaccination against disease
          999.5
      smallpox vaccination NEC 999.5
    toxic NEC 695.0
  tooth, teeth
    accelerated 520.6
    delayed 520.6

Eruption—*continued*
  tooth, teeth—*continued*
    disturbance of 520.6
    in abnormal sequence 520.6
    incomplete 520.6
    late 520.6
    partial 520.6
    premature 520.6
  vesicular 709.9
Erysipelas (gangrenous) (infantile)
      (newborn) (phlegmonous)
      (suppurative) 035
  puerperal, postpartum, childbirth 670
Erysipelatoid, Rosenbach's 027.1
Erysipeloid, Rosenbach's 027.1
Erythema, erythematous (infectional)
      695.9
  ab igne 692.7
  annulare
    centrifugum 695.0
    rheumaticum 695.0
  arthriticum epidemicum 026.1
  brucellum (*see also* Brucellosis) 023.9
  due to
    chemical (contact) 692.4
      internal - *see* Table of adverse
          effects
    drug - *see* Dermatitis, due to drug
  elevatum diutinum 695.9
  endemic 262
  epidemic, arthritic 026.1
  figuratum perstans 695.0
  gluteal 692.9
  heat 692.9
  ichthyosiforme congenitum 757.2
  induratum (primary) (scrofulosorum)
      017.0
    late effect or sequela 019.9
    non-tuberculous 695.2
  infectiosum 057.0
  inflammation NEC 695.9
  intertrigo 709.9
  iris 695.1
  lupus (local) (*see also* Lupus) 695.4
  marginatum 695.0
  medicamentosum - *see* Dermatitis, due
      to drug
  migrans 529.1
  multiforme 695.1
    bullosum 695.1
    conjunctiva 695.1
    exudativum (hebra) 695.1
    pemphigoides 694
  napkin 692.9
  neonatorum 695.9

Erythema, etc. — *continued*
  nodosum 695.2
    tuberculous 017.0
      late effect or sequela 019.9
  palmar 695.0
  pernio 443.2
  rash, newborn 695.9
  scarlatiniform (recurrent) (exfoliative)
      695.0
  solare 692.7
  streptogenes 696.5
  toxic, toxicum NEC 695.0
    newborn 695.0
  tuberculous (primary) 017.0
    late effect or sequela 019.9
Erythematosus - *see* condition
Erythematous - *see* condition
Erythermalgia (primary) 443.8
Erythralgia 443.8
Erythrasma 111.8
  scrotal 111.8
Erythredema 985.0
  polyneuritica 985.0
  polyneuropathy 985.0
Erythremia (chronic) 208
  acute 207.2
  secondary 289.0

Erythroblastemia 208
Erythroblastoma 208
Erythroblastopenia 284
Erythroblastosis (fetalis) (newborn) (*see
    also* Disease, hemolytic) 775.9
Erythrocyanosis (crurum) 443.8
Erythrocythemia - *see* Erythremia
Erythrocytosis (megalosplenic) 208
  oval, hereditary (*see also* Elliptocytosis)
      282.1

Erythroderma (*see also* Erythema) 695.9
  desquamativum 695.9
  exfoliative 695.9
  ichthyosiform, congenital 757.2
  maculopapular 696.2
  neonatorum 695.9
  psoriaticum 696.1
Erythrogenesis imperfecta 284

Erythroleukemia 207.2
Erythroleukosis 289.9
Erythromelalgia 443.8
Erythrophagocytosis 289.9
Erythrophobia 300.2
Erythroplakia
  oral mucosa 528.7
Erythroplasia
  buccal 528.7
  cervix 621.1
  of Queyrat 702

Erythroplasia — *continued*
  penis 607.1
  tongue 529.7
  vagina 629.1
  vulva 629.1
Eso-enteritis - *see* Enteritis
Esophagectasis 530.9
  due to cardiospasm 530.0
Esophagismus 530.9
Esophagitis (acute) (chronic) (infectional)
      (necrotic) (peptic) (reflux) 530.1
  tuberculous 017.9
    late effect or sequela 019.9

Esophagomalacia 530.9
Esophagostomiasis 127.4
Esophagotracheal - *see* condition
Esophagus - *see* condition
Esophoria 373.0
  convergence, excess 373.0
  divergence, insufficiency 373.0
Esotropia (accommodative) (alternating)
      (nonaccommodative) (periodic)
      373.0

Espundia 085.2
Essential - *see* condition
Esthesioneuroblastoma 160.0
Esthiomene 099.1
Estivo-autumnal
  fever 084.0
  malaria 084.0
Estriasis 134.0
Ethanolism (*see also* Alcoholism) 303.9
Etherism 304.8
Ethmoid, ethmoidal - *see* condition
Ethmoiditis (chronic) (purulent)
      (nonpurulent) (*see also* Sinusitis)
      503.9
Ethylism (*see also* Alcoholism) 303.9
Eulenburg's disease 330.9
Eunuchism 257.1
Eunuchoidism 257.1
  hypogonatropic 257.1
European blastomycosis 116.0

Eustachian - *see* condition
Euthyroidism 793.8
Eventration
  with congenital defect of diaphragm -
      see Hernia, diaphragm
  colon into chest - *see* Hernia,
      diaphragm
  diaphragm (congenital) - *see* Hernia,
      diaphragm
Eversion
  bladder 596.9
  cervix (uteri) 623.4

Eversion—*continued*
  cervix (uteri)—*continued*
    complicating delivery - *see*
        Obstetrical trauma
    due to lacerations (old)   621.4
    infectional   623.4
  foot NEC   738.6
    congenital   755.7
  lachrymal, lacrimal apparatus   378.3
  punctum lacrimale (postinfectional)
      (senile)   378.3
  ureter (meatus)   593.5
  urethra (meatus)   599.9
  uterus   623.4
    complicating delivery - *see*
        Obstetrical trauma
Evisceration
  birth injury (*see also* Birth injury NEC)
      772.9
  bowel (congenital) (*see also* Hernia,
      abdomen)   551.2
  congenital (*see also* Hernia, abdomen)
      551.2
  operative wound   998.3
  traumatic NEC   869.1
    eye   871
Evulsion - *see* Avulsion
Ewing's
  angio-endothelioma - *see* Neoplasm,
      bone, malignant
  sarcoma - *see* Neoplasm, bone,
      malignant
  tumor - *see* Neoplasm, bone, malignant
Exaggerated lumbosacral angle (with
    impinging spine)   756.1
Examination (without complaint or illness)
    Y00.9
  with complaints or symptoms - *see*
      Observation
  annual   Y00.0
  child care (routine)   Y00.5
  clinical research investigation (normal
      control patient)   Y00.8
  donor   Y09.9
  eye (routine)   Y00.6
  false positive serology   Y00.7
  follow-up - *see* Follow-up
  general, negative findings   Y00.0
  laboratory   Y00.3
  medical (general) (insurance) (routine)
      (school) (survey)   Y00.0
  periodic   Y00.0
  postoperative - *see* Follow-up,
      postoperative
  pregnancy, unconfirmed   Y00.4
  prenatal   Y06

Examination, etc.—*continued*
  psychiatric (general)   Y00.1
    follow-up not needing further care
        Y03.4
  radiological   Y00.2
  specified type NEC   Y00.9
  well baby   Y00.5
Exanthem, exanthema (*see also* Rash)
    788.2
  Boston   046
  epidemic with meningitis   046
  subitum   057.1
  viral, virus NEC   057.9
Excess, excessive, excessively
  carbohydrate tissue, localized   279
  carotin (dietary)   278.1
  cold   991.9
  convergence   373.0
  development, breast   611.1
  divergence   373.1
  drinking (alcohol)   303.9
    continual   303.1
    episodic   303.0
    habitual   303.1
    periodic   303.0
  eyelid fold   744.7
  fat   277
    in heart (*see also* Insufficiency,
        myocardial)   428
    tissue, localized   279
  foreskin   605
  heat NEC (*see also* Heat)   992.9
  large
    colon   569.9
      congenital   751.2
    organ or site, congenital NEC - *see*
        Anomaly, specified type NEC
  lid fold   744.7
  long
    colon   569.9
      congenital   751.4
    organ or site, congenital NEC - *see*
        Anomaly, specified type NEC
    umbilical cord - *see* Complications,
        umbilical cord
  menstruation   626.2
  number of teeth   520.1
    causing crowding   524.3
  nutrient (dietary) NEC   278.9
  salivation (*see also* Ptyalism)   527.7
  secretion milk   678
  short
    organ or site, congenital NEC - *see*
        Anomaly, specified type NEC
    umbilical cord - *see* Complications,
        umbilical cord

Excess, excessive — *continued*
  skin, eyelid   744.7
    acquired   378.2
  sputum   783.4
  thirst   994.3
  vitamin A (dietary)   278.0
    administered as drug   963.6
  vitamin D (dietary)   278.2
    administered as drug   963.6
Excitability, abnormal, under minor stress
    307
Excitation
  psychogenic   298.1
  reactive (from emotional stress,
    psychological trauma)   298.1
Excitement
  manic   296.1
  mental   306.9
    reactive (from emotional stress,
      psychological trauma)   298.1
  state   306.9
    reactive (from emotional stress,
      psychological trauma)   298.1
Excluded pupils   378.6
Excoriation (traumatic) (*see also* Injury,
    superficial)   918.0
  neurotic   698.4
Excyclophoria   373.1
Excyclotropia   373.1
Excencephalus   743.0
Exfoliative - *see also* condition
  dermatitis   695.9
Exfoliatrix   695.9
Exhaustion, exhaustive (physical NEC)
    790.1
  battle   307
  cardiac (*see also* Failure, heart)   782.4
  delirium   299
  due to
    cold   991.9
    excessive exertion   994.5
    exposure   994.4
  fetus or newborn   778.9
  heart (*see also* Failure, heart)   782.4
  heat - *see* Heat, exhaustion
  manic   296.1
  maternal, complicating delivery   657.9
    fetus or newborn - *see* categories
      768.0-768.9
  mental   300.5
  myocardium, myocardial (*see also*
    Failure, heart)   782.4
  nervous   300.5
  old age   794
  postinfectional NEC   790.1
  psychogenic   300.5

Exhaustion, exhaustive — *continued*
  psychosis   299
  senile   794
    dementia   290.0
Exhibitionism   302.4
Exomphalos   551.1
  gangrenous, incarcerated, irreducible,
    strangulated or with obstruction
    (intestinal)   553.1
Exophoria   373.1
  convergence, insufficiency   373.1
  divergence, excess   373.1
Exophthalmia gonorrheal   098.2
Exophthalmos   781.1
  congenital   744.8
  hyperthyroidism   242.0
  intermittent NEC   378.9
  malignant   242.0
  pulsating   781.1
  thyroid   242.0
Exostosis   213.0
  congenital   756.5
  gonococcal   098.8
  jaw (bone)   526.9
  multiple (cancellous) (cartilaginous)
    (hereditary) (osteocartilaginous)
    756.5
  syphilitic   095
Exothelioma - *see* Meningioma
Exotropia (alternating) (intermittent)
    (periodic)   373.1
Exposure   994.4
  cold   991.9
  effects of   994.4
  exhaustion due to   994.4
  to infective or parasitic disease   Y04.9
    poliomyelitis   Y04.1
    rabies   Y04.2
    tuberculosis   Y04.0
Extensive - *see* condition
Extra - *see also* Accessory
  rib   756.4
    cervical   756.3
Extraction
  with hook   773
  breech
    fetus or newborn (*see also* Birth
      injury NEC)   772.9
  manual
    fetus or newborn (*see also* Birth
      injury NEC)   772.9
Extrasystole (atrial) (ventricular) (*see also*
    Action, heart, irregular)   427.9
Extra-uterine gestation or pregnancy - *see*
    Pregnancy, ectopic

F

Faber's syndrome 280

Fabry's disease 272.2

Face, facial - *see* condition

Facet of cornea - *see* Opacity, cornea

Faciocephalalgia, autonomic 358.9

Facioscapulohumeral myopathy 330.3

Factor
  IX deficiency 286.1
  V deficiency (*see also* Defect,
    coagulation) 286.9
  VII deficiency (*see also* Defect,
    coagulation) 286.9
  VIII deficiency NEC 286.0
  X deficiency (*see also* Defect,
    coagulation) 286.9
  XI deficiency 286.2
  XII deficiency (*see also* Defect,
    coagulation) 286.9
  XIII deficiency (*see also* Defect,
    coagulation) 286.9

Fahr-Volhard disease (*see also*
    Hypertension, malignant with renal
    involvement) 400.3

Failed - *see also* Failure
  induction (of labor) (with postmature
    pregnancy) 634.9

Failure
  cardiac (*see also* Failure, heart) 782.4
  cardiorenal (chronic) (*see also* Failure,
    heart) 782.4
  cardiorespiratory (*see also* Failure,
    heart) 782.4
  cardiovascular (chronic) (*see also*
    Failure, heart) 782.4
  cerebrovascular (*see also* Disease,
    cerebrovascular NEC) 438.9
  circulation, circulatory 796.0
    fetus or newborn 778.9
    peripheral 782.9
  compensation - *see* Disease, heart
  congestive (*see also* Failure, heart,
    congestive) 427.0
  coronary (*see also* Insufficiency,
    coronary) 411.9
  descent of head
    complicating delivery 655
    fetus or newborn - *see* categories
      765.0-765.9

Failure - *continued*
  heart (acute) (sudden) 782.4
    with
      acute pulmonary edema - *see*
        Failure, ventricular, left
      decompensation (*see also* Failure,
        heart, congestive) 427.0
      dilatation - *see* Disease, heart
    arteriosclerotic 440.9
    congestive 427.0
      with
        hypertension (benign) (conditions
          in 401) (*see also*
          Hypertension, heart) 402
        malignant (*see also*
          Hypertension, malignant
          with heart involvement)
          400.1
        rheumatic fever (conditions in
          390)
          active 391.9
          inactive or quiescent (with
            chorea) 398
      fetus or newborn 778.9
      rheumatic (chronic) (inactive) (with
        chorea) 398
        active or acute 391.9
        with chorea 392.0
    degenerative (*see also* Insufficiency,
      myocardial) 428
    fetus or newborn 778.9
    high output - *see* Disease, heart
    hypertensive (*see also* Hypertension,
      heart) 402
    left (ventricular) (*see also* Failure,
      ventricular, left) 427.1
    organic - *see* Disease, heart
    rheumatic (chronic) (inactive) 398
    right (ventricular) (*see also* Failure,
      heart, congestive) 427.0
    senile 794
    thyrotoxic (*see also* Thyrotoxicosis)
      242.2
    valvular - *see* Endocarditis
  hepatic 573.9
  hepatorenal 573.9
  involution, thymus (gland) 254
  kidney - *see* Failure, renal
  liver 573.9
  medullary 796.0

Failure — *continued*
  myocardial, myocardium (*see also*
      Failure, heart) 782.4
    chronic (*see also* Failure, heart,
        congestive) 427.0
    congestive (*see also* Failure, heart,
        congestive) 427.0
  ovarian 615.9
  ovulation 615.9
  renal 593.2
    with
      abortion - *see* Abortion, by type,
          with toxemia
      edema (*see also* Nephrosis) 581
      hypertension (benign) (conditions in
          401) (*see also* Hypertension,
          kidney) 403
      malignant (*see also*
          Hypertension, malignant
          with renal involvement)
          400.3
    acute (anuric) (oliguric) - *see*
        Nephritis, acute
    arising during pregnancy 636
      fetus or newborn 762.0
    chronic - *see* Nephritis, chronic
    following crushing 995.6
    hypertensive (*see also* Hypertension,
        kidney) 403
      malignant (*see also* Hypertension,
          malignant with renal
          involvement) 400.3
    puerperal, postpartum 636
  respiration, respiratory 796.0
    center 347.9
      newborn (*see also* Asphyxia,
          newborn) 776.9
    newborn (*see also* Asphyxia,
        newborn) 776.9
  rotation
    cecum 751.1
    colon 751.1
    intestine 751.1
    kidney 753.3
  segmentation - *see also* Fusion
    fingers 755.1
    toes 755.1
  senile (general) 794
  testis, primary (seminal) 257.1
  to thrive 778.9
  urinary 796.0
  ventricular (*see also* Failure, heart)
      782.4
    left 427.1

Failure — *continued*
  ventricular — *continued*
    left — *continued*
      with
        hypertension (benign) (conditions
            in 401) (*see also*
            Hypertension, heart) 402
        malignant (*see also*
            Hypertension, malignant
            with heart involvement)
            400.1
        rheumatic fever (conditions in
            390)
          active 391.9
          inactive or quiescent (with
              chorea) 398
        rheumatic (chronic) (inactive) (with
            chorea) 398
          active or acute 391.9
            with chorea 392.0
    right (*see also* Failure, heart,
        congestive) 427.0
  vital centers
    fetus or newborn 778.9
Fainting (fit) 782.5
Falciform hymen 752.6
Fall, maternal, affecting fetus or newborn
    761.5
Fallen arches 736
Falling, any organ or part - *see* Prolapse
Fallopian tube - *see* condition
Fallot's tetrad or tetralogy 746.2
Fallout, radioactive (adverse effect)
    990.0
False - *see also* condition
  joint - *see* Pseudarthrosis
  labor (pains) (undelivered) 634.7
  opening, urinary 752.8
  passage, urethra (prostatic) 599.9
  pregnancy 300.1
Family, familial - *see* condition
Famine 994.2
  edema 269.9
Fanconi(-de Toni)(-Debre) syndrome
    270.2
Fanconi's anemia 284
Farcin 024
Farcy 024
Farmers'
  lung 516.1
  skin 709.9
Farsightedness 370.1
Fascia - *see* condition
Fasciculation 780.3
Fasciculitis optica 367
Fasciitis (nodular) (plantar) 732

Fasciitis— *continued*
  perirenal   593.3
  traumatic (old)   732
    current - *code by* site under Sprain,
      strain
Fascioliasis   121.3
Fasciolopsiasis   121.4
Fasciolopsis, small intestine   121.4
Fat
  embolism (cerebral) (pulmonary)
      (systemic)   995.1
    complicating delivery - *see*
      Obstetrical trauma
  excessive   277
    in heart (*see also* Insufficiency,
      myocardial)   428
  general   277
  hernia, herniation   733.9
  indigestion   269.0
  localized (pad)   277
    heart (*see also* Insufficiency,
      myocardial)   428
    knee   729.8
    retropatellar   729.8
  necrosis - *see also* Fatty degeneration
    breast (aseptic)   611.0
    mesentery   569.9
    pancreas   577.9
    peritoneum   569.9
Fatal syncope   782.5
Fatigue   790.1
  auditory deafness (*see also* Deafness)
      389.9
  combat   307
  heat (transient)   992.6
  muscle   733.9
    ciliary   378.6
  myocardium (*see also* Failure, heart)
      782.4
  nervous   300.5
  neurosis   300.5
  operational   300.8
  posture   733.9
  psychogenic (general)   300.5
  senile   794
  syndrome   300.5
  undue   790.1
  voice   783.5
Fatness   277
Fatty - *see also* condition
  apron   277
  degeneration (diffuse) (general) NEC
      279
    liver - *see* Cirrhosis, portal
    localized - *see* Degeneration by site,
      fatty

Fatty— *continued*
  degeneration, etc. — *continued*
    placenta - *see* Placenta, abnormal
    disease (diffuse) (general) - *see* Fatty
      degeneration
    heart (enlarged) (*see also* Insufficiency,
      myocardial)   428
    infiltration (diffuse) (general) - *see* Fatty
      degeneration
    liver - *see* Cirrhosis, portal
    metamorphosis (diffuse) (general) - *see*
      Fatty degeneration
    necrosis - *see* Fatty degeneration
    phanerosis   279
    tumor (embryonal) (*see also* Lipoma)
      214.9
Fauces - *see* condition
Faucitis   508.9
Faulty - *see also* condition
  position of teeth   524.3
Favism   282.2
  anemia   282.2
Favus - *see* Dermatophytosis
Fear
  complex   300.2
  reaction   300.2
Febricula (continued) (simple) (*see also*
      Pyrexia)   788.6
Febrile (*see also* Pyrexia)   788.6
Febris (*see also* Fever)   788.6
  aestiva - *see* Fever, hay
  flava (*see also* Fever, yellow)   060.9
  melitensis   023.0
  pestis (*see also* Plague)   020.9
  puerperalis   670
  recurrens (*see also* Fever, relapsing)
      088.9
    pediculo vestimenti, causa   088.0
  rubra   034.1
  typhoidea   001
  typhosa   001
Fecal - *see also* condition
  abscess   569.9
  fistula   569.3
  impaction or mass   560.3
    with hernia - *see* Hernia, by site, with
      obstruction
Fecalith (impaction)   560.3
  with hernia - *see* Hernia, by site, with
    obstruction
  appendix   543
Feeble rapid pulse due to shock following
    injury   995.5
Feeble-mindedness - *see* Retardation,
    mental, mild

Feeding
  case   269.9
    routine formula check   Y00.5
  faulty   269.9
  improper   269.9
  problem (infant) (newborn)   269.9
Feer's disease   985.0
Feet - *see* condition
Feil-Klippel syndrome   756.2
Felix's disease   722.2
Felon (any digit) (with lymphangitis)   681
Felty's syndrome   712.1
Feminization, testicular   257.9
Femur, femoral - *see* condition
Fenestration, fenestrated - *see also*
        Imperfect closure
  aorta-pulmonary   746.0
  aortic or pulmonic cusps   746.6
  aorticopulmonary   746.0
  cusps, heart valve (any)   746.6
  hymen   752.6
Fermentation (gastric) (gastro-intestinal)
        (stomach)   536.9
  intestine   564.9
    psychogenic   305.5
  psychogenic   305.5
Fetalis uterus   752.5
Fetid
  sweat   705.9
Fetishism   302.1
Fetus, fetal - *see also* condition
  blood loss before birth   778.0
  distress syndrome (*see also* Distress,
        fetal)   776.3
  type lung tissue (*see also* Syndrome,
        respiratory distress)   776.2
Fever   788.6
  with chills   788.9
    in malarial regions   084.9
  abortus NEC   023.9
  Aden   061
  African tick-borne   088.1
  American
    mountain tick   068.1
    spotted   082.0
  and ague   084.9
  aphthous   079.4
  Assam   085.0
  Australian A or Q   083.1
  Bangkok hemorrhagic   067.4
  bilious, hemoglobinuric   084.4
  blackwater   084.4
    nonmalarial   283.0
  blister   054
  boutonneuse   082.1
  brain   323

Fever—*continued*
  brain—*continued*
    late effects   324
  breakbone   061
  Bullis   082.9
  Burdwan   085.0
  Bwamba   068.2
  Cameroon   084.9
  Canton   081.9
  cat scratch   079.3
  catarrhal (acute)   460
    chronic   502.1
    lung - *see* Pneumonia, broncho
  cerebral   323
    late effects   324
  cerebrospinal (meningococcal) - *see*
        Meningitis, cerebrospinal
  Chagres   084.0
  Charcot's (biliary) (hepatic)
        (intermittent) (*see also*
        Cholelithiasis)   574.9
  Chikungunya   068.2
  childbed   670
  Chitral   068.0
  Colombo   002.9
  Colorado tick (virus)   068.1
  congestive
    malarial (*see also* Malaria)   084.9
    remittent (*see also* Malaria)   084.9
  continued
    malarial   084.0
  Corsican   084.9
  Crimean hemorrhagic   067.0
  Cyprus (*see also* Brucellosis)   023.9
  dandy   061
  deer fly   021
  dehydration, newborn   778.9
  dengue   061
    virus hemorrhagic   067.4
  desert   114
  due to heat   992.0
  Dumdum   085.0
  enteric   001
  ephemeral (of unknown origin) (*see also*
        Pyrexia)   788.6
  epidemic, hemorrhagic of the Far East
        067.0
  erysipelatous (*see also* Erysipelas)   035
  estivo-autumnal (malarial)   084.0
  famine - *see* Fever, relapsing
    meaning typhus - *see* Typhus
  Far Eastern hemorrhagic   067.0
  Fort Bragg   100.8
  gastro-enteric   001
  gastromalarial (*see also* Malaria)   084.9
  Gibraltar (*see also* Brucellosis)   023.9

Fever—*continued*
glandular 075
Haverhill 026.1
hay (allergic) (any cause) (grass) (pollen)
(ragweed) (tree) 507
with
asthma (bronchial) 493
conjunctivitis 507
rhinitis 507
heat (effects) 992.0
hematuric, bilious 084.4
hemoglobinuric (malarial) 084.4
bilious 084.4
nonmalarial 283.0
hemorrhagic (arthropod-borne) NEC
067.9
with renal syndrome 067.5
Argentinian 067.9
Bangkok 067.4
Bolivian 067.9
Crimean 067.0
dengue virus 067.4
epidemic 067.5
of Far East 067.0
Far Eastern 067.0
Korean 067.5
Machupo virus 067.9
mite-borne 067.9
mosquito-borne 067.4
Omsk 067.1
Philippine 067.4
Russian (Yaroslav) 067.5
Singapore 067.4
Southeast Asia 067.4
Thailand 067.4
tick-borne NEC 067.3
Yunin virus 067.9
hepatic (*see also* Cholecystitis) 575
intermittent (*see also* Cholelithiasis)
574.9
herpetic 054
Hyalomma tick 067.0
inanition 788.6
infective NEC 136
intermittent (bilious) (*see also* Malaria)
084.9
hepatic (Charcot) (*see also*
Cholelithiasis) 574.9
of unknown origin (*see also* Pyrexia)
788.6
pernicious 084.0
iodide 977.0
specified iodide - *see* Table of
adverse effects
Japanese river 081.2
jungle yellow 060.0

Fever—*continued*
Kedani 081.2
Kenya 082.1
Lone Star 082.9
lung - *see also* Pneumonia
catarrhal - *see* Pneumonia, broncho
malaria, malarial (*see also* Malaria)
084.9
Malta (*see also* Brucellosis) 023.9
Marseilles 082.1
marsh (*see also* Malaria) 084.9
Mediterranean (*see also* Brucellosis)
023.9
familial 276
tick 082.1
meningeal - *see* Meningitis
metal fumes 985.9
Meuse 083.2
Mexican - *see* Typhus, Mexican
mianeh 088.1
miasmatic (*see also* Malaria) 084.9
miliary 136
milk, female 678
mill 516.1
Monday 516.1
mosquito-borne NEC 068.2
hemorrhagic NEC 067.4
mountain
meaning
Rocky Mountain spotted 082.0
undulant fever (*see also*
Brucellosis) 023.9
tick (American) 068.1
mud 100.8
nine-mile 083.1
non-exanthematous tick 068.1
North Asian tick-borne typhus 082.2
O'nyong-nyong 068.2
Omsk hemorrhagic 067.1
Oroya 089.0
paludal (*see also* Malaria) 084.9
Panama 084.0
pappataci 068.0
paratyphoid 002.9
A 002.0
B 002.1
C 002.2
parrot 073
periodic 276
pernicious, acute 084.0
persistent (of unknown origin) (*see also*
Pyrexia) 788.6
petechial 036.0
pharyngoconjunctival 078.2
Philippine hemorrhagic 067.4
phlebotomus 068.0

Fever—*continued*
  Plasmodium ovale   084.3
  pleural (*see also* Pleurisy)   511.0
  pretibial   100.8
  puerperal, postpartum   670
  putrid - *see* Septicemia
  pyemic - *see* Septicemia
  Q   083.1
  quadrilateral   083.1
  quartan (malaria)   084.2
  Queensland (costal)   083.1
    seven day   100.8
  quotidian   084.0
  rabbit   021
  rat-bite   026.9
    due to Spirochaeta morsus muris
        026.0
    due to Streptobacillus moniliformis
        026.1
    spirillary   026.0
    Spirillum minus   026.0
  recurrent - *see* Fever, relapsing
  relapsing   088.9
    Carter's (Asiatic)   088.0
    Dutton's (West African)   088.1
    Koch's   088.9
    louse-borne   088.0
    Novy's (American)   088.1
    Obermeyer's (European)   088.0
    spirillum NEC   088.9
    tick-borne   088.1
  remittent (bilious) (congestive) (gastric)
        (*see also* Malaria)   084.9
  rheumatic (active) (acute) (chronic)
        (subacute)   390
    active with heart involvement - *see*
        Category 391
    inactive or quiescent with
      cardiac hypertrophy   398
      carditis   398
      congestive heart failure (conditions
          in 427.0)   398
      endocarditis   397.9
        aortic (valve)   395.0
          with mitral (valve) disease
              396.0
        mitral (valve)   394.0
          with aortic (valve) disease
              396.0
        pulmonary (valve)   397.9
        tricuspid (valve)   397.0
      heart disease NEC (conditions in
          429)   398
      left ventricular failure (conditions
          in 427.1)   398

Fever—*continued*
  rheumatic—*continued*
    inactive or quiescent with—*continued*
      myocardial insufficiency (condition
          in 428)   398
      myocarditis   398
      pancarditis   398
      pericarditis   393
  Rift Valley   068.2
  Rocky Mountain spotted   082.0
  rose   507
  San Joaquin   114
  sandfly   068.0
  Sao Paulo   082.0
  scarlet   034.1
    puerperal, postpartum, childbirth
        670
  septic - *see* Septicemia
  seven day   061
    of
      Japan   100.8
      Queensland   100.8
  shin bone   083.2
  Singapore hemorrhagic   067.4
  solar   061
  sore   054
  South African tick-bite   088.1
  Southeast Asia hemorrhagic   067.4
  spinal - *see* Meningitis
  splenic   022
  spotted (Rocky Mountain)   082.0
    American   082.0
    Brazilian   082.0
    Colombian   082.0
    meaning
      cerebrospinal meningitis   036.0
      typhus   082.9
  steroid   962.0
  streptobacillary   026.1
  subtertian   084.0
  Sumatran mite   081.2
  sun   061
  swamp   100.8
  sweating   136
  swine   003.9
    due to food   003.0
  tertian - *see* Malaria, tertian
  Thailand hemorrhagic   067.4
  thermic   992.0
  three-day   068.0
    with Coxsackie exanthem   074.9
  tick-bite NEC   068.1
  tick-borne NEC   068.1
    hemorrhagic NEC   067.3
  transitory of newborn   778.9
  trench   083.2

Fever—*continued*
 tsutsugamushi 081.2
 typhogastric 001
 typhoid (abortive) (ambulant) (any site)
   (hemorrhagic) (infection)
   (intermittent) (malignant)
   (rheumatic) 001
 typhomalarial 084.9
 typhus - *see* Typhus
 undulant (*see also* Brucellosis) 023.9
 unknown origin (*see also* Pyrexia)
   788.6
 uremic - *see* Uremia
 uveoparotid 135
 valley 114
 Venezuelan equine 068.2
 West African 084.4
 West Nile 068.2
 Whitmore's 025
 Wolhynian 083.2
 worm 128.9
 yellow 060.9
  jungle 060.0
  sylvatic 060.0
  urban 060.1
Fibrillation
 atrial or auricular (established)
   (paroxysmal) 427.4
 with
   hypertension (benign) (conditions in
     401) (*see also* Hypertension,
     heart) 402
   malignant (*see also*
     Hypertension, malignant
     with heart involvement)
     400.1
 cardiac (*see also* Action, heart,
   irregular) 427.9
 coronary (*see also* Infarct, myocardium)
   410.9
 heart (*see also* Action, heart, irregular)
   427.9
 muscular 733.9
 ventricular 427.6
 with
   hypertension (benign) (conditions in
     401) (*see also* Hypertension,
     heart) 402
   malignant (*see also*
     Hypertension, malignant
     with heart involvement)
     400.1
Fibrin
 ball or bodies, pleural (sac) 511.0
 chamber, anterior (eye) (gelatinous
   exudate) 378.6

Fibrinogenolysis - *see* Fibrinolysis
Fibrinogenopenia (*see also* Defect,
   coagulation) 286.9
Fibrinolysis (hemorrhagic) 286.4
 causing hemorrhage of pregnancy
   632.4
 fetus or newborn 769.9
 following childbirth 675
 newborn 778.2
Fibrinopenia (hereditary) (*see also* Defect,
   coagulation) 286.9
Fibrinopurulent - *see* condition
Fibrinous - *see* condition
Fibro-adenoma (breast) 217
 prostate 600
 specified site NEC - *see* Neoplasm,
   benign
Fibro-adenosis, breast 610
Fibro-angioma (juvenile) (nasopharynx)
   227.1
Fibroblastoma - *see also* Neoplasm,
   connective tissue
 arachnoid - *see* Fibroblastoma,
   meningeal
 benign - *see* Neoplasm, connective
   tissue, benign
 malignant - *see* Neoplasm, connective
   tissue, malignant
 meningeal 225.9
  brain 225.2
  spinal cord 225.4
  perineural 225.5
  perineurial 225.5
Fibrocarcinoma - *see* Neoplasm,
   malignant
Fibrochondroma (*see also* Neoplasm,
   cartilage, benign) 213.9
Fibrochondro-osteoma 213.9
Fibrochondrosarcoma - *see* Neoplasm,
   cartilage, malignant
Fibrocyst - *see* Fibroma
Fibrocystic
 disease 273.0
  bone NEC 723.9
  breast 610
  jaw 526.2
  kidney (congenital) 753.1
  liver 751.6
  lung (congenital) 748.4
  pancreas 273.0
 kidney (congenital) 753.1
Fibroelastosis (cordis) (endocardial)
   (endomyocardial) 746.7
 acquired 425
Fibro-endothelioma - *see also* Fibroma

Fibro-endothelioma—*continued*
  malignant - *see* Neoplasm, connective
    tissue, malignant
Fibro-epithelioma - *see also* Epithelioma,
  benign
  malignant - *see* Epithelioma, malignant
  ovary 220.9
  uterus 219.0
Fibroid (tumor) (uterus) 218
  bleeding 218
  cervix (stump) (uterus) 218
  complicating delivery 657.9
    fetus or newborn - *see* categories
      764.0-764.9
  disease, lung (chronic) (*see also*
    Fibrosis, lung) 517
  heart (disease) (*see also* Insufficiency,
    myocardial) 428
  induration, lung (chronic) (*see also*
    Fibrosis, lung) 517
  liver - *see* Cirrhosis, liver
  lung (*see also* Fibrosis, lung) 517
  malignant change in 182.9
  multiple 218
  not of uterus (*see also* Neoplasm,
    connective tissue, benign) 215
  noted during pregnancy (undelivered)
    634.9
  ovary 220.2
  pneumonia (chronic) (*see also* Fibrosis,
    lung) 517
  submucous 218
  subserous 218
Fibrolipoma (*see also* Lipoma) 214.9
Fibroliposarcoma - *see* Neoplasm,
  connective tissue, malignant
Fibroma (*see also* Neoplasm, connective
  tissue, benign) 215
  bone 213.9
  cervix (stump) (uterus) 218
  chondromyxoid (*see also* Chondroma)
    213.2
  corpus albicans 220.2
  durum (*see also* Dermatofibroma)
    216.8
  fungoides 202.1
  mandible, ossifying 213.9
  myometrium 218
  nasopharynx, nasopharyngeal (juvenile)
    227.1
  nonosteogenic (nonossifying) 213.9
  ovary 220.2
  periosteum 213.9
  polypoid (cervix) (uterus) 218
    not of uterus - *see* Neoplasm,
      connective tissue, benign

Fibroma—*continued*
  prostate 600
  skin (molle) (soft) (*see also*
    Dermatofibroma) 216.8
  spermatic cord 222.8
  tunica vaginalis 222.8
  uterus 218
  vulva 221.2
Fibromatosis
  gingival 523.9
  subcutaneous pseudosarcomatous 732
Fibromyeloid reticulosis 209
  Robb-Smith's 201
Fibromyoma (cervix) (stump) (uterus,
  uterine) 218
  complicating delivery 657.9
    fetus or newborn - *see* categories
      764.0-764.9
  not of uterus (*see also* Neoplasm,
    connective tissue, benign) 215
  noted during pregnancy (undelivered)
    634.9
Fibromyositis 717.9
  scapulohumeral 717.1
Fibromyxoma (*see also* Neoplasm,
  connective tissue, benign) 215
Fibromyxosarcoma - *see* Neoplasm,
  connective tissue, malignant
Fibroneuroma 225.5
Fibro-osteochondroma 213.9
Fibro-osteoma 213.9
  sinus, nasal 212.0
Fibroplasia, retrolental 377.0
Fibropurulent - *see* condition
Fibrosarcoma (*see also* Neoplasm,
  connective tissue, malignant)
  171.9
  odontogenic - *see* Ameloblastoma,
    malignant
Fibrosclerosis, penis (corpora cavernosa)
  607.9
Fibrosis, fibrotic
  adrenal (gland) 255.9
  amnion - *see* Placenta, abnormal
  anal papillae 569.2
  anus 569.2
  appendix, appendiceal, noninflammatory
    543
  arteriocapillary - *see* Arteriosclerosis
  bauxite (of lung) 516.0
  bladder 596.9
    panmural (*see also* Cystitis) 595
  bone marrow 209
  bone, diffuse 756.7

Fibrosis, fibrotic—*continued*
  breast 611.9
  capillary - *see also* Arteriosclerosis
    lung (chronic) (*see also* Fibrosis, lung)
      517
  cardiac (*see also* Insufficiency,
    myocardial) 428
  cervix 621.9
  chorion - *see* Placenta, abnormal
  choroidea corrugans 378.6
  corpus cavernosum 607.9
  cystic (of pancreas) 273.0
  ejaculatory duct 607.9
  endocardium (*see also* Endocarditis)
    424.9
  endomyocardial 425
  epididymis 607.9
    postinfectional 607.9
  eye muscle 378.9
  eyelid 378.2
  graphite (of lung) 516.0
  heart (*see also* Insufficiency,
    myocardial) 428
  hepatolienal - *see* Cirrhosis, liver
  hepatosplenic - *see* Cirrhosis, liver
  intrascrotal 607.9
  kidney (*see also* Sclerosis, renal) 584
  liver - *see* Cirrhosis, liver
  lung (atrophic) (capillary) (chronic)
    (confluent) (massive) 517
    with
      anthracosilicosis 515.1
      anthracosis 515.1
      asbestosis 515.2
      bagassosis 516.1
      berylliosis 516.0
      byssinosis 516.1
      calcicosis 515.0
      chalicosis 515.0
      dust reticulation 515.9
      farmers' lung 516.1
      gannister disease 515.0
      pneumonoconiosis 515.9
      pneumosiderosis 516.0
      siderosis 516.0
      silicosis 515.0
      tuberculosis (*see also* Tuberculosis,
        pulmonary) 011.9
        with pneumoconiosis (conditions
          in 515) 010
        late effect or sequela 019.0
      silicotic 515.0
      tuberculous (*see also* Tuberculosis,
        pulmonary) 011.9
        with pneumoconiosis (conditions in
          515) 010

Fibrosis, fibrotic—*continued*
  lymphatic gland 289.3
  median bar 600
  mediastinum (idiopathic) 519.9
  meninges (*see also* Meningitis) 320.9
  myocardium, myocardial (*see also*
    Insufficiency, myocardial) 428
  oviduct 615.9
  pancreas 577.9
  penis 607.9
  peri-appendiceal 543
  placenta - *see* Placenta, abnormal
  pleura 511.0
  prostate (chronic) 600
  pulmonary (*see also* Fibrosis, lung)
    517
  rectal sphincter 569.2
  retroperitoneal, idiopathic 593.3
  scrotum 607.9
  seminal vesicle 607.9
    postinfectional 607.9
  senile 794
  skin NEC 709.9
  spermatic cord 607.9
  spleen 289.5
  submucous NEC 709.9
    oral 528.8
  syncytium - *see* Placenta, abnormal
  testis 607.9
    chronic, due to syphilis 095
  thymus (gland) 254
  tunica vaginalis 607.9
  uterus (non neoplastic) 625.9
  vagina 629.9
  valve, heart (*see also* Endocarditis)
    424.9
  vas deferens 607.9
  vein 458.9
    lower extremities 458.9
Fibrositis (periarticular) (rheumatoid)
  717.9
  humeroscapular region 717.1
  nodular, chronic
    Jaccoud 712.5
    rheumatoid 712.5
  scapulohumeral 717.1
Fibrothorax 511.0
Fibrotic - *see* Fibrosis
Fibrous - *see* condition
Fiedler's
  disease 100.0
  myocarditis (acute) 422
Fifth disease 057.0
Filaria, filarial - *see* Infestation, filarial
Filariasis (*see also* Infestation, filarial)
  125.9

Filariasis — *continued*
  due to
    bancrofti 125.0
    Brugia (Wuchereria) (malayi) 125.1
    malayi 125.1
    Wuchereria (bancrofti) 125.0
Filatov's disease 075
File-cutters' disease 984
Fimbrial cyst 752.5
Fimbriated hymen 752.6
Finger - *see* condition
Fire, St. Anthony's (*see also* Erysipelas)
    035
Fish hook stomach 537.9
Fissure
  anus, anal 565.0
    congenital 751.4
  buccal cavity 528.9
  ear, lobule (congenital) 745.2
  epiglottis (congenital) 748.3
  larynx 508.3
    congenital 748.3
  lip 528.5
    congenital 749.1
      with cleft palate 749.2
  nipple 611.2
    puerperal, postpartum 678
  palate (congenital) 749.0
    with cleft lip 749.2
  postanal 565.0
  rectum 565.0
  skin 709.9
    streptococcal 686.9
  spine (congenital) 741.9
    with hydrocephalus 741.0
  tongue (congenital) 750.0
    acquired 529.5
Fissured tongue 529.5
  congenital 750.0
Fistula 686.9
  abdomen (wall) 569.3
    bladder 596.0
    intestine 569.3
    ureter 593.5
    uterus 616.9
  abdominopelvo-intestinovaginal 616.9
  abdominorectal 569.3
  abdominosigmoidal 569.3
  abdominothoracic 510
  abdomino-uterine 616.9
    congenital 752.5
  abdomino-uterinecolonic 616.9
  abdominovesical 596.0
  accessory sinuses (*see also* Sinusitis)
    503.9
  actinomycotic 113

Fistula — *continued*
  alveolar
    antrum (*see also* Sinusitis, antrum)
      503.0
    process 522.7
  anorectal 565.1
  antrobuccal (*see also* Sinusitis, antrum)
    503.0
  antrum (*see also* Sinusitis, antrum)
    503.0
  anus, anal (recurrent) (infectional)
    565.1
    congenital 751.4
    tuberculous 014
      late effect or sequela 019.9
  aorta-duodenal 447
  appendix, appendicular 543
  arteriovenous (acquired) 442
    congenital 747.6
    coronary
      congenital 746.8
    pulmonary
      congenital 747.6
  aural 387.9
    congenital 745.4
  auricle 387.9
    congenital 745.4
  Bartholin's gland 629.9
  bile duct (*see also* Fistula, gallbladder)
    576.1
  biliary (*see also* Fistula, gallbladder)
    576.1
  bladder (sphincter) 596.0
    into seminal vesicle 596.0
  bone 723.9
  brain 347.9
  branchial (cleft) 745.4
  branchiogenous 745.4
  breast 611.9
    puerperal, postpartum 678
  bronchial 510
  bronchocutaneous, bronchomediastinal,
      bronchopleural,
      bronchopleuromediastinal
      (infective) 510
    tuberculous (*see also* Tuberculosis,
      pulmonary) 011.9
  broncho-esophageal 530.9
    congenital 750.2
  buccal cavity (infective) 528.3
  canal ear 387.9
  carotid-cavernous 447
  cecosigmoidal 569.3
  cecum 569.3
  cerebrospinal (fluid) 347.9

Fistula—*continued*
cervical, lateral 745.4
cervico-aural 745.4
cervicosigmoidal 616.9
cervicovesical 596.0
cervix 621.9
chest (wall) 510
cholecystocolic (*see also* Fistula,
  gallbladder) 576.1
cholecystocolonic (*see also* Fistula,
  gallbladder) 576.1
cholecystoduodenal (*see also* Fistula,
  gallbladder) 576.1
cholecysto-enteric (*see also* Fistula,
  gallbladder) 576.1
cholecystogastric (*see also* Fistula,
  gallbladder) 576.1
cholecysto-intestinal (*see also* Fistula,
  gallbladder) 576.1
choledochoduodenal (*see also* Fistula,
  gallbladder) 576.1
cholocolic (*see also* Fistula, gallbladder)
  576.1
coccyx 685
colon 569.3
colostomy 998.7
common duct (*see also* Fistula,
  gallbladder) 576.1
complicating delivery (any site in pelvis)
  657.9
  fetus or newborn - *see* categories
    764.0-764.9
congenital, site not listed - *see*
  Anomaly, specified type NEC
cornea 378.4
costal region 510
cul-de-sac, Douglas' 616.9
cutaneous 686.9
cystic duct (*see also* Fistula,
  gallbladder) 576.1
  congenital 751.6
dental 522.7
diaphragm 510
  bronchovisceral 510
  pleuroperitoneal 510
  pulmonoperitoneal 510
duodenum 537.9
ear (external) 387.9
enterocolic 569.3
entero-uterine 616.9
  congenital 752.5
enterovaginal 616.9
  congenital 752.6
epididymis 607.9
  tuberculous 016.2
esophagobronchial 530.9

Fistula—*continued*
esophagobronchial—*continued*
  congenital 750.2
esophagocutaneous 530.9
esophagopleural-cutaneous 530.9
esophagotracheal 530.9
  congenital 750.2
esophagus 530.9
  congenital 750.8
ethmoid (*see also* Sinusitis) 503.9
eyelid 378.2
fallopian tube (external) 615.9
fecal 569.3
  congenital 751.4
from periapical lesion 522.7
frontal sinus (*see also* Sinusitis, frontal)
  503.1
gallbladder 576.1
  with calculus, cholelithiasis, stones
    574.9
gastric 537.9
gastrocolic 537.9
  congenital 750.8
  tuberculous 014
    late effect or sequela 019.9
gastro-enterocolic 537.9
gastrojejunal 537.9
gastrojejunocolic 537.9
hepatopleural 510
hepatopulmonary 510
ileorectal 569.3
ileosigmoidal 569.3
ileovesical 596.0
ileum 569.3
in ano 565.1
  tuberculous 014
    late effect or sequela 019.9
inner ear (labyrinth) 387.9
intestine 569.3
intestinocolonic (abdominal) 569.3
intestino-ureteral 593.5
intestino-uterine 616.9
intestinovesical 596.0
ischiorectal (fossa) 566
jejunum 569.3
joint (*see also* Disease, joint) 729.9
  tuberculous - *see* Tuberculosis, joint
kidney (*see also* Lesion, kidney) 593.2
labium (majus) (minus) 629.9
labyrinth 387.9
lachrymal, lacrimal (gland) (sac) 368
lachrymonasal, lacrimonasal duct 368
laryngotracheal 748.3
larynx 508.3

Fistula—*continued*
  lip 528.5
    congenital 750.8
  lumbar, tuberculous 015.0
    late effect or sequela 019.3
  lung 510
  lymphatic 457
  malignant - *see* Neoplasm, malignant
  mammary (gland) 611.9
    puerperal, postpartum 678
  mastoid (process) (region) (*see also*
        Mastoiditis) 383.9
  maxillary (*see also* Sinusitis, maxillary)
        503.0
  mediastinal 510
  mediastinobronchial 510
  mediastinocutaneous 510
  middle ear 387.9
  mouth 528.3
  nasal 508.9
    duct 368
    sinus (*see also* Sinusitis) 503.9
  nasopharynx 508.9
  nipple - *see* Fistula, breast
  nose 508.9
  oral (cutaneous) 528.3
    maxillary sinus (*see also* Sinusitis,
        maxillary) 503.0
    nasal (with cleft palate) 749.0
  orbit, orbital 378.9
  oro-antral (*see also* Sinusitis, antrum)
        503.0
  oviduct (external) 615.9
  pancreatic 577.9
  pancreaticoduodenal 577.9
  parotid (gland) 527.4
    region 528.3
  pelvo-abdomino-intestinal 569.3
  penis 607.9
  peri-anal 565.1
  pericardium (pleura) (sac) - *see*
        Pericarditis
  pericecal 569.3
  perineorectal 569.2
  perineosigmoidal 569.3
  perineo-urethroscrotal 607.9
  perineum, perineal NEC 599.1
    tuberculous 017.9
      late effect or sequela 019.9
    ureter 593.5
  perirectal 569.2
    tuberculous 014
      late effect or sequela 019.9
  peritoneum (*see also* Peritonitis) 567.9
  peri-urethral 599.1
  pharyngo-esophageal 508.9

Fistula—*continued*
  pharynx 508.9
    branchial cleft (congenital) 745.4
  pilonidal (infected) (rectum) 685
  pleura, pleural, pleurocutaneous,
        pleuroperitoneal 510
    stomach 510
    tuberculous 012.1
      with pneumoconiosis (conditions in
        515) 010
      late effect or sequela 019.0
  postauricular 387.9
  postoperative, persistent 998.6
  pre-auricular (congenital) 745.4
    acquired 387.9
  prostate 602
  pulmonary 510
    tuberculous (*see also* Tuberculosis,
        pulmonary) 011.9
  pulmonoperitoneal 510
  rectolabial 616.9
  rectosigmoid 569.2
    intercommunicating 569.2
  recto-ureteral 593.5
  recto-urethral 599.1
    congenital 753.8
  recto-uterine 616.9
    congenital 752.5
  rectovaginal 629.8
    congenital 752.6
    old, postpartal 629.8
    tuberculous 014
      late effect or sequela 019.9
  rectovesical 596.0
    congenital 753.8
  rectovesicovaginal 596.0
  rectovulval 616.9
    congenital 752.6
  rectum 569.2
    tuberculous 014
      late effect or sequela 019.9
  renal (*see also* Lesion, kidney) 593.2
  retroauricular 387.9
  salivary duct or gland 527.4
    congenital 750.8
  sclera 378.6
  scrotum (urinary) 607.9
    tuberculous 016.2
      late effect or sequela 019.2
  semicircular canals 387.9
  sigmoid 569.3
    vesico-abdominal 596.0
  skin 686.9
    ureter 593.5
    vagina 629.9

Fistula—*continued*
  sphenoidal sinus (*see also* Sinusitis)
      503.9
  splenocolic 289.5
  stercoral 569.3
  stomach 537.9
  sublingual gland 527.4
      congenital 750.8
  submaxillary
      gland 527.4
          congenital 750.8
      region 528.3
  thoracic 510
      duct 457
  thoracico-abdominal 510
  thoracicogastric 510
  thoracico-intestinal 510
  thoracogastric 510
  thorax 510
  thyroglossal duct 758.2
  thyroid 246
  trachea (congenital) (external) (internal)
      748.3
  tracheo-esophageal 530.9
      congenital 750.2
  tuberculous - *code by* site under
      Tuberculosis
  typhoid 001
  umbilical 758.8
  umbilico-urinary 753.8
  urachus 753.8
  ureter (persistent) 593.5
  uretero-abdominal 593.5
  ureterocervical 593.5
  ureterorectal 593.5
  ureterosigmoido-abdominal 593.5
  ureterovaginal 629.9
  ureterovesical 596.0
  urethra 599.1
      congenital 753.8
      tuberculous 016.1
          late effect or sequela 019.2
  urethroperineal 599.1
  urethroperineovesical 596.0
  urethrorectal 599.1
      congenital 753.8
  urethroscrotal 607.9
  urethrovaginal 629.9
  urethrovesical 596.0
  urinary (persistent) (recurrent) 599.1
      tract 599.1
  utero-abdominal 616.9
      congenital 752.5
  utero-enteric 616.9
  uterofecal 616.9

Fistula—*continued*
  utero-intestinal 616.9
      congenital 752.5
  uterorectal 616.9
      congenital 752.5
  uterovaginal 625.9
  uterovesical 596.0
      congenital 752.5
  uterus 625.9
  vagina (wall) 629.9
      postpartal, old 629.9
  vaginocutaneous (postpartal) 629.9
  vesical 596.0
  vesico-abdominal 596.0
  vesicocervicovaginal 596.0
  vesicocolic 596.0
  vesico-enteric 596.0
  vesico-intestinal 596.0
  vesicometrorectal 596.0
  vesicoperineal 596.0
  vesicorectal 596.0
      congenital 753.8
  vesicosigmoidal 596.0
  vesicosigmoidovaginal 596.0
  vesico-ureteral 596.0
  vesico-ureterovaginal 596.0
  vesico-urethral 596.0
  vesico-urethrorectal 596.0
  vesico-uterine 596.0
      congenital 752.5
  vesicovaginal 596.0
  vulvorectal 616.9
      congenital 752.6
Fit 780.2
  apoplectic (*see also* Disease,
          cerebrovascular, acute) 436.9
  epileptic (*see also* Epilepsy) 345.9
  fainting 782.5
  hysterical 300.1
  parietal 780.2
  uncinate 780.2
Fitting of prosthetic device Y12.9
  artifical
      arm(s) Y12.0
      eye(s) Y12.2
      leg(s) Y12.1
  colostomy belt or other abdominal
          appliance Y12.4
  dental Y12.3
  specified type NEC Y12.9
Fitzhugh-Curtis syndrome 098.8
Fixation
  joint - *see* Ankylosis
  larynx 508.3
  pupil 378.6
  stapes 386

Fixation—*continued*
  stapes—*continued*
    deafness (*see also* Deafness) 389.9
  uterus (acquired) - *see* Malposition,
      uterus
  vocal cord 508.3
Flaccid - *see also* condition
  foot 738.6
  forearm 738.2
  palate, congenital 750.8
Flail
  chest NEC - *see also* Fracture, rib(s)
    newborn (*see also* Birth injury, bone
        or nerve) 772.2
  joint (paralytic) 729.9
    ankle 729.9
    elbow 729.3
    finger 729.9
    hip 729.5
    knee 729.8
    postpoliomyelitic 044
    shoulder 729.2
    spine 729.1
    toe 729.9
    wrist 729.9
Flajani's disease 242.0
Flap
  liver 573.9
Flat
  chamber (eye) 378.6
  chest, congenital 756.4
  foot (acquired) (fixed type) (painful)
      (postural) (spastic) 736
    congenital 755.7
    rachitic 265.1
  organ or site, congenital NEC - *see*
      Anomaly, specified type NEC
  pelvis 738.8
    complicating delivery 654.2
      fetus or newborn - *see* categories
          764.0-764.9
    congenital 755.7
    noted during pregnancy (undelivered)
        634.9
Flatau-Schilder disease 341
Flattening
  head, femur 723.9
  hip 723.9
  lip (congenital) 745.8
  nose (congenital) 748.1
Flatulence 785.4
  colic 785.5
Flatus 785.4
  vaginalis 629.9
Flax-dressers' disease 516.1
Flea bite - *see* Injury, superficial

Fleischer-Kayser ring 273.3
Fleischer's ring 273.3
Fleischner's disease 722.2
Fleshy mole (abortion) (*see also* Abortion,
    other) 645.9
  undelivered 634.9
Flexibilitas cerea - *see* Catalepsy
Flexion
  cervix (*see also* Malposition, uterus)
      624.9
  deformity, joint (*see also* Contraction,
      joint) 729.9
    hip, congenital 755.6
  uterus (*see also* Malposition, uterus)
      624.9
  lateral - *see* Lateroversion, uterus
Flexner-Boyd dysentery 004.2
Flexner's
  bacillus 004.1
  diarrhea (ulcerative) 004.1
  dysentery 004.1
Flexure - *see* condition
Floater 796.2
Floating
  cartilage (joint) - *see* Loose bodies in
      joint
  gallbladder (congenital) 751.6
  kidney (*see also* Lesion, kidney) 593.2
    congenital 753.3
  rib 756.4
  spleen 289.5
Flooding 626.2
Floor - *see* condition
Flu - *see* Influenza
Fluctuating blood pressure 458.9
Fluid
  abdomen 785.3
  chest (*see also* Pleurisy, with effusion)
      012.2
  heart (*see also* Failure, heart,
      congestive) 427.0
  joint (*see also* Disease, joint) 729.9
  loss (acute) 788.0
  lung - *see also* Edema, lung
    encysted 511.2
  of re-expansion 511.2
  peritoneal cavity 785.3
  pleural cavity (*see also* Pleurisy, with
      effusion) 012.2
Flukes NEC (*see also* Infestation, flukes)
    121.9
  blood NEC (*see also* Infestation,
      Schistosoma) 120.9
Fluor (vaginalis) 629.3
  trichomonal or due to Trichomonas
      (vaginalis) 131

Fluorosis 520.3
  dental (chronic) 520.3
Flushing 782.3
Flutter
  atrial or auricular (*see also* Fibrillation,
    atrial) 427.4
  heart (*see also* Action, heart, irregular)
    427.9
  ventricular (*see also* Fibrillation,
    ventricular) 427.6
Flux
  bloody 009.0
  serosanguineous 009.0
Fochier's abscess 682.9
  specified site - *code by* site under
    Abscess
Focus, Assmann's (with symptoms) - *see*
    Tuberculosis, pulmonary
Fogo selvagem 694
Folds, anomalous - *see also* Anomaly,
    specified type NEC
  epicanthic 744.8
  heart 746.8
Follicle
  cervix (nabothian) (ruptured) (*see also*
    Cervicitis, chronic) 620.0
  graafian, ruptured, with hemorrhage
    615.9
  nabothian (*see also* Cervicitis, chronic)
    620.0
Folliclis (primary) 017.0
  late effect or sequela 019.9
Follicular - *see* condition
Folliculitis 704
  abscedens et suffodiens 704
  decalvans 704
  gonorrheal (acute) 098.0
    chronic or duration of 2 months or
      over 098.1
  keloid, keloidalis 706.1
  pustular 704
  ulerythematosa reticulata 701.9
Folliculoma (ovary) 256.0
  malignum ovarii - *see* Teratoma
Folling's disease 270.0
Follow-up (examination) (not needing
    further care) (needing only
    prophylactic care) Y03.9
  disease NEC Y03.9
  inactive tuberculosis
    pulmonary (after treatment) Y03.0
      chemotherapy, prophylactic
        Y03.0
      not known to have been active
        Y03.1

Follow-up - *continued*
  inactive tuberculosis - *continued*
    pulmonary - *continued*
      status following surgical collapse of
        lung Y03.0
      without treatment Y03.1
    site other than lung Y03.2
  injury Y03.9
  neoplasm after treatment Y03.3
  operation NEC Y03.9
  postoperative Y03.9
    neoplasm Y03.3
    tuberculosis, pulmonary Y03.0
  psychiatric Y03.4
Food
  asphyxia (from aspiration or inhalation)
    (*see also* Asphyxia, food) 933
  choked on (*see also* Asphyxia, food)
    933
  deprivation 994.2
    particular kind of food NEC 269.9
  improper 269.9
  lack of 994.2
  refusal or rejection NEC 306.5
  strangulation or suffocation (*see also*
    Asphyxia, food) 933
Foot - *see* condition
Foramen ovale (nonclosure) (patent)
    (persistent) 746.4
Forbe's glycogen storage disease 271.1
Forbes-Albright syndrome 253.9
Forced birth or delivery
  fetus or newborn (*see also* Birth injury
    NEC) 772.9
Forceps
  application delivery
    fetus or newborn (*see also* Birth
      injury NEC) 772.9
  injury (*see also* Birth injury NEC)
    772.9
Fordyce-Fox disease 705.9
Fordyce's disease (mouth) 750.8
Forearm - *see* condition
Foreign body
  entering through orifice (current) (old)
    accessory sinus 932
    air passage (upper) 933
      lower 934
    alimentary canal 938
    alveolar process 935
    anterior chamber (eye) 930
    antrum (Highmore) 932
    anus 937
    appendix 936
    asphyxia due to (*see also* Asphyxia,
      food) 933

Foreign body—*continued*
  entering through, etc.—*continued*
    auditory canal 931
    auricle 931
    bladder 939
    bronchioles 934
    bronchus 934
    buccal cavity 935
    canthus (inner) 930
    cecum 936
    cervix (canal) 939
    ciliary body (eye) 930
    coil, ileocecal 936
    colon 936
    conjunctiva 930
    conjunctival sac 930
    cornea 930
    digestive organ or tract NEC 938
    duodenum 936
    ear (external) 931
    esophagus 935
    eye, eyeball, eyelid (adnexa) 930
    frontal sinus 932
    gastro-intestinal tract 938
    genito-urinary tract 939
    globe 930
    gum 935
    Highmore's antrum 932
    hypopharynx 933
    ileocecal coil 936
    ileum 936
    intestine 936
    iris 930
    lacrimal apparatus, duct, gland, or sac 930
    larynx 933
    lens 930
    lid, eye 930
    lung 934
    maxillary sinus 932
    mouth 935
    nasal sinus 932
    nasopharynx 933
    nose (passage) 932
    nostril 932
    ocular muscle 930
    oral cavity 935
    orbit 930
    palate 935
    penis 939
    pharynx 933
    pyriform sinus 933
    rectosigmoid 937
     junction 937
    rectum 937
    respiratory tract 933
    retina 930

Foreign body—*continued*
  entering through, etc.—*continued*
    sclera 930
    sinus 932
     accessory 932
     frontal 932
     maxillary 932
     nasal 932
     pyriform 933
    small intestine 936
    stomach (hairball) 935
    suffocation by 933
    tear ducts or glands 930
    throat 933
    tongue 935
    tonsil, tonsillar 933
     fossa 933
    trachea 934
    ureter 939
    urethra 939
    vagina 939
    vitreous (humor) (humour) 930
  granuloma (old) 733.6
  in open wound - *see* Wound, open,
    complicated
  in tissue or bone (residual) 733.6
  inadvertently left in operation wound
    998.4
  ingestion, ingested NEC 938
  inhalation or inspiration (*see also*
    Asphyxia, food) 933
  internal organ, not entering through a
    natural orifice - code as Injury,
    internal, by site, with open
    wound
  old or residual (in tissue or bone)
    733.6
  operation wound 998.4
  swallowed NEC 938
Form, teeth, abnormal 520.2
Formation
  connective tissue in vitreous 378.9
  hyalin in cornea - *see* Opacity, cornea
  sequestrum in bone (due to infection)
    720.1
  valve
    colon, congenital 751.4
    ureter (congenital) 753.2
Fort Bragg fever 100.8
Fossa - *see also* condition
  pyriform - *see* condition
Fothergill disease 351
  meaning scarlatina anginosa 034.1
Foul breath 788.9
Found dead (cause unknown) 796.2

Fournier's disease 607.9
Fourth
  cranial nerve - *see* condition
  disease 057.8
Foville's syndrome 344.9
Fox-Fordyce disease 705.9
Fox's
  disease 705.9
  impetigo 684
Fracture (abduction) (adduction) (avulsion)
    (compression) (crush) (dislocation)
    (oblique) (separation) 829

Note — For fracture of any of the following sites with fracture of other bones — *see* Fracture, multiple.

The following fourth-digit subdivisions indicated below are for use with those categories in 800–829 for which a more detailed fourth-digit subdivision is not shown in the index listing:
  .0 Closed
  .1 Open
  .9 Late effect
"Closed" includes the following descriptions of fractures, with or without delayed dealing, unless they are specified as open or compound:

comminuted	linear
depressed	march
elevated	simple
fissured	slipped epiphysis
greenstick	spiral
impacted	unspecified

"Open" includes the following descriptions of fractures, with or without delayed healing:

compound	puncture
infected	with foreign body
missile	

"Late effect" includes malunion and nonunion.

Fracture, etc. — *continued*
  acetabulum (with visceral injury) 808
  acromion (process) 811
  ankle (malleolus) (external) (internal)
        (lateral) (medial) 824
    bone 825
    talus 825
  antrum 801
  arm 818
    and leg(s) (any bones) 828
    both (any bones) (with ribs) (with
        sternum) 819

Fracture, etc. — *continued*
  arm — *continued*
    upper - *see* Fracture, humerus
  astragalus 825
  axis - *see* Fracture, vertebra, cervical
  back - *see* Fracture, vertebra
  Barton's - *see* Fracture, radius, lower
      end
  basal (skull) 801
  Bennett's (*see also* Fracture,
        metacarpus) 815
  bone
    due to birth injury (*see also* Birth
          injury, bone or nerve) 772.2
    pathological (cause unknown) 723.2
  boot top - *see* Fracture, fibula
  breast bone - *see* Fracture, sternum
  bucket handle (semilunar cartilage) - *see*
        Dislocation, knee
  calcaneus 825
  capitellum (humerus) - *see* Fracture,
        humerus, lower end
  carpal bone(s) 814
  cartilage, knee (semilunar) - *see*
        Dislocation, knee
  cervical - *see* Fracture, vertebra,
        cervical
  chauffeurs' - *see* Fracture, ulna, lower
        end
  clavicle (acromial end)
        (interligamentous) (shaft) 810
  clay-shovellers' - *see* Fracture,
        vertebra, cervical
  coccyx - *see* Fracture, vertebra, coccyx
  collar bone 810
  Colles' (reversed) *see* Fracture, radius,
        lower end
  congenital 756.9
  costochondral junction - *see* Fracture,
        rib
  costosternal junction - *see* Fracture, rib
  cranium - *see* Fracture, skull
  cricoid cartilage - *see* Fracture, larynx
  cuboid (ankle) 825
  cuneiform
    foot 825
    wrist 814
  due to
    gunshot - code as Fracture, open
    neoplasm- *see* Neoplasm, bone
  Dupuytren's 824
  elbow (supracondylar) - *see also*
        Fracture, humerus, lower end
    olecranon - *see* Fracture, ulna, upper
        end

Fracture, etc. — *continued*
  humerus, etc. — *continued*
    lower
        end (articular process)   812.4
          late effect   812.9
          open   812.5
        extremity - *see* Fracture, humerus,
              lower end
        open NEC   812.3
        proximal end - *see* Fracture,
              humerus, upper end
        shaft   812.2
          late effect   812.9
          open   812.3
        surgical neck - *see* Fracture,
              humerus, upper end
        T-shaped - *see* Fracture, humerus,
              lower end
        tuberosity - *see* Fracture, humerus,
              upper end
    upper
        end   812.0
          late effect   812.9
          open   812.1
        extremity - *see* Fracture, humerus,
              upper end
  hyoid bone - *see* Fracture, larynx
  hyperextension - *see* Fracture, radius,
        lower end
  Illum (with visceral injury)   808
  incus   801
  innominate bone (with visceral injury)
        808
  instep, of one foot   825
    with toe(s) of same foot   827
  internal
      ear   801
      semilunar cartilage, knee (current) -
            see Dislocation, knee
  intra-uterine (*see also* Birth injury, bone
        or nerve)   772.2
  ischium (with visceral injury)   808
  jaw (bone) (condyle) (coronoid (process))
        (ramus) (symphysis) (lower)
        (closed) - *see also* Fracture,
        mandible
    upper - *see* Fracture, maxilla
  knee
      cap   822
      cartilage (semilunar) (current) - *see*
            Dislocation, knee
  larynx (closed)   807.4
    late effect   807.9
    open   807.5
  leg   827
    with rib(s) or sternum   828
    both (any bones)   828

Fracture, etc. — *continued*
  leg — *continued*
      lower - *see* Fracture, tibia
      upper - *see* Fracture, femur, shaft
  limb
      lower (multiple) NEC   827
      upper (multiple) NEC   818
  malar bone (closed)   802.4
    late effect   802.9
    open   802.5
  Malgaigne's   808
  malleolus (external) (internal) (lateral)
        (medial)   824
  malleus   801
  malunion - code as Fracture, late effect
  mandible (condylar) (lower jaw) (closed)
        802.2
    late effect   802.9
    open   802.3
  manubrium - *see* Fracture, sternum
  march   825
  maxilla (superior) (upper jaw) (closed)
        802.4
      inferior - *see* Fracture, mandible
      late effect   802.9
      open   802.5
  meniscus (internal, lateral, medial) knee
        (current) - *see* Dislocation, knee
  metacarpus, metacarpal (bone(s)), of one
        hand   815
    with phalanx, phalanges, hand
          (finger(s)) (thumb) of same hand
          817
  metatarsus, metatarsal (bone(s)), (with
        tarsus) of one foot   825
  Monteggia's - *see* Fracture, ulna, upper
        end
  multiple

Note — Multiple fractures of sites classifiable to the same three- or four-digit category are coded to that category, except for sites classifiable to 810–818 or 820–827 in different limbs.

Multiple fractures of sites classifiable to different fourth-digit subdivisions within the same three-digit category should be dealt with according to the coding rules.

Multiple fractures of sites classifiable to different three-digit categories (identifiable from the listing under "Fracture"), and of sites classifiable to 810–818 or 820–827 in different limbs should be coded according to the following list, which should be referred to in the following priority orders: skull or face bones, pelvis or vertebral column, legs, arms.

Fracture, etc. — *continued*
  multiple — *continued*
    arm (multiple bones in same arm
        except in hand alone) (site(s)
        classifiable to 810-817 with
        site(s) classifiable to a different
        three-digit category in that
        range in same arm) 818
    arms, both or arm(s) with rib(s) or
        sternum (site(s) classifiable to
        810-818 with site(s) classifiable
        to same range of categories in
        other limb or to 807) 819
    bones of trunk NEC 809
    hand, metacarpal bone(s) with
        phalanx or phalanges of same
        hand (site(s) classifiable to 815
        with site(s) classifiable to 816
        in same hand) 817
    leg (multiple bones in same leg)
        (site(s) classifiable to 820-826
        with site(s) classifiable to a
        different three-digit category in
        that range in same leg) 827
    legs, both or leg(s) with arm(s), rib(s)
        or sternum (site(s) classifiable
        to 820-827 with site(s)
        classifiable to same range of
        categories in other leg or to
        807 or 810-819) 828
    pelvis with other bone(s) except skull
        or face bone(s) (site(s)
        classifiable to 808 with site(s)
        classifiable to 805, 806, 807 or
        810-829) 809
    skull, specified or unspecified bone(s),
        or face bone(s) with any other
        bone(s) (site(s) classifiable to
        800-803 with site(s) classifiable
        to 805-829) 804
    vertebral column with other bone(s)
        except skull or face bone(s)
        (site(s) classifiable to 805 or
        806 with site(s) classifiable to
        807, 808 or 810-829) 809
  nasal sinus 801
  navicular
    tarsal 825
    wrist 814
  neck - *see* Fracture, vertebra, cervical
  neural arch - *see* Fracture, vertebra
  nose, nasal (bone) (septum) (closed)
      802.0
    late effect 802.9

Fracture, etc. — *continued*
  nose, etc. — *continued*
    open 802.1
  occiput 801
  odontoid process - *see* Fracture,
      vertebra, cervical
  olecranon (ulna) - *see* Fracture, ulna,
      upper end
  orbit (blow-out) (bone) (region) (closed)
      802.4
    late effect 802.9
    open 802.5
  os calcis 825
  os magnum 814
  os pubis (with visceral injury) 808
  osseous
    auditory meatus 801
    labyrinth 801
  ossicles, auditory 801
  palate (closed) 802.4
    late effect 802.9
    open 802.5
  parietal bone 800
  patella 822
  pathological (cause unknown) 723.2
  pedicle (of vertebral arch) - *see*
      Fracture, vertebra
  pelvis, pelvic (bone(s)) (multiple) (rim)
      (with visceral injury) 808
  phalanx, phalanges, of one
    foot 826
    hand 816
  pisiform 814
  pond 800
  Pott's 824
  pubis (with visceral injury) 808
  radius (with ulna) (closed) 813.0
    distal end - *see* Fracture, radius,
        lower end
    epiphysis
      lower - *see* Fracture, radius, lower
          end
      upper - *see* Fracture, radius, upper
          end
    head - *see* Fracture, radius, upper
        end
    late effect 813.9
    lower
      end 813.4
        late effect 813.9
        open 813.5
      extremity - *see* Fracture, radius,
          lower end
    neck - *see* Fracture, radius, upper
        end
    open NEC 813.1

Fracture, etc. — *continued*
  radius, etc. — *continued*
    proximal end - *see* Fracture, radius,
        upper end
    shaft 813.2
      late effect 813.9
      open 813.3
    upper
      end 813.0
        late effect 813.9
        open 813.1
  ramus
    inferior or superior (with visceral
        injury) 808
    mandible - *see* Fracture, mandible
  rib(s) (closed) 807.0
    late effect 807.9
    open 807.1
  root, tooth - *see* Wound, open, face
  sacrum - *see* Fracture, vertebra, sacrum
  scaphoid
    ankle 825
    wrist 814
  scapula (acromial process) (body)
    (glenoid (cavity)) (neck) 811
  semilunar
    bone, wrist 814
    cartilage (knee) (interior) (current) -
      see Dislocation, knee
  sesamoid bone - *code by* site under
    Fracture
  shoulder - *see also* Fracture, humerus,
    upper end
    blade 811
  sinus (ethmoid) (frontal) (maxillary)
    (nasal) (sphenoidal) 801
  skull (multiple NEC) 803
    base 801
    due to birth injury (*see also* Birth
        injury, bone or nerve) 772.2
    face bones - *see* Fracture, face bones
    vault 800
  Smith's - *see* Fracture, radius, lower
    end
  sphenoid 801
  spine - *see* Fracture, vertebra
  spinous process - *see* Fracture, vertebra
  spontaneous (cause unknown) 723.2
  stapes 801
  stave (*see also* Fracture, metacarpus)
    815
  sternum (closed) 807.2
    late effect 807.9
    open 807.3
  supracondylar, elbow - *see* Fracture,
    humerus, lower end

Fracture, etc. — *continued*
  symphysis pubis (with visceral injury)
    808
  talus (ankle bone) 825
  tarsus, tarsal bone(s) (with metatarsus)
    of one foot 825
    astragalus 825
    calcaneous 825
    cuboid 825
    cuneiform 825
    heel bone 825
    navicular 825
    os calcis 825
    scaphoid 825
  temporal bone (styloid) 801
  tendon - *see* Sprain, strain
  thigh - *see* Fracture, femur, shaft
  thumb (and finger(s)) of one hand 816
    with metacarpal bone(s) of same hand
      817
  thyroid cartilage - *see* Fracture, larynx
  tibia (with fibula) (closed) 823.0
    condyles - *see* Fracture, tibia, upper
      end
    distal end 824
    epiphysis
      lower 824
      upper - *see* Fracture, tibia, upper
        end
    head (involving knee joint) - *see*
      Fracture, tibia, upper end
    intercondyloid eminence - *see*
      Fracture, tibia, upper end
    involving ankle 824
    late effect 823.9
    lower
      end 824
      extremity (anterior lip) (posterior
        lip) 824
    malleolus (internal) (medial) 824
    open NEC 823.1
    proximal end - *see* Fracture, tibia,
      upper end
    shaft 823.2
      late effect 823.9
      open 823.3
    spine - *see* Fracture, tibia, upper end
    tuberosity - *see* Fracture, tibia, upper
      end
    upper
      end 823.0
        late effect 823.9
        open 823.1
      extremity - *see* Fracture, tibia,
        upper end
  toe(s), of one foot 826

Fracture, etc. — *continued*
  vertebra, vertebral — *continued*
    sacrum — *continued*
      open 805.5
    thoracic, thoracolumbar 805.2
      with spinal cord lesion 806.2
        late effect 806.9
        open 806.3
      late effect 805.9
      open 805.3
    vertex 800
    vomer (bone) - *see* Fracture, nose
    wrist 814
    xiphoid (process) - *see* Fracture,
      sternum
    zygoma (closed) 802.4
      late effect 802.9
      open 802.5
Fragilitas
  crinium 704
  ossium 756.6
    with blue sclerotics 756.6
  unguium 703.9
    congenital 757.4
Fragility
  bone 756.6
    with deafness and blue sclera 756.6
  capillary 448
    hereditary 287.9
  hair 704
  nails 703.9
Fragmentation - *see* Fracture
Fragments
  endometrial 625.9
  myometrium 625.9
Frambesia, frambesial (tropica) (*see also*
    Yaws) 102.9
  initial lesion or ulcer 102.0
  primary 102.0
Frambeside
  gummatous 102.4
  of early yaws 102.2
Frambesioma 102.1
Franceschetti syndrome 756.0
Francis' disease 021
Francois' syndrome 378.4
Frank's essential thrombocytopenia (*see
    also* Thrombocytopenia) 287.1

Franklin's disease 275.9

Freckle 709.9
  melanotic (of Hutchinson) 702

Freezing 991.9

Frei's disease 099.1

Freiberg's
  disease 722.2

Freiberg's — *continued*
  infraction of metatarsal head 722.2
  osteochondrosis 722.2
Frenulum linguae 750.0
Frenum
  external os 752.5
  tongue 750.0
Frequency
  micturition (nocturnal) 786.3
    psychogenic 305.6
Frey's syndrome 356
Friction burn - *see* Burn
Friderichsen-Waterhouse syndrome or
    disease - *see* Meningococcemia
Friedlander's B (bacillus) NEC (*see also*
    condition) 039.9
  sepsis or septicemia 038.8
Friedreich's
  ataxia 332.0
  combined systemic disease 332.0
  disease 347.9
  sclerosis (spinal cord) 332.0
Frigidity 781.6
  psychic or psychogenic 305.6
Frohlich's syndrome 253.1
Froin's syndrome 349.9
Frommel-Chiari syndrome 678
Frommel's disease 678
Frontal - *see* condition
Frostbite 991.3
  face 991.0
  foot 991.2
  hand 991.1
Frozen 991.9
  pelvis 616.9
  shoulder 717.1
Fructosemia 271.3
Fructosuria (essential) 271.3
Fuchs' black spot 370.0
Fugue 780.7
  hysterical 300.1
Fulminant, fulminating - *see* condition

Functional - *see also* condition
  bleeding (uterus) 626.6

Fundus - *see* condition

Fungemia 117.9

Fungus, fungous
  cerebral 347.9
    following brain abscess 324
  disease NEC 117.9
  growth, uterus NEC 234.9
  hematodes - *see* Neoplasm, nervous
      system, malignant
  infection - *see* Infection, fungus
  malignant - *see* Neoplasm, malignant

Fungus, fungous — *continued*
  testis 016.2
    late effect or sequela 019.2
  tumor - *see* Neoplasm
Funiculitis (acute) 607.5
  chronic 607.5
  endemic 607.5
  gonococcal 098.0
    chronic or duration of 2 months or
      over 098.1
  tuberculous 016.2
    late effect or sequela 019.2
Funis wound around fetus - *see*
    Complications, umbilical cord
Funnel
  breast (acquired) 738.8
    congenital 756.4
    late effect of rickets 265.1
  chest (acquired) 738.8
    congenital 756.4
    late effect of rickets 265.1
  pelvis (acquired) 738.8
    complicating delivery - *see*
        Deformity, pelvis, complicating
        delivery
    congenital 755.7
    noted during pregnancy (undelivered)
        634.9
Furfur 690
  microsporon 110.0
Furor, paroxysmal (idiopathic) 345.9
Furrowed tongue 529.5
  congenital 750.0
Furrowing nail(s) (transverse) 703.9
  congenital 757.4

Furuncle 680.9
  abdominal wall 680.2
  ankle 680.6
  anus 680.5
  arm (any part, above wrist) 680.3
  axilla 680.3
  back (any part) 680.2
  breast 680.2
  buttock 680.5
  chest wall 680.2
  corpus cavernosum 607.5
  ear (any part) (external) 680.0
  eyelid 362
  face (any part, except eye) 680.0
  finger (any) 680.4
  foot (any part) 680.6
  forearm 680.3
  gluteal (region) 680.5
  groin 680.2
  hand (any part) 680.4
  head (any part, except face) 680.8

Furuncle — *continued*
  heel 680.6
  hip 680.6
  kidney (*see also* Abscess, kidney)
      590.2
  knee 680.6
  labia (minora) (*see also* Vulvitis) 622.1
  lachrymal, lacrimal gland or sac 368
  leg (any part) 680.6
  lower extremity 680.6
  malignant 022
  multiple sites NEC 680.8
  neck 680.1
  nose (septum) 680.0
  orbit, orbital 369.0
  partes posteriores 680.5
  penis 607.5
  scalp (any part) 680.8
  scrotum 607.5
  seminal vesicle 607.4
  shoulder 680.3
  skin NEC 680.9
  specified site NEC 680.8
  spermatic cord 607.5
  temple (region) 680.0
  testis 607.5
  thigh 680.6
  thumb 680.4
  toe (any) 680.6
  trunk 680.2
  tunica vaginalis 607.5
  upper arm 680.3
  vas deferens 607.5
  vulva (*see also* Vulvitis) 622.1
  wrist 680.4

Furunculosis (*see also* Furuncle) 680.9

Fusion, fused (congenital)
  anal (and urogenital canal) 751.4
  aorta and pulmonary artery 746.0
  aortic cusps 746.6
  astragalo-scaphoid 755.7
  atria 746.4
  atrium and ventricle 746.5
  auditory canal 745.0
  auricles, heart 746.4
  bone 756.9
  cervical spine - *see* Fusion, spine
  choanal 748.0
  cusps, heart valve (any) 746.6
  ear ossicles 745.0
  fingers 755.1
  hymen 752.6
  joint (acquired) - *see also* Ankylosis
    congenital 755.9
  kidneys (incomplete) 753.3
  labium (majus) (minus) 752.6

Fusion, fused — *continued*
  larynx and trachea   748.3
  limb   755.9
    lower   755.7
    upper   755.5
  lobes, lung   748.6
  lumbosacral (acquired)   727.0
    congenital   756.1
    surgical   729.1
  nares   748.0
  nose, nasal   748.0
  nostril(s)   748.0
  organ or site not listed - *see* Anomaly,
    specified type NEC
  ossicles   756.9
    auditory   745.0
  pulmonary valve segment   746.6
  pulmonic cusps   746.6
  ribs   756.4
  sacro-iliac (joint) (acquired)   726
    congenital   755.7

Fusion, fused — *continued*
  sacro-iliac — *continued*
    surgical   729.1
  spine (acquired)   727.0
    arthrodesis status   729.1
    congenital   756.2
    postoperative status   729.1
  sublingual duct with submaxillary duct
    at opening in mouth   750.8
  testis   752.8
  toes   755.1
  tooth, teeth   520.2
  trachea and esophagus   750.2
  twins   759.1
  vagina   752.6
  valve cusps   746.6
  ventricles, heart   746.3
  vertebra (arch) - *see* Fusion, spine
  vulva   752.6
Fusospirillosis (mouth) (tongue) (tonsil)
  101

G

Gafsa boil   085.1
Gaisbock's disease   289.0
Gait
  abnormality   787.6
    hysterical   300.1
  ataxic   787.6
    hysterical   300.1
  disturbance   787.6
    hysterical   300.1
  paralytic   787.6
  spastic   787.6
  staggering   787.6
    hysterical   300.1
Galactocele (breast) (infected)   610
  puerperal, postpartum   678
Galactophoritis   611.0
  puerperal, postpartum   678
Galactorrhea   678
Galactosemia   271.2
Galactosuria   279
Galacturia   789.2
  bilharziasis   120.0
Galen's vein - see condition
Gall duct - see condition
Gallbladder - see also condition
  acute (see also Disease, gallbladder)
      576.9
Gallop rhythm (see also Action, heart,
      irregular)   427.9
Gallstone (cholemic) (colic) (impacted)
      (see also Cholelithiasis)   574.9
  causing intestinal obstruction (see also
      Impaction, intestine)   560.3

Gamna's disease   289.5

Gandy-Nanta disease   289.5

Ganglioma - see Ganglioneuroma

Ganglion (compound) (diffused) (joint)
      (tendon) (sheath)) (see also Bursitis)
      731.9
  of yaws (early) (late)   102.6
  tuberculous   015.9
    late effect or sequela   019.6

Ganglioneurofibroma - see
      Ganglioneuroma

Ganglioneuroma   225.6
  adrenal gland   225.6
  ciliary nerve   225.6
  cranial nerves, any except ciliary
      225.1

Ganglioneuroma—continued
  malignant   192.5
    adrenal gland   192.5
    ciliary nerve   192.5
    cranial nerves, any except ciliary
        192.0
    parasympathetic, sympathetic (nerve)
        192.5
  parasympathetic, sympathetic (nerve)
      225.6

Ganglionitis
  fifth nerve   351
  gasserian   351
  geniculate   350
    newborn (see also Birth injury, bone
        or nerve)   772.2
  herpes zoster   053.9
  herpetic geniculate   053.1

Gangliosidosis   333.0

Gangosa   102.5

Gangrene, gangrenous (cutaneous) (dry)
      (infected) (local) (moist) (septic)
      (skin) (spreading cutaneous) (stasis)
      (ulcer) (ulcerative)   445.9
  with
    arteriosclerosis (conditions in 440) -
        see Gangrene, arteriosclerotic
    diabetes (mellitus) - see category 250
  abdomen (wall)   445.9
    arteriosclerotic   445.0
  alveolar   526.5
  anus   569.2
  appendices epiploicae - see Gangrene,
      mesentery
  appendix   540.9
    with perforation, peritonitis, or
        rupture   540.0
  arteriosclerotic (general) (senile) (of site
      classifiable to 445.9)   445.0
  auricle   445.9
  Bacillus welchii (see also Gangrene,
      gas)   039.0
  bile duct (see also Cholecystitis)   575
  bladder (see also Cystitis)   595
  bowel, cecum, or colon - see Gangrene,
      intestine
  bubonocele   552
  Clostridium perfringens or welchii (see
      also Gangrene, gas)   039.0
  connective tissue   445.9

Gangrene, etc. — *continued*
  cornea (*see also* Keratitis) 363.9
  corpora cavernosa 607.5
    noninfective 607.9
  decubital 445.9
  diabetic (any site) - *see* category 250
  dropsical 445.9
  emphysematous (*see also* Gangrene,
      gas) 039.0
  enterocele 553.9
  epidemic (ergotized grain) 988.2
  epididymis (infectional) (*see also*
      Epididymitis) 604
  epigastrocele 553.2
  epiplocele 553.9
  exomphalos 553.1
  extremity (lower) (upper) 445.9
  gallbladder or duct (*see also*
      Cholecystitis) 575
  gas (bacillus) 039.0
    with
      abortion - *see* Abortion, by type,
          with sepsis
      ectopic gestation - *see* categories
          631.0-631.3
      puerperal, postpartum, childbirth
          670
  gum 523.9
  hernia (*see also* Hernia, by site, with
      obstruction) 553.9
  intestine, intestinal 569.9
    with
      intestinal obstruction (*see also*
          Obstruction, intestine)
          560.9
      mesenteric embolism or infarction
          (conditions in 444.2) 444.2
  liver 573.9
  lung 513
  Meleney's 686.0
  merocele 553.0
  mesentery 569.9
    with
      intestinal obstruction (*see also*
          Obstruction, intestine)
          560.9
      mesenteric embolism or infarction
          (conditions in 444.2) 444.2
  mouth 528.1
  omentocele 553.9
  omentum - *see* Gangrene, mesentery
  omphalocele 553.1
  ovary (*see also* Salpingo-oophoritis)
      614
  pancreas 577.0
  penis 607.5

Gangrene, etc. — *continued*
  penis — *continued*
    noninfective 607.9
  perineum 445.9
  pharynx 462
  presenile 443.1
  pulmonary 513
  pulp 522.1
  Raynaud's 443.0
  rectum 569.2
  retropharyngeal 508.9
  rupture (meaning hernia) (*see also*
      Hernia, by site, with obstruction)
      553.9
  sarco-epiplocele 553.9
  sarco-epiplomphalocele 553.1
  scrotum 607.5
    noninfective 607.9
  senile (of site classifiable to 445.9)
      445.0
  spermatic cord 607.5
    noninfective 607.9
  spine 445.9
  spirochetal NEC 104.9
  stomach 537.9
  symmetrical 443.0
  testicle (infectional) (*see also* Orchitis)
      604
    noninfective 607.9
  throat 462
    diphtheritic 032
  thyroid (gland) 246
  tuberculous NEC (*see also*
      Tuberculosis) 011.9
  tunica vaginalis 607.5
    noninfective 607.9
  umbilicus 445.9
  uterus (*see also* Endometritis) 622.0
  vas deferens 607.5
    noninfective 607.9
  vulva (*see also* Vulvitis) 622.1
Gannister disease - *see* Disease, gannister
Ganser's syndrome 300.1
  psychotic NEC 299
  reaction to exceptional stress (transient)
      307
    psychotic NEC 298.9
Gardner-Diamond syndrome 283.9
Gargoylism 273.8
Garre's
  disease 720.1
  osteitis (sclerosing) 720.1
  osteomyelitis 720.1
Garrulity, vulva 629.9
Gartner's duct
  cyst 752.8

Gartner's duct — *continued*
persistent 752.8
Gas
asphyxia, asphyxiation, inhalation,
poisoning, suffocation NEC
987.9
specified gas - *see* Table of adverse
effects
bacillus gangrene or infection - *see* Gas
gangrene
cyst, mesentery 569.9
gangrene 039.0
with
abortion - *see* Abortion, by type,
with sepsis
ectopic gestation - *see* categories
631.0-631.3
puerperal, postpartum, childbirth
670
on stomach 785.4
pains 785.4
Gastralgia 536.9
psychogenic 305.5
Gastrectasis 536.1
psychogenic 305.5
Gastric - *see* condition
Gastritis (acute) (atrophic) (bilious)
(catarrhal) (chronic) (diarrheal)
(dietetic) (exogenous) (glandular)
(hemorrhagic) (hypertrophic)
(infectional) (infective)
(phlegmonous) (sclerotic) (septic)
(simple) (subacute) (suppurative)
(toxic) (ulcerative) 535
alcoholic 303.2
acute 303.9
allergic 535
due to diet deficiency 269.9
giant hypertrophic 535
nervous 305.5
spastic 535
tuberculous 017.9
late effect or sequela 019.9
Gastrocarcinoma (*see also* Neoplasm,
stomach, malignant) 151.9
Gastrocolic - *see* condition
Gastrocolitis - *see* Enteritis
Gastrodisciasis 121.9
Gastroduodenal ulcer - *see* Ulcer, peptic
Gastroduodenitis (*see also* Gastritis) 535
catarrhal 535
infectional 535
virus, viral 008.9
Gastrodynia 536.9

Gastro-enteritis (acute) (catarrhal)
(congestive) (epidemic)
(hemorrhagic) (infectious) (septic)
(zymotic) (*see also* Enteritis)
009.2
alcoholic 303.2
acute 303.9
allergic 561
chronic 563.9
dietetic 561
due to food poisoning (*see also*
Poisoning, food) 005.9
noninfectious 561
toxic 561
Gastro-enterocolitis - *see* Enteritis
Gastro-enteroptosis 569.9
Gastrohepatitis (acute) (chronic)
(catarrhal) (*see also* Gastritis) 535
Gastro-intestinal - *see* condition
Gastrojejunal - *see* condition
Gastrojejunitis 535
Gastrojejunocolic - *see* condition
Gastroliths 537.9
Gastromalacia 537.9
Gastropathy, exudative 269.9
Gastroptosis 537.9
Gastrorrhagia (*see also* Hematemesis)
784.5
Gastrorrhea 536.0
psychogenic 305.5
Gastroschisis (congenital) 758.8
acquired 569.9
Gastrospasm (neurogenic) (reflex) 536.1
neurotic 305.5
psychogenic 305.5
Gastrostaxis (*see also* Hematemesis)
784.5
Gastrostenosis 537.9
Gastrosuccorrhea (continuous)
(intermittent) 536.0
neurotic 305.5
psychogenic 305.5
Gaucher's
disease (adult) (infantile) 272.2
splenomegaly 272.2
Gee-Herter disease 269.0
Gee-Thaysen disease 269.0
Gee's disease 269.0
Gelineau's syndrome 347.0
Gemination
tooth, teeth 520.2
General, generalized - *see* condition
Genital - *see* condition
Genito-anorectal syndrome 099.1
Genito-urinary system - *see* condition
Genu
congenital 755.7

Genu — *continued*
  extrorsum, introrsum, recurvatum,
      valgum, varum (acquired) 738.5
    congenital 755.7
    late effect of rickets 265.1
    postpoliomyelitic 044
  postpoliomyelitic 044
  rachitic (old) 265.1
Geographic tongue 529.1
Geotrichosis 117.8
  intestine 117.8
  lung 117.8
  mouth 117.8
Gephyrophobia 300.2
Gerhardt's syndrome 508.0
Gerlier's disease 079.8
German measles 056
Germinoma - *see* Dysgerminoma
Gerontoxon 378.4
Gerstmann's syndrome 781.5
Gestation (period) - *see also* Pregnancy
  ectopic - *see* Pregnancy, ectopic
  incomplete, liveborn infant 777
    for classification of births in hospital
      - *see* Newborn
  less than
    28 weeks, with delivery
      dead fetus - *see* Abortion, by type
      liveborn infant - *see* Delivery
    37 wks. or approximately 8 1/2 mos.
      liveborn infant 777
  28 weeks or more, with delivery,
      liveborn infant or dead fetus -
    see Delivery
Ghon tubercle primary infection (with
    symptoms) 012.0
  late effect or sequela 019.0
Ghoul hand 102.3
Giant
  cell tumor - *see also* Neoplasm, benign
    malignant - *see* Neoplasm, malignant
    peripheral (gingiva) 523.9
  colon (congenital) 751.2
  esophagus (congenital) 750.8
  follicular lymphoma 202.0
  kidney 753.3
  urticaria 708.0
Giardiasis 007.1
Gibert's disease 696.3
Giddiness 780.5
  hysterical 300.1
  psychogenic 305.9
Gierke's disease 271.0
Gigantism (hypophyseal) 253.0
Gilbert's disease 273.5

Gilchrist's disease 116.1
Gilford-Hutchinson disease 258.9
Gilles de la Tourette's disease 347.9
Gingivitis 523.1
  acute 523.0
    necrotizing 101
  catarrhal 523.0
  chronic 523.1
  desquamative 523.1
  expulsiva 523.4
  hyperplastic 523.1
  marginal, simple 523.1
  pellagrous 262
  ulcerative 523.1
    acute necrotizing 101
  Vincent's 101
Gingivoglossitis 529.0
Gingivopericementitis 523.4
Gingivosis 523.1
Gingivostomatitis 523.1
  herpetic 054
Giovannini's disease 117.9
Gland, glandular - *see* condition
Glanders 024
Glanzmann's disease or thrombasthenia
    287.3
Glass-blowers' disease 527.1
Glaucoma (congestive) (hemorrhagic)
    (inflammatory) (noninflammatory)
    (primary) 375.9
  absolute 375.1
  acute 375.0
    narrow angle 375.0
    secondary 375.2
  arrested, follow-up examination Y03.9
  capsulare 375.2
  chronic 375.1
    noncongestive 375.1
    open angle 375.1
    simple 375.1
  closed angle 375.0
  congenital 744.2
  infantile 744.2
  malignant 375.0
  narrow angle 375.0
  newborn 744.2
  noncongestive (chronic) 375.1
  nonobstructive 375.1
  obstructive 375.2
  open angle 375.1
  postinfectious 375.2
  secondary 375.2
  simple (chronic) 375.1
  simplex 375.1
  syphilitic 095
  tuberculous 017.2
    late effect or sequela 019.9

Gleet 098.1
Glenard's disease 569.9
Glioblastoma (multiforme) - *see also*
    Neoplasm, nervous system,
    malignant
  eye 190
  nose 212.0
  parietal 191
Glioma (astrocytic) (cystic) (*see also*
    Neoplasm, nervous system,
    malignant) 192.9
  benign (*see also* Neoplasm, nervous
    system, benign) 225.9
  brain stem 191
  choroid 190
  eye 190
  nose 212.0
  optic nerve 192.0
  retina 190
Glioneuroma - *see* Neoplasm, nervous
    system, malignant
Gliosarcoma - *see* Neoplasm, nervous
    system, malignant
Gliosis 347.9
  cerebral 347.9
    with degeneration 347.9
  spinal 349.0
Glisson's
  cirrhosis - *see* Cirrhosis, portal
  disease (*see also* Rickets) 265.0
Glissonitis 573.0
Globinuria 279
Globus 305.5
  hystericus 300.1
Glomangioma (skin) (subcutaneous tissue)
    227.0
  not of skin or subcutaneous tissue
    227.1
Glomerular nephritis (*see also* Nephritis)
    583
Glomerulitis (*see also* Nephritis) 583
Glomerulonephritis (*see also* Nephritis)
    583
  membranous - *see* Nephritis, subacute
Glomerulosclerosis (*see also* Sclerosis,
    renal) 584
  intercapillary - *see* category 250
Glomus tumor - *see* Glomangioma
Glossalgia 529.6
Glossitis 529.0
  areata exfoliativa 529.1
  atrophic 529.0
  benign migratory 529.1
  gangrenous 529.0
  Hunter's 529.4
  median rhomboid 529.2

Glossitis—*continued*
  Moeller's 529.4
  pellagrous 262
Glossodynia 529.6
  exfoliativa 529.4
Glossophytia 529.3
Glossoplegia 781.4
Glossopyrosis 529.6
Glossy skin 701.9
Glottis - *see* condition
Glottitis - *see* Glossitis
Glucoglycinuria 270.8
Glue sniffing (airplane glue) 304.8
Glycemia - *see* category 250
Glycinemia 270.8
Glycinuria 270.2
Glycogen
  infiltration (*see also* Disease, glycogen
    storage) 271.1
  storage disease (*see also* Disease,
    glycogen storage) 271.1
Glycogenosis (diffuse) (generalized) (with
    hepatic cirrhosis) (*see also* Disease,
    glycogen storage) 271.1
Glycopenia 251
Glycosuria 789.5
  renal 273.8
Gnathostoma spinigerum (infection)
    (infestation) 128.8
  wandering swellings from 128.8
Gnathostomiasis 128.8
Gogomon 110.9
Goiter (adolescent) (colloid) (diffuse)
    (dipping) (due to iodine deficiency)
    (heart) (hyperplastic) (internal)
    (intrathoracic) (juvenile) (mixed
    type) (nontoxic) (parenchymatous)
    (plunging) (simple) (subclavicular)
    (substernal) 240.9
  with
    hyperthyroidism (recurrent) 242.0
      adenomatous 242.1
      nodular 242.1
    thyrotoxicosis 242.0
      adenomatous 242.1
      nodular 242.1
  adenomatous (*see also* Goiter, nodular)
    241.9
  cancerous 193
  congenital 243
  cystic (*see also* Goiter, nodular) 241.9
  endemic 240.0
    adenomatous 241.0
    nodular 241.0
  exophthalmic 242.0
  fibrous 245.1

Goiter, etc. — *continued*
  lingual 758.2
  lymphadenoid 245.1
  malignant 193
  nodular 241.9
    with
      hyperthyroidism 242.1
      thyrotoxicosis 242.1
    endemic 241.0
    exophthalmic 242.1
    sporadic 241.1
    toxic 242.1
  nonendemic (*see also* Goiter, sporadic)
    240.1
  pulsating 242.0
  sporadic 240.1
    adenomatous 241.1
    nodular 241.1
  toxic 242.0
    adenomatous 242.1
    nodular 242.1
Goldberg-Maxwell syndrome 257.9
Goldblatt
  hypertension (*see also* Arteriosclerosis,
    renal, artery) 440.1
  kidney (*see also* Arteriosclerosis, renal,
    artery) 440.1
Goldflam-Erb disease or syndrome
  733.0
Goldscheider's disease 757.2
Goldstein's disease 448
Gonecystitis (*see also* Vesiculitis) 607.4
Gongylonemiasis 125.8
  mouth 125.8

Gonococcemia 098.8

Gonococcus, gonococcal (disease)
    (infection) (*see also* condition)
    098.9
  bursa 098.3
  chronic NEC 098.9
  conjunctiva, conjunctivitis (neonatorum)
    098.2
  endocardium 098.8
  eye (newborn) 098.2
  fallopian tubes (chronic) 098.1
    acute 098.0
  genito-urinary (organ) (system) (tract)
    (acute) (*see also* Gonorrhea)
    098.0
  heart 098.8
  joint 098.3
  lymphatic (gland) (node) 098.8
  meninges 098.8
  pelvis (acute) 098.0
    chronic or duration of 2 months or
      over 098.1

Gonococcus, etc. — *continued*
  pyosalpinx (chronic) 098.1
    acute 098.0
  rectum 098.8
  skin 098.8
  specified site NEC 098.8
  tendon sheath 098.3
  urethra (acute) 098.0
    chronic or duration of 2 months or
      over 098.1
  vulva (acute) 098.0
    chronic or duration of 2 months or
      over 098.1
Gonorrhea 098.0
  acute 098.0
  Bartholin's gland (acute) 098.0
    chronic or duration of 2 months or
      over 098.1
  bladder (acute) 098.0
    chronic or duration of 2 months or
      over 098.1
  cervix (acute) 098.0
    chronic or duration of 2 months or
      over 098.1
  chronic 098.1
  conjunctiva, conjunctivitis (neonatorum)
    098.2
  Cowper's gland (acute) 098.0
    chronic or duration of 2 months or
      over 098.1
  duration two months or over 098.1
  fallopian tube (chronic) 098.1
    acute 098.0
  genito-urinary (organ) (system) (tract)
    (acute) 098.0
    chronic 098.1
    duration two months or over 098.1
  kidney (acute) 098.0
    chronic or duration of 2 months or
      over 098.1
  late effects NEC 098.9
  ovary (acute) 098.0
    chronic or duration of 2 months or
      over 098.1
  pelvis (acute) 098.0
    chronic or duration of 2 months or
      over 098.1
  penis (acute) 098.0
    chronic or duration of 2 months or
      over 098.1
  prostate (acute) 098.0
    chronic or duration of 2 months or
      over 098.1
  seminal vesicle (acute) 098.0
    chronic or duration of 2 months or
      over 098.1

Gonorrhea—*continued*
 specified site not listed - *see*
  Gonococcus
 spermatic cord (acute) 098.0
  chronic or duration of 2 months or
   over 098.1
 urethra (acute) 098.0
  chronic or duration of 2 months or
   over 098.1
  late effects 098.1
 vagina (acute) 098.0
  chronic or duration of 2 months or
   over 098.1
 vas deferens (acute) 098.0
  chronic or duration of 2 months or
   over 098.1
 vulva (acute) 098.0
  chronic or duration of 2 months or
   over 098.1
Goodpasture's syndrome 446.1
Goodwin-Harrison syndrome 426
Gopalan's syndrome 261
Gordon's enteropathy, exudative 269.9
Goundou 102.6
Gout, gouty (any site) 274
 lead 984
 saturnine 984
 syphilitic 095
Gower's
 muscular dystrophy 330.3
 syndrome 782.5
Gradenigo's syndrome 382.0
Grain mite 133.9
Grand mal (idiopathic) 345.1
Granite workers' lung 515.0
 tuberculous 010
Granular - *see also* condition
 kidney (contracting) (*see also* Sclerosis,
   renal) 584
 liver - *see* Cirrhosis, liver
 nephritis - *see* Nephritis
Granulation tissue - *see* Granuloma
Granulocytopenia, granulocytopenic
   (primary) 288
 malignant 288
 ulcer
  colon 288
  intestine 288

Granuloma 686.1
 abdomen 569.9
 amebic 006.9
  with liver abscess 006.0
 annulare 695.9
 apical 522.6
 aural 380
 beryllium (skin) 709.9

Granuloma—*continued*
 bone 720.2
  eosinophilic 279
  from residual foreign body 733.6
 canaliculus lachrymalis, lacrimalis 368
 cerebral 322
  late effects 324
 coccidioidal 114
  lung 114
  meninges 114
 colon 569.9
 conjunctiva 360
 dental 522.6
 ear, middle (*see also* Otitis, media)
   381.9
 eosinophilic 279
  bone 279
  lung 279
 eyelid 361
 facial
  lethal midline 446.3
  malignant 446.3
 foot NEC 686.1
 foreign body (in bone or tissue) NEC
   733.6
  in operation wound 998.4
  skin 709.9
 fungoides 202.1
 gangraenescens 446.3
 giant cell reparative (jaw) 526.3
  gingiva 523.9
  peripheral (gingiva) 523.9
 gland (lymph) 289.3
 Hodgkin's 201
 ileum 569.9
 infectious NEC 136
 inguinale (Donovan) 099.2
  venereal 099.2
 intestine 569.9
 jaw (bone) 526.3
  reparative giant cell 526.3
 kidney (*see also* Infection, kidney)
   590.9
 lachrymal, lacrimal sac (nonspecific)
   368
 larynx 508.3
 lethal midline 446.3
 lipid 999.9
 liver 572
 lung (infectious) (*see also* Fibrosis, lung)
   517
  coccidioidal 114
  eosinophilic 279
 malignant of face 446.3
 mandible 526.3

Granuloma—*continued*
  midline 446.3
  monilial 112
  operation wound 998.5
    foreign body 998.4
    stitch 998.4
    talc 998.4
  oral mucosa, pyogenic 528.9
  orbit, orbital 369.9
  paracoccidioidal 116.2
  penis 099.2
  periapical 522.6
  peritoneum 569.9
    due to ova of helminths NEC (*see
        also* Infestation, helminth)
        128.9
  prostate 601
  pudendorum (ulcerative) 099.2
  pulp, internal (tooth) 521.4
  pyogenic, pyogenicum (skin) 686.1
    of maxillary alveolar ridge 522.6
    oral mucosa 528.9
  rectum 569.2
  rubrum nasi 705.9
  Schistosoma 120.9
  septic (skin) 686.1
  silica (skin) 709.9
  sinus (infectional) - see Sinusitis
  skin (pyogenicum) 686.1
    from foreign body or material 709.9
  spine
    syphilitic (epidural) 094.9
    tuberculous 015.0
      late effect or sequela 019.3
  stitch (post-operative) 998.4
  suppurative (skin) 686.1
  swimming pool 031.9
  telangiectaticum (skin) 686.1
  tropicum 102.4
  umbilicus 686.1
  urethra 599.9
  uveitis 366
  vagina 099.2
  venereum 099.2
Granulomatosis NEC 686.1
  infantiseptica 027.0
  miliary 027.0
  necrotizing
    respiratory 446.3
  Wegener's 446.3

Granulomatous tissue - see Granuloma

Granulosa cell tumor 256.0
  malignant 183.0

Granulosis rubra nasi 705.9

Graphite fibrosis (of lung) 516.0

Graphospasm 300.8
Grating scapula 723.9
Gravel (urinary) (*see also* Calculus) 594
Graves' disease 242.0
Gravis - see condition
Grawitz's
  cachexia 281.9
  tumor 189.0
    ovary 256.0
      malignant 183.0
Gray syndrome 960.2
Grayness, hair (premature) 704
  congenital 757.3
Green sickness 280
Greenfield's disease 333.1
Greenstick fracture - code as Fracture,
    closed
Greesley disease 078.2
Griesinger's disease (*see also*
    Ancylostomiasis) 126.9
Grinders'
  asthma 515.0
    tuberculous 010
  lung 515.0
    tuberculous 010
  phthisis 010
Grip
  Dabney's 074.1
  devil's 074.1
Grippe, grippal - see also Influenza
  Balkan 083.1
  summer 074.9
Grippy cold 472
Groin - see condition
Growing pains, children 787.1
Growth (neoplastic) (new) (*see also*
    Neoplasm) 239.9
  adenoid 500
  benign - see Neoplasm, benign
  fibroid (uterus) 218
    not of uterus (*see also* Neoplasm,
        connective tissue, benign)
        215
  fungoid - see Neoplasm
  fungous, uterus 234.9
  malignant - see Neoplasm, malignant
  multiple (malignant), without
      specification of site 199.0
    benign - see Neoplasm, benign
  nonmalignant - see Neoplasm, benign
  secondary - see Secondary neoplasm
Gruber's hernia - see Hernia, Gruber's
Gruby's disease 110.0
Gubler-Millard paralysis 344.1
Guerin-Stern syndrome 755.8
Guillain-Barre syndrome 354

Guinea worms (infection) (infestation) 125.8
Gull and Sutton's disease - *see* Hypertension, kidney
Gull's disease 244
Gum - *see* condition
Gumboil 522.7
Gumma (syphilitic) 095
  artery 093.9
    cerebral or spinal 094.9
  bone 095
    of yaws (late) 102.6
  brain 094.9
  cauda equina 094.9
  central nervous system 094.9
  ciliary body 095
  congenital 090.5
    testicle 090.5
  eyelid 095
  heart 093.9
  intracranial 094.9
  iris 095
  kidney 095
  larynx 095
  leptomeninges 094.9
  liver 095
  meninges 094.9
  myocardium 093.9
  nasopharynx 095
  neurosyphilitic 094.9
  nose 095
  orbit 095

Gumma (syphilitic) — *continued*
  palate (soft) 095
  penis 095
  pericardium 093.9
  pharynx 095
  pituitary 095
  scrofulous 017.0
    late effect or sequela 019.9
  skin 095
  specified site NEC 095
  spinal cord 094.9
  tongue 095
  tonsil 095
  trachea 095
  tuberculous 017.0
    late effect or sequela 019.9
  ulcerative due to yaws 102.4
  ureter 095
  yaws 102.4
Gunn's syndrome 743.8
Gunshot wound - *see also* Wound, open fracture - code as Fracture, open
  internal organs (abdomen, chest or pelvis) - *see* Injury, internal, by site, with open wound
  intracranial 851.1
Gynandrism 752.0
Gynandroblastoma 256.0
  malignant 183.0
Gynecoid pelvis, male 738.8
Gynecomastia 611.1
Gyrate scalp 757.2

H

H disease 270.2
Habit, habituation
chorea 306.2
disturbance, child 308
drug - *see* Dependence
spasm 306.2
tic 306.2
Haff disease 988.9
Hageman factor deficiency (*see also*
Defect, coagulation) 286.9
Hailey-Hailey disease 757.2
Hair - *see* condition
Hairball in stomach 935
Hairy black tongue 529.3
Half vertebra 756.2
Halitosis 788.9
Hallerman-Streiff syndrome 756.0
Hallervorden-Spatz syndrome 331.9
Hallopeau's
acrodermatitis 686.9
disease 701.0

Hallucination (auditory) (gustatory)
(olfactory) (tactile) (visual) 781.8
Hallucinosis 299
alcoholic (acute) 291.2
Hallus - *see* Hallux
Hallux 737.0
malleus (acquired) (*see also* Hammer
toe) 738.7
rigidus (acquired) 738.7
congenital 755.7
late effects of rickets 265.1
residual of poliomyelitis 044
valgus (acquired) 737.0
congenital 755.7
residual of poliomyelitis 044
varus (acquired) 737.1
congenital 755.7
residual of poliomyelitis 044

Hamartoblastoma - *see* Neoplasm, benign

Hamartoma - *see* Neoplasm, benign

Hamman-Rich syndrome (*see also*
Fibrosis, lung) 517

Hammer toe (acquired) 738.7
congenital 755.7
late effects of rickets 265.1
residual of poliomyelitis 044

Hand - *see* condition

Hand-Schuller-Christian disease 279

Hanging (asphyxia) (strangulation)
(suffocation) 994.7
judicial 806.0
Hangnail (with lymphangitis) 681
Hanot-Chauffard(-Troisier) syndrome
273.2
Hanot's cirrhosis or disease - *see*
Cirrhosis, biliary
Hansen's disease 030.9
benign form 030.1
malignant form 030.0
Harada's syndrome 366
Hardening
artery - *see* Arteriosclerosis
brain 341
liver - *see* Cirrhosis, liver
Hare eye 378.2
Harelip (complete) (incomplete) 749.1
with cleft palate 749.2
Harlequin (fetus) (color change syndrome)
757.2
Harley's disease 283.9
Harris' lines 723.9
Hartnup's disease 270.2
Hashimoto's disease 245.1
Hass' disease 722.2
Haut mal 345.1
Haverhill fever 026.1
Hawkins' keloid 701.3
Hayem-Widal syndrome 283.9

Haygarth's nodosities 713.0

Hb (abnormal)
disease - *see* Disease, hemoglobin
trait - *see* Trait

Head - *see* condition

Headache 791
allergic 346
emotional 306.8
histamine 346
lumbar puncture 997.0
migraine 346
nonorganic origin 306.8
postspinal 997.0
psychogenic 306.8
sick 346
spinal fluid loss 997.0
tension 306.8
vascular 791
migraine type 346
vasomotor 346

Health audit (negative findings)   Y00.0
Healthy
  donor   Y09.9
  person   Y09.9
    accompanying sick relative   Y08
    admitted for sterilization (operation)
        Y09.0
    receiving prophylactic inoculation or
        vaccination   Y02
Heart - *see* condition
Heartburn   784.3
  psychogenic   305.5
Heat (effects)   992.9
  allergy, allergic reaction (skin)   692.9
  apoplexy   992.0
  burn - *see also* Burn
    from sun   692.8
  collapse   992.1
  cramps   992.2
  dermatitis or eczema   692.9
  edema   992.7
  erythema NEC   692.9
  excessive NEC   992.9
  exhaustion   992.5
    anhydrotic   992.3
    due to
      salt (and water) depletion   992.4
      water depletion   992.3
  fatigue (transient)   992.6
  fever   992.0
  hyperpyrexia   992.0
  prickly   705.1
  prostration - *see* Heat, exhaustion
  pyrexia   992.0
  rash   705.1
  stroke   992.0
  sunburn   692.8
  syncope   992.1
Hebephrenia, hebephrenic (acute)   295.1
  dementia (praecox)   295.1
  schizophrenia   295.1
Heberden's
  disease   713.0
  nodes   713.0
Hebra-Jadassohn disease   695.0
Hebra, nose   039.1
Hebra's
  disease   695.9
    meaning erythema multiforme
        exudativum   695.1
  pityriasis   695.9
  prurigo   698.2
Heel - *see* condition
Heerfordt's disease   135
Hegglin's anomaly (*see also*
        Thrombocytopenia)   287.1

Heidenhain's disease   290.1
  with dementia   290.1
Heine-Medin disease   043
  late effects   044
Heinz-body anemia, congenital   282.2
Heller's disease or syndrome   295.8
Helminthiasis (*see also* Infestation)
      128.9
  Ancylostoma (*see also* Ancylostoma)
      126.9
  intestinal NEC   127.9
  mixed types (intestinal) (types
      classifiable to more than one of
      the titles 120-127.4)   127.5
  Necator (americanus)   126.1
  specified type NEC   128.8
Heloma   700
Hemangio-ameloblastoma (*see also*
      Ameloblastoma)   210.4
Hemangioblastoma - *see* Neoplasm,
      connective tissue, malignant
Hemangioblastomatosis - *see also*
      Neoplasm, connective tissue,
      malignant
  cerebelloretinal   759.8
Hemangioendothelioma   227.1
  bone (diffuse) - *see* Neoplasm, bone,
      malignant
  brain   225.0
    malignant   191
  central nervous system NEC   225.9
    malignant   192.9
  dural - *see* Hemangioendothelioma,
      meninges
  malignant - *see* Neoplasm, connective
      tissue, malignant
  meninges (diffuse)   225.9
    brain   225.2
      malignant   192.1
    malignant   192.9
    spinal cord   225.4
      malignant   192.3
  retina   224
    malignant   190
  skin   227.0
  spinal cord   225.3
    malignant   192.2
Hemangio-endotheliosarcoma - *see*
      Neoplasm, connective tissue,
      malignant
Hemangiofibroma (*see also*
      Dermatofibroma)   216.8
Hemangioma (arterial) (arteriovenous)
      (benign) (capillary) (cavernous)
      (congenital) (plexiform) (skin)
      (venous)   227.0

Hemangioma, etc. — *continued*
  brain 225.0
  cavernous diffuse 759.8
  central nervous system NEC 225.9
  choroid 224
  iris 224
  malignant NEC - *see* Neoplasm,
      connective tissue, malignant
  meninges 225.9
    brain 225.2
    spinal cord 225.4
  placenta (complicating pregnancy) - *see*
      Placenta, abnormal
  retina 224
  sclerosing (*see also* Dermatofibroma)
      216.8
  specified site NEC 227.1
  spinal cord 225.3
Hemangiomatosis (systemic) 759.8
  involving single site - *see* Hemangioma
Hemangiopericytoma (*see also* Neoplasm,
    connective tissue, malignant)
    171.9
  benign - *see* Hemangioma
Hemangiosarcoma - *see* Neoplasm,
    connective tissue, malignant
Hemarthrosis (nontraumatic) (*see also*
    Disease, joint) 729.9
  traumatic (skin surface intact) - *see*
    Contusion
Hematemesis 784.5
  with ulcer (*see also* Ulcer, peptic)
      533.9
    duodenum - *see* Ulcer, duodenum,
      with hemorrhage
    stomach - *see* Ulcer, stomach, with
      hemorrhage
  newborn 778.2
Hematidrosis 705.9
Hematinuria (*see also* Hemoglobinuria)
    789.4
  malarial 084.4
  paroxysmal 283.9
Hematite miners' lung 516.0
Hematocele 607.9
  cord, male 607.9
  female NEC 629.9
  ischiorectal 569.2
  male NEC 607.9
  ovary 615.9
  pelvis, pelvic
    female 629.9
      with ectopic pregnancy - *see*
        Pregnancy, tubal
      associated with pregnancy - *see*
        Pregnancy, tubal

Hematocele — *continued*
  pelvis, pelvic — *continued*
    male 607.9
  peri-uterine 616.9
  retro-uterine 616.9
  scrotum 607.9
  spermatic cord (diffuse) 607.9
  testis 607.9
  tunica vaginalis 607.9
  uterine ligament 616.9
Hematocephalus 743.2
Hematochyluria (*see also* Infestation,
    filarial) 125.9
Hematocolpos 626.9
Hematogenous - *see* condition
Hematoma (traumatic) (skin surface intact)
    - *see also* Contusion
  with
    fracture - *see* Fracture
    injury of internal organs - *see* Injury,
      internal, by site
    nerve injury - *see* Injury, nerve
    open wound - *see* Wound, open
  amnion - *see* Placenta, abnormal
  aorta, dissecting 441.0
  arterial (complicating trauma) 995.3
  birth injury (*see also* Birth injury NEC)
      772.9
  brain (without skull fracture) 853.0
    with
      cerebral laceration or contusion
        (*see also* Laceration,
          cerebral) 851.0
      open intracranial wound 853.1
    fetus or newborn (*see also* Birth
      injury, brain) 772.0
    late effect 853.9
    nontraumatic (*see also* Hemorrhage,
      brain) 431.9
    newborn 778.2
    subarachnoid, arachnoid or
      meningeal (*see also*
        Hemorrhage, subarachnoid)
        430.9
    subdural, epidural or extradural
      (*see also* Hemorrhage,
        subdural) 431.9
  subarachnoid, arachnoid or meningeal
      - *see* Hematoma, subarachnoid
  subdural, epidural or extradural - *see*
      Hematoma, subdural
  breast (nontraumatic) 611.9
  broad ligament (nontraumatic) 616.9
    traumatic - *see* Injury, internal, broad
      ligament
  calcified NEC 996.9

Hematoma—*continued*
  capitis - *see also* Contusion, scalp
    due to birth injury (*see also* Birth
        injury NEC) 772.9
  cerebral - *see* Hematoma, brain
  chorion - *see* Placenta, abnormal
  complicating delivery NEC - *see*
        Obstetrical trauma
  corpus
    cavernosum (nontraumatic)   607.9
    luteum (ruptured) 615.9
  dura (mater) - *see* Hematoma, subdural
  epididymis (nontraumatic) 607.9
  epidural - *see also* Hematoma, subdural
    spinal - *see* Injury, spinal, by region
  extradural - *see* Hematoma, subdural
  genital organ NEC (nontraumatic)
    female 629.9
    male 607.9
    traumatic (external site) - *see*
        Contusion, trunk
      internal - *see* Injury, internal, pelvis
  graafian follicle (ruptured) 615.9
  internal organs (abdomen, chest or
        pelvis) - *see* Injury, internal, by
        site
  kidney, cystic (*see also* Lesion, kidney)
        593.2
  mediastinum - *see* Injury, internal,
        mediastinum
  meninges, meningeal (brain) - *see also*
        Hematoma, subarachnoid
    spinal - *see* Injury, spinal
  mesosalpinx (nontraumatic) 615.9
    traumatic - *see* Injury, internal, pelvis
  muscle - *code by* site as Contusion
  orbit, orbital (nontraumatic) 378.9
    with injury 921
  ovary (corpus luteum) (nontraumatic)
        615.9
    traumatic - *see* Injury, internal, ovary
  pelvis (female) nontraumatic 629.9
    male 607.9
    traumatic - *see* Injury, internal, pelvis
  penis (nontraumatic) 607.9
  pericranial - *see also* Contusion, scalp
    due to birth injury (*see also* Birth
        injury NEC) 772.9
  perirenal, cystic (*see also* Lesion,
        kidney) 593.2
  placenta - *see* Placenta, abnormal
  postoperative 998.1
  puerperal, postpartum, delayed
        complication 677.9
  retroperitoneal (nontraumatic) 569.9

Hematoma—*continued*
  retroperitoneal—*continued*
    traumatic - *see* Injury, internal,
        retroperitoneal
  scalp - *see also* Contusion, scalp
    fetus or newborn (*see also* Birth
        injury NEC) 772.9
  scrotum (nontraumatic) 607.9
  seminal vesicle (nontraumatic) 607.9
    traumatic - *see* Injury, internal,
        seminal vesicle
  spermatic cord - *see also* Injury,
        internal, spermatic cord
    nontraumatic 607.9
  spinal (cord) (meninges) - *see also*
        Injury, spinal, by region
    fetus or newborn (*see also* Birth
        injury, spinal cord) 772.1
  sternocleidomastoid originating at birth
        (*see also* Birth injury NEC)
        772.9
  sternomastoid originating at birth (*see
        also* Birth injury NEC) 772.9
  subarachnoid (without skull fracture)
        852.0
    with
      cerebral laceration or contusion
          (*see also* Laceration,
          cerebral) 851.0
      open intracranial wound 852.1
    fetus or newborn (*see also* Birth
        injury, brain) 772.0
    late effect 852.9
    nontraumatic (*see also* Hemorrhage,
        subarachnoid) 430.9
    newborn 778.2
  subdural (without skull fracture) 852.0
    with
      cerebral laceration or contusion
          (*see also* Laceration,
          cerebral) 851.0
      open intracranial wound 852.1
    fetus or newborn (*see also* Birth
        injury, brain) 772.0
    late effect 852.9
    nontraumatic (*see also* Hemorrhage,
        subdural) 431.9
    newborn 778.2
  syncytium - *see* Placenta, abnormal
  testis (nontraumatic) 607.9
  tunica vaginalis (nontraumatic) 607.9
  uterine ligament (nontraumatic) 616.9
    traumatic - *see* Injury, internal, pelvis
  vagina (ruptured) nontraumatic 629.9
  vas deferens (nontraumatic) 607.9

Hematoma—*continued*
  vas deferens—*continued*
    traumatic - *see* Injury, internal, vas
      deferens
  vitreous   377.0
  vocal cord - *see* Contusion, vocal cord
  vulva (nontraumatic)   629.9
    complicating delivery - *see*
      Obstetrical trauma
    during pregnancy (undelivered)
      634.9
Hematometra   625.9
Hematomyelia   349.9
  with fracture, vertebra (conditions in
    805) - *code by* region under
    Fracture, vertebra, with spinal
    cord lesion
  fetus or newborn (*see also* Birth injury,
    spinal cord)   772.1
Hematomyelitis   323
  late effects   324
Hematoperitoneum - *see*
  Hemoperitoneum
Hematopneumothorax (*see also*
  Hemothorax)   511.2
Hematoporphyria (congenital)   273.1
  acquired   279
Hematoporphyrinuria (congenital)   273.1
  acquired   279
Hematorachis, hematorrhachis   349.9
  fetus or newborn (*see also* Birth injury,
    spinal cord)   772.1
Hematosalpinx   615.9
  infectional (*see also* Salpingo-oophoritis)
    614
Hematospermia   607.9
Hematothorax (*see also* Hemothorax)
  511.2
Hematuria (essential) (idiopathic)   789.3
  endemic   120.0
  intermittent   789.3
  malarial   084.4
  paroxysmal   789.3
  sulphonamide, sulfonamide   961.0
  tropical   120.0
  tuberculous   016.1
    late effect or sequela   019.2
Hemendothelioma - *see*
  Hemangioendothelioma
Hemeralopia   378.9
  vitamin A deficiency   260.8
Hemi-abiotrophy   796.0
Hemi-analgesia (*see also* Disturbance,
  sensation)   781.6
Hemianencephaly   740

Hemi-anesthesia (*see also* Disturbance,
  sensation)   781.6
Hemi-anopia, hemianopsia (binasal)
  (bitemporal) (nasal) (peripheral)
  781.0
  syphilitic   095
Hemi-athetosis   780.3
Hemi-atrophy   796.0
  cerebellar   347.1
  face   356
    progressive   356
  fascia   733.9
  leg   733.9
  postpoliomyelitic   044
  tongue   529.9
Hemiballismus   347.9
Hemicardia   746.8
Hemicephalus, hemicephaly   740
Hemichorea   347.9
Hemicrania   346
  congenital malformation   740
Hemidystrophy - *see* Hemi-atrophy
Hemi-ectromelia   755.4
Hemihypalgesia (*see also* Disturbance,
  sensation)   781.6
Hemihypertrophy (congenital)   759.8
  cranial   756.0
Hemihypesthesia (*see also* Disturbance,
  sensation)   781.6
Hemimelia   755.4
  lower limb   755.3
  upper limb   755.2
Hemiparalysis (*see also* Hemiplegia)
  344.1
Hemiparesis (*see also* Hemiplegia)   344.1
Hemiparesthesia (*see also* Disturbance,
  sensation)   781.6
Hemiplegia   344.1
  acute (*see also* Disease,
    cerebrovascular, acute)   436.9
  alternans facialis   344.1
  apoplectic (*see also* Disease,
    cerebrovascular, acute)   436.9
    late effect or residual   344.1
  arteriosclerotic (*see also* Disease,
    cerebrovascular NEC)   438.9
    late effect or residual   344.1
  ascending (spinal) NEC   349.2
  attack (*see also* Disease,
    cerebrovascular, acute)   436.9
  brain, cerebral (current episode) (*see
    also* Disease, cerebrovascular
    NEC)   438.9
  fetus or newborn (*see also* Birth
    injury, brain)   772.0

Hemiplegia—*continued*
  brain, cerebral—*continued*
    late effect or residual NEC   344.1
      due to specified lesion - *see*
          Hemiplegia, late effect of
    cerebral - *see* Hemiplegia, brain
    congenital (cerebral) (spastic) (spinal) -
        see Hemiplegia, infantile
    cortical - *see* Hemiplegia, brain
    embolic (current episode) (*see also*
        Embolism, brain)   434.9
      late effect or residual   344.1
    hereditary - *see* Hemiplegia, infantile
  hypertensive (current episode) (*see also*
      Disease, cerebrovascular NEC,
      with hypertention)   438.0
    late effect or residual   344.1
  hysterical   300.1
  infantile (cerebral) (spastic) (spinal)
      343.0
    with other types of motor disturbance
        (e.g., ataxic, athetoid, atonic,
        rigidity, or tremor)   343.9
    athetoid   343.2
      with other types of motor
          disturbance (e.g., ataxic,
          atonic, rigidity, spastic, or
          tremor)   343.9
    specified type NEC   343.9
  late effect or residual of
    acute poliomyelitis (conditions in 040-
        043)   044
    birth injury, intracranial or spinal
        (conditions in 764-768 or 772
        with fourth digit .0 or .1) - *see*
        Hemiplegia, infantile
    cerebral laceration or contusion
        (conditions in 851.0, 851.1)
        851.9
    fracture or fracture dislocation of
        vertebral column with spinal
        cord lesion (conditions in
        806.0-806.7)   806.9
    intracranial
      abscess or pyogenic infection
          (conditions in 320-323)   324
      hemorrhage following injury
          (conditions in 853.0, 853.1)
          853.9
      vascular lesion (conditions in 430-
          438)   344.1
    spinal cord lesion (nontraumatic)
        NEC   349.2
      traumatic (conditions in 958.0-
          958.7)   958.9

Hemiplegia—*continued*
  late, effect, etc.—*continued*
    subarachnoid, subdural or extradural
        hemorrhage, following injury
        (conditions in 852.0, 852.1)
        852.9
    viral encephalitis (conditions in 062-
        065)   066
  middle alternating NEC   344.1
  old or longstanding NEC   344.1
    due to specified lesion - *see*
        Hemiplegia, late effect of
  residual NEC   344.1
    due to specified lesion- *see*
        Hemiplegia, late effect of
  seizure (current episode) (*see also*
      Disease, cerebrovascular, acute)
      436.9
    late effect or residual   344.1
  spastic (cerebral) (infantile) (spinal)
      343.0
    with other types of motor disturbance
        (e.g., ataxic, athetoid, atonic,
        rigidity, or tremor)   343.9
    not infantile or congenital (cerebral)
        344.1
      late effect or residual NEC   344.1
        due to specified lesion - *see*
            Hemiplegia, late effect of
    spinal   349.2
      late effect or residual NEC
          349.2
        due to specified lesion - *see*
            Hemiplegia, late effect
            of
  spinal (cord)   349.2
    late effect or residual NEC   349.2
      due to specified lesion - *see*
          Hemiplegia, late effect of
  thrombotic (current episode) (*see also*
      Thrombosis, brain)   433.9
    late effect or residual   344.1
Hemisection, spinal cord - *code by* region
    under Fracture, vertebra, with
    spinal cord lesion
Hemispasm   780.3
  facial   781.4
Hemisporosis   117.8
Hemitremor   780.3
Hemivertebra   756.2
Hemochromatosis   273.2
  with refractory anemia   285.0
  diabetic   273.2
  hereditary   273.2
  liver   273.2
  myocardium   273.2

Hemorrhage, etc. — *continued*
  brain — *continued*
    due to — *continued*
      rupture of aneurysm — *continued*
        mycotic - code as Hemorrhage,
          brain
      syphilis   094.9
      fetus (*see also* Birth injury, brain)
        772.0
      newborn (*see also* Birth injury, brain)
        772.0
      nontraumatic   778.2
      puerperal, postpartum, childbirth
        674
      punctate   850.9
      subarachnoid, arachnoid or meningeal
        - *see* Hemorrhage,
        subarachnoid
      subdural, epidural or extradural - *see*
        Hemorrhage, subdural
      traumatic (without skull fracture)
        NEC   853.0
        with
          cerebral laceration or contusion
            (*see also* Laceration,
            cerebral)   851.0
          open intracranial wound   853.1
        late effect   853.9
        subarachnoid, subdural or
          extradural - *see*
            Hemorrhage, subarachnoid,
            traumatic
  breast   458.9
  bronchial tube - *see* Hemorrhage, lung
  bronchopulmonary - *see* Hemorrhage,
    lung
  bronchus - *see* Hemorrhage, lung
  bulbar (*see also* Hemorrhage, brain)
    431.9
  capillary   448
    primary   287.9
  cardiovascular - *see* Disease, heart
  cecum   569.9
  cephalic (*see also* Hemorrhage, brain)
    431.9
  cerebellar (*see also* Hemorrhage, brain)
    431.9
  cerebellum (*see also* Hemorrhage,
    brain)   431.9
  cerebral (*see also* Hemorrhage, brain)
    431.9
  cerebrospinal (*see also* Hemorrhage,
    brain)   431.9
  cerebrum (*see also* Hemorrhage, brain)
    431.9
  . cervix (uteri) (stump) NEC   621.9

Hemorrhage, etc. — *continued*
  chamber anterior (eye)   378.6
  childbirth - *see* Hemorrhage,
    complicating delivery
  choroid   378.6
  cochlea   387.9
  colon - *see* Hemorrhage, intestine
  complicating delivery (intrapartum)
    (postpartum) (puerperal)   653
    due to
      placenta previa   651.0
        fetus or newborn   770.0
      premature separation of placenta
        651.1
        fetus or newborn   770.1
      retained placenta or secundines
        652
    fetus or newborn   769.9
  concealed NEC   458.9
  congenital   778.2
  conjunctiva   378.3
    newborn   778.2
  cord, newborn - *see also* Complications,
    umbilical cord
    stump   778.9
  corpus luteum (ruptured)   615.9
  cortical (*see also* Hemorrhage, brain)
    431.9
  cranial (*see also* Hemorrhage, brain)
    431.9
  cutaneous   287.0
    newborn   778.2
  cystitis (*see also* Cystitis)   595
  diathesis (familial) ' 287.9
    newborn   778.2
  disease   287.9
    newborn   778.2
  duodenum, duodenal   537.9
    ulcer - *see* Ulcer, duodenum, with
      hemorrhage
  dura mater - *see* Hemorrhage, subdural
  endotracheal - *see* Hemorrhage, lung
  epidural - *see* Hemorrhage, subdural
  esophagus   530.9
    varix   456.0
  external   458.9
  extradural - *see* Hemorrhage, subdural
  eye   378.9
    fundus   377.0
  face   458.9
  fallopian tube   615.9
  fetus before birth   778.0
  fibrinogenolysis (*see also* Fibrinolysis)
    286.4
  fibrinolysis (*see also* Fibrinolysis)
    286.4

Hemorrhage, etc. — *continued*

fontanel (*see also* Birth injury, bone or nerve) 772.2

fundus, eye 377.0

funis - *see* Complications, umbilical cord

gastric (*see also* Hemorrhage, stomach) 784.5

gastritis 535

gastro-enteric 569.9
 newborn 778.2

gastro-intestinal (tract) 569.9
 newborn 778.2

genito-urinary (tract) NEC 599.9

globe (eye) 378.9

gravidarum - *see* Hemorrhage, pregnancy

gum 523.9

heart see Disease, heart

hypopharyngeal (throat) 458.9

intermenstrual 626.6

internal (organs) 458.9
 capsule (*see also* Hemorrhage, brain) 431.9
 ear 387.9
 newborn 778.2

intestine 569.9
 congenital 778.2
 newborn 778.2

into
 bursa - *see* Bursitis
 corpus Luysii (*see also* Hemorrhage, brain) 431.9

intra-abdominal 458.9

intracranial NEC (*see also* Hemorrhage, brain) 431.9

intramedullary NEC 349.9

intra-ocular 378.9

intrapartum - *see* Hemorrhage, complicating delivery

intrapelvic
 female 629.9
 male 458.9

intraperitoneal 458.9

intrapontine (*see also* Hemorrhage, brain) 431.9

intra-uterine 625.9
 complicating delivery - *see* Hemorrhage, complicating delivery
 puerperal, postpartum, childbirth - *see also* Hemorrhage, complicating delivery
 delayed 677.2

intraventricular (*see also* Hemorrhage, brain) 431.9

Hemorrhage, etc. — *continued*

intravesical 596.9

iris (postinfectional) (postinflammatory) (toxic) 378.6

joint (nontraumatic) (*see also* Disease, joint) 729.9

kidney (*see also* Lesion, kidney) 593.2

knee (joint) 729.8

labyrinth 387.9

leg NEC 458.9

lenticular striate artery (*see also* Hemorrhage, brain) 431.9

ligature, vessel 458.9

liver 573.9

lower extremity 458.9

lung 783.1
 newborn 778.2
 tuberculous (*see also* Tuberculosis, pulmonary) 011.9

lymphatic gland 458.9

mediastinum - *see* Hemorrhage, lung

medulla (*see also* Hemorrhage, brain) 431.9

membrane (brain) (*see also* Hemorrhage, subarachnoid) 430.9
 spinal cord - *see* Hemorrhage, spinal cord

meninges, meningeal (brain) (middle) (*see also* Hemorrhage, subarachnoid) 430.9
 spinal cord - *see* Hemorrhage, spinal cord

mesentery 569.9

metritis 625.9

midbrain (*see also* Hemorrhage, brain) 431.9

mole (abortion) (*see also* Abortion, other) 645.9
 undelivered 634.9

mouth 528.9

mucous membrane NEC 458.9
 newborn 778.2

muscle 733.9

nail (subungual) 703.9

nasal turbinate 783.0
 newborn 778.2

nasopharynx 508.9

navel 778.9

neck 458.9
 newborn 778.2

nipple 611.9

nose 783.0
 newborn 778.2

omentum 569.9
 newborn 778.2

Hemorrhage, etc. — *continued*
  optic nerve (sheath)   377.6
  orbit, orbital   378.9
  ovary   615.9
  oviduct   615.9
  pancreas   577.9
  parathyroid (gland) (spontaneous)
    252.9
  parturition - *see* Hemorrhage,
    complicating delivery
  penis   607.9
  pericardium, pericarditis - *see*
    Pericarditis
  peritoneum, peritoneal   458.9
  peritonsillar tissue
    due to infection   501
  petechial   287.0
  pituitary (gland)   253.9
  placenta (complicating delivery)   651.1
    fetus or newborn   770.1
    undelivered NEC   632.1
  pleura - *see* Hemorrhage, lung
  polio-encephalitis superior   263.9
  polymyositis - *see* Polymyositis
  pons (*see also* Hemorrhage, brain)
    431.9
  pontine (*see also* Hemorrhage, brain)
    431.9
  popliteal   458.9
  postmenopausal   626.7
  postnasal   783.0
  postoperative   998.1
  postpartum (*see also* Hemorrhage,
    complicating delivery)   653
    delayed   677.2
  pregnancy (before onset of labor)
    (concealed)   632.9
    accidental (due to premature
      separation of placenta)   632.1
      complicating delivery   651.1
      fetus or newborn   770.1
    complicating delivery   651.9
      fetus or newborn   769.9
    due to
      afibrinogenemia, or other
        coagulation defect
        (conditions in category 286)
        632.4
        complicating delivery   651.9
        fetus or newborn   769.9
      marginal sinus (rupture)   632.2
        complicating delivery   651.1
        fetus or newborn   770.1
      placenta previa   632.0
        complicating delivery   651.0
        fetus or newborn   770.0

Hemorrhage, etc. — *continued*
  pregnancy — *continued*
    due to — *continued*
      premature separation placenta
        (normally implanted)   632.1
        complicating delivery   651.1
        fetus or newborn   770.1
      threatened abortion   632.3
        complicating delivery   651.9
        fetus or newborn   769.9
    fetus or newborn   769.9
    unavoidable - *see* Hemorrhage,
      pregnancy due to placenta
      previa
  prepartum - *see* Hemorrhage,
    pregnancy
  preretinal   377.0
  prostate   602
  puerperal - *see also* Hemorrhage,
    complicating delivery
    delayed   677.2
  pulmonary - *see* Hemorrhage, lung
  purpura (primary) (*see also*
    Thrombocytopenia)   287.1
  rectum (sphincter)   569.2
  recurring, following initial hemorrhage
    at time of injury   995.2
  renal (*see also* Lesion, kidney)   593.2
  respiratory tract - *see* Hemorrhage, lung
  retina, retinal (vessels)   377.0
    diabetic - *see* category 250
  retroperitoneal   458.9
  retroplacental (*see also* Placenta,
    separation)   651.1
  scalp   458.9
    due to injury at birth (*see also* Birth
      injury NEC)   772.9
  scrotum   607.9
  secondary (nontraumatic)   458.9
    following initial hemorrhage at time
      of injury   995.2
  seminal vesicle   607.9
  skin   287.0
    newborn   778.2
  spermatic cord   607.9
  spinal (cord)   349.9
    aneurysm   349.9
      ruptured   349.9
      syphilitic   094.9
    due to or with birth injury (*see also*
      Birth injury, spinal cord)
      772.1
    fetus or newborn (*see also* Birth
      injury, spinal cord)   772.1
  spleen   289.5
  stomach   784.5

Hemorrhage, etc. — *continued*
  stomach — *continued*
    newborn 778.2
    ulcer - *see* Ulcer, stomach, with
       hemorrhage
  subarachnoid (nontraumatic) 430.9
  with
    hypertension (benign) (conditions in
       401) 430.0
      malignant (*see also*
         Hypertension, malignant
         with cerebrovascular
         involvement) 400.2
    fetus (*see also* Birth injury, brain)
       772.0
    newborn (*see also* Birth injury, brain)
       772.0
    nontraumatic 778.2
    puerperal, postpartum, childbirth
       674
    traumatic (without skull fracture)
       852.0
    with
      cerebral laceration or contusion
         (*see also* Laceration,
         brain) 851.0
      open intercranial wound 852.1
      late effect 852.9
  subconjunctiva 378.3
  subcortical (*see also* Hemorrhage,
     brain) 431.9
  subcutaneous 458.9
  subdiaphragmatic 458.9
  subdural (nontraumatic) 431.9
  with
    hypertension (benign) (conditions in
       401) 431.0
      malignant (*see also*
         Hypertension, malignant,
         with cerebrovascular
         involvement) 400.2
    due to birth injury (*see also* Birth
       injury, brain) 772.0
    fetus (*see also* Birth injury, brain)
       772.0
    newborn (*see also* Birth injury, brain)
       772.0
    nontraumatic 778.2
    spinal 349.9
    traumatic (without skull fracture)
       852.0
    with
      cerebral laceration or contusion
         (*see also* Laceration,
         cerebral) 851.0
      open intracranial wound 852.1

Hemorrhage, etc. — *continued*
  subdural, etc. — *continued*
    traumatic, etc. — *continued*
      late effect 852.9
  subhyaloid 377.0
  subperiosteal 723.9
  subretinal 377.0
  subtentorial (*see also* Hemorrhage,
     brain) 431.9
  subungual 703.9
  suprarenal (capsule) (gland) 255.9
    due to injury at birth (*see also* Birth
       injury NEC) 772.9
  tentorium (traumatic) (without skull
     fracture) NEC 853.0
    due to birth injury (*see also* Birth
       injury, brain) 772.0
    fetus or newborn (*see also* Birth
       injury, brain) 772.0
    late effect 853.9
    nontraumatic - *see* Hemorrhage, brain
  testicle 607.9
  thigh 458.9
  thorax - *see* Hemorrhage, lung
  throat 458.9
  thrombocythemia 287.2
  thymus (gland) 254
  thyroid (gland) 246
    cyst 246
  tongue 529.9
  tonsil 500
  trachea - *see* Hemorrhage, lung
  traumatic - *see also* nature of injury
    brain - *see* Hemorrhage, brain,
       traumatic
    recurring or secondary (following
       initial hemorrhage at time of
       injury) 995.2
  tuberculous NEC (*see also*
     Tuberculosis) 011.9
  ulcer NEC - *see* Ulcer, peptic
  umbilical
    cord - *see* Complications, umbilical
       cord
    stump 778.9
  unavoidable (complicating delivery) (due
     to placenta previa) 651.0
    fetus or newborn 770.0
    undelivered 632.0
  upper extremity 458.9
  urethra (idiopathic) 599.9
  uterus, uterine (abnormal) 626.9
    after parturition (*see also*
       Hemorrhage, complicating
       delivery) 653
    delayed 677.2

Hemorrhage, etc. — *continued*
  uterus, uterine — *continued*
    climacteric 627
    during parturition (*see also*
        Hemorrhage, complicating
        delivery) 653
    functional or dysfunctional 626.6
    intermenstrual 626.6
    postmenopausal 626.7
    postpartum (*see also* Hemorrhage,
        complicating delivery) 653
    prepubertal 626.9
    pubertal 626.9
    traumatic, obstetrical, complicating
        delivery - *see* Obstetrical
        trauma
  vagina 629.5
  vas deferens 607.9
  ventricular (*see also* Hemorrhage, brain)
      431.9
  vesical 596.9
  viscera 458.9
    newborn 778.2
  vitreous (humor) (intra-ocular) 377.0
  vulva 629.9
Hemorrhoids (bleeding) (external)
        (internal) (prolapsed) (rectum)
        (strangulated) (thrombosed)
        (ulcerated) 455
Hemosalpinx 615.9
Hemosiderosis 279
  dietary 279
  pulmonary
    idiopathic 279
  transfusion 999.8
Hemothorax 511.2
  newborn 778.2
  nontuberculous 511.2
    bacterial 511.1
  pneumococcal 511.1
  staphylococcal 511.1
  streptococcal 511.1
  traumatic 860.0
    with open wound into thorax 860.1
    late effect 860.9
  tuberculous 012.1
    with pneumoconiosis (conditions in
        515) 010
    late effect or sequela 019.0
Henle's warts 378.4
Henoch(-Schonlein)
  disease or syndrome 287.0
  purpura 287.0
Henpue, henpuye 102.6
Hepar lobatum 095
Hepatalgia 573.9

Hepatic - *see also* condition
  flexure syndrome 569.9
Hepatitis 573.0
  acute (*see also* Necrosis, liver) 570
    infective 070
  alcoholic 571.0
  amebic 006.0
  anicteric
    acute 070
  catarrhal (acute) 070
    chronic - *see* Cirrhosis, postnecrotic
    newborn 070
  cholangiolitic 573.0
  cholestatic 573.0
  chronic - *see* Cirrhosis, liver
  diffuse 573.0
  due to toxoplasmosis 130.9
    acquired 130.0
    congenital (active) 130.1
      late effects 130.2
  epidemic 070
  fetus or newborn 778.9
  fibrous (chronic) - *see also* Cirrhosis,
      liver
    acute 573.0
  from injection, inoculation or
      transfusion (blood) (plasma)
      (serum) (other substance) for
      immunization or other
      prophylactic or therapeutic
      purpose (onset within 8 months
      after administration) 999.2
  fulminant 070
  hemorrhagic 573.0
  homologous serum 999.2
  hypertrophic (chronic) - *see also*
      Cirrhosis, liver
    acute 573.0
  infectious, infective (acute) (chronic)
      (subacute) 070
  inoculation 999.2
  interstitial (chronic) - *see also* Cirrhosis,
      liver
    acute 573.0
  lupoid 573.0
  malarial NEC (*see also* Malaria) 084.9
  malignant (*see also* Necrosis, liver)
      570
  neonatal (toxic) 778.9
  parenchymatous (acute) (*see also*
      Necrosis, liver) 570
  peliosis 573.0
  plasma cell 573.0
  post-immunization 999.2
  post-transfusion 999.2

Hepatitis—*continued*
  septic 573.0
  serum 999.2
  subacute (*see also* Necrosis, liver) 570
  suppurative (diffuse) 572
  syphilitic (late) 095
    congenital 090.0
  toxic 573.0
    fetus or newborn 778.9
  tuberculous 017.9
    late effect or sequela 019.9
  virus 070
Hepatization lung (acute) - *see also*
    Pneumonia, lobar
  chronic (*see also* Fibrosis, lung) 517
Hepatoblastoma 155.0
Hepatocarcinoma 197.8
  primary 155.0
Hepatocholangitis 573.0
Hepatocystitis (*see also* Cholecystitis)
  575
Hepatolenticular degeneration 273.3
Hepatolienal cirrhosis or fibrosis - *see*
  Cirrhosis, liver
Hepatoma 155.0
  benign 211.5
  embryonal 155.0
Hepatomegalia glycogenica diffusa 271.1
Hepatomegaly (*see also* Hypertrophy,
  liver) 785.1
  congenital 751.6
  syphilitic 090.0
Hepatoptosis 573.9
Hepatosis (toxic) 573.9
Hepatosplenomegaly - *see also* Cirrhosis,
  liver
  hyperlipemic (Buerger-Grutz type)
    272.0
Hereditary - *see* condition
Heredodegeneration 333.9
  macular 377.1
Heredopathia atactica polyneuritiformis
  332.9
Heredosyphilis (*see also* Syphilis,
  congenital) 090.9
Hermaphroditism (true) 752.0
Hernia, hernial (acquired) (congenital)
  (recurrent) 551.9
  with obstruction 553.9
  abdomen (wall) 551.2
    with obstruction 553.2
  abdominal, specified site NEC 551.8
    with obstruction 553.8
  appendix 551.8
    with obstruction 553.8
  bilateral (inguinal) 550

Hernia, hernial—*continued*
  bilateral (inguinal)—*continued*
    with obstruction 552
  bladder (sphincter)
    congenital (female) (male) 753.8
    female 623.0
    male 596.9
  brain 347.9
    congenital 743.0
  cartilage, vertebra - *see* Displacement,
    intervertebral disc
  cerebral 347.9
    congenital 743.0
    endaural 743.0
  ciliary body 378.6
  colic 551.9
    with obstruction 553.9
  colon 551.9
    with obstruction 553.9
  Cooper's 551.8
    with obstruction 553.8
  crural - *see* Hernia, femoral
  diaphragm, diaphragmatic 551.3
    with obstruction 553.3
    due to gross defect of diaphragm
      756.8
  direct (inguinal) 550
    with obstruction 552
  diverticulum, intestine 551.9
    with obstruction 553.9
  double (inguinal) 550
    with obstruction 552
  due to
    gross congenital defect of diaphragm
      756.8
  en glissade - *see* Hernia, sliding
  epigastric 551.2
    with obstruction 553.2
  esophageal hiatus 551.3
    with obstruction 553.3
  external (inguinal) 550
    with obstruction 552
  fallopian tube 615.9
  fascia 733.9
  fat 733.9
  femoral 551.0
    with obstruction 553.0
  foramen magnum 347.9
    congenital 743.0
  funicular (umbilical) 551.1
    with obstruction 553.1
    spermatic (cord) 550
      with obstruction 552
  gangrenous (*see also* Hernia, by site,
      with obstruction) 553.9
  gastro-intestinal tract 551.9

Hernia, hernial — *continued*
spigelian 551.2
  with obstruction 553.2
spinal 741.9
  with hydrocephalus 741.0
strangulated (*see also* Hernia, by site,
    with obstruction) 553.9
supra-umbilicus 551.2
  with obstruction 553.2
tendon 733.9
testis (nontraumatic) 095
Treitz's (fossa) 551.8
  with obstruction 553.8
tunica vaginalis 752.8
umbilicus, umbilical 551.1
  with obstruction 553.1
ureter 593.5
  with obstruction 593.3
uterus 625.9
  pregnant (undelivered) 634.9
vaginal (posterior) 623.3
Velpeau's 551.0
  with obstruction 553.0
ventral 551.2
  with obstruction 553.2
vesical
  congenital (female) (male) 753.8
  female 623.0
  male 596.9
vitreous (into anterior chamber) 378.9
Herniation - *see also* Hernia
gastric mucosa (into duodenal bulb)
    537.9
mediastinum 519.9
nucleus pulposus - *see* Displacement,
    intervertebral disc
Herpangina 074.0
Herpes 054
circinatus bullosus 693
circine 110.9
conjunctiva (zoster) 053.0
  simplex 054
cornea (zoster) 053.0
  simplex 054
encephalitis 054
eye (zoster) 053.0
  simplex 054
febrilis (any site) 054
genital, genitalis 054
gestationis 693
iris (any site) 695.1
keratitis 054
labialis 054
  meningococcal 036.8
larynx 054

Herpes — *continued*
lip 054
ophthalmicus (zoster) 053.0
  simplex 054
penis 054
scrotum 054
simplex (any site) 054
tonsurans 110.0
  maculosus (of Hebra) 696.3
vulva 054
zoster 053.9
  abdomen 053.2
  auricularis 053.1
  conjunctiva 053.0
  cornea 053.0
  eye 053.0
  face, except eye 053.1
  ophthalmicus 053.0
  oticus 053.1
  specified site NEC 053.9
  trunk 053.2
zosteriform, intermediate type 053.9
Herpetic
fever 054
geniculate ganglionitis 053.1
Herrick's anemia (*see also* Disease, sickle
    cell) 282.5
Hers' disease 271.1
Herter-Gee syndrome 269.0
Herxheimer's reaction 999.4
Hesselbach's hernia - *see* Hernia,
    Hesselbach's
Heterochromia (congenital) 744.8
cataract 374.1
cyclitis 364
iritis 364
retained metallic foreign body 930
uveitis 366
Heteromorphic tumor - *see* Neoplasm
Heterophoria (*see also* Strabismus)
    373.9
Heterophyes, small intestine 121.9
Heterophyiasis 121.9
Heteropsia 370.9
Heterotopia, heterotopic - *see also*
    Malposition, congenital
cerebralis 743.2
spinalis 743.3
Heterotropia (*see also* Strabismus) 373.9
Heubner's disease 094.9
Hexadactylism 755.0
Heyd's syndrome 573.9
Hibernoma (*see also* Lipoma) 214.9
Hiccough 784.6
epidemic 079.8
psychogenic 305.2

Hiccup (*see also* Hiccough)   784.6

Hicks(-Braxton) contractures (undelivered)
   634.7

Hidradenitis (suppurative) (axillaris)
   705.9

Hidradenoma (skin) (*see also* Adenoma,
   sweat glands)   216.2

Hidrocystoma (*see also* Adenoma, sweat
   glands)   216.2

High
  altitude effects   993.2
    anoxia   993.2
    on ears   993.0
    on sinuses   993.1
    polycythemia   289.0
  arch
    foot   755.7
    palate   750.8
  arterial tension (*see also* Hypertension)
      401
  basal metabolic rate   788.9
  blood pressure (*see also* Hypertension)
      401
  diaphragm (congenital)   756.8
  grade defect - *see* Retardation, mental,
      mild
  palate   750.8
  temperature (of unknown origin) (*see
      also* Pyrexia)   788.6
  thoracic rib   756.4

Hildenbrand's disease   081.9

Hill diarrhea   269.0

Hilliard's lupus   017.0
  late effect or sequela   019.9

Hilum - *see* condition

Hip - *see* condition

Hippel's disease   224

Hippus   378.6

Hirschsprung's disease or megacolon
   751.2

Hirsuties (*see also* Hypertrichosis)   704

Hirsutism (*see also* Hypertrichosis)   704

Hirudiniasis (external) (internal)   134.3

His-Werner disease   083.2

Hiss-Russel dysentery   004.1

Histamine cephalgia or headache   346

Histidinemia   270.8

Histidinuria   270.8

Histiocytoma (*see also* Dermatofibroma)
   216.8

Histiocytosis   279
  cholesterol   279
  essential   279
  lipid, lipoid (essential)   272.2
  X   279

Histoplasmosis (Darling's)   115
  lung   115

Hives (bold) (*see also* Urticaria)   708.9

Hoarseness   783.5

Hobnail liver - *see* Cirrhosis, portal

Hoboism   301.7

Hodgkin's
  disease   201
  granuloma   201
  lymphoblastoma   201
  lymphogranulomatosis   201
  lymphoma   201
  lymphosarcoma   201
  pseudoleukemia   201
  sarcoma   201

Hodgson's disease   441.9

Hole
  retina (macula)   377.1
  vitreous humor   378.9

Holla disease (*see also* Spherocytosis)
   282.0

Hollow foot (congenital)   754.0
  acquired   738.6

Holmes's syndrome   781.0

Homesickness   307

Homocystinemia   270.8

Homocystinuria   270.8

Homologous serum jaundice
   (prophylactic) (therapeutic)   999.2

Homosexuality   302.0

Honeycomb lung   748.4

Hong Kong ear   117.3

Hooded
  clitoris   752.6
  penis   752.8

Hookworm (anemia) (disease) (infection)
   (infestation) - *see* Ancylostomiasis

Hordeolum (eyelid) (external) (internal)
   (recurrent)   362

Horn
  cutaneous   702
    cheek   702
    eyelid   702
  nail   703.9
    congenital   757.4
  papillary   700

Horner's syndrome   358.0
  traumatic - *see* Injury, nerve, cervical
      sympathetic

Horseshoe kidney (congenital)   753.3

Horton's
  disease   446.4
  syndrome   346

Hospital
  gangrene, noma   528.1
  putrefaction, noma   528.1

Hourglass contraction, contracture
  bladder 596.2
    congenital 753.8
  gallbladder (see also Disease,
      gallbladder) 576.9
    congenital 751.6
  stomach 536.1
    congenital 750.8
    psychogenic 305.5
  uterus, complicating delivery 657.9
    fetus or newborn - see categories
      767.0-767.9
Housemaid's knee 731.6
Hudson-Stahli line 378.9
Huebner-Herter disease 269.0
Huguier's disease 218
Human bite (open wound) - see also
    Wound, open
  intact skin surface - see Contusion
Humpback (acquired) 735.1
  congenital 756.2
Hunchback (acquired) 735.1
  congenital 756.2
Hunger 994.2
  air, psychogenic 305.2
Hunner's ulcer (see also Cystitis) 595
Hunt's
  disease 347.9
  neuralgia 053.1
  syndrome 053.1
Hunter
  glossitis 529.4
Hunter-Hurler syndrome 273.8
Huntington's
  chorea 331.0
  disease 331.0
Huppert's disease 203
Hurler's
  disease 273.8
  syndrome (in bones) 273.8
Hurthle cell
  carcinoma (thyroid) 193
  tumor - see Adenoma, thyroid
Hutchinson-Boeck disease or syndrome
    135
Hutchinson-Gilford disease or syndrome
    258.9
Hutchinson's
  disease, summer eruption, or summer
    prurigo 709.9
  syndrome 194.0
  teeth or incisors (congenital syphilis)
    090.5
Hyalin plaque, sclera, senile 378.6

Hyaline
  degeneration (diffuse) (generalized)
    734.9
    localized - see Degeneration, by site
  membrane (disease) (lung) 776.1
  with
    abnormality of bones, organs or
      tissues of pelvis - see
      categories 764.0-764.4
    abnormality of forces of labor - see
      categories 767.0-767.4
    difficult labor NEC - see categories
      768.0-768.4
    disproportion, fetopelvic - see
      categories 765.0-765.4
    with abnormality of bones,
      organs or tissues of pelvis
      - see categories 764.0-
      764.4
    malposition of fetus - see categories
      766.0-766.4
Hyalinosis
  cutis et mucosae 279
Hyalitis (asteroid) 369.9
  syphilitic 095
Hydatid
  cyst or tumor - see Hydatidosis
  mole - see Hydatidiform mole
  Morgagni 752.8
Hydatidiform mole (benign) (complicating
    pregnancy) (delivered) (undelivered)
    634.0
  malignant (change) 181
Hydatidosis 122.9
  liver 122.0
  lung 122.1
  specified site NEC 122.8
Hyde's disease 697.9
Hydradenitis - see Hidradenitis
Hydradenoma (skin) (see also Adenoma,
    sweat glands) 216.2
Hydramnios (complicating pregnancy)
    (undelivered) 634.3
  with delivery 661.8
  fetus or newborn 769.2
Hydrancephaly 742
  with spina bifida 741.0
Hydranencephaly 742
  with spina bifida 741.0
Hydrargyrism NEC 985.0
Hydrarthrosis (intermittent) (see also
    Disease, joint) 729.9
  gonococcal 098.3
  of yaws (early) (late) 102.6
  syphilitic 095
    congenital 090.5

Hydrops 782.6
 abdominis 785.3
 amnii (complicating pregnancy) (*see also*
  Hydramnios) 634.3
 articulorum intermittens (*see also*
  Hydrarthrosis) 729.9
 cardiac (*see also* Failure, heart,
  congestive) 427.0
 congenital (*see also* Disease, hemolytic)
  775.9
 fetal or newborn (*see also* Disease,
  hemolytic) 775.9
  not due to hemolytic disease 778.9
 gallbladder (*see also* Disease,
  gallbladder) 576.9
 joint (*see also* Hydrarthrosis) 729.9
 labyrinth 385
 meningeal 347.9
 nutritional 269.9
 pericardium - *see* Pericarditis
 pleura (*see also* Hydrothorax) 511.2
 renal (*see also* Nephrosis) 581
 spermatic cord (*see also* Hydrocele)
  603
Hydropyonephrosis (*see also* Pyelitis)
  590.1
 chronic 590.0
Hydrorrhachis 743.3
Hydrorrhea (nasal) 508.9
 gravidarum 634.9
 pregnancy 634.9
Hydrosadenitis - *see* Hidradenitis
Hydrosalpinx (fallopian tube) (follicularis)
  615.1
Hydrothorax (double) (pleura) 511.2
 chylous (nonfilarial) 457
  filarial (*see also* Infestation, filarial)
   125.9
 nontuberculous 511.2
  bacterial 511.1
 pneumococcal 511.1
 staphylococcal 511.1
 streptococcal 511.1
 traumatic 860.0
  with open wound into thorax 860.1
  late effect 860.9
 tuberculous 012.1
  with pneumoconiosis (conditions in
   515) 010
  late effect or sequela 019.0
Hydro-ureter 593.4
 congenital 753.2
Hydro-ureteronephrosis (*see also*
  Hydronephrosis) 591
Hydro-urethra 599.9
Hydroxykynureninuria 270.8

Hydroxyprolinemia 270.8
Hygroma (cystic) (congenital) 227.2
 praepatellare, prepatellar 731.6
Hymen - *see* condition
Hymenolepiasis (diminuta) (infection)
  (infestation) (nana) 123.6
Hymenolepis (diminuta) (infection)
  (infestation) (nana) 123.6
Hypalgesia (*see also* Disturbance,
  sensation) 781.6
Hyperacidity (gastric) 536.0
 psychogenic 305.5
Hyperactive, hyperactivity
 basal cell
  uterine cervix 621.9
  cervix epithelial (basal) 621.9
 child 308
 gastro-intestinal 536.1
  psychogenic 305.5
 nasal mucous membrane 508.9
 stomach 536.1
 thyroid (gland) (*see also*
  Hyperthyroidism) 242.2
Hyperadrenalism 255.0
Hyperadrenocorticism 255.0
 congenital 273.6
 iatrogenic 962.0
Hyperaffectivity 301.1
Hyperaldosteronism (primary) 255.0
Hyperalgesia (*see also* Disturbance,
  sensation) 781.6
Hyperalimentation 278.9
 carotin 278.1
 vitamin A 278.0
 vitamin D 278.2
Hyperaminoaciduria
 arginine 270.1
 cystine 270.1
 lysine 270.1
 ornithine 270.1
Hyperammoniemia, congenital 270.8
Hyperazotemia - *see* Uremia
Hyperbetalipidproteinemia, familial
  272.0
Hyperbetalipoproteinemia, familial 272.0
Hyperbilirubinemia 785.2
 congenital 273.5
 constitutional 273.5
 newborn NEC 778.9
  prolonged (*see also* Disease,
   hemolytic) 775.9
Hyperbilirubinemica encephalopathia,
  newborn (*see also* Disease,
  hemolytic, by type, with
  kernicterus) 774.9
Hypercalcemia 788.9

Hypercapnia   783.2
Hypercementosis   521.5
Hyperchloremia   788.0
Hyperchlorhydria   536.0
  neurotic   305.5
  psychogenic   305.5
Hypercholesterinemia   279
  essential   272.0
  familial (essential)   272.0
  hereditary   272.0
  primary   272.0
Hypercholesterolemia - *see*
    Hypercholesterinemia
Hypercholesterolosis   279
Hyperchylia gastrica   536.0
  psychogenic   305.5
Hyperchylomicronemia
  familial   272.0
    with hyperbetalipoproteinemia   272.0
Hypercorticosteronism   962.0
Hypercortisonism   962.0
Hyperelectrolythemia   788.0
Hyperemesis   536.9
  with abortion - *see* Abortion, by type,
      with toxemia
  arising during pregnancy - *see*
      Hyperemesis, gravidarum
  gravidarum   638.9
    with neuritis   638.0
      fetus or newborn   762.4
    fetus or newborn   762.4
  psychogenic   305.5
Hyperemia (acute)   788.9
  anal mucosa   569.2
  cerebral (*see also* Disease,
      cerebrovascular NEC)   438.9
  conjunctiva   360
  ear internal, acute   384.9
  enteric   569.9
  eye   378.9
  eyelid (active) (passive)   361
  intestine   569.9
  iris   378.6
  kidney (*see also* Lesion, kidney)   593.2
  labyrinth   384.9
  liver (active) (passive)   573.9
  lung   514
  passive   788.9
  pulmonary   514
  renal (*see also* Lesion, kidney)   593.2
  retina   377.0
  stomach   537.9
Hyperesthesia (body surface) (*see also*
      Disturbance, sensation)   781.6
  larynx (reflex)   508.3
    hysterical   300.1

Hyperesthesia—*continued*
  pharynx (reflex)   508.9
    hysterical   300.1
Hyperextension, joint (*see also* Disease,
      joint)   729.9
Hyperfructosemia   271.3
Hyperfunction
  adrenal (cortex)   255.0
    medulla   255.2
    virilism   255.0
  ovarian   256.0
  pancreas   577.9
  parathyroid (gland)   252.0
  pituitary (gland) (anterior)   253.0
  testicular   257.0
Hypergammaglobulinemia   289.9
Hyperglobulinemia   275.9
Hyperglycemia - *see* category 250
  maternal
    affecting fetus or newborn   761.1
    manifest diabetes in infant - *see*
        category 250
Hyperglyceridemia   279
  essential   272.0
  familial   272.0
  hereditary   272.0
Hypergonadism
  ovarian   256.0
  testicular (primary)   257.0
    infantile   257.0
Hyperheparinemia (*see also* Circulating
      anticoagulants)   286.5
Hyperhidrosis, hyperidrosis   788.1
  psychogenic   305.0
Hyperinsulinism NEC   251
  therapeutic misadventure (from
      administration of insulin)   962.3
Hyperkalemia   788.0
Hyperkeratosis (*see also* Keratosis)
      701.1
  cervix   621.9
  congenital   757.2
  due to yaws (early) (late) (palmar or
      plantar)   102.3
  excentrica   757.2
  figurata centrifuga atrophica   757.2
  follicularis   757.2
    in cutem penetrans   704
  palmoplantaris climacterica   701.1
  senile (with pruritus)   702
  universalis congenita   757.2
  vocal cord   508.3
  vulva   629.9
Hyperkinesia, child   308
Hyperkinetic heart (disease) (syndrome)
    - *see* Disease, heart

Hyperlipemia 279
  combined fat and carbohydrate induced
    272.0
  congenital 272.0
  essential 272.0
  familial (carbohydrate-induced)
    (essential) (fat-induced) 272.0
  hereditary 272.0
  idiopathic 272.0
  in familial hypercholesterolemic
    xanthomatosis 272.0
  mixed 272.0
Hyperlipidosis 272.9
  hereditary 272.9
Hyperlipoproteinemia
  familial 272.0
Hypermaturity (fetus or newborn) 778.1
Hypermenorrhea 626.2
Hypermetropia (congenital) 370.1
Hypermobility
  cecum 564.1
  coccyx 723.9
  colon 564.1
    psychogenic 305.5
  ileum 564.9
  meniscus (knee) 724.5
  scapula 723.9
  stomach 536.1
    psychogenic 305.5
Hypermotility
  gastro-intestinal 536.1
  intestine 564.1
    psychogenic 305.5
  stomach 536.1
Hypermyopia 370.1
Hypernatremia 788.0
Hypernephroma 189.0
Hypernephromatosis 189.0

Hyperopia 370.1
Hyperosmia (see also Disturbance,
  sensation) 781.6

Hyperostosis 723.9
  cortical 723.9
    infantile 756.7
  frontal, internal 723.4
  interna frontalis 723.4
  monomelic 723.9
  skull 723.4
    congenital 756.0
Hyperovarianism 256.0
Hyperovarism 256.0
Hyperoxaluria 271.8
  primary 271.8
Hyperoxia 987.9
Hyperparathyroidism 252.0

Hyperpathia (see also Disturbance,
  sensation) 781.6
Hyperperistalsis 785.8
  psychogenic 305.5
Hyperpermeability, capillary 448
Hyperphagia 278.9
Hyperphoria 373.2
Hyperphosphatemia 788.9
Hyperpiesia (see also Hypertension) 401
Hyperpiesis (see also Hypertension) 401
Hyperpigmentation - see Pigmentation
Hyperpinealism 258.9
Hyperpituitarism 253.0
Hyperplasia, hyperplastic
  adrenal (capsule) (cortex) (gland) 255.9
    with
      sexual precocity 255.0
      virilism, adrenal 255.0
      virilization (female) 255.0
    congenital 273.6
  appendix (lymphoid) 542
  bone 723.9
    marrow 289.9
  breast (see also Hypertrophy, breast)
    611.1
  cementum (tooth) (teeth) 521.5
  cervical gland 782.7
  cervix (uteri) 621.9
    basal cell 621.9
    congenital 752.5
    endometrium 621.2
    polypoid 621.9
  clitoris, congenital 752.6
  dentin 521.5
  endocervicitis 621.2
  endometrium, endometrial
    (adenomatous) (atypical) (cystic)
      (polypoid) (uterus) 625.2
    cervix 621.2
  epithelial 709.9
    nipple 611.1
    skin 709.9
    vaginal wall 629.9
  erythroid 289.9
  generalized, giant, of lymph nodes and
    spleen 202.0
  genital
    female 629.9
    male 607.9
  giant lymph follicle of spleen 202.0
  gingiva 523.9
  glandularis
    cystica uteri 625.2
    interstitialis uteri 625.2
  gum 523.9
  hymen, congenital 752.6

Hyperplasia, etc. — *continued*
  kidney (congenital) 753.3
  liver (congenital) 751.6
  lymph
    gland 782.7
    nodes 782.7
  mandible, mandibular 524.0
    unilateral condylar 526.9
  Marchand multiple nodular (liver) - *see*
      Cirrhosis, postnecrotic
  maxilla, maxillary 524.0
  myometrium, myometrial 625.9
  ·nose
    lymphoid 508.9
    polypoid 508.9
  oral mucosa (inflammatory) 528.9
  organ or site, congenital NEC - *see*
      Anomaly, specified type NEC
  ovary 615.9
  parathyroid (gland) 252.0
  persistent (primary)
    vitreous 744.8
  pharynx
    lymphoid 508.9
  placenta - *see* Placenta, abnormal
  prostate (adenofibromatous) (nodular)
      600
  reticulo-endothelial (cell) 289.9
  salivary gland (any) 527.1
  Schimmelbusch's 610
  suprarenal (capsule) (gland) 255.9
  thymus (gland) 254
  thyroid (gland) (*see also* Goiter) 240.9
  tonsil (lymphoid tissue) 500
  uterus, uterine 625.9
    endometrium 625.2
  vulva 629.9
Hyperpnea (*see also* Hyperventilation)
      783.2
Hyperpotassemia 788.0
Hyperprebetalipoproteinemia
    familial 272.0
Hyperprolinemia 270.8
Hyperproteinemia 275.9
Hyperpyrexia 788.6
  heat (effects) 992.0
  malarial (*see also* Malaria) 084.9
  rheumatic - *see* Fever, rheumatic
  unknown origin (*see also* Pyrexia)
      788.6
Hyper-reactor vascular 782.5
Hyper-reflexia 780.3
Hypersalivation (*see also* Ptyalism)
      527.7
Hypersecretion
  gastric 536.0

Hypersecretion — *continued*
  gastric — *continued*
    psychogenic 305.5
  lachrymal, lacrimal glands 378.3
  meibomian glands 378.2
  milk 678
  upper respiratory 508.9
Hypersensitive, hypersensitiveness,
      hypersensitivity - *see also* Allergy
  carotid sinus 358.1
  colon 564.1
    psychogenic 305.5
  esophagus 530.9
  insect bites - *see* Injury, superficial
  pain (*see also* Disturbance, sensation)
      781.6
  reaction - *see* Allergy
  stomach (allergic) (nonallergic) 536.9
    psychogenic 305.5
Hypersomnia 306.4
Hypersplenia 289.4
Hypersplenism 289.4
Hypersuprarenalism 255.0
Hypersusceptibility - *see* Allergy
Hypertelorism 756.0
Hypertension, hypertensive (arterial)
      (arteriolar) (benign) (degeneration)
      (disease) (essential) (fluctuating)
      (idiopathic) (intermittent) (labile)
      (orthostatic) (paroxysmal) (primary)
      (vascular) 401
  with
    abortion - *see* Abortion, by type, with
        toxemia
    angina (cardiac) (pectoris) (vasomotor)
        (conditions in 413.9) 413.0
    cerebral
      embolism (conditions in 434.9)
          434.0
      hemorrhage (conditions in 431.9)
          431.0
      ischemia (conditions in 437.9)
          437.0
        transient (cOnditions in 435.9)
            435.0
      thrombosis (conditions in 433.9)
          433.0
    cerebrovascular disease (conditions
        in 438.9) 438.0
      acute (conditions in 436.9) 436.0
      ischemic (conditions in 437.9)
          437.0
    coronary insufficiency (acute)
        (conditions in 411.9) 411.0
      chronic 412.0

Hypertension, etc. — *continued*
  with — *continued*
    heart involvement (conditions in 427-429) (*see also* Hypertension, heart) 402
    hemorrhage
      brain (conditions in 431.9) 431.0
      subarachnoid (conditions in 430.9) 430.0
    ischemic heart disease (chronic) (conditions in 412.9) 412.0
      acute or with a stated duration of 8 weeks or less 410.0
      asymptomatic 414.0
    myocardial infarction (acute) (conditions in 410.9) 410.0
      chronic or with a stated duration of over 8 weeks 412.0
    occlusion of precerebral arteries (conditions in 432.9) 432.0
    renal sclerosis (conditions in 584) (*see also* Hypertension, kidney) 403
  arising during pregnancy (with pre-eclampsia) ·637.0
    with eclampsia 637.1
      fetus or newborn 762.2
    fetus or newborn 762.1
  cardiorenal (disease) 404
    with
      malignant hypertension (*see also* Hypertension, malignant with multiple organ involvement) 400.9
      malignant (*see also* Hypertension, malignant with multiple organ involvement) 400.9
  cardiovascular disease (arteriosclerotic) (malignant) (sclerotic) 412.0
  cardiovascular renal (disease) (sclerosis) (*see also* Hypertension, cardiorenal) 404
  cerebrovascular disease NEC 438.0
    malignant (*see also* Hypertension, malignant with cerebrovascular involvement) 400.2
  chronic maternal, affecting fetus or newborn 760.2
  Goldblatt's (*see also* Arteriosclerosis, renal, artery) 440.1
  heart (disease) 402
    with
      hypertension, kidney (conditions in 403) (*see also* Hypertension, cardiorenal) 404

Hypertension, etc. — *continued*
  heart (disease) — *continued*
    with — *continued*
      renal sclerosis (conditions in 584) (*see also* Hypertension, cardiorenal) 404
      malignant (*see also* Hypertension, malignant with heart involvement) 400.1
  intracranial 347.9
  kidney 403
    with
      heart involvement (conditions in 427-429) (*see also* Hypertension, cardiorenal) 404
      hypertension, heart (conditions in 402) (*see also* Hypertension, cardiorenal) 404
      malignant (*see also* Hypertension, malignant with renal involvement) 400.3
  lesser circulation 426
  malignant 400.0
    with
      angina (cardiac) (pectoris) (vasomotor) (conditions in 413.9) 413.0
      cardiorenal disease (conditions in 404) 400.9
      cardiovascular disease (arteriosclerotic) (sclerotic) 412.0
      cerebrovascular involvement (conditions in 430-438) 400.2
        with
          heart involvement (conditions in 400.1, 402, 427-429) 400.9
          renal involvement (conditions in 400.3, 403, 580-584, 593.2, 792) 400.9
      coronary insufficiency (acute) (conditions in 411.9) 411.0
        chronic 412.0
      heart involvement (conditions in 402, 427-429) 400.1
        with
          cerebrovascular involvement (conditions in 400.2, 430-438) 400.9
          renal involvement (conditions in 400.3, 403, 580-584, 593.2, 792) 400.9

Hypertension, etc. — *continued*
  malignant — *continued*
    with — *continued*
      ischemic heart disease (chronic)
          (conditions in 412.9)   412.0
        acute or with a stated duration of
            8 weeks or less   410.0
        asymptomatic   414.0
        multiple organ involvement (any
            combination of conditions in
            400.1, 400.2, and 400.3)
            400.9
        myocardial infarction (acute)
            (conditions in 410.9)   410.0
        chronic or with a stated duration
            of over 8 weeks   412.0
        renal involvement (conditions in
            403, 580-584, 593.2, 792)
            400.3
        with
          cerebrovascular involvement
              (conditions in 400.2,
              430-438)   400.9
          heart involvement (conditions
              in 400.1, 402, 427-429)
              400.9
  portal (due to cirrhosis) - *see* Cirrhosis,
      liver
  psychogenic   305.3
  pulmonary (artery)   426
  renal (*see also* Hypertension, kidney)
      403
  secondary NEC   401
Hyperthecosis ovary   256.9
Hyperthermia (of unknown origin) (*see
    also* Pyrexia)   788.6
Hyperthymergasia   296.1
  reactive (from emotional stress,
      psychological trauma)   298.1
Hyperthymism   254
Hyperthyroid (recurrent) - *see*
    Hyperthyroidism
Hyperthyroidism (recurrent) (latent) (pre-
    adult)   242.2
  with
    adenoma, thyroid (gland)   242.1
    goiter (diffuse)   242.0
      adenomatous   242.1
      nodular   242.1
Hypertonia - *see* Hypertonicity
Hypertonicity   780.4
  bladder   596.9
  fetus or newborn   778.9
  gastro-intestinal (tract)   536.1
  muscle   733.9
  stomach   536.1

Hypertonicity — *continued*
  stomach — *continued*
    psychogenic   305.5
Hypertony - *see* Hypertonicity
Hypertrichosis   704
  congenital   757.3
  lanuginosa   757.3
  acquired   704
Hypertriglyceridemia, essential   272.0
Hypertrophy, hypertrophic
  adenoids (and tonsils) (infectional)   500
  adrenal   255.9
  alveolar process or ridge   525.9
  anal papillae   569.2
  artery   447
    congenital NEC   747.6
  arthritis (chronic)   713.0
    spine   713.1
  asymmetrical (heart)   425
  auricular - *see* Hypertrophy, cardiac
  Bartholin's gland   629.9
  bile duct (*see also* Disease, gallbladder)
      576.9
  bladder (sphincter) (trigone)   596.9
  blind spot, visual field   377.4
  bone   723.9
  brain   347.9
  breast   611.1
    cystic   610
    fetus or newborn   778.9
    puerperal, postpartum   678
    senile (parenchymatous)   611.1
  cardiac (chronic) (idiopathic)   429.0
    with
      hypertension (benign) (conditions in
          401) (*see also* Hypertension,
          heart)   402
        malignant (*see also*
            Hypertension, malignant
            with heart involvement)
            400.1
      rheumatic fever (conditions in 390)
        active   391.9
        inactive or quiscent (with chorea)
            398
    congenital NEC   746.8
    fatty (*see also* Insufficiency,
        myocardial)   428
    rheumatic (with chorea)   398
      active or acute   391.9
        with chorea   392.0
    valve (*see also* Endocarditis)   424.9
      congenital   746.6
  cartilage (joint) (*see also* Disease, joint)
      729.9

Hypertrophy, hypertrophic — *continued*
cecum 569.9
cervix (uteri) 621.9
  congenital 752.5
ciliary body 378.6
clitoris (cirrhotic) 629.9
  congenital 752.6
colon 569.9
  congenital 751.2
conjunctiva, lymphoid 360
corpora cavernosa 607.9
duodenum 537.9
endometrium (uterus) 625.9
  cervix 621.9
epididymis 607.9
esophageal hiatus (congenital) 756.8
  with hernia - *see* Hernia, diaphragm
eyelid 378.2
falx, skull 723.9
fat pad
  infrapatellar 729.8
  knee 729.8
  popliteal 729.8
  prepatellar 729.8
  retropatellar 729.8
foot (congenital) 755.7
frenum (tongue) 529.9
  lip 528.5
gallbladder or duct (*see also* Disease,
    gallbladder) 576.9
gland, glandular (general) NEC 782.7
gum (mucous membrane) 523.9
heart (idiopathic) - *see also*
      Hypertrophy, cardiac
  valve - *see also* Endocarditis
    congenital 746.6
hepatic - *see* Hypertrophy, liver
hiatus (esophageal) (congenital) 756.8
  with hernia - *see* Hernia, diaphragm
hilus gland 782.7
hymen, congenital 752.6
ileum 569.9
infrapatellar fat pad 729.8
intestine 569.9
jejunum 569.9
kidney (compensatory) (*see also* Lesion,
    kidney) 593.2
  congenital 753.3
labium (majus) (minus) 629.9
ligament (articular) (*see also* Disease,
    joint) 729.9
lingual tonsil (infectional) 500
lip 528.5
  congenital 745.8
liver 785.1
  acute 573.9

Hypertrophy, hypertrophic — *continued*
liver — *continued*
  chronic - *see* Cirrhosis, liver
  cirrhotic - *see* Cirrhosis, liver
  congenital 751.6
  fatty - *see* Cirrhosis, portal
lymph, lymphatic gland 782.7
  tuberculous - *see* Tuberculosis, lymph
      gland
mammary gland - *see* Hypertrophy,
    breast
Meckel's diverticulum (congenital)
    751.0
median bar 600
mediastinum 519.9
meibomian gland 378.2
meniscus, knee, congenital 755.7
metatarsal head 723.9
metatarsus 723.9
mouth 528.9
mucous membrane
  alveolar process 523.9
  nose 508.9
  of turbinate 508.9
muscle 733.9
muscular coat, artery 447
myocardium (*see also* Hypertrophy,
    cardiac) 429.0
  idiopathic 425
myometrium 625.9
nail 703.9
  congenital 757.4
nasal 508.9
  alae 508.9
  bone 738.0
  cartilage 508.9
  mucous membrane (septum) 508.9
  sinus (*see also* Sinusitis) 503.9
nasopharynx, lymphoid (infectional)
    (tissue) (wall) 508.9
neck uterus 621.9
nipple 611.1
normal aperture diaphragm (congenital)
    756.8
  with hernia - *see* Hernia, diaphragm
nose 508.9
organ or site, congenital NEC - *see*
    Anomaly, specified type NEC
ovary 615.9
palate (hard) 526.9
  soft 528.9
papillae anal 569.2
parathyroid (gland) 252.0
parotid gland 527.1
penis 607.9
phallus 607.9

Hypertrophy, hypertrophic — *continued*
phallus — *continued*
   female 629.9
pharyngeal tonsil 500
pharynx 508.9
  lymphoid (infectional) (tissue) (wall)
    508.9
pituitary (fossa) (gland) 253.9
popliteal fat pad 729.8
prepuce (congenital) 605
  female 629.9
prostate (adenofibromatous)
    (asymptomatic) (benign) (early)
    (recurrent) 600
  congenital 752.8
pseudomuscular 330.3
pylorus (muscle) (sphincter) 537.0
  congenital 750.1
  infantile 750.1
rectal sphincter 569.2
rectum 569.2
rhinitis (turbinate) 502.1
salivary duct or gland 527.1
  congenital 750.8
scaphoid (tarsal) 723.9
scar 701.3
scrotum 607.9
sella turcica 253.9
seminal vesicle 607.9
sigmoid 569.9
spermatic cord 607.9
spleen - *see* Splenomegaly
spondylitis 713.1
stomach 537.9
sublingual gland 527.1
  congenital 750.8
submaxillary gland 527.1
suprarenal (gland) 255.9
tendon 733.9
testis 607.9
  congenital 752.8
thymic, thymus (gland) (congenital)
    254
thyroid (gland) (*see also* Goiter) 240.9
toe (congenital) 755.7
  acquired 738.7
tongue 529.9
  congenital 750.0
  papillae (foliate) 529.3
tonsils (and adenoids) (faucial)
    (infectional) (lingual) (lymphoid)
    (pharyngeal) 500
tunica vaginalis 607.9
ureter 593.5
urethra 599.9
uterus 625.9

Hypertrophy, hypertrophic — *continued*
uvula 528.9
vagina 629.9
vas deferens 607.9
vein 458.9
ventricle, ventricular (heart) - *see also*
    Hypertrophy, cardiac
  congenital 746.8
  right with ventricular septal defect,
    pulmonary stenosis or atresia,
    and dextraposition of aorta
    746.2
verumontanum 599.9
vocal cord 508.3
vulva 629.9
  stasis (nonfilarial) 629.9
Hypertropia (periodic) 373.2
Hyperuricemia 274
Hyperventilation (tetany) 783.2
  hysterical 300.1
  psychogenic 305.2
Hyperviscidosis 273.0
Hypervitaminosis (dietary) NEC 278.9
  A 278.0
  D 278.2
  from excessive administration or use of
    vitamin preparations 963.6
    vitamin K 964.3
Hypervolemia 289.0
Hypesthesia (*see also* Disturbance,
    sensation) 781.6
Hyphema - *see* Hyphemia
Hyphemia (anterior chamber) (aqueous)
    (choroid) (ciliary body) (iris) 378.6
  traumatic 921
Hypo-acidity gastric 536.0
  psychogenic 305.5
Hypo-adrenalism, hypo-adrenia 255.1
  tuberculous 017.9
    late effect or sequela 019.9
Hypoadrenocorticism 255.1
  pituitary 253.9
Hypoalbuminemia 275.9
Hypobarism 993.2
Hypobaropathy 993.2
Hypocalcemia 788.5
  dietary 269.9
Hypochloremia 788.0
Hypochlorhydria 536.0
  neurotic 305.5
  psychogenic 305.5
Hypocholesteremia 279
Hypochondria (reaction) 300.7
Hypochondriac 300.7
Hypochondriasis 300.7
Hypochromasia blood cells 280

Hypodontia (*see also* Anodontia) 520.0
Hypo-eosinophilia 289.9
Hypo-esthesia (*see also* Disturbance,
    sensation) 781.6
Hypofibrinogenemia (*see also* Defect,
    coagulation) 286.9
Hypofunction
  adrenal cortical 255.1
  cerebral 347.9
  intestinal 564.9
  ovary 256.1
  pituitary (gland) (anterior) 253.1
  testicular 257.1
Hypogammaglobulinemia 275.1
Hypogenitalism (male) (female)
  (congenital) 752.8
Hypoglycemia (spontaneous) 251
  with diabetes (mellitus) 250.9
  coma 251
  due to insulin (therapeutic
    misadventure) 962.3
  infantile 251
  leucine-induced 270.8
  reactive 251
Hypogonadism
  female 256.1
  male 257.1
  ovarian (primary) 256.1
  pituitary 253.9
  testicular (primary) 257.1
Hypohematosalpinx 615.9
Hypohidrosis 705.0
Hypoidrosis 705.0
Hypokalemia 788.0
Hypoleukia splenica 288
Hypoleukocytosis 289.9
Hypomania, hypomanic reaction 296.1
Hypomenorrhea 626.1
Hypometabolism 788.9
Hypomotility
  gastro-intestinal tract 536.1
    psychogenic 305.5
  intestine 564.9
    psychogenic 305.5
  stomach 536.1
    psychogenic 305.5
Hyponatremia 788.0
Hypo-ovarianism 256.1
Hypo-ovarism 256.1
Hypoparathyroidism 252.1
Hypopharyngitis 462
Hypophoria 373.2
Hypophosphatasia 273.4
Hypophosphatemia (acquired)
  (nonfamilial) 279
  congenital 273.4

Hypophosphatemia—*continued*
  familial 273.4
  renal 273.4
Hypophyseal, hypophysis - *see also*
  condition
  dwarfism 253.1
  gigantism 253.0
Hypopiesis 458.0
Hypopinealism 258.9
Hypopituitarism (juvenile) 253.1
  postpartum hemorrhage 253.1
  von Bergmann's 253.1
Hypoplasia, hypoplasis 758.8
  adrenal (gland) 758.1
  alimentary tract 751.8
    lower 751.4
    upper 750.8
  anus, anal (canal) 751.3
  aorta, aortic 747.2
    arch (tubular) 747.1
  appendix 751.4
  areola 757.2
  arm 755.2
  artery (peripheral) 747.6
    brain 747.8
    coronary 746.8
    pulmonary 747.3
    retinal 744.8
    umbilical 747.5
  auditory canal 745.2
    causing impairment of hearing 745.0
  biliary duct or passage 751.5
  bone NEC 756.9
    face 756.0
    mandible 524.0
    marrow 284
    maxilla 524.0
    skull (*see also* Hypoplasia, skull)
      756.0
  brain 743.1
    gyri 743.2
    specified part 743.2
  breast (areola) 757.2
  bronchus 748.3
  cardiac 746.8
    valve (any) 746.6
  carpus 755.2
  cartilaginous 756.9
  cecum 751.4
  cementum 520.4
  cephalic 743.1
  cerebellum 743.2
  cervix (uteri) 752.5
  clavicle 755.5
  coccyx 756.2

Hypoplasia, hypoplasis — *continued*
  colon 751.4
  corpus callosum 743.2
  cricoid cartilage 748.3
  digestive organ(s) or tract NEC 751.8
    lower 751.4
    upper 750.8
  ear (auricle) (lobe) 745.2
    middle 745.0
  enamel of teeth 520.4
  endocrine (gland) NEC 758.3
  endometrium 625.9
  epididymis 752.8
  epiglottis 748.3
  erythroid, congenital 284
  esophagus 750.3
  eustachian tube 745.2
  eye 744.1
    lid 744.8
  face 745.8
    bone(s) 756.0
  fallopian tube 752.5
  femur 755.3
  fibula 755.3
  finger 755.2
  foot 755.3
  gallbladder 751.6
  genitalia, genital organ(s)
    female 752.8
      external 752.6
      internal NEC 752.5
    in adiposogenital dystrophy 253.1
    male 752.8
  glottis 748.3
  hair 757.3
  hand 755.2
  heart 746.8
    valve (any) 746.6
  humerus 755.2
  hymen 752.6
  intestine (large) (small) 751.4
  iris 744.5
  jaw 524.0
  kidney(s) 753.0
  labium (majus) (minus) 752.6
  labyrinth, membranous 745.0
  larynx 748.3
  leg 755.3
  limb 755.4
    lower 755.3
    upper 755.2
  liver 751.6
  lung (lobe) 748.6
  mammary (areola) 757.2
  mandible 524.0
  mandibular 524.0

Hypoplasia, hypoplasis — *continued*
  maxillary 524.0
  metacarpus 755.2
  metatarsus 755.3
  muscle 756.8
    eye 744.8
  nail(s) 757.4
  nervous system NEC 743.8
  neural 743.8
  nose, nasal 748.1
  ophthalmic 744.1
  organ
    of Corti 745.0
    or site not listed - *see* Anomaly,
          specified type NEC
  osseous meatus (ear) 745.2
  ovary 752.5
  oviduct 752.5
  pancreas 751.7
  parathyroid (gland) 758.3
  parotid gland 750.8
  patella 755.7
  pelvis, pelvic girdle 755.7
  penis 752.8
  peripheral vascular system 747.6
  pituitary (gland) 758.3
  pulmonary 748.6
    artery 747.3
    valve 746.6
  radio-ulnar 755.2
  radius 755.2
  rectum 751.3
  respiratory system NEC 748.9
  rib 756.4
  sacrum 756.1
  scapula 755.5
  shoulder girdle 755.5
  skin 757.2
  skull (bone) 756.0
    with
      anencephalus 740
      encephalocele 743.0
      hydrocephalus 742
        with spina bifida 741.0
      microcephalus 743.1
  spinal (cord) (ventral horn cell) 743.3
    vessel 747.6
  spine 756.2
  spleen 758.0
  sternum 756.4
  tarsus 755.3
  testis, testicle 752.8
  thymus (gland) 758.3
  thyroid (gland) 243
    cartilage 748.3
  tibio-fibular 755.3

Hypoplasia, hypoplasis — *continued*
  toe 755.3
  tongue 750.0
  trachea (cartilage) (rings) 748.3
  Turner's 520.4
  ulna 755.2
  umbilical artery 747.5
  ureter 753.2
  uterus 752.5
  vagina 752.6
  vascular NEC 747.6
    brain 747.8
  vein(s) (peripheral) 747.6
    brain 747.8
    great 747.4
    portal 747.4
    pulmonary 747.4
  vena cava (inferior) (superior) 747.4
  vertebra 756.2
  vulva 752.6
  zonule (ciliary) 744.8
Hypopotassemia 788.0
Hypoproconvertinemia, congenital (*see
    also* Defect, coagulation) 286.9
Hypoproteinemia 275.9
Hypoproteinosis 267
Hypoprothrombinemia (congenital)
    (idiopathic) (*see also* Defect,
    coagulation) 286.9
  newborn 778.2
Hypopyon (eye) (anterior chamber) 366
  iritis 364
  ulcer (cornea) 363.0
Hypopyrexia 788.9
Hyporeflex 780.3
Hyposecretion
  ACTH 253.1
  ovary 256.1
Hyposiderinemia 280
Hyposomnia 306.4
Hypospadias (male) 752.2
  female 753.8
Hypospermatogenesis 606
Hypostasis pulmonary 514
Hypostatic - *see* condition
Hyposthenuria (*see also* Lesion, kidney)
    593.2

Hyposuprarenalism 255.1
Hypotension (arterial) (constitutional)
    (orthostatic) (permanent idiopathic)
    (postural) 458.0
Hypothermia 788.9
Hypothymergasia 296.2
Hypothyroidism (acquired) 244
  congenital 243
Hypotonia, hypotonicity, hypotony
    780.4
  bladder 596.9
  congenital 778.9
  eye 378.9
  following loss of aqueous or vitreous
    378.9
  muscle 733.9
Hypotrichosis 704
  congenital 757.3
  lid, congenital 757.3
  postinfectional NEC 704
Hypotropia 373.2
Hypoventilation 783.2
Hypovitaminosis (*see also* Deficiency,
    vitamin) 266.9
Hypovolemia 782.9
  surgical shock 998.0
  traumatic (shock) 995.5
Hypoxia - *see also* Anoxia
  myocardial (*see also* Insufficiency,
    coronary) 411.9
  newborn (*see also* Asphyxia, newborn)
    776.9
Hypsarhythmia 345.1
Hysteralgia, pregnant uterus 634.9
Hysterectomy
  fetus or newborn (*see also* Birth injury
    NEC) 772.9
Hysteria, hysterical (conversion)
    (dissociative state) (any
    manifestation) 300.1
  anxiety 300.0
  psychosis, acute 298.1
Hystero-epilepsy 300.1
Hysteromyoma 218
Hysterotomy
  fetus or newborn (*see also* Birth injury
    NEC) 772.9

I

Ichthyosis (congenita) 757.2
 acquired 701.1
 fetalis gravior 757.2
 follicularis 757.2
 hystrix 757.2
 palmaris and plantaris 757.2
 simplex 757.2
 vera 757.2
Ichthyotoxism 988.0
 bacterial (*see also* Poisoning, food)
  005.9
Ictero-anemia, hemolytic (acquired)
  283.9
 congenital (*see also* Sperocytosis)
  282.0
Icterus (*see also* Jaundice) 785.2
 catarrhal 070
 conjunctiva 785.2
  fetus or newborn 778.9
 encephalomyelopathy (*see also* Disease,
  hemolytic, by type, with
  kernicterus) 774.9
 epidemic - *see* Icterus, infectious
 febrilis - *see* Icterus, infectious
 fetus or newborn NEC 778.9
 gravis (*see also* Necrosis, liver) 570
  fetus or newborn (*see also* Disease,
   hemolytic) 775.9
 hematogenous (acquired) 283.9
  fetus or newborn (*see also* Disease,
   hemolytic) 775.9
 hemolytic (acquired) 283.9
  congenital (*see also* Spherocytosis)
   282.0
  fetus or newborn (*see also* Disease,
   hemolytic) 775.9
 hemorrhagic (acute) 100.0
  leptospiral 100.0
  newborn 778.2
  spirochetal 100.0
 infectious 070
  leptospiral 100.0
  spirochetal 100.0
 intermittens juvenilis 273.5
 malignant (*see also* Necrosis, liver)
  570
 pernicious (*see also* Necrosis, liver)
  570
 praecox (*see also* Disease, hemolytic)
  775.9
 spirochetal 100.0
Ictus solaris, solis 992.0

Id reaction (due to bacteria) 692.9
Idioglossia 306.0
Idiopathic - *see* condition
Idiosyncrasy
 food (*see also* Allergy, food) 692.5
 to substances - *see* Allergy
Idiot, idiocy (congenital) - *see also*
  Retardation, mental, profound
 amaurotic (Bielschowsky(-Jansky))
  (family) (infantile (late)) (juvenile
  (late)) (Vogt-Spielmeyer) 333.0
Ileitis - *see also* Enteritis
 regional (ulcerative) 563.0
 terminal (ulcerative) 563.0
Ileocolitis - *see* Enteritis
Ileotyphus 001
Ileum - *see* condition
Ileus (adynamic) (bowel) (colon)
  (inhibitory) (intestine) (neurogenic)
  (paralytic) 560.1
 with hernia - *see* Hernia, by site, with
  obstruction
 arteriomesenteric duodenal 537.9
 due to gallstone (in intestine) 560.3
 duodenal, chronic 537.9
 mechanical 560.9
 meconium 273.0
Iliac - *see* condition
Illness - *see also* Disease
 manic-depressive (*see also* Psychosis,
  manic-depressive) 296.9
Illusions 306.9
Imbalance 780.4
 autonomic 358.9
 electrolyte 788.0
 endocrine 258.9
 eye muscle 373.9
  cyclophoria 373.9
  esophoria 373.0
  exophoria 373.1
  hyperphoria 373.2
 hormone 258.9
 hysterical 300.1
 labyrinth 385
 posture 733.9
 sympathetic 358.9
Imbecile, imbecility
 moral 301.7
 old age 290.0
 senile 290.0
 specified I.Q. - *see* I.Q.

Imbecile, imbecility — *continued*
  unspecified I.Q. - *see* Retardation,
    mental, severe
Imbibition, cholesterol (gallbladder) (*see
    also* Disease, gallbladder) 576.9

Immature - *see also* Immaturity
  personality 301.8

Immaturity 777
  for classification of births in hospital -
    see Newborn
  lung, fetus or newborn (*see also*
    Syndrome, respiratory distress)
    776.2
  organ or site NEC - *see* Hypoplasia
  reaction 301.8
  sexual (female) (male) 258.9

Immersion 994.1
  foot 991.4
  hand 991.4

Immobile, immobility
  intestine 569.9
  joint - *see* Ankylosis

Immunization
  complication - *see* Complications,
    vaccination
  to Rh factor
    from transfusion 999.7
    noted during pregnancy 634.5
      fetus 775.0
      newborn 775.0
        with kernicterus or nervous
          affection 774.0

Impaction, impacted
  bowel, colon, rectum (fecal) 560.3
    with hernia - *see* Hernia, by site, with
      obstruction
  calculus - *see* Calculus
  cerumen (ear) (external) 387.1
  cuspid 520.6
    with abnormal position (same or
      adjacent tooth) 524.3
  dental 520.6
    with abnormal position (same or
      adjacent tooth) 524.3
  fecal, feces 560.3
    with hernia - *see* Hernia, by site, with
      obstruction
  fracture - code as Fracture, closed
  gallbladder (*see also* Cholelithiasis)
    574.9
  gallstone(s) (*see also* Cholelithiasis)
    574.9
  in intestine (any part) 560.3
    with hernia - *see* Hernia, by site,
      with obstruction

Impaction, impacted — *continued*
  intestine (calculous) (fecal) (gallstone)
    560.3
    with hernia - *see* Hernia, by site, with
      obstruction
  molar 520.6
    with abnormal position (same or
      adjacent tooth) 524.3
  tooth, teeth 520.6
    with abnormal position (same or
      adjacent tooth) 524.3
  turbinate 723.9

Impaired, impairment (function)
  hearing - *see* Deafness, partial
  heart - *see* Disease, heart
  kidney (*see also* Lesion, kidney) 593.2
  liver 573.9
  mastication 524.9
  myocardium, myocardial (*see also*
    Insufficiency, myocardial) 428
  rectal sphincter 569.2
  renal (*see also* Lesion, kidney) 593.2
  vision NEC 378.9

Impaludism - *see* Malaria
Impediment, speech NEC 306.0
  secondary to organic lesion 781.5
Imperception auditory (acquired)
  (congenital) (*see also* Deafness)
    389.9

Imperfect
  aeration, lung (newborn) (*see also*
    Asphyxia, newborn) 776.9
  closure (congenital)
    alimentary tract NEC 751.8
      lower 751.4
      upper 750.8
    atrioventricular ostium 746.5
    branchial cleft or sinus 745.4
    choroid 744.4
    cricoid cartilage 748.3
    cusps, heart valve (any) 746.6
    ductus
      arteriosus 747.0
      botalli 747.0
    ear drum 745.2
    epiglottis 748.3
    esophagus with communication to
      bronchus or trachea 750.2
    eustachian valve 746.8
    eyelid 744.4
    foramen
      botalli 746.4
      ovale 746.4
    genitalia, genital organ(s) or system
      female 752.8
        external 752.6
        internal NEC 752.5

Imperfect—*continued*
  closure, etc.—*continued*
    genitalia, etc.—*continued*
      male 752.8
    glottis 748.3
    interatrial ostium or septum 746.4
    interauricular ostium or septum
      746.4
    interventricular ostium or septum
      746.3
    iris 744.4
    kidney 753.3
    larynx 748.3
    lens 744.4
    lip 749.1
      with cleft palate 749.2
    nasal septum or sinus 748.1
    nose 748.1
    omphalomesenteric duct 751.0
    optic nerve entry 744.4
    organ or site not listed - *see*
      Anomaly, specified type NEC
    palate 749.0
      with cleft lip 749.2
    preauricular sinus 745.4
    retina 744.4
    roof of orbit 743.0
    sclera 744.4
    septum
      aortic 746.0
      aorticopulmonary 746.0
      atrial 746.4
      between aorta and pulmonary
        artery 746.0
      heart 746.8
      interatrial 746.4
      interauricular 746.4
      interventricular 746.3
        with pulmonary stenosis or
          atresia, dextraposition of
          aorta, and hypertrophy of
          right ventricle 746.2
      nasal 748.1
      ventricular 746.3
        with pulmonary stenosis or
          atresia, dextraposition of
          aorta, and hypertrophy of
          right ventricle 746.2
    skull 756.0
      with
        anencephalus 740
        encephalocele 743.0
        hydrocephalus 742
          with spina bifida 741.0
        microcephalus 743.1
    spine (with meningocele) 741.9
      with hydrocephalus 741.0

Imperfect—*continued*
  closure, etc.—*continued*
    thyroid cartilage 748.3
    trachea 748.3
    tympanic membrane 745.2
    uterus (with communication to
      bladder, intestine or rectum)
      752.5
    uvula 749.0
      with cleft lip 749.2
    vitelline duct 751.0
  erection 607.9
  fusion - *see* Imperfect closure
  inflation, lung (newborn) (*see also*
    Asphyxia, newborn) 776.9
  intestinal canal 751.4
  poise 733.9
  rotation - *see* Malrotation
  septum
    ventricular 746.3

Imperfectly descended testis 752.1

Imperforate (congenital) - *see also* Atresia
  anus 751.3
  cervix (uteri) 752.5
  esophagus 750.3
  hymen 752.6
  jejunum 751.4
  pharynx 750.8
  rectum 751.3
  urethra 753.6
  vagina 752.6

Impervious (congenital) - *see also* Atresia
  anus 751.3
  bile duct 751.5
  esophagus 750.3
  intestine (large) (small) 751.4
  rectum 751.3
  ureter 753.2
  urethra 753.6

Impetigo (any organism) (any site)
    (bullous) (circinate) (contagiosa)
    (neonatorum) (simplex) 684
  Bockhart's 684
  Fox's 684
  furfuracea 696.5
  herpetiformis 693
  staphylococcal infection 684
  ulcerative 686.9
  vulgaris 684

Implant
  endometrial (any site) 625.3

Implantation
  anomalous - *see also* Anomaly,
    specified type NEC
    ureter 753.4

Implantation — *continued*
  cyst
    external area or site (skin) NEC
      709.9
    iris 378.6
    vagina or vulva 629.9
  dermoid (cyst)
    external area or site (skin) NEC
      709.9
    iris 378.6
    vagina or vulva 629.9
  placenta, low or marginal - *see* Placenta
    previa
Impotence (sexual) (psychogenic) 305.6
  organic origin NEC 607.9
Impoverished blood 285.9
Impression
  basilar 756.0
Improper
  care (child) (newborn) 994.9
  food 269.9
Improperly tied umbilical cord 778.9
Impulses, obsessional 300.3
Impulsive neurosis 300.3
Inaction, kidney (*see also* Lesion, kidney)
  593.2
Inactive - *see* condition
Inadequate, inadequacy
  biologic, constitutional, functional, or
    social 301.6
  cardiac and renal (*see also*
    Hypertension, cardiorenal) 404
  development 778.9
    genitalia
      after puberty NEC 258.9
      congenital - *see* Hypoplasia,
        genitalia
    lungs 748.6
    organ or site not listed - *see*
      Hypoplasia
  dietary 269.9
  mental (*see also* Retardation, mental)
    315.9
  nervous system 790.0
  personality 301.6
  pulmonary
    function 783.2
      newborn (*see also* Asphyxia,
        newborn) 776.9
    ventilation (newborn) (*see also*
      Asphyxia, newborn) 776.9
  respiration 783.2
    newborn (*see also* Asphyxia,
      newborn) 776.9
Inanition 269.9
  with edema 269.9

Inanition — *continued*
  due to
    deprivation of food 994.2
    malnutrition 269.9
  fever 788.6
Inattention after or at birth 994.9
Incarceration, incarcerated
  bubonocele 552
  colon (by hernia) - *see* Hernia, by site,
    with obstruction
  enterocele 553.9
  epigastrocele 553.2
  epiplocele 553.9
  exomphalos 553.1
  hernia - *see* Hernia, by site, with
    obstruction
  iris 378.6
  lens 378.8
  merocele 553.0
  omentocele 553.9
  omentum (by hernia) - *see* Hernia, by
    site, with obstruction
  omphalocele 553.1
  rupture (meaning hernia) (*see also*
    Hernia, by site, with obstruction)
    553.9
  sarco-epiplocele 553.9
  sarco-epiplomphocele 553.1
  uterus 625.9
    gravid (undelivered) 634.9
Incident
  cerebrovascular (*see also* Disease,
    cerebrovascular, acute) 436.9
Incineration (entire body) (from fire or
    conflagration) 948.3
  electricity, electric current 994.8
  lightning 994.0
Incised wound
  external - *see* Wound, open
  internal organs (abdomen, chest or
    pelvis) - *see* Injury, internal, by
    site, with open wound
Incision, incisional
  hernia - *see* Hernia, incisional
  surgical, complication - *see*
    Complications, surgical
    procedure
  traumatic
    external - *see* Wound, open
    internal organs (abdomen, chest or
      pelvis) - *see* Injury, internal, by
      site, with open wound
Inclusion
  cyst - *see* Cyst, inclusion
  gallbladder in liver (congenital) 751.6
  iris 378.6

Incompatibility
  ABO
    fetus 775.1
    infusion or transfusion reaction
      999.6
    newborn 775.1
      with kernicterus or nervous
        affection 774.1
    blood (group) (M, N, P) NEC
    fetus 775.2
    infusion or transfusion reaction
      999.6
    newborn 775.2
      with kernicterus or nervous
        affection 774.2
    Rh (blood group) (factor)
    fetus 775.0
    infusion or transfusion reaction
      999.7
    newborn 775.0
      with kernicterus or nervous
        affection 774.0
    noted during pregnancy 634.5
    due to infusion or transfusion
      634.5
    rhesus - *see* Incompatibility, Rh
Incompetency, incompetent
  annular
    aortic (valve) (*see also* Endocarditis,
      aortic) 395.9
    mitral (valve) (*see also* Endocarditis,
      mitral) 394.9
    pulmonary valve (heart) (*see also*
      Endocarditis, pulmonary)
      424.9
  aortic (valve) (*see also* Endocarditis,
    aortic) 395.9
  cardiac (orifice) 530.0
    valve - *see* Endocarditis
  cervix, cervical (os) 621.9
    causing abortion - *see* Abortion,
      spontaneous
    complicating pregnancy 634.9
    fetus or newborn 769.0
  mitral (valve) - *see* Endocarditis, mitral
  pulmonary valve (heart) (*see also*
    Endocarditis, pulmonary) 424.9
  tricuspid (annular) (valve) (*see also*
    Endocarditis, tricuspid) 397.0
  valvular - *see* Endocarditis
Incomplete - *see also* condition
  expansion lungs (newborn) (*see also*
    Asphyxia, newborn) 776.9
  rotation - *see* Malrotation
Incontinence 786.2
  anal sphincter 785.6

Incontinence — *continued*
  feces 785.6
    due to hysteria 300.1
    nonorganic origin 306.7
  hysterical 300.1
  stress 786.2
  urethral sphincter 786.2
  urine (stress) 786.2
    neurogenic 786.2
    nonorganic origin 306.6
Incontinentia pigmenti 757.2
Incoordinate
  uterus, complicating delivery 657.9
    fetus or newborn - *see* categories
      767.0-767.9
Incoordination, muscular 780.4
Increase, increased
  abnormal, in development 279
  cold sense (*see also* Disturbance,
    sensation) 781.6
  estrogen 256.0
  function
    adrenal (cortex) 255.0
      medulla 255.2
    pituitary (gland) (anterior) (lobe)
      253.0
  heat sense (*see also* Disturbance,
    sensation) 781.6
  intracranial pressure 347.9
  permeability
    capillaries 448
  sphericity, lens 744.8
  splenic activity 289.4
  venous pressure 458.9
Incrustation, cornea, lead or zinc 930
Incyclophoria 373.0
Incyclotropia 373.0
Indeterminate sex 752.0
India rubber skin 757.2
Indigestion (bilious) (functional) 536.9
  acid 536.0
  catarrhal 535
  due to decomposed food NEC 005.9
  fat 269.0
  nervous 305.5
  psychogenic 305.5
Indirect - *see* condition
Induced
  abortion - *see* Abortion, induced
  birth
    fetus or newborn (*see also* Birth
      injury NEC) 772.9
    mother - *see* Delivery
Induration, indurated
  brain 340
  breast (fibrous) 611.9
    puerperal, postpartum 678

Induration, indurated — *continued*
  broad ligament 616.9
  corpora cavernosa (penis) (plastic)
      607.9
  liver (chronic) - *see also* Cirrhosis, liver
    acute 573.9
    cyanotic - *see* Cirrhosis, cardiac
  lung (black) (brown) (chronic) (fibroid)
      (*see also* Fibrosis, lung) 517
    essential 279
  penile 607.9
  phlebitic - *see* Phlebitis
  stomach 537.9
Inebriety 303.9
Inefficiency, kidney (*see also* Lesion,
    kidney) 593.2
Inequality, leg (length) (acquired) 738.5
  congenital 755.3
Inertia
  bladder 596.9
    due to nervous system lesion 596.9
  stomach 536.1
    psychogenic 305.5
  uterus, uterine (hypertonic) (hypotonic)
    (intrapartum)
    complicating delivery 657.1
      fetus or newborn - *see* categories
        767.0-767.9
  vesical 596.9
    due to nervous system lesion 596.9
Infancy, infantile *see also* condition
  genitalia, genitals 258.9
    complicating delivery 657.9
      fetus or newborn - *see* categories
        764.0-764.9
    noted during pregnancy (undelivered)
      634.9
  heart 746.9
  kidney 753.3
  lack of care 994.9
  os, uterus (*see also* Infantile genitalia)
    258.9
  pelvis 738.8
    complicating delivery - *see*
        Deformity, pelvis, complicating
        delivery
    noted during pregnancy (undelivered)
      634.9
  penis 258.9
  testicle 257.1
  uterus (*see also* Infantile genitalia)
    258.9
  vulva 752.6
Infant - *see also* Infancy
  for classification of births in hospital
    see Newborn

Infantilism (with dwarfism) 258.9
  Brissaud's 244
  celiac 269.0
  intestinal 269.0
  pancreatic 577.9
  pituitary 253.1
  renal 593.0
  sex (with obesity) 258.9
Infarct, infarction
  adrenal (capsule) (gland) 255.9
  amnion - *see* Infarct, placenta
  anterior NEC (*see also* Infarct,
    myocardium) 410.9
  appendices epiploicae - *see* Infarct,
    mesentery
  bowel - *see* Infarct, intestine
  brain (thrombotic) (*see also*
    Thrombosis, brain) 433.9
    embolic (*see also* Embolism, brain)
      434.9
  breast 611.9
  cardiac (*see also* Infarct, myocardium)
    410.9
  cerebellar (thrombotic) (*see also*
    Thrombosis, brain) 433.9
    embolic (*see also* Embolism, brain)
      434.9
  cerebral (hemorrhagic) (thrombotic) (*see*
    also Thrombosis, brain) 433.9
    embolic (*see also* Embolism, brain)
      434.9
  chorion - *see* Infarct, placenta
  colon (embolic) (thrombotic) (with
    gangrene) 444.2
  coronary artery (*see also* Infarct,
    myocardium) 410.9
  embolic (*see also* Embolism) 444.9
  fallopian tube 615.9
  heart (*see also* Infarct, myocardium)
    410.9
  hypophysis (anterior lobe) 253.1
  intestine (embolic) (thrombotic) (with
    gangrene) 444.2
  kidney - *see* Infarct, renal
  liver 573.9
  lung (embolic) (thrombotic) 450
    with
      abortion - *see* Abortion, by type,
        with sepsis
      ectopic gestation - *see* categories
        631.0-631.3
      complicating pregnancy 634.9
      puerperal, postpartum, childbirth
        673.9
  lymph node 457
  meibomian gland (eyelid) 378.2

Infarct, infarction — *continued*
  mesentery, mesenteric (embolic)
      (thrombotic) (with gangrene)
      444.2
  myocardium, myocardial (acute or with
      a stated duration of 8 weeks or
      less)   410.9
    with hypertensive disease (conditions
        in 400-404)   410.0
    chronic or with a stated duration of
        over 8 weeks   412.9
      with hypertensive disease
          (conditions in 400-404)
          412.0
    healed or old - *see* Infarct,
        myocardium, chronic
    repeat during current hospitalization
        410.1
    syphilitic   093.9
  omentum - *see* Infarct, mesentery
  ovary   615.9
  papillary muscle - *see* Infarct,
      myocardium
  pituitary (gland)   253.1
  placenta (complicating pregnancy)
      634.1
    causing complicated delivery   661.8
    fetus or newborn   770.2
  posterior NEC (*see also* Infarct,
      myocardium)   410.9
  prostate   602
  pulmonary (artery) (vein) (hemorrhagic)
      450
    with
      abortion - *see* Abortion, by type,
          with sepsis
      ectopic gestation - *see* categories
          631.0-631.3
      complicating pregnancy   634.9
      puerperal, postpartum, childbirth
          673.9
  renal (*see also* Lesion, kidney)   593.2
    embolic or thrombotic   444.3
  retina, retinal (artery)   377.0
  spleen   289.5
    embolic or thrombotic   444.9
  subchorionic - *see* Infarct, placenta
  subendocardial (*see also* Insufficiency,
      coronary)   411.9
  suprarenal (capsule) (gland)   255.9
  syncytium - *see* Infarct, placenta
  thrombotic (*see also* Thrombosis)   453
    artery, arterial - *see* Embolism
  ventricle (heart) (*see also* Infarct,
      myocardium)   410.9
Infecting - *see* condition

Infection, infected   136
  with lymphangitis - *see* Lymphangitis
  abortion - *see* Abortion, by type, with
      sepsis
  abscess (skin) - *code by* site under
      Abscess
  Acanthocheilonema
    perstans   125.4
    streptocera   125.8
  accessory sinus (chronic) (*see also*
      Sinusitis)   503.9
  achorion - *see* Dermatophytosis
  acromioclavicular   729.2
  Actinomyces   113
    israeli   113
    muris-ratti   026.1
  adenoid (and tonsil) (chronic)   500
  adenovirus NEC   079.9
  aerogenes capsulatus (*see also* Gas
      gangrene)   039.0
  aertrycke   003.9
    due to food   003.0
  alimentary canal NEC   009.9
  alveolus, alveolar (process)   522.4
  ameba, amebic (histolytica)   006.9
    with liver abscess   006.0
    coli   006.9
      with liver abscess   006.0
    gingivalis   006.9
      with liver abscess   006.0
  amniotic fluid
    causing complicated delivery   661.8
    complicating pregnancy (delivered)
        (undelivered)   634.9
    fetus or newborn   763.9
  anal canal   569.2
  anthrax   022
  antrum (chronic) (*see also* Sinusitis,
      antrum)   503.0
  anus (papillae) (sphincter)   569.2
  arbor virus, arbovirus NEC   068.9
  argentophil-rod   027.0
  arising during pregnancy NEC   634.9
    fetus or newborn   763.9
  Ascaris lumbricoides   127.0
  Aspergillus (fumigatus)   117.3
  atypical
    acid-fast (bacilli) (pulmonary)   031.0
      nonpulmonary   031.9
    mycobacteria (pulmonary)   031.0
      nonpulmonary   031.9
  auditory meatus (circumscribed)
      (diffuse) (external)   380
  auricle (ear)   380
  axillary gland   683

Infection, infected — *continued*
Bacillus 039.9
abortus 023.1
anthracis 022
coli - *see* Infection. Escherichia coli
coliform NEC 039.9
Ducrey's (any location) 099.0
Flexner's 004.1
Friedlander's NEC 039.9
fusiformis 101
gas (gangrene) (*see also* Gas
gangrene) 039.0
mallei 024
melitensis 023.0
paratyphoid, paratyphosus 002.9
A 002.0
B 002.1
C 002.2
Shiga 004.0
suipestifer 003.9
due to food 003.0
swimming pool 031.9
typhosa 001
welchii (*see also* Gas gangrene)
039.0
bacterial NEC 039.9
Bacterium
paratyphosum 002.9
A 002.0
B 002.1
C 002.2
typhosum 001
Bacteroides 039.9
Bartholin's gland (*see also* Vaginitis)
622.1
bile duct (*see also* Cholecystitis) 575
bladder (*see also* Cystitis) 595
Blastomyces, blastomycotic 116.9
brasiliensis 116.2
dermatitidis 116.1
European 116.0
North American 116.1
South American 116.2
blood stream - *see* Septicemia
bone - *see* Osteomyelitis
brain 323
late effects 324
membranes - *see* Meningitis
septic 322
late effects 324
meninges - *see* Meningitis
branchial cyst 745.4
breast 611.0
puerperal, postpartum 678
bronchus (*see also* Bronchitis) 490
fungus NEC 117.9

Infection, infected — *continued*
Brucella 023.9
abortus 023.1
melitensis 023.0
suis 023.2
Brugia malayi 125.1
bursa - *see* Bursitis
buttocks (skin) 686.9
Candida albicans (any site) 112
cartilage (joint) (*see also* Disease, joint)
729.9
cat liver fluke 121.0
cellulitis - *code by* site under Cellulitis
Cercomonas hominis (intestinal) 007.9
cerebellar artery 323
late effects 324
cerebrospinal (*see also* Encephalitis)
323
late effects 324
cervical gland 683
cervix (*see also* Cervicitis) 620.9
Chilomastix (intestinal) 007.9
Cladosporium
mansonii 111.1
werneckii 111.1
Clonorchis (sinensis) (liver) 121.1
Clostridium
botulinus 005.1
perfringens (*see also* Gas gangrene)
039.0
due to food 005.2
welchii (*see also* Gas gangrene)
039.0
due to food 005.2
colon (*see also* Enteritis) 009.2
bacillus - *see* Infection, Escherichia
coli
common duct (*see also* Cholecystitis)
575
congenital NEC 136
corpus luteum (*see also* Salpingo-
oophoritis) 614
Coxsackie NEC (*see also* Coxsackie)
079.9
meninges 045.0
myocardium 074.2
pericardium 074.2
pharynx 074.0
specified disease NEC 074.9
Cryptococcus neoformans 116.0
cyst - *see* Cyst
Cysticercus cellulosae 123.1
dental 522.4
diabetic - *see* category 250
diphtherial 032
Diphyllobothrium (latum) 123.4

Infection, infected—*continued*
  Gnathostoma (spinegerum) 128.8
  Gongylonema 125.8
  gonococcal NEC (*see also* Gonococcus)
      098.9
  gram-negative bacilli NEC 039.9
  guinea worm 125.8
  gum 523.1
  heart - *see* Disease, heart
  helminths NEC 128.9
    intestinal 127.9
      mixed (types classifiable to more
          than one of the titles 120-
          127.4) 127.5
  Hemophilus influenzae NEC 039.9
  Heterophyes 121.9
  Histoplasma capsulatum 115
  hookworm (*see also* Ancylostomiasis)
      126.9
  Hymenolepis 123.6
  hypopharynx 508.9
  inguinal glands 683
    due to soft chancre 099.0
  intestine, intestinal (*see also* Enteritis)
      009.2
  intrauterine
    fetus or newborn NEC 763.9
  jaw (bone) (lower) (upper) 526.4
  joint - *see* Arthritis, infectious or
      infective
  kidney (cortex) (hematogenous) 590.9
    with
      abortion - *see* Abortion, by type,
          with sepsis
      calculus 592
      ectopic gestation - *see* categories
          631.0-631.3
      arising during pregnancy 635.0
      fetus or newborn 763.0
      puerperal, postpartum 635.0
  knee (skin) NEC 686.9
    joint - *see* Arthritis, infectious or
        infective
  Koch's (*see also* Tuberculosis,
      pulmonary) 011.9
  labia (majora) (minora) (*see also*
      Vulvitis) 622.1
  lachrymal, lacrimal (apparatus) (glands)
      368
  larynx NEC 508.3
  leg (skin) NEC 686.9
  Leishmania 085.9
    braziliensis 085.2
    donovani 085.0
    furunculosa 085.1

Infection, infected—*continued*
  Leishmania—*continued*
    infantum 085.0
    tropica 085.1
  leptospirochetal NEC (*see also*
      Leptospirosis) 100.9
  Leptothrix 117.9
  Listeria
    monocytogenes 027.0
  Loa loa 125.2
  local, skin (staphylococcal)
      (streptococcal) NEC 686.9
    abscess - *code by* site under Abscess
    cellulitis - *code by* site under
        Cellulitis
    ulcer (*see also* Ulcer, skin) 707.9
  Loefflerella
    mallei 024
    whitmori 025
  lung 519.2
    atypical Mycobacterium 031.0
    tuberculous (*see also* Tuberculosis,
        pulmonary) 011.9
    basilar 519.2
    chronic (*see also* Fibrosis, lung) 517
    fungus NEC 117.9
    spirochetal 104.9
    virus - *see* Pneumonia, virus
  lymph gland (axillary) (cervical)
      (inguinal) 683
    mesenteric 289.2
  lymphoid tissue, base of tongue or
      posterior pharynx, NEC 500
  malarial - *see* Malaria
  Malassezia furfur 111.0
  Malleomyces
    mallei 024
    pseudomallei 025
  mammary gland 611.0
    puerperal, postpartum 678
  Mansonella (ozzardi) 125.5
  mastoid (suppurative) - *see* Mastoiditis
  maxilla, maxillary 526.4
    sinus (chronic) (*see also* Sinusitis,
        maxillary) 503.0
  mediastinum 519.9
  medina 125.8
  meibomian
    cyst 362
    gland 362
  meninges (*see also* Meningitis) 320.9
  meningococcal 036.9
    brain 036.0
    cerebrospinal 036.0
    endocardium 036.8

Infection, infected — *continued*
  meningococcal — *continued*
    generalized 036.1
      with meningitis 036.0
    meninges 036.0
    specified site NEC 036.8
  mesenteric lymph nodes or glands NEC
    289.2
  metatarsophalangeal 729.9
  mixed flora NEC 039.9
  Monilia (albicans) (any site) 112
  mouth NEC 528.9
    parasitic 112
  muscle NEC 732
  mycelium NEC 117.9
  Mycobacterium - *see* Mycobacterium
  mycotic NEC 117.9
    skin 111.9
    systemic 117.9
  myocardium NEC 422
  nail (chronic) (with lymphangitis) 681
    ingrowing 703.0
  nasal sinus (chronic) (*see also* Sinusitis)
    503.9
  nasopharynx (chronic) 508.9
    acute 460
  navel (newborn) 686.9
  Neissera - *see* Gonococcus
  nipple 611.0
    puerperal, postpartum 678
  nose 508.9
  nostril 508.9
  Oesophagostomum 127.4
  Oestrus ovis 134.0
  Oidium albicans (any site) 112
  Onchocerca (volvulus) 125.3
  operation wound 998.5
  Opisthorchis (felineus) (viverrini)
    121.0
  orbit 369.0
  ovary (*see also* Salpingo-oophoritis)
    614
  overwhelming NEC 039.9
  Oxyuris vermicularis 127.3
  pancreas 577.0
  Paracoccidioides brasiliensis 116.2
  Paragonimus westermani 121.2
  parainfluenza NEC 470
  parameningococcus NEC 036.9
    with meningitis 036.0
  parasitic NEC 136
  para-urethral ducts - *see* Infection,
    urinary
  parotid gland 527.2
  Pasteurella NEC 027.9
    pestis (*see also* Plague) 020.9

Infection, infected — *continued*
  Pasteurella NEC — *continued*
    pseudotuberculosis 027.9
  pelvic, female (*see also* Disease, pelvis,
    inflammatory) 616.0
  penis (glans) (preputial) (retention) NEC
    607.5
  periapical 522.4
  peridental 523.3
  periorbital 369.0
  perirectal 569.2
  perirenal (*see also* Infection, kidney)
    590.9
  peritoneal (*see also* Peritonitis) 567.9
  peri-ureteral 593.5
  pharynx 508.9
    Coxsackie virus 074.0
    phlegmonous 462
    posterior, lymphoid 500
  Piedraia hortai 111.8
  pinworm 127.3
  pneumococcal NEC 481
    generalized (purulent) 038.2
      with pneumonia - *see* Pneumonia,
        pneumococcal
  postoperative wound 998.5
  post-traumatic, local, of wound NEC -
    code as Wound, open,
    complicated
  postvaccinal 999.3
  prepuce NEC 607.5
  prostate (capsule) (*see also* Prostatitis)
    601
  Proteus vulgaris NEC 039.9
  protozoal NEC 136
    intestinal NEC 007.9
  puerperal, postpartum, childbirth 670
  pulmonary - *see* Infection, lung
  purulent - *see* Abscess
  putrid, generalized - *see* Septicemia
  pyemic - *see* Septicemia
  rectum (sphincter) 569.2
  renal (*see also* Infection, kidney)
    590.9
  respiratory 519.9
    chronic (*see also* Fibrosis, lung) 517
    neonatal (*see also* Pneumonia) 486
    upper (acute) (multiple sites) NEC
      465
      with flu, grippe, or influenza 472
      influenzal 472
      streptococcal 034.0
      viral NEC 465
  resulting from insertion of shunt or
    other internal prosthetic device
    997.6

Infection, infected — *continued*
Rhinocladium 117.8
Rhinosporidium (seeberi) 117.0
rhinovirus 460
Saccharomyces 112
salivary duct or gland (any) 527.2
Salmonella 003.9
  choleraesuis 003.9
    due to food 003.0
  due to food 003.0
  enteritidis 003.9
    due to food 003.0
  hirschfeldii 002.2
  paratyphi 002.9
    A 002.0
    B 002.1
    C 002.2
  schottmuelleri 002.1
  typhi 001
  typhimurium 003.9
    due to food 003.0
saprophytic 136
Schistosoma - *see* Infestation,
    Schistosoma
scratch or other superficial injury - *see*
    Injury, superficial, infected
scrotum (acute) NEC 607.5
seminal vesicle (*see also* Vesiculitis)
    607.4
septic
  generalized - *see* Septicemia
  localized, skin (*see also* Abscess)
    682.9
septicemic - *see* Septicemia
Shigella NEC 004.9
sinus - *see also* Sinusitis
  pilonidal 685
  skin NEC 686.9
Skene's duct or gland (*see also*
    Urethritis) 597
skin (local) (staphylococcal)
    (streptococcal) NEC 686.9
  abscess - *code by* site under Abscess
  cellulitis - *code by* site under
    Cellulitis
  due to fungus NEC 111.9
  mycotic NEC 111.9
  ulcer (*see also* Ulcer, skin) 707.9
Sparganum mansoni 123.5
specific (*see also* Syphilis) 097.9
spermatic cord NEC 607.5
sphenoidal (sinus) (*see also* Sinusitis)
    503.9
spinal cord NEC 323
  abscess 322
    late effects 324

Infection, infected — *continued*
spinal cord NEC — *continued*
  late effects 324
  meninges - *see* Meningitis
  streptococcal 323
Spirillum
  minus 026.0
  obermeieri 088.0
spirochetal NEC 104.9
  lung 104.9
spleen 289.5
Sporotrichum (schenckii) 117.1
Sporozoa 136
staphylococcal NEC 039.9
  generalized (purulent) 038.1
steatoma 706.2
streptococcal NEC 039.9
  generalized (purulent) 038.0
streptotrichosis 113
Strongyloides (stercoralis) 127.1
stump (amputation) (surgical) 997.2
  traumatic - code as Amputation,
    traumatic, complicated
subcutaneous tissue, local NEC 686.9
submaxillary region 528.9
suipestifer 003.9
  due to food 003.0
systemic - *see* Septicemia
Taenia - *see* Infestation, Taenia
tapeworm - *see* Infestation, tapeworm
tendon (sheath) 732
Ternidens diminutus 127.4
testis (*see also* Orchitis) 604
thigh (skin) 686.9
threadworm 127.1
throat 508.9
  pneumococcal 462
  staphylococcal 462
  streptococcal 034.0
  viral 462
thyroglossal duct 529.9
toe (skin) 686.9
  abscess (with lymphangitis) 681
  cellulitis (with lymphangitis) 681
tongue NEC 529.0
  parasitic 112
tonsil (and adenoid) (faucial) (lingual)
    (pharyngeal) 500
  acute or subacute 463
  tag 500
tooth, teeth 522.4
  periapical 522.4
  peridental 523.3
  socket 526.5
Torula histolytica 116.0
Toxocara (cani) (felis) 128.0

Infection, infected — *continued*
Toxoplasma (generalized) - *see*
  Toxoplasmosis
trachea, chronic 491
  fungus 117.9
trematode NEC 121.9
Treponema pallidum (*see also* Syphilis)
  097.9
Trichinella (spiralis) 124
Trichomonas (urogenital) 131
  cervix 131
  intestine 007.9
  prostate 131
  specified site NEC 136
  urethra 131
  vagina 131
  vulva 131
Trichophyton, trichophytid - *see*
  Dermatophytosis
Trichosporon beigellii 111.2
Trichuris trichiura 127.2
Trombicula (irritans) 133.9
Trypanosoma (*see also*
  Trypanosomiasis) 087.9
tubal (*see also* Salpingo-oophoritis)
  614
tuberculous NEC (*see also*
  Tuberculosis) 011.9
tubo-ovarian (*see also* Salpingo-
  oophoritis) 614
tunica vaginalis 607.9
tympanic membrane - *see* Otitis media
typhoid (abortive) (ambulant) (bacillus)
  001
umbilicus (newborn) 686.9
ureter 593.5
urethra - *see* Infection, urinary
urinary (tract) NEC 599.0
  with
    abortion - *see* Abortion, by type,
      with sepsis
    ectopic gestation - *see* categories
      631.0-631.3
    arising during pregnancy 635.9
    fetus or newborn 763.1
    puerperal, postpartum, childbirth
      635.9
    tuberculous 016.1
    late effect or sequela 019.2
uterus, uterine (*see also* Endometritis)
  622.0
utriculus masculinus NEC 607.5
vaccination 999.3
vagina (granulation tissue) (wall) (*see
  also* Vaginitis) 622.1
varicose veins - *see* Varicose vein

Infection, infected — *continued*
vas deferens NEC 607.5
verumontanum - *see* Infection, urinary
vesical (*see also* Cystitis) 595
Vincent's (gums) (mouth) (tonsil) 101
virus NEC 079.9
  central nervous system NEC 079.9
    enterovirus 046
      meningitis - *see* Meningitis,
        aseptic
    chest 519.9
    Coxsackie - *see* Coxsackie
    intestine (*see also* Enteritis, viral)
      008.9
    lung - *see* Pneumonia, virus
  vulva (*see also* Vulvitis) 622.1
  whipworm 127.2
  wound (local) (post-traumatic) NEC -
    code as Wound, open,
    complicated
  with
    dislocation - code as Dislocation,
      compound
    fracture - code as Fracture, open
    surgical 998.5
  Wuchereria 125.0
    bancrofti 125.0
    malayi 125.1
  yeast 112
  Zeis' gland 362
Infective, infectious - *see* condition
Infertility
  female 628
  male 606
Infestation 134.9
  Acanthocheilonema
    perstans 125.4
    streptocera 125.8
  Agamofilaria streptocera 125.8
  Ancylostoma 126.9
    americanum 126.1
    braziliense 126.8
    caninum 126.8
    ceylonicum 126.8
    duodenale 126.0
  arthropod NEC 134.2
  Ascaris lumbricoides 127.0
  Bacillus fusiformis 101
  Balantidium coli 007.0
  beef tapeworm 123.2
  Bothriocephalus (latus) 123.4
    larval 123.5
  broad tapeworm 123.4
    larval 123.5
  Brugia malayi 125.1
  cat liver flukes 121.0

Infestation—*continued*
  Cercomonas hominis (intestinal) 007.9
  cestodes NEC 123.9
  chigger 133.9
  chigoe 134.2
  Chilomastix 007.9
  Clonorchis (sinensis) (liver) 121.1
  coccidia 007.2
  Cysticercus cellulosae 123.1
  Demodex folliculorum 133.9
  Dermatobia (hominis) 134.0
  Dibothriocephalus (latus) 123.4
  Diphyllobothrium (latum) (intestinal)
      123.4
    larval 123.5
  Dipylidium (caninum) 123.9
  Distoma hepaticum 121.3
  dog tapeworm 123.9
  Dracunculus medinensis 125.8
  dwarf tapeworm 123.6
  Echinococcus (granulosus)
      (multilocularis) (*see also* Cyst,
      hydatid) 122.9
  Embadomonas 007.9
  Endameba (histolytica) - *see* Infection,
      ameba
  Enterobius vermicularis 127.3
  Epidermophyton - *see* Dermatophytosis
  Fasciola
    gigantica 121.3
    hepatica 121.3
  Fasciolopsis (buski) (small intestine)
      121.4
  filarial 125.9
    due to
      Acanthocheilonema perstans
          125.4
      Brugia (Wuchereria) malayi 125.1
      Dracunculus medinensis 125.8
      guinea worms 125.8
      Monsonella (ozzardi) 125.5
      Onchocerca volvulus 125.3
      Wuchereria bancrofti 125.0
  fish tapeworm 123.4
  fluke 121.9
    blood NEC (*see also* Schistosomiasis)
        120.9
    cat liver 121.0
    intestinal 121.4
    liver 121.3
      due to clonorchiasis 121.1
    lung (oriental) 121.2
  fly larvae 134.0
  Gasterophilus (intestinalis) 134.0
  Giardia lamblia 007.1
  Gongylonema 125.8

Infestation—*continued*
  guinea worm 125.8
  helminth NEC 128.9
    intestinal 127.9
      mixed (types classifiable to more
          than one of the titles 120-
          127.4) 127.5
  Heterophyes (small intestine) 121.9
  hookworm (*see also* Infestation,
      Ancylostoma) 126.9
  Hymenolepis (diminuta) (nana) 123.6
  intestinal NEC 129
  leeches (aquatic) (land) 134.3
  Leishmania - *see* Leishmaniasis
  lice, louse (body) (head) 132
    pubic 134.1
  linguatulids Pentastomata 134.2
  Loa loa 125.2
  maggots 134.0
  Mansonella (ozzardi) 125.5
  medina 125.8
  Metagonimus (small intestine) 121.9
  microfilaria streptocera 125.3
  Microsporon furfur 111.0
  mites 133.9
    scabic 133.0
  Monilia (albicans) 112
    vulva 112
  mouth 112
  Necator americanus 126.1
  nematode NEC 127.9
    Ancylostoma (*see also* Ancylostoma)
        126.9
    conjunctiva NEC 128.9
    intestinal NEC 127.4
  Oesophagostomum 127.4
  Oestrus ovis 134.0
  Onchocerca (volvulus) 125.3
  Opisthorchis (felineus) (viverrini)
      121.0
  Oxyuris vermicularis 127.3
  Paragonimus westermanii 121.2
  parasite, parasitic NEC 136
    intestinal 129
    skin 134.9
  Pediculus (humanus) (capitis) (corporis)
      132
    pubis 134.1
  Phthirus (pubis) 134.1
  pinworm 127.3
  pork tapeworm 123.0
  protozoal NEC 136
  pubic louse 134.1
  rat tapeworm 123.6
  roundworm (large) NEC 127.0
  sand flea 134.2

Infestation—*continued*
  saprophytic NEC   136
  Sarcoptes scabiei   133.0
  scabies   133.0
  Schistosoma   120.9
    bovis   120.8
    cercariae   120.3
    hematobium   120.0
    intercalatum   120.8
    japonicum   120.2
    mansoni   120.1
    specified
      site - *see* Schistosomiasis
      type NEC   120.8
    spindale   120.8
  screw worms   134.0
  skin NEC   134.9
  Sparganum (mansoni) (proliferum)
      123.5
  Sporozoa NEC   136
  Strongyloides stercoralis   127.1
  Strongylus (gibsoni)   127.4
  Taenia   123.3
    diminuta   123.6
    echinococcus (*see also* Cyst, hydatid)
      122.9
    mediocanellata   123.2
    nana   123.6
    Saginata   123.2
    solium (intestinal form)   123.0
      larval form   123.1
  tapeworm   123.9
    beef   123.2
    broad   123.4
      larval   123.5
    dog   123.9
    dwarf   123.6
    fish   123.4
    pork   123.0
    rat   123.6
  Ternidens diminutus   127.4
  Tetranychus molestissimus   133.9
  threadworm   127.1
  tongue   112
  Toxocara (cani) (felis)   128.0
  trematode(s) NEC   121.9
  Trichina spiralis   124
  Trichinella spiralis   124
  Trichocephalus   127.2
  Trichomonas (urogenital)   131
    cervix   131
    intestine   007.9
    prostate   131
    specified site NEC   136
    urethra   131
    vagina   131
    vulva   131

Infestation—*continued*
  Trichophyton - *see* Dermatophytosis
  Trichostrongylus instabilis   127.1
  Trichuris trichiura   127.2
  Trombicula (irritans)   133.9
  Trypanosoma - *see* Trypanosomiasis
  Tunga penetrans   134.2
  Uncinaria americana   126.1
  whipworm   127.2
  worms NEC   128.9
  Wuchereria   125.0
    bancrofti   125.0
    malayi   125.1
Infiltrate, infiltration
  with an iron compound   279
  amyloid (any site) (generalized)   276
  calcareous NEC   279
    localized - *see* Degeneration by site
  calcium salt   279
  corneal   378.6
  eyelid   378.2
  fatty (diffuse) (generalized)   279
    localized - *see* Degeneration by site,
      fatty
  glycogen, glycogenic (*see also* Disease,
      glycogen storage)   271.1
  heart, cardiac
    fatty (*see also* Insufficiency,
      myocardial)   428
    glycogenic   271.1
  inflammatory in vitreous   369.9
  kidney (*see also* Lesion, kidney)   593.2
  leukemic (*see also* Leukemia)   207.9
  liver - *see also* Cirrhosis, liver
    fatty - *see* Cirrhosis, portal
    glycogen (*see also* Disease, glycogen
      storage)   271.1
  lung (eosinophilic)   519.2
  lymphatic (*see also* Leukemia,
      lymphatic)   204.9
    gland, pigmentary   289.3
  muscle, fatty   733.9
  myelogenous (*see also* Leukemia,
      myeloid)   205.9
  myocardium, myocardial
    fatty (*see also* Insufficiency,
      myocardial)   428
    glycogenic   271.1
  Ranke's primary (with symptoms)
      012.0
    with pneumoconiosis (conditions in
      515)   010
    late effect or sequela   019.0
  thymus (gland) (fatty)   254
  urine   596.9
  vitreous humor   378.9

Infirmity   796.0
  senile   794
Inflammation, inflamed, inflammatory
    (with exudation)
  abducens (nerve)   369.9
  accessory sinus ((chronic) (see also
      Sinusitis)   503.9
  adrenal (gland)   255.9
  alimentary canal - see Enteritis
  alveoli NEC   526.5
    scorbutic   264
    teeth   526.5
  amnion - see Amnionitis
  anal canal   569.2
  antrum (chronic) (see also Sinusitis,
      antrum)   503.0
  anus   569.2
  appendix (see also Appendicitis)   541
  arachnoid - see Meningitis
  areola   611.0
    puerperal, postpartum   678
  areolar tissue NEC   686.9
  artery - see Arteritis
  auditory meatus (external)   380
  Bartholin's gland (see also Vaginitis)
      622.1
  bile duct or passage (see also
      Cholecystitis)   575
  bladder (see also Cystitis)   595
  bone - see Osteomyelitis
  bowel - see Enteritis
  brain (see also Encephalitis)   323
    late effects   324
    membrane - see Meningitis
    softening   323
      late effects   324
  breast   611.0
    puerperal, postpartum   678
  broad ligament (see also Disease,
      pelvis, inflammatory)   616.0
  bronchi - see Bronchitis
  bursa - see Bursitis
  catarrhal (see also Catarrh)   460
  cecum (see also Appendicitis)   541
  cerebral (see also Encephalitis)   323
    late effects   324
    membrane - see Meningitis
  cerebrospinal   320.9
    H. influenzae   320.0
      late effects   324
    influenzal   320.0
      late effects   324
    late effects   324
    meningococcal   036.0
    pneumococcal   320.1
      late effects   324

Inflammation, etc. - continued
  cerebrospinal - continued
    specified organism NEC   320.8
      late effects   324
    tuberculous   013.9
      late effect or sequela   019.1
  cervix (uteri) (see also Cervicitis)
      620.9
  chest   519.9
  choroid NEC   365
  colon - see Enteritis
  connective tissue (diffuse) NEC   734.9
  cornea (see also Keratitis)   363.9
  corpora cavernosa   607.5
  cranial nerve - see Neuritis, cranial
      nerve
  diarrhea - see Diarrhea
  duodenum   535
  dura mater - see Meningitis
  ear (middle) (septic) - see also Otitis
      media
    external   380
    inner   384.0
  esophagus   530.1
  ethmoidal (chronic) (see also Sinusitis)
      503.9
  eustachian tube (catarrhal)   384.0
  extrarectal   569.2
  eyelid   361
  fallopian tube (see also Salpingo-
      oophoritis)   614
  fascia   732
  fetal membranes (acute)
    causing complicated delivery   661.8
    complicating pregnancy (delivered)
        (undelivered)   634.9
    fetus or newborn   763.9
  frontal (chronic) (sinus) (see also
      Sinusitis, frontal)   503.1
  gall duct (see also Cholecystitis)   575
  gallbladder (see also Cholecystitis)
      575
  gastro-intestinal - see Enteritis
  genital organ (internal) (diffuse) NEC
    female   629.4
      with
        abortion - see Abortion, by type,
            with sepsis
        ectopic gestation - see categories
            631.0-631.3
      arising during pregnancy   630
        fetus or newborn   763.1
      puerperal, postpartum, childbirth
          670
    male   607.5

Inflammation, etc. — *continued*
sphenoidal (sinus) (*see also* Sinusitis)
503.9
spinal
cord (*see also* Myelitis) 323
late effects 324
membrane - *see* Meningitis
nerve - *see* Compression, nerve
spine (*see also* Spondylitis) 713.1
spleen (capsule) 289.5
stomach - *see* Gastritis
subcutaneous tissue NEC 686.9
suprarenal (gland) 255.9
synovial (fringe) (membrane) - *see*
Bursitis
tendon (sheath) NEC 732
testicle (*see also* Orchitis) 604
thigh 686.9
throat (*see also* Sore throat) 462
diphtheritic 032
thymus (gland) 254
thyroid (gland) (*see also* Thyroiditis)
245.9
tongue 529.0
tonsil - *see* Tonsillitis
trachea - *see* Tracheitis
trochlear (nerve) 369.9
tubal (*see also* Salpingo-oophoritis)
614
tuberculous NEC (*see also*
Tuberculosis) 011.9
tubo-ovarian (*see also* Salpingo-
oophoritis) 614
tunica vaginalis 607.5
tympanum - *see* Otitis media
umbilicus (newborn) 686.9
uterine ligament (*see also* Disease,
pelvis, inflammatory) 616.0
uterus (catarrhal) (*see also*
Endometritis) 622.0
uveal tract (sympathetic) NEC 366
vagina (*see also* Vaginitis) 622.1
vas deferens 607.5
vein (*see also* Phlebitis) 451.9
thrombotic 451.9
cerebral (*see also* Thrombosis,
brain) 433.9
leg 451.0
lower extremity 451.0
vocal cord 508.3
vulva (*see also* Vulvitis) 622.1
Inflation, lung imperfect (newborn) (*see
also* Asphyxia, newborn) 776.9
Influenza, influenzal 470
with
bronchiolitis 472

Influenza, influenzal — *continued*
with — *continued*
bronchitis 472
bronchopneumonia 471
cold (any type) 472
digestive symptoms but no
respiratory symptoms 473
ethmoiditis 472
hemorrhage, lung 472
laryngitis 472
laryngotracheitis 472
nervous symptoms but no digestive
or respiratory symptoms 474
pharyngitis 472
pleurisy 472
pneumonia (any form) 471
respiratory symptoms NEC 472
sinusitis 472
sore throat 472
tonsillitis 472
tracheitis 472
tracheobronchitis 472
upper respiratory infection 472
abdominal 473
arachnoiditis (brain or spinal) 320.0
late effects 324
Asian 470
bronchial 472
bronchopneumonia 471
catarrhal 472
cerebral 474
ventriculitis 320.0
late effects 324
cerebrospinal 474
meningitis (purulent) 320.0
late effects 324
encephalitis 474
lethargica 065
late effects 066
encephalomeningomyelitis, disseminated
320.0
late effects 324
ependymitis (chronic) 320.0
late effects 324
epidemic 470
gastric 473
gastrointestinal 473
infection
brain, septic 320.0
late effects 324
meninges 320.0
late effects 324
intestinal 473
leptomeningitis 320.0
late effects 324

Influenza, influenzal — *continued*
  maternal
    affecting fetus or newborn   761.2
    manifest influenza in infant - *see*
        categories 470-474
  meningitis (cerebral) (cerebrospinal)
      (nonmeningococcal)
      (postinfectious) (purulent) (serosa
      circumscripta) (spinal)   320.0
    late effects   324
  meningomyelitis   320.0
    late effects   324
  pachymeningitis (adhesive) (fibrous)
      (hemorrhagic) (hypertrophic)
      (spinal)   320.0
    late effects   324
  pneumonia (any form)   471
  respiratory   472
  stomach   473
Influenza-like disease   470
Infraction, Freiberg's (metatarsal head)
    722.2
Infusion
  complication, misadventure, or reaction
      - *see* Complications, infusion
Ingestion
  chemical or drug - *see* Table of adverse
      effects
  foreign body NEC   938
Ingrowing
  hair   704
  nail (finger) (toe)   703.0
Inguinal - *see also* condition
  testicle   752.1
Inhalation
  carbon monoxide   986
  flame (asphyxia)   949.0
  food or foreign body (*see also*
      Asphyxia, food or foreign body)
      933
  gas, fumes, or vapor   987.9
    specified agent - *see* Table of adverse
        effects
  mucus (*see also* Asphyxia, mucus)   933
  oil (causing suffocation) (*see also*
      Asphyxia, food or foreign body)
      933
  smoke   987.9
  steam   987.9
Iniencephalus   759.2
Injury   996.9
  abdomen, abdominal (viscera) - *see also*
      Injury, internal, abdomen
    muscle or wall   996.1
  acoustic, resulting in deafness - *see*
      Injury, nerve, acoustic

Injury — *continued*
  adenoid   996.0
  adrenal (gland) - *see* Injury, internal,
      adrenal
  alveolar (process)   996.0
  ankle (and knee) (and leg, except thigh)
      (and foot)   996.7
  anterior chamber, eye - *see* Injury, eye
  anus - *see* Injury, internal, anus
  aorta - *see* Injury, internal, aorta
  appendix - *see* Injury, internal,
      appendix
  arm, upper (and shoulder)   996.2
  artery (complicating trauma)   995.3
    cerebral or meningeal (*see also*
        Hemorrhage, subdural,
        traumatic)   852.0
  auditory canal (external) (meatus)
      996.0
  auricle, auris, ear   996.0
  axilla   996.2
  back   996.1
  bile duct - *see* Injury, internal, bile duct
  birth - *see also* Birth injury
    canal, complicating delivery - *see*
        Obstetrical trauma
  bladder (sphincter) - *see* Injury, internal,
      bladder
  blast (air) (hydraulic) (immersion)
      (underwater) NEC   869.0
    abdomen or thorax - *see* Injury,
        internal, by site
    brain - *see* Concussion, brain
    ear (acoustic nerve trauma) - *see also*
        Injury, nerve, acoustic
      with perforation of tympanic
          membrane - *see* Wound,
          open, ear
  brachial plexus - *see* Injury, nerve, arm,
      upper
  brain NEC (*see also* Injury,
      intracranial)   854.0
  breast   996.1
  broad ligament - *see* Injury, internal,
      broad ligament
  bronchus, bronchi - *see* Injury, internal,
      bronchus
  brow   996.0
  buttock   996.1
  canthus, eye - *see* Injury, eye
  cauda equina - *see* Injury, spinal, sacral
  cavernous sinus (*see also* Injury,
      intracranial)   854.0
  cecum - *see* Injury, internal, cecum

Injury—*continued*
  cerebellum (*see also* Injury, intracranial)
    854.0
  cervix (uteri) - *see* Injury, internal,
    cervix
  cheek 996.0
  chest - *see also* Injury, internal, chest
    wall 996.1
  childbirth - *see* Birth injury NEC
  chin 996.0
  choroid (eye) - *see* Injury, eye
  clitoris 996.1
  coccyx 996.1
  colon - *see* Injury, internal, colon
  common duct - *see* Injury, internal,
    common duct
  conjunctiva - *see* Injury, eye
  cord
    spermatic - *see* Injury, internal,
      spermatic cord
    spinal - *see* Injury, spinal, by region
  cornea 921
    abrasion - *see* Injury, superficial,
      cornea
  cortex (cerebral) (*see also* Injury,
    intracranial) 854.0
  costal region 996.1
  costochondral 996.1
  cranial
    bones - *see* Fracture, skull
    cavity (*see also* Injury, intracranial)
      854.0
  delivery - *see also* Birth injury
    maternal NEC - *see* Obstetrical
      trauma
  Descemet's membrane - *see* Injury eye
  diaphragm - *see* Injury, internal,
    diaphragm
  duodenum - *see* Injury, internal,
    duodenum
  ear (auricle) (external) (drum) (canal)
    996.0
  elbow (and forearm) (and wrist) 996.3
  epididymis 996.1
  epigastric region 996.1
  epiglottis 996.0
  epiphyseal, current - *see* Fracture
  esophagus - *see* Injury, internal,
    esophagus
  eustachian tube 996.0
  extremity (lower) (upper) 996.8
  eye (lid) (muscle) (globe) 921
    superficial - *see* Injury, superficial,
      eye
  eyeball 921
    superficial - *see* Injury, superficial,
      eye

Injury—*continued*
  eyebrow 996.0
  face (and neck) 996.0
  fallopian tube - *see* Injury, internal,
    fallopian tube
  finger(s) (nail) 996.5
  flank 996.1
  foot (and knee) (and leg, except thigh)
    (and ankle) 996.7
  forceps (*see also* Birth injury NEC)
    772.9
  forearm (and elbow) (and wrist) 996.3
  forehead 996.0
  gallbladder - *see* Injury, internal,
    gallbladder
  gasserian ganglion - *see* Injury, nerve,
    trigeminal
  gastro-intestinal tract - *see* Injury,
    internal, gastro-intestinal tract
  genital organ(s)
    complicating delivery - *see*
      Obstetrical trauma
    external 996.1
    internal - *see* Injury, internal, genital
      organs
  gland
    lacrimal 921
    parathyroid 996.0
    salivary 996.0
    thyroid 996.0
  globe (eye) - *see* Injury, eye
  groin 996.1
  gum 996.0
  hand(s) (except fingers) 996.4
  head NEC (*see also* Injury, intracranial)
    854.0
  heart - *see* Injury, internal, heart
  heel 996.7
  hip (and thigh) 996.6
  hymen 996.1
  ileum - *see* Injury, internal, ileum
  iliac region 996.1
  infrared rays - *see* Effect, adverse,
    infrared
  instrumental (during surgery) 998.2
    delivery (*see also* Birth injury NEC)
      772.9
    nonsurgical (*see also* Injury, by site)
      996.9
  internal 869

Note—Categories 860–869 include internal injuries with fractures in the same region, except visceral injury with fracture of pelvis.

For injury of internal organ(s) by foreign body entering through a natural ori-

fice (e.g., inhaled, ingested, or swallowed) –
see Foreign body, entering through orifice.

For internal injury of any of the following sites with internal injury of any other
of the sites – *see* Injury, internal, multiple.

The following fourth-digit subdivisions
are for use with categories 860 and 862–
869:

> .0 *Without mention of open wound*
>   *into cavity*
> .1 *With open wound into cavity*
> .9 *Late effect*

"With open wound" includes internal injury with mention of infection or foreign
body.

Injury – *continued*
  internal – *continued*
    with fracture, pelvis - *see* Fracture,
      pelvis
    abdomen, abdominal (viscera) NEC
      868
      with fracture, pelvis - *see* Fracture,
        pelvis
    adrenal (gland) 868
    anus 863
    aorta (thoracic) 862
      abdominal 868
    appendix 863
    bile duct 868
    bladder (sphincter) 867
    broad ligament 867
    bronchus, bronchi 862
    cecum 863
    cervix (uteri) 867
      complicating delivery - *see*
        Obstetrical trauma
    chest 862
    colon 863
    common duct 868
    diaphragm 862
    duodenum 863
    esophagus 862
    fallopian tube 867
    gallbladder 868
    gastro-intestinal tract NEC 863
    genital organs (any) 867
    heart 861.0
      with open wound into thorax
        861.1
      late effect 861.9
    ileum 863
    intestine (any part) (large) (small)
      863
    intra-abdominal (organs) (multiple)
      NEC 868

Injury – *continued*
  internal – *continued*
    intrathoracic organs (multiple) 862
      heart (only) - *see* Injury, internal,
        heart
      lung (only) - *see* Injury, internal,
        lung
    intra-uterine 867
      complicating delivery - *see*
        Obstetrical trauma
    jejunum 863
    kidney (subcapsular) 866
    liver 864
    lung 861.2
      with open wound into thorax
        861.3
      hemothorax - *see* Hemothorax,
        traumatic
      late effect 861.9
      pneumothorax - *see* Pneumothorax,
        traumatic
    mediastinum 862
    mesentery 863
    mesosalpinx 867
    multiple 869

Note – Multiple internal injuries of sites
classifiable to the same three- or four-digit
category should be classified to that
category.

Multiple injuries classifiable to different
fourth-digit subdivisions of 861 (heart and
lung injuries) should be dealt with according to the coding rules.

Multiple injuries of sites classifiable to
different three-digit categories should be
coded according to the following list.

---

    intra-abdominal organ (site
      classifiable to 863-868)
    with
      intrathoracic organ(s) (site(s)
        classifiable to 861, 862)
        869
      other intra-abdominal organ(s)
        (site(s) classifiable to
        863-868, except where
        classifiable to the same
        three-digit category)
        868
    intrathoracic organ (site classifiable
      to 861, 862)
    with
      intra-abdominal organ(s) (site(s)
        classifiable to 863-868)
        869

Injury—*continued*
  internal—*continued*
    multiple—*continued*
      intrathoracic organ—*continued*
        with—*continued*
          other intrathoracic organ(s)
            (site(s) classifiable to
            861, 862, except where
            classifiable to the same
            three-digit category)
            862
    myocardium - *see* Injury, internal,
      heart
    ovary 867
    pancreas 863
    pelvis, pelvic (organs) (viscera) 867
      with fracture, pelvis - *see* Fracture,
        pelvis
    peritoneum 868
    pleura 862
    prostate 867
    rectum 863
    retroperitoneal 868
    round ligament 867
    seminal vesicle 867
    spermatic cord 867
    spleen 865
    stomach 863
    suprarenal gland (multiple) 868
    thorax, thoracic (cavity) (organs)
      (multiple) 862
    thymus (gland) 862
    trachea 862
    ureter 867
    urethra (sphincter) 867
    uterus 867
      complicating delivery - *see*
        Obstetrical trauma
    vas deferens 867
    vesical (sphincter) 867
    viscera (abdominal) 868
      with fracture, pelvis - *see* Fracture,
        pelvis
      thoracic NEC 862
  interscapular region 996.1
  intervertebral disc 996.1
  intestine (any part) (large) (small) - *see*
    Injury, internal, intestine
  intra-abdominal (organs) NEC - *see*
    Injury, internal, intra-abdominal
  intracranial (without skull fracture)
    854.0
    with open intracranial wound 854.1
    late effect 854.9
  intra-ocular - *see* Injury eye

Injury—*continued*
  intrathoracic organs NEC (multiple) -
    see Injury, internal, intrathoracic
  intra-uterine - *see* Injury, internal, intra-
    uterine
  iris - *see* Injury, eye
  jaw 996.0
  jejunum - *see* Injury, internal, jejunum
  joint NEC 996.9
    old or residual 729.9
  kidney - *see* Injury, internal, kidney
  knee (and leg, except thigh) (and ankle)
    (and foot) 996.7
  labium (majus) (minus) 996.1
  labyrinth, ear 996.0
  lacrimal apparatus, gland, or sac - *see*
    Injury, eye
  larynx 996.0
  leg except thigh (and knee) (and ankle)
    (and foot) 996.7
    upper or thigh 996.6
  lens, eye - *see* Injury, eye
  lip 996.0
  liver - *see* Injury, internal, liver
  lobe
    occipital or parietal (*see also*
      Contusion, brain) 851.0
  lumbar (region) 996.1
    plexus - *see* Injury, nerve, lumbar
      plexus
  lumbosacral (region) 996.1
    plexus - *see* Injury, nerve,
      lumbosacral plexus
  lung - *see* Injury, internal, lung
  malar region 996.0
  mastoid region 996.0
  maternal, during pregnancy
    fetus or newborn 761.5
  maxilla 996.0
  mediastinum - *see* Injury, internal,
    mediastinum
  membrane
    brain (*see also* Injury, intracranial)
      854.0
    tympanic 996.0
  meningeal artery (*see also* Hemorrhage,
    subdural, traumatic) 852.0
  meninges (cerebral) (*see also* Injury,
    intracranial) 854.0
  mesentery - *see* Injury, internal,
    mesentery
  mesosalpinx - *see* Injury, internal,
    mesosalpinx
  middle ear 996.0
  midthoracic region 996.1
  mouth 996.0

Injury—*continued*
  nerve—*continued*
    tibial 959.2
      with open wound 959.3
      ankle and foot 957
      late effect 959.9
      lower leg 956
    toe 957
    trigeminal 951
    trochlear 951
    ulnar 959.2
      with open wound 959.3
      forearm 953
      late effect 959.9
      wrist (and hand) 954
    upper arm (brachial plexus)
      (musculospiral) 952
    vagus 951
    wrist and hand (digital) (median)
      (radial) (ulnar) 954
  nervous system diffuse 959.2
    with open wound(s) 959.3
    late effect 959.9
  nose (septum) 996.0
  occipital (region) (scalp) 996.0
    lobe (*see also* Injury, intracranial)
      854.0
  optic chiasm - *see* Injury, nerve, optic
  orbit, orbital (region) - *see* Injury, eye
  ovary - *see* Injury, internal, ovary
  palate (soft) 996.0
  pancreas *see* Injury, internal, pancreas
  parathyroid (gland) 996.0
  parietal (region) (scalp) 996.0
    lobe (*see also* Injury, intracranial)
      854.0
  pelvic
    floor 996.1
    organs - *see* Injury, internal, pelvic
      organs
  pelvis 996.1
  penis 996.1
  perineum 996.1
  peritoneum - *see* Injury, internal,
    peritoneum
  phalanges
    foot 996.7
    hand 996.5
  pharynx 996.0
  pleura - *see* Injury, internal, pleura
  popliteal space 996.7
  prepuce 996.1
  prostate - *see* Injury, internal, prostate
  pubic region 996.1
  pudenda 996.1
  radiation - *see* Effect, adverse, radiation

Injury—*continued*
  radioactive substance or radium - *see*
    Effect, adverse, radioactive
    substance
  rectovaginal septum 996.1
  rectum - *see* Injury, internal, rectum
  retina - *see* Injury, eye
  retroperitoneal - *see* Injury, internal,
    retroperitoneal
  roentgen rays - *see* Effect, adverse, x-
    rays
  round ligament - *see* Injury, internal,
    round ligament
  sacral (region) 996.1
    plexus - *see* Injury, nerve, sacral
  sacro-iliac ligament NEC 996.1
  sacrum 996.1
  salivary ducts or glands 996.0
  scalp 996.0
  scapular region 996.2
  sclera - *see* Injury, eye
  scrotum 996.1
  seminal vesicle - *see* Injury, internal,
    seminal vesicle
  shoulder (and upper arm) 996.2
  sinus
    cavernous (*see also* Injury,
      intracranial) 854.0
    nasal 996.0
  skin NEC 996.9
  skull - *see* Fracture, skull
  soft tissue (severe) (of external sites) -
    see Wound, open
  spermatic cord - *see* Injury, internal,
    spermatic cord
  spinal (cord) 958.6
    with
      fracture, vertebra (conditions in
        805) - *code by* region under
        Fracture, vertebra, with
        spinal cord lesion
      open wound 958.7
    cervical 958.0
      with open wound 958.1
    dorsal 958.2
      with open wound 958.3
    late effect (any part) 958.9
    lumbar 958.2
      with open wound 958.3
    nerve (root) NEC - *see* Injury, nerve,
      spinal
    sacral 958.4
      with open wound 958.5
    thoracic 958.2
      with open wound 958.3
  spleen - *see* Injury, internal, spleen

Injury — *continued*
  sternal region 996.1
  stomach - *see* Injury, internal, stomach
  subconjunctival - *see* Injury, eye
  subcutaneous NEC 996.9
  submaxillary region 996.0
  submental region 996.0
  subungual
    fingers 996.5
    toes 996.7
  superficial 918

Note — The following fourth-digit subdi-
·visions are for use with categories 910–918:
  .0 Without mention of infection
  .1 Infected
  .9 Late effect

---

abdomen, abdominal (muscle) (wall)
    (and other part(s) of trunk)
    911
ankle (and hip) (and thigh) (and leg)
    (and knee) 916
anus (and other part(s) of trunk) 911
arm 918
  upper (and shoulder) 912
auditory canal (external) (meatus) (and
    other part(s) of face, neck, or
    scalp) 910
axilla (and upper arm) 912
back (and other part(s) of trunk) 911
breast (and other part(s) of trunk)
    911
brow (and other part(s) of face, neck,
    or scalp) 910
buttock (and other part(s) of trunk)
    911
canthus eye (and other part(s) of face,
    neck, or scalp) 910
cheek(s) (and other part(s) of face,
    neck, or scalp) 910
chest wall (and other part(s) of trunk)
    911
chin (and other part(s) of face, neck,
    or scalp) 910
clitoris (and other part(s) of trunk)
    911
conjunctiva (and other part(s) of face,
    neck, or scalp) 910
cornea (and other part(s) of face,
    neck, or scalp) 910
costal region (and other part(s) of
    trunk) 911
ear(s) (auricle) (canal) (drum)
    (external) (and other part(s) of
    face, neck, or scalp) 910

Injury — *continued*
  superficial — *continued*
    elbow (and forearm) (and wrist) 913
    epididymis (and other part(s) of trunk)
      911
    epigastric region (and other part(s) of
      trunk) 911
    epiglottis (and other part(s) of face,
      neck, or scalp) 910
    eye(s) (lid) (muscle) (globe) (and other
      part(s) of face, neck, or scalp)
      910
    face (and neck or scalp) (any part(s))
      910
    finger(s) (nail) (any) 915
    flank (and other part(s) of trunk) 911
    foot (phalanges) (and toe(s)) 917
    forearm (and elbow) (and wrist) 913
    forehead (and other part(s) of face,
      neck, or scalp) 910
    globe (eye) (and other part(s) of face,
      neck, or scalp) 910
    groin (and other part(s) of trunk) 911
    gum(s) (and other part(s) of face,
      neck, or scalp) 910
    hand(s) (except fingers alone) 914
    head (and other part(s) of face, neck,
      or scalp) 910
    heel (and toe) (and foot) 917
    hip (and thigh) (and leg) (and ankle)
      (and knee) 916
    iliac region (and other part(s) of trunk)
      911
    interscapular region (and other part(s)
      of trunk) 911
    iris (and other part(s) of face, neck, or
      scalp) 910
    knee (and hip) (and thigh) (and leg)
      (and ankle) 916
    labium (majus) (minus) (and other
      part(s) of trunk) 911
    lacrimal (apparatus) (gland) (sac) (and
      other part(s) of face, neck, or
      scalp) 910
    leg (upper) (lower) (and hip) (and
      thigh) (and ankle) (and knee)
      916
    lip(s) (and other part(s) of face, neck,
      or scalp) 910
    lower extremity (except foot) 916
    lumbar region (and other part(s) of
      trunk) 911
    malar region (and other part(s) of
      face, neck, or scalp) 910
    mastoid region (and other part(s) of
      face, neck, or scalp) 910

Injury — *continued*
  superficial — *continued*
    midthoracic region (and other part(s) of trunk) 911
    mouth (and other part(s) of face, neck, or scalp) 910
    multiple sites (not classifiable to the same three-digit category) 918
    nasal (septum) (and other part(s) of face, neck, or scalp) 910
    neck (and face or scalp) (any part(s)) 910
    nose (septum) (and other part(s) of face, neck, or scalp) 910
    occipital region (and other part(s) of face, neck, or scalp) 910
    orbital region (and other part(s) of face, neck, or scalp) 910
    palate (soft) (and other part(s) of face, neck, or scalp) 910
    parietal region (and other part(s) of face, neck, or scalp) 910
    penis (and other part(s) of trunk) 911
    perineum (and other part(s) of trunk) 911
    pharynx (and other part(s) of face, neck, or scalp) 910
    popliteal space (and ankle) (and hip) (and leg) (and thigh) 916
    prepuce (and other part(s) of trunk) 911
    pubic region (and other part(s) of trunk) 911
    pudenda (and other part(s) of trunk) 911
    sacral region (and other part(s) of trunk) 911
    salivary (ducts) (glands) (and other part(s) of face, neck, or scalp) 910
    scalp (and other part(s) of face or neck) 910
    scapular region (and upper arm) 912
    sclera (and other part(s) of face, neck, or scalp) 910
    scrotum (and other part(s) of trunk) 911
    shoulder (and upper arm) 912
    skin NEC 918
    specified site(s) NEC 918
    sternal region (and other part(s) of trunk) 911
    subconjunctival (and other part(s) of face, neck, or scalp) 910

Injury — *continued*
  superficial — *continued*
    subcutaneous NEC 918
    submaxillary region (and other part(s) of face, neck, or scalp) 910
    submental region (and other part(s) of face, neck, or scalp) 910
    supra-orbital (and other part(s) of face, neck, or scalp) 910
    supraclavicular fossa - *see* Injury superficial, neck
    temple (and other part(s) of face, neck, or scalp) 910
    temporal region (and other part(s) of face, neck, or scalp) 910
    testicle (and other part(s) of trunk) 911
    thigh (and hip) (and leg) (and ankle) (and knee) 916
    thorax, thoracic (external) (and other part(s) of trunk) 911
    throat (and other part(s) of face, neck, or scalp) 910
    thumb(s) (nail) 915
    toe(s) (nail) (subungual) (and foot) 917
    tongue (and other part(s) of face, neck, or scalp) 910
    tooth, teeth 521.2
    trunk (any part(s)) 911
    tunica vaginalis (and other part(s) of trunk) 911
    tympanum, tympanic membrane (and other part(s) of face, neck, or scalp) 910
    upper extremity NEC 918
    uvula (and other part(s) of face, neck, or scalp) 910
    vagina (and other part(s) of trunk) 911
    vulva (and other part(s) of trunk) 911
    wrist (and elbow) (and forearm) 913
  supraclavicular fossa 996.1
  supra-orbital 996.0
  surgical complication (external or internal site) 998.2
  symphysis pubis 996.1
  temple 996.0
  temporal region 996.0
  testicle 996.1
  thigh (and hip) 996.6
  thorax, thoracic (external) 996.1
    cavity - *see* Injury, internal, thorax
    internal - *see* Injury, internal, thorax
  throat 996.0

Injury—*continued*
thumb(s) (nail)   996.5
thymus - *see* Injury, internal, thymus
thyroid (gland)   996.0
toe (any) (nail)   996.7
tongue   996.0
tonsil   996.0
tooth NEC   873.7
trachea - *see* Injury, internal, trachea
trunk   996.1
tunica vaginalis   996.1
tympanum, tympanic membrane   996.0
ultraviolet rays - *see* Effect, adverse,
    ultraviolet
ureter - *see* Injury, internal, ureter
urethra (sphincter) - *see* Injury, internal,
    urethra
uterus - *see also* Injury, internal, uterus
    complicating delivery - *see*
        Obstetrical trauma
uvula   996.0
vagina   996.1
vas deferens - *see* Injury, internal, vas
    deferens
vesical (sphincter) - *see* Injury, internal,
    vesical
viscera (abdominal) - *see also* Injury,
    internal, viscera
    with fracture, pelvis - *see* Fracture,
        pelvis
vitreous (humor)   921
vulva   996.1
whiplash (cervical spine)   847.0
wrist (and elbow) (and forearm)   996.3
x-ray - *see* Effect, adverse, x-rays
Inoculation   Y02
    complication or reaction - *see*
        Complications, vaccination
    prophylactic   Y02
Insanity, insane (*see also* Psychosis)   299
    adolescent (*see also* Schizophrenia)
        295.9
    alternating   296.3
    circular   296.3
    climacteric   296.0
    confusional   299
    delusional   299
    menopausal   296.0
    puerperal   294.4
    senile   290.0
Insect
    bite - *see* Injury, superficial
    venomous, poisoning by   989.4
Insertion
    cord (umbilical) lateral or velamentous
        - *see* Placenta, abnormal

Insertion—*continued*
    placenta, vicious - *see* Placenta previa
Insolation   992.0
    meaning sunstroke   992.0
Insomnia   306.4
Inspiration
    food or foreign body (*see also*
        Asphyxia, food)   933
    mucus (*see also* Asphyxia, mucus)   933
        newborn (*see also* Aspiration, content
            of birth canal)   776.0
        vaginal (*see also* Aspiration, content
            of birth canal)   776.0
Instability
    emotional (excessive)   306.9
    joint (post-traumatic) (*see also* Disease,
        joint)   729.9
    lumbosacral   729.1
    sacro-iliac   726
    nervous   301.8
    personality (emotional)   301.5
    vasomotor   782.5
Instrumental
    birth
        fetus or newborn (*see also* Birth
            injury NEC)   772.9
    delivery
        injury by (*see also* Birth injury NEC)
            772.9
Insufficiency, insufficient
    accommodation   370.9
    adrenal (gland)   255.9
        primary   255.9
    anus   569.2
    aortic (valve) (*see also* Endocarditis,
        aortic)   395.9
        congenital   746.6
        syphilitic   093.9
    arterial   447
        basilar artery (*see also* Occlusion,
            precerebral artery)   432.9
        carotid arteries (*see also* Occlusion,
            precerebral artery)   432.9
        cerebral (*see also* Ischemia, cerebral)
            437.9
        peripheral   443.9
        vertebral artery (*see also* Occlusion,
            precerebral artery)   432.9
    arteriovenous   458.9
    biliary (*see also* Disease, gallbladder)
        576.9
    cardiac (*see also* Insufficiency,
        myocardial)   428
    cardiorenal - *see* Hypertension,
        cardiorenal

Insufficiency, insufficient — *continued*
cardiovascular - *see also* Ischemia,
   heart
  renal - *see* Hypertension, cardiorenal
cerebral (vascular) (*see also* Ischemia,
   cerebral) 437.9
cerebrovascular (*see also* Ischemia,
   cerebral) 437.9
circulatory NEC 458.9
  fetus or newborn 778.9
convergence 373.1
coronary (acute or subacute) 411.9
  with hypertensive disease (conditions
    in 400-404) 411.0
  chronic (*see also* Ischemia, heart)
    412.9
cortico-adrenal 255.1
dietary 269.9
divergence 373.0
food 994.2
gastro-esophageal 537.9
gonadal
  ovary 256.1
  testicle 257.1
heart - *see also* Insufficiency,
   myocardial
  fetus or newborn 778.9
  valve (*see also* Endocarditis) 424.9
    congenital 746.6
hepatic 573.9
kidney (*see also* Lesion, kidney) 593.2
liver 573.9
lung 519.2
  newborn (*see also* Asphyxia,
    newborn) 776.9
mental (congenital) (*see also*
   Retardation, mental) 315.9
mitral - *see also* Endocarditis, mitral
  congenital 746.6
muscle
  heart - *see* Insufficiency, myocardial
  ocular (*see also* Strabismus) 373.9
myocardial, myocardium 428
  with
    arteriosclerosis (conditions in 440)
      (*see also* Ischemia, heart)
      412.9
    hypertension (benign) (conditions in
      401) (*see also* Hypertension,
      heart) 402
    malignant (*see also*
      Hypertension, malignant
      with heart involvement)
      400.1
    rheumatic fever (conditions in 390)
      active 391.2

Insufficiency, insufficient — *continued*
myocardial, myocardium — *continued*
  with — *continued*
    rheumatic fever — *continued*
      active — *continued*
        with chorea 392.0
      inactive or quiescent (with
        chorea) 398
  arteriolar (*see also* Ischemia, heart)
    412.9
  arteriosclerotic (*see also* Ischemia,
    heart) 412.9
  congenital 746.8
  fetus or newborn 778.9
  hypertensive (*see also* Hypertension,
    heart) 402
    malignant (*see also* Hypertension,
      malignant with heart
      involvement) 400.1
  rheumatic 398
    active, acute, or subacute 391.2
  syphilitic 093.9
nourishment 994.2
organic 796.0
ovary 256.1
pancreatic 577.9
parathyroid (gland) 252.1
peripheral vascular 443.9
pituitary 253.1
placental - *see* Placenta, insufficiency
progressive pluriglandular 258.1
pulmonary 519.2
  newborn (*see also* Asphyxia,
    newborn) 776.9
  valve (*see also* Endocarditis,
    pulmonary) 424.9
  congenital 746.6
pyloric 537.9
renal (*see also* Lesion, kidney) 593.2
respiratory 796.0
  newborn (*see also* Asphyxia,
    newborn) 776.9
rotation - *see* Malrotation
suprarenal 255.9
tarso-orbital fascia, congenital 744.8
testicle 257.1
thyroid (gland) (acquired) 244
  congenital 243
tricuspid (*see also* Endocarditis,
    tricuspid) 397.0
  congenital 746.6
urethral sphincter 786.2
valve, valvular (heart) (*see also*
    Endocarditis) 424.9
vascular 458.9
  peripheral 443.9

Insufficiency, insufficient — *continued*
vascular — *continued*
renal (*see also* Hypertension, kidney)
403
venous 458.9
ventricular - *see* Insufficiency,
myocardial
Insufflation
meconium (*see also* Aspiration, content
of birth canal) 776.0
Insular - *see* condition
Insuloma 251
Insult
brain (*see also* Disease, cerebrovascular
NEC) 438.9
cerebral (*see also* Disease,
cerebrovascular NEC) 438.9
cerebrovascular (*see also* Disease,
cerebrovascular NEC) 438.9
vascular NEC (*see also* Disease,
cerebrovascular NEC) 438.9
Intelligence, borderline - *see* Retardation,
mental, borderline
Intemperance - *see* Alcoholism
Intermenstrual
bleeding 626.6
hemorrhage 626.6
pain(s) 626.3
Intermittent - *see* condition
Internal - *see* condition
Interruption
bundle of His (*see also* Block, heart)
427.3
Interstitial - *see* condition
Intertrigo 709.9
Intervertebral disc - *see* condition
Intestine, intestinal - *see* condition
Intolerance
disaccharide (hereditary) 271.8
fat NEC 269.0
foods NEC 269.9
fructose (hereditary) 271.3
lactose (hereditary) (infantile) 271.8
lysine 270.8
milk NEC 269.9
starch NEC 269.0
Intoxicated NEC 303.9
Intoxication
acid 788.0
acute NEC 303.9
alcoholic (acute) (*see also* Alcoholism)
303.9
alimentary canal 561
chronic, specified drug or chemical -
see listing under Dependence, if
not listed, see Table of adverse
effects

Intoxication — *continued*
drug or chemical - *see* Table of adverse
effects
enteric - *see* Intoxication, intestinal
food - *see* Poisoning, food
gastro-intestinal 561
intestinal 569.9
due to putrefaction of food 005.9
methyl alcohol (*see also* Alcoholism)
303.9
pathologic 291.9
septic
with
abortion - *see* Abortion, by type,
with sepsis
ectopic gestation - *see* categories
631.0-631.3
general - *see* Septicemia
puerperal, postpartum, childbirth
670
serum (prophylactic) (therapeutic)
999.5
uremic - *see* Uremia
urinary 596.9
water 788.0
Intracranial - *see* condition
Intrahepatic gallbladder 751.6
Intraligamentous - *see also* condition
pregnancy - *see* Pregnancy, ectopic
Intrathoracic - *see also* condition
kidney 753.3
stomach - *see* Hernia, diaphragm
Intra-uterine - *see also* condition
death of fetus, complicating pregnancy
(undelivered) 634.2
Intraventricular - *see* condition
Intrinsic deformity - *see* Deformity
Intumescence
lens (eye) (*see also* Cataract) 374.9
Intussusception (colon) (intestine) (rectum)
560.0
with hernia - *see* Hernia, by site, with
obstruction
appendix 543
congenital 751.4
ureter 593.5
Invagination
colon or intestine 560.0
with hernia - *see* Hernia, by site, with
obstruction
Invalid (since birth) 796.0
Invalidism (chronic) 796.0
Inversion
albumin-globulin (A-G) ratio 275.9
bladder 596.9
cecum (*see also* Intussusception)
560.0

Inversion—*continued*
  cervix (*see also* Malposition, uterus)
    624.9
  nipple 611.9
    congenital 757.2
    puerperal, postpartum 678
  optic papilla 744.8
  organ or site, congenital NEC - *see*
    Anomaly, specified type NEC
  sleep rhythm 780.6
  testis (congenital) 752.1
  uterus (postinfectional) (postpartal, old)
    (*see also* Malposition, uterus)
    624.9
    during delivery - *see* Obstetrical
      trauma
  vagina 623.9
Investigation
  allergens Y01
  negative findings (*see also* Examination)
    Y00.9
Inviability 777
Involuntary movement, abnormal 780.3
Involution, involutional - *see also*
  condition
  breast, cystic 610
  ovary, senile 615.9
I.Q.
  under 20 - *see* Retardation, mental,
    profound
  20-35 - *see* Retardation, mental, severe
  36-51 - *see* Retardation, mental,
    moderate
  52-67 - *see* Retardation, mental, mild
  68-85 - *see* Retardation, mental,
    borderline
Irideremia 744.5
Iridis
  rubeosis 378.6
Iridochoroiditis 364
Iridocyclitis (granulomatous)
    (nongranulomatous) 364
  gonococcal 098.2
Iridocyclochoroiditis 364
Iridodonesis 378.6
Iridoplegia (complete) (partial) (reflex)
  378.6
Iris - *see* condition
Iritis 364
  diabetic - *see* category 250
  due to
    allergy 364
    herpes simplex 054
    leprosy 030.9
  endogenous 364
  gonococcal 098.2

Iritis—*continued*
  gouty 274
  hypopyon 364
  papulosa 095
  rheumatic 364
  sympathetic 364
  syphilitic (late) 095
    congenital 090.0
  tuberculous 017.2
    late effect or sequela 019.9
Iron
  deficiency anemia 280
  metabolism disease 279
  storage disease 273.2
Iron-miner lung 516.0
Irradiated
  enamel (tooth, teeth) 521.8
Irradiation
  effects, adverse - *see* Effect, adverse,
    radiation
Irreducible, irreducibility - *see also*
    condition
  bubonocele 552
  enterocele 553.9
  epigastrocele 553.2
  epiplocele 553.9
  exomphalos 553.1
  hernia (*see also* Hernia, by site, with
    obstruction) 553.9
  merocele 553.0
  omentocele 553.9
  omphalocele 553.1
  rupture (meaning hernia) (*see also*
    Hernia, by site, with obstruction)
    553.9
  sarco-epiplocele 553.9
  sarco-epiplomphalocele 553.1
Irrefraction
  diabetic - *see* category 250
Irregular, irregularity
  action, heart (*see also* Action, heart,
    irregular) 427.9
  alveolar process 525.9
  breathing 783.2
  colon 569.9
  contour of cornea 744.8
  dentin in pulp 522.3
  menstruation (cause unknown) 626.5
  pupil 378.6
  respiratory 783.2
  septum (nasal) 504
  shape, organ or site, congenital NEC -
    see Distortion
  vertebra 723.9
Irritability
  bladder 596.9

Irritability—*continued*
  bowel 564.1
  bronchial (*see also* Bronchitis) 490
  colon 564.1
    psychogenic 305.5
  duodenum 564.9
  heart 305.3
  ileum 564.9
  jejunum 564.9
  myocardium 305.3
  rectum 564.9
  stomach 536.9
    psychogenic 305.5
  sympathetic 358.9
  urethra 599.9
Irritable - *see* Irritability
Irritation
  anus 569.2
  bladder 596.9
  brachial plexus 357.0
  brain (traumatic) (*see also* Injury,
      intracranial) 854.0
    by scar tissue 854.9
  bronchial (*see also* Bronchitis) 490
  cerebral (traumatic) (*see also* Injury,
      intracranial) 854.0
    nontraumatic - *see* Encephalitis
  cervical plexus 357.0
  cervix (*see also* Cervicitis) 620.9
  choroid, sympathetic 365
  cranial nerve, unqualified (*see also*
      Neuritis, cranial nerve) 355.0
  digestive tract 536.9
  duodenal bulb 537.9
  gastric 536.9
    psychogenic 305.5
  gastro-intestinal (tract) 536.9
    psychogenic 305.5
  globe, sympathetic 369.9
  intestinal 564.1
  labyrinth 387.9
  lumbosacral plexus 357.9
  meninges (traumatic) (*see also* Injury,
      intracranial) 854.0
    nontraumatic - *see* Meningitis
  nerve - *see* Compression, nerve
  nervous 790.0
  nose 508.9
  optic nerve (sympathetic) 367
  penis 607.9
  perineum NEC 709.9
  peripheral
    autonomic nervous system 358.9
    nerve - *see* Compression, nerve
  peritoneum (*see also* Peritonitis) 567.9
  pharynx 508.9

Irritation—*continued*
  spinal (cord) (traumatic) - *see also*
      Injury, spinal, by region
    nerve - *see also* Compression, nerve
        root NEC 728.9
      traumatic - *see* Injury, nerve, spinal
      nontraumatic - *see* Myelitis
  stomach 536.9
    psychogenic 305.5
  sympathetic nerve NEC 358.9
  uvea (sympathetic) 366
  vagina 629.9
Ischemia, ischemic 458.9
  brain - *see also* Ischemia, cerebral
    recurrent focal (*see also* Ischemia,
        cerebral, transient) 435.9
  cardiac (*see also* Ischemia, heart)
      412.9
  cerebral (arteriosclerotic) (generalized)
      437.9
    with hypertension (benign) (conditions
        in 401) 437.0
      malignant (*see also* Hypertension,
          malignant with
          cerebrovascular
          involvement) 400.2
    intermittent 435.9
      with hypertension (benign)
          (conditions in 401) 435.0
        malignant (*see also*
            Hypertension, malignant
            with cerebrovascular
            involvement) 400.2
    puerperal, postpartum, childbirth
        674
    transient 435.9
      with hypertension (benign)
          (conditions in 401) 435.0
        malignant (*see also*
            Hypertension, malignant
            with cerebrovascular
            involvement) 400.2
  coronary (*see also* Ischemia, heart)
      412.9
  heart (chronic or with a stated duration
      of over 8 weeks) 412.9
    with hypertensive disease (conditions
        in 400-404) 412.0
    acute or with a stated duration of 8
        weeks or less 410.9
      with hypertensive disease
          (conditions in 400-404)
          410.0
  intestine 569.9
  myocardial (*see also* Ischemia, heart)
      412.9

Ischemia, ischemic — *continued*
  retina, retinal 377.0
  subendocardial (*see also* Insufficiency,
    coronary) 411.9
Ischial spine - *see* condition
Ischialgia (*see also* Sciatica) 353
Ischiopagus 759.1
Ischium, ischial - *see* condition
Ischuria 786.5
Islands of
  parotid tissue in
    lymph nodes 750.8
    neck structures 750.8
  submaxillary glands in
    fascia 750.8
    lymph nodes 750.8
    neck muscles 750.8
Islet cell tumor, pancreas 251
  malignant 157.9
Itch (*see also* Pruritus) 698.9
  bakers' 692.9
  barbers' 110.0
  bricklayers' 692.9
  cheese 133.9
  clam digger 120.3
  coolie 126.9
  copra 133.9

Itch — *continued*
  Cuban 050.1
  dew 126.9
  dhobie 110.9
  filarial (*see also* Infestation, filarial)
    125.9
  grain 133.9
  grocers' 133.9
  ground 126.9
  harvest 133.9
  jock 110.9
  Malabar - *see* Dermatophytosis
  meaning scabies 133.0
  Norwegian 133.0
  poultrymen's 133.9
  sarcoptic 133.0
  scrub 134.2
  seven-year 133.0
  straw 133.9
  swimmers' 120.3
  washerwomen's 692.4
  water 120.3
  winter 698.9
Itching (*see also* Pruritus) 698.9
Ixodes 133.9
Ixodiasis 133.9

J

Jaccoud's nodular fibrositis, chronic
    712.5
Jackson's
    membrane   751.1
    paralysis or syndrome   344.9
    veil   751.1
Jacksonian
    epilepsy - *see* Epilepsy, jacksonian
    seizures (focal) - *see* Epilepsy,
        jacksonian
Jacob's ulcer - *see* Neoplasm, skin,
        malignant
Jacquet's dermatitis   692.9
Jadassohn-Tieche nevus   757.1
Jadassohn's disease   695.0
Jaffe-Lichtenstein syndrome   723.9
Jakob-Creutzfeldt disease   333.9
    with dementia   290.1
Jaksch-Luzet disease   285.8
Janet's disease   300.8
Janiceps   759.1
Jansky-Bielschowsky amaurotic familial
        idiocy   333.0
Jaundice (yellow)   785.2
    acholuric (familial) (splenomegalic) (*see*
            also Spherocytosis)   282.0
        acquired   283.9
        breast-milk   778.9
    catarrhal (acute)   070
        chronic - *see* Cirrhosis, postnecrotic
        epidemic - *see* Jaundice, epidemic
    chronic idiopathic   273.5
    epidemic (catarrhal)   070
        leptospiral   100.0
        spirochetal   100.0
    febrile (acute)   070
        leptospiral   100.0
        spirochetal   100.0
    fetus or newborn NEC   778.9
    from injection, inoculation or
            transfusion (blood) (plasma)
            (serum) (other substance) for
            immunization or other
            prophylactic or therapeutic
            purpose (onset within 8 months
            after administration)   999.2
    hematogenous   283.9
        fetus or newborn (*see also* Disease,
            hemolytic)   775.9
    hemolytic (acquired)   283.9
        congenital (*see also* Spherocytosis)
            282.0

Jaundice (yellow) — *continued*
    hemolytic (acquired) — *continued*
        fetus or newborn (*see also* Disease,
            hemolytic)   775.9
        hemorrhagic (acute)   100.0
            leptospiral   100.0
            newborn   778.2
            spirochetal   100.0
        hepato-cellular   573.9
        homologous (serum)   999.2
        idiopathic
            chronic   273.5
        infectious (acute) (subacute)   070
            leptospiral   100.0
            spirochetal   100.0
        leptospiral   100.0
        malignant (*see also* Necrosis, liver)
            570
        newborn (physiological) NEC   778.9
            with incompatibility blood (group) -
                see Disease, hemolytic
        nonfamilial, newborn (*see also* Disease,
            hemolytic)   775.9
            with kernicterus or nervous affection
                774.9
        nonhemolytic
            congenital familial (Gilbert)   273.5
        nuclear
            newborn (*see also* Disease,
                hemolytic, by type, with
                kernicterus)   774.9
        obstructive (*see also* Obstruction,
            gallbladder)   576.0
        post-immunization   999.2
        post-transfusion   999.2
        regurgitation (*see also* Obstruction,
            gallbladder)   576.0
        serum (homologous) (prophylactic)
            (therapeutic)   999.2
        spirochetal (hemorrhagic)   100.0
        symptomatic   785.2
            newborn   778.9
Jaw - *see* condition
Jaw-winking phenomenon   743.8
Jealousy, childhood   308
Jejunitis - *see* Enteritis
Jejunum, jejunal - *see* condition
Jensen's disease   365
Jerks, myoclonic   780.3
Jigger disease   134.2

Joint - *see also* condition
  mice - *see* Loose bodies in joint
  sinus to bone (*see also* Disease, joint)
    729.9
Jungling's disease   135

Justo minor pelvis
  complicating delivery - *see* Deformity,
    pelvis, complicating delivery
  noted during pregnancy (undelivered)
    634.9
Juvenile - *see* condition

K

Keratolysis exfoliativa (congenital) 757.2
  acquired 705.9
  neonatorum 695.9
Keratoma 701.1
  congenital 757.2
  malignum congenitale 757.2
  palmaris and plantaris hereditarium

    757.2
  senile 702
Keratomalacia 378.4
  vitamin A deficiency 260.1
Keratomegaly 744.8
Keratomycosis 111.1
  nigricans palmaris 111.1
Keratopathy 378.4
  band (see also Keratitis) 363.9
  bullous (see also Keratitis) 363.9
Keratoscleritis, tuberculous 017.2
  late effect or sequela 019.9
Keratosis 701.1
  arsenical 692.4
  blenorrhagica 701.1
    gonococcal 098.8
  congenital (any type) 757.2
  female genital (external) 629.9
  follicular, vitamin A deficiency 260.8
  follicularis 757.2
    acquired 701.1
    congenita (acneiformis) (Siemen's)
      757.2
    spinulosa (decalvans) 757.2
  gonococcal 098.8
  larynx 508.3
  male genital (external) 607.9
  nigricans 701.1
    congenital 757.2
  obturans 387.9
  palmaris et plantaris (symmetrical)
    757.2
  pharyngeus 508.9
  pilaris 757.2
    acquired 701.1
  punctata (palmaris et plantaris) 701.1
  scrotal and penile 607.9
  seborrheic 216.0
    breast 217
    external area or site NEC 216.0
    genital organ NEC - code as
      Neoplasm, benign, by site
    scrotum 216.0
  senile 702
  suprafollicularis 757.2
  tonsillaris 508.9
  vegetans 757.2
Kerato-uveitis 366
Keraunoparalysis 994.0

Kerion 110.0
  celsi 110.0
Kernicterus of newborn (see also Disease,
    hemolytic, by type, with
    kernicterus) 774.9
  not due to hemolytic disease 778.9
Keto-acidosis 788.0
  diabetic 250.0
Ketonuria 789.6
Ketosis 788.0
  diabetic 250.0
Kidney - see condition
Kienbock's
  disease 722.2
  osteochondrosis 722.2
Kimmelstiel(-Wilson) disease - see
    category 250
Kink
  appendix 543
  artery 447
  cystic duct, congenital 751.5
  ileum or intestine (see also Obstruction,
    intestine) 560.9
  Lane's (see also Obstruction, intestine)
    560.9
  organ or site, congenital NEC - see
    Anomaly, specified type NEC
  ureter (pelvic junction) 593.3
    congenital 753.2
  vein(s) 458.9
    caval 458.1

Kinking hair (acquired) 704
Klebs' disease (see also Nephritis) 583
Klein-Wardenburg syndrome 270.8
Kleine-Levin syndrome 347.9
Kleptomania 300.3
Klinefelter's syndrome 759.5
Klippel-Feil syndrome 756.2
Klippel-Trenaunay syndrome 759.8
Klippel's disease 715
Klumpke(-Dejerine) palsy, paralysis (birth)
    (newborn) (see also Birth injury,
    bone or nerve) 772.2
Knee - see condition
Knifegrinders' rot 010
Knock knee (acquired) 738.5
  congenital 755.7
Knot (true), umbilical cord - see
    Complications, umbilical cord
Knots, surfer 918.0
Knotting of hair 704
Koch-Weeks' conjunctivitis 360
Koch's
  infection (see also Tuberculosis,
    pulmonary) 011.9
  relapsing fever 088.9

Koebner's disease 757.2
Kohler's disease 722.2
Koilonychia 703.9
  congenital 757.4
Kojevnikov's, Kojewnikoff's epilepsy
    345.2
Koniophthisis 010
Koplik's spots 055
Kopp's asthma 254
Korsakoff's disease, psychosis, or
    syndrome (alcoholic) 291.1
  nonalcoholic 299
Korsakov's - *see* Korsakoff's
Korsakow's - *see* Korsakoff's
Krabbe's disease 333.1
Kraepelin-Morel disease (*see also*
    Schizophrenia) 295.9
Kraft-Weber-Dimitri disease 759.8
Kraurosis
  ani 569.2
  penis 607.0
  vagina 629.2
  vulva 629.2
Kreotoxism - *see* Poisoning, food
Krompecher's tumor - *see* Neoplasm,
    skin, malignant
Krukenberg's
  spindle 378.6
  tumor (malignant) (secondary) 198.9
Kuf's disease 333.0

Kulchistzky's cell carcinoma 258.9
Kummell's disease or spondylitis 713.2
Kundrat's disease 200.1
Kunekune - *see* Dermatophytosis
Kunkel syndrome 573.0
Kuru 347.9
Kussmaul's
  coma 250.0
  disease 446.0
Kwashiorkor (marasmus type) 267
Kyasanur Forest disease 067.2
Kyphoscoliosis, kyphoscoliotic (acquired)
    735.2
  congenital 756.2
  heart (disease) 426
  late effect of rickets 265.1
  tuberculous 015.0
    late effect or sequela 019.3
Kyphosis, kyphotic (adolescent postural)
      (acquired) 735.1
  congenital 756.2
  late effect of
    acute poliomyelitis 044
    rickets 265.1
  Morquio-Brailsford type (spinal) 273.8
  pelvis 735.1
  syphilitic, congenital 090.5
  tuberculous 015.0
    late effect or sequela 019.3
Kyrle's disease 704

L

La grippe - *see* Influenza
Labia, labium - *see* condition
Labiated hymen   752.6
Labile
    blood pressure   458.9
    vasomotor system   443.9
Labioglossal paralysis   348.1
Labium leporinum   749.1
    with cleft palate   749.2
Labor (*see also* Delivery)   650
    abnormal NEC   661.9
        fetus or newborn - *see* categories
            768.0-768.9
    desultory, complicating delivery   657.9
        fetus or newborn - *see* categories
            767.0-767.9
    difficult, affecting fetus or newborn
        with
            abnormality of bones, organs or
                tissues of pelvis - *see*
                categories 764.0-764.9
            abnormality of forces of labor - *see*
                categories 767.0-767.9
            disproportion, fetopelvic - *see*
                categories 765.0-765.9
            with abnormality of bones,
                organs or tissues of pelvis
                - *see* categories 764.0-
                764.9
            malposition of fetus - *see* categories
                766.0-766.9
            other and unspecified complications
                - *see* categories 768.0-768.9
    false (undelivered)   634.7
    forced or induced
        fetus or newborn (*see also* Birth
            injury NEC)   772.9
    irregular, complicating delivery   657.9
        fetus or newborn - *see* categories
            767.0-767.9
    missed (at or near term) (undelivered)
        634.2
    obstructed, complicating delivery
        657.9
        fetus or newborn - *see* categories
            768.0-768.9
    pains, spurious (undelivered)   634.7
    precipitate, complicating delivery
        661.1
        fetus or newborn - *see* categories
            767.0-767.9

Labor—*continued*
    premature
        with delivery
            dead fetus
                less than 28 weeks gestation -
                    see Abortion, by type
                28 weeks or more gestation - *see*
                    Delivery
            liveborn infant - *see* Delivery
        prolonged or protracted, complicating
            delivery   657.9
        fetus or newborn - *see* categories
            768.0-768.9
    undelivered   634.7
Labored breathing (*see also*
    Hyperventilation)   783.2
Labyrinthitis (circumscribed) (destructive)
    (diffuse) (inner ear) (latent)
    (purulent) (suppurative)   384.0
    syphilitic   095
Laceration - *see also* Wound, open
    accidental, complicating surgery   998.2

    Achilles tendon   845.0
        with open wound   892.2
    anus (sphincter) - *see also* Injury,
        internal, anus
        complicating delivery (*see also*
            Laceration, perineum,
            complicating delivery)   658.2
        nontraumatic, nonpuerperal   565.0
    bladder (urinary), complicating delivery
        - *see* Obstetrical trauma
    brain (any part) (cortex) (membrane)
        (*see also* Laceration, cerebral)
        851.0
        during birth (*see also* Birth injury,
            brain)   772.0
    capsule, joint - *see* Sprain
    causing eversion of cervix uteri (old)
        621.4
    cerebellum (*see also* Laceration,
        cerebral)   851.0
    cerebral (without skull fracture)   851.0
        with open intracranial wound   851.1
        during birth (*see also* Birth injury,
            brain)   772.0
        late effect   851.9
    cervix (uteri)
        complicating delivery   660.1
        fetus or newborn - *see* categories
            768.0-768.9

Laceration — *continued*
  cervix (uteri) — *continued*
    nonpuerperal, nontraumatic   621.4
    old (postpartal)   621.4
  chordae heart - *see* Disease, heart
  cortex (cerebral) (*see also* Laceration,
        cerebral)   851.0
  fourchette, complicating delivery (*see
        also* Laceration, perineum,
        complicating delivery)   658.0
  hernial sac - *see* Hernia, by site
  internal organ (abdomen, chest, or
        pelvis) - *see* Injury, internal, by
        site
  ligament - *see* Sprain
  meninges (*see also* Laceration, cerebral)
        851.0
  meniscus (lateral) (medial) (knee)
        (current injury) (*see also*
        Dislocation, knee)   836.0
    late effect   836.9
    old   724.5
    site other than knee - code as Sprain
    old - *see* category 724
  muscle - *see* Sprain
  nerve - *see* Injury, nerve, by site
  pelvic
    floor
      complicating delivery (*see also*
            Laceration, perineum,
            complicating delivery)
            658.1
      nonpuerperal   629.6
      old (postpartal)   629.6
    organ NEC, complicating delivery -
          see Obstetrical trauma
  perineum   629.6
    complicating delivery (without other
          laceration)   658.9
      fetus or newborn - *see* categories
            768.0-768.9
      first degree (fourchette) (hymen)
            (vagina) (vulva)   658.0
      fourth degree   658.2
      second degree (pelvic floor)
            (perineal muscles) (vaginal,
            deep)   658.1
      third degree (anal sphincter)
            (rectovaginal septum)   658.2
    nonpuerperal   629.6
    old (postpartal)   629.6
  peritoneum, complicating delivery - *see*
        Obstetrical trauma

Laceration — *continued*
  rectovaginal (septum)
    complicating delivery (*see also*
          Laceration, perineum,
          complicating delivery)   658.2
    nonpuerperal   629.6
    old (postpartal)   629.6
  spinal cord (meninges) - *see also* Injury,
        spinal, by region
    during birth (*see also* Birth injury,
          spinal cord)   772.1
    fetus or newborn (*see also* Birth
          injury, spinal cord)   772.1
  tentorium cerebelli (*see also* Laceration,
        cerebral)   851.0
    during birth (*see also* Birth injury,
          brain)   772.0
  urethra
    complicating delivery   660.0
      fetus or newborn - *see* categories
            768.0-768.9
    nonpuerperal, nontraumatic   599.9
  uterus
    complicating delivery - *see*
          Obstetrical trauma
    nonpuerperal, nontraumatic   625.9
    old (postpartal)   625.9
  vagina
    complicating delivery (*see also*
          Laceration, perineum,
          complicating delivery)   658.0
    nonpuerperal, nontraumatic   629.6
    old (postpartal)   629.6
  valve, heart - *see* Endocarditis
  vulva
    complicating delivery (*see also*
          Laceration, perineum,
          complicating delivery)   658.0
    nonpuerperal, nontraumatic   629.6
    old (postpartal)   629.6
Lachrymal - *see* condition
Lachrymonasal duct - *see* condition
Lack of
  appetite (*see also* Anorexia)   784.0
  care (at or after birth) (infant)   994.9
  development - *see* Hypoplasia
  food   994.2
  medical attention   796.0
  memory (*see also* Amnesia)   780.7
  ovulation   615.9
  water   994.3
Lacrimal - *see* condition
Lacrimation, eye   378.3
Lacrimonasal duct - *see* condition

Lactation, lactating (breast) (puerperal, postpartum)
  defective 678
  disorders 678
  excessive 678
  failed 678
  mastitis 678
  nonpuerperal 611.9
Lactosuria 271.8
Lacunar skull 756.0
Laennec's cirrhosis (alcoholic) 571.0
  nonalcoholic - *see* Cirrhosis, portal
Lafora's disease 331.2
Lag, lid (nervous) 378.2
Lagleyze-von Hippel disease 224
Lagophthalmos (eyelid) (nervous) 378.2
  keratitis (*see also* Keratitis) 363.9
Lalling 306.0
Lambliasis 007.1
Lame back 728.9
Lancereaux's diabetes - *see* category 250
Landouzy-Dejerine dystrophy or
    fascioscapulohumeral atrophy
    330.3
Landry's disease or paralysis 354
Lane's
  disease 569.9
  kink (*see also* Obstruction, intestine)
    560.9
Langdon Down's syndrome 759.3
Laparotomy for ectopic gestation
  fetus or newborn (*see also* Birth injury
    NEC) 772.9
Lardaceous
  degeneration (any site) 276
  kidney 276
  liver 276
Large
  ear 745.2
  fetus
    complicating delivery 655
    fetus or newborn - *see* categories
      765.0-765.9
  physiological cup 744.8
  waxy liver 276
  white kidney (*see also* Nephrosis) 581
Larsen-Johansson disease 722.2
Larva migrans
  cutaneous NEC 126.8
  of Diptera in vitreous 128.0
  visceral NEC 128.0
Laryngismus (stridulus) 508.3
  congenital 748.3
  diphtheric 032

Laryngitis (acute) (croupous) (edematous)
    (fibrinous) (gangrenous) (infective)
    (infiltrative) (malignant)
    (membranous) (obstructive)
    (phlegmonous) (pneumococcal)
    (pseudomembranous) (septic)
    (subglottic) (suppurative)
    (ulcerative) (viral) (with tracheitis)
    464
  with
    influenza, flu, or grippe 472
  atrophic 506
  Borrelia vincenti 101
  catarrhal 506
  chronic 506
  diphtheritic 032
  H. influenzae 464
  hypertrophic 506
  influenzal 472
  pachydermic 508.3
  sicca 506
  spasmodic 508.3
    acute 464
  streptococcal 034.0
  stridulous 508.3
  syphilitic 095
    congenital 090.5
  tuberculous 012.3
    with pneumoconiosis (conditions in
      515) 010
  late effect or sequela 019.0
  Vincent's 101
Laryngocele (congenital) (ventricular)
    748.3
Laryngofissure 508.3
Laryngoplegia 508.0
Laryngoptosis 508.3
Laryngospasm 508.3
Laryngostenosis 508.3
Laryngotracheitis (acute) (infectional) (*see
    also* Laryngitis) 464
Laryngotracheobronchiolitis (*see also*
    Bronchitis) 490
  acute 466
Laryngotracheobronchitis (*see also*
    Bronchitis) 490
  acute 466
  chronic 491
Laryngotracheobronchopneumonitis - *see*
    Pneumonia, broncho
Larynx, laryngeal - *see* condition
Lasegue's disease 306.9
Lassitude - *see* Weakness
Late, latent - *see* condition
Laterocession - *see* Lateroversion
Lateroflexion - *see* Lateroversion

Lateroversion
  cervix - *see* Lateroversion, uterus
  uterus, uterine (cervix) (postinfectional)
        (postpartal, old)   624.1
    complicating
      delivery   657.9
        fetus or newborn - *see* categories
            764.0-764.9
        pregnancy (undelivered)   634.9
    congenital   752.5
    pregnant or gravid (undelivered)
        634.9
Lathyrism   988.2
Launois' syndrome   253.0
Laurell and Ericson's disease   273.8
Laurence-Moon-Biedl syndrome   759.8
Lax, laxity - *see also* Relaxation
  skin (acquired)   701.9
    congenital   757.2
Lead miner's lung   516.0
Leakage
  amniotic fluid (undelivered)   634.4
    complicating delivery   661.0
      fetus or newborn - *see* categories
          768.0-768.9
Leaky heart - *see* Endocarditis
Learning defect, specific (reading)
        (mathematics) (strephosymbolia)
        306.1
Leatherbottle stomach   151.9
Leber's optic atrophy (congenital)   377.9
Lederer's anemia   283.0
Leeches (aquatic) (land)   134.3
Leg - *see* condition
Legg-Calve-Perthes disease, syndrome, or
        osteochondrosis   722.1
Legg-Perthes
  disease   722.1
  osteochondrosis   722.1
Leiner's disease   695.9
Leiofibromyoma (*see also* Neoplasm,
        connective tissue, benign)   215
  uterus   218
 .Leiomyoma (*see also* Neoplasm,
        connective tissue, benign)   215
  prostate (polypoid)   600
  skin (*see also* Dermatofibroma)   216.8
  uterus   218
Leiomyomata, uterus   218
Leiomyosarcoma (*see also* Neoplasm,
        connective tissue, malignant)
        171.9
Leishmaniasis   085.9
  American   085.2
  Brazilian   085.2
  cutaneous   085.1
  dermal   085.1

Leishmaniasis—*continued*
  dermal—*continued*
    post-kala-azar   085.0
  infantile   085.0
  Mediterranean   085.0
  mucocutaneous   085.2
  naso-oral   085.2
  nasopharyngeal   085.2
  visceral   085.0
Leishmanoid, dermal   085.1
  post-kala-azar   085.0
Lengthening, leg   738.5
Lens - *see* condition
Lenticonus (anterior) (posterior)
        (congenital)   744.8
Lenticular degeneration, progressive
        273.3
Lentiglobus (posterior) (congenital)   744.8
Lentigo (congenital)   709.9
  maligna   702
Leontiasis
  ossium   723.4
  syphilitic   095
    congenital   090.5
Lepothrix   111.8
Lepra   030.9
  Willan's   696.1
Leprechaunism   258.1
Leprosy   030.9
  anesthetic   030.1
  beriberi   030.1
  borderline   030.3
  cornea   030.9
  dimorphous (lepromatous) (tuberculoid)
        030.3
  indeterminate   030.2
  leonine   030.0
  lepromatous   030.0
  macular (early) (neuritic) (simple)
        030.2
  maculo-anesthetic   030.1
  mixed   030.0
  neuro   030.1
  nodular   030.0
  primary neuritic   030.3
  tubercular   030.1
  tuberculoid (major and minor)   030.1
Leptocytosis, hereditary (*see also*
        Thalassemia)   282.4
Leptomeningitis (circumscribed) (chronic)
        (hemorrhagic) (nonsuppurative)
        (purulent) (suppurative) (*see also*
        Meningitis)   320.9
Leptomeningopathy (*see also* Meningitis)
        320.9
Leptospiral - *see* condition
Leptospirochetal - *see* condition

Leptospirosis 100.9
  canicula 100.8
  grippotyphosa 100.8
  icterohemorrhagica 100.0
  pomona 100.8
Leptothricosis 117.9
  conjunctiva 117.9
  cornea 117.9
Leptothrix infestation 117.9
Leriche's syndrome 444.0
Lermoyez's syndrome 389.9
Lesbianism 302.0
Lesion
  alveolar process 525.9
  anorectal 569.2
  aortic (valve) - see Endocarditis, aortic
  auditory nerve 387.9
  basal ganglion 347.9
  bile duct (see also Disease, gallbladder)
      576.9
  bone 723.9
  brain 347.9
    congenital 743.9
    vascular (see also Disease,
        cerebrovascular NEC) 438.9
    degenerative (see also Ischemia,
        cerebral) 437.9
  buccal 528.9
  calcified - see Calcification
  canthus 378.2
  carate - see Pinta, lesions
  cardia 537.9
  cardiac - see also Disease, heart
    congenital 746.9
    valvular - see Endocarditis
  cauda equina 349.9
  cecum 569.9
  cerebral - see Lesion, brain
  cerebrovascular (see also Disease,
      cerebrovascular NEC) 438.9
    degenerative (see also Ischemia,
        cerebral) 437.9
  chiasmal 377.6
  chorda tympani 350
  coin, lung 519.2
  colon 569.9
  congenital - see Anomaly
  conjunctiva 378.3
  coronary artery (see also Ischemia,
      heart) 412.9
  cranial nerve (see also Atrophy, nerve,
      cranial) 356
  cystic - see Cyst
  degenerative - see Degeneration
  duodenum 537.9
  eyelid 378.2
  gasserian ganglion 356

Lesion—continued
  gastric 537.9
  gastroduodenal 537.9
  gastro-intestinal 569.9
  heart (organic) - see Disease, heart
  helix (ear) 709.9
  hyperkeratotic (see also
      Hyperkeratosis) 701.1
  hypopharynx 508.9
  hypothalamic 347.9
  ileocecal (coil) 569.9
  ileum 569.9
  in continuity - see Injury, nerve, by site
  inflammatory - see Inflammation
  intestine 569.9
  intracerebral - see Lesion, brain
  intrachiasmal (optic) 377.6
  joint (see also Disease, joint) 729.9
    sacro-iliac (old) 726
  keratotic - see Keratosis
  kidney 593.2
    with
      hypertension, malignant (see also
          Hypertension, malignant
          with renal involvement)
          400.3
  laryngeal nerve (recurrent) 356
  lip 528.5
  liver 573.9
  lung (coin) 519.2
  mitral - see Endocarditis, mitral
  motor cortex 347.9
  nerve (see also Neuropathy) 357.9
  nervous system
    congenital 743.9
  nose (internal) 508.9
  obstructive - see Obstruction
  organ or site NEC - see Disease, by
      site
  osteolytic 723.9
  paramacular - see Opacity, cornea
  peptic 537.9
  perirectal 569.2
  pigmented (skin) 709.9
  pinta - see Pinta, lesions
  polypoid - see Polyp
  prechiasmal (optic) 377.6
  primary - see also Syphilis, primary
    carate 103.0
    pinta 103.0
    yaws 102.0
  pulmonary 519.2
    valve (see also Endocarditis,
        pulmonary) 424.9
  pylorus 537.9
  radiation - see Effect, adverse, radiation

Lesion—*continued*
  radium - *see* Effect, adverse,
      radioactive substance
  rectosigmoid 569.2
  retina, retinal 377.4
    vascular 377.0
  sacro-iliac (joint) (old) 726
  salivary gland 527.9
    benign lympho-epithelial 527.8
  secondary - *see* Syphilis, secondary
  sigmoid 569.9
  sinus - *see* Sinusitis
  skin 709.9
    suppurative 686.0
  spinal cord 349.9
    congenital 743.9
    traumatic (complete) (incomplete)
        (transverse) - *see also* Injury,
        spinal, by region
      with
        broken
          back - *code by* region under
              Fracture, vertebra, with
              spinal cord lesion
          neck (closed) 806.0
            late effect 806.9
            open 806.1
          fracture, vertebra (conditions in
              805) - *code by* region
              under Fracture, vertebra,
              with spinal cord lesion
  spleen 289.5
  stomach 537.9
  syphilitic - *see* Syphilis
  tertiary - *see* Syphilis, tertiary
  tonsillar fossa 500
  tooth, teeth 525.9
    white spot 521.0
  traumatic NEC (*see also* nature and site
      of injury) 996.9
  tricuspid (valve) - *see* Endocarditis,
      tricuspid
  trigeminal nerve 356
  ulcerated or ulcerative - *see* Ulcer
  uterus 625.9
    complicating delivery - *see*
        Obstetrical trauma
  valvular - *see* Endocarditis
  vascular 458.9
    affecting central nervous system (*see
        also* Disease, cerebrovascular
        NEC) 438.9
    following trauma 995.3
    retina, retinal 377.0
  warty - *see* Verruca
  x-ray - *see* Effect, adverse, x-rays

Lethargic - *see* condition
Lethargy, negro 087.8
Letterer-Siwe disease 279
Leuc(o)-for any term beginning thus - *see*
    Leuk(o)
Leukamide - *see* Leukemia
Leukasmus 270.8
Leukemia, leukemic (aleukemic)
        (aleupenic) (atypical) (compound)
        (congenital) (cutis) (labyrinth)
        (leukopenic) (myeloproliferative)
        (splenic) (subleukemic) (true)
        207.9
  acute 207.0
  adenia 204.9
    acute 204.0
    chronic 204.1
  adenitis 204.9
    acute 204.0
    chronic 204.1
  basophilic 205.9
    acute 205.0
    chronic 205.1
  blast cell (acute) 207.0
    chronic 207.1
  blastic (acute) 207.0
    chronic 207.1
  chronic 207.1
  embryonal (acute) 207.0
    chronic 207.1
  eosinophilic 205.9
    acute 205.0
    chronic 205.1
  giant cell 207.9
    acute 207.0
    chronic 207.1
  granulocytic 205.9
    acute 205.0
    chronic 205.1
  hemoblastic (acute) 207.0
    chronic 207.1
  histiocytic 206.9
    acute 206.0
    chronic 206.1
  lymphatic 204.9
    acute 204.0
    chronic 204.1
    lachrymal, lacrimal gland 204.9
      acute 204.0
      chronic 204.1
  lymphoblastic (acute) 204.0
    chronic 204.1
  lymphocytic 204.9
    acute 204.0
    chronic 204.1
  lymphogenous 204.9
    acute 204.0

Leukemia, etc. — *continued*
  lymphogenous — *continued*
    chronic   204.1
  lymphoid   204.9
    acute   204.0
    chronic   204.1
  lymphoidocytic (acute)   207.0
    chronic   207.1
  mast cell   207.9
    acute   207.0
    chronic   207.1
  megakaryocytic   207.9
    acute   207.0
    chronic   207.1
  mixed (cell)   205.9
    acute   205.0
    chronic   205.1
  monoblastic (acute)   206.0
    chronic   206.1
  monocytic   206.9
    acute   206.0
    chronic   206.1
    Naegeli type   205.1
  monocytoid myelogenous   205.9
    acute   205.0
    chronic   205.1
  monomyelocytic (chronic)   205.1
    acute   205.0
  myeloblastic (acute)   205.0
    chronic   205.1
  myelocytic (chronic)   205.1
    acute   205.0
  myelogenous   205.9
    acute   205.0
    chronic   205.1
  myeloid   205.9
    acute   205.0
    chronic   205.1
  myelosclerotic   205.9
    acute   205.0
    chronic   205.1
  Naegeli type monocytic   205.1
  plasma-cell   207.9
    acute   207.0
    chronic   207.1
  plasmacytic   207.9
    acute   207.0
    chronic   207.1
  reticular cell   206.9
    acute   206.0
    chronic   206.1
  Rieder-cell   207.9
    acute   207.0
    chronic   207.1
  splenolymphatic   204.9
    acute   204.0

Leukemia, etc. — *continued*
  splenolymphatic — *continued*
    chronic   204.1
  splenomedullary   205.9
    acute   205.0
    chronic   205.1
  splenomyelogenous   205.9
    acute   205.0
    chronic   205.1
  stem cell (acute)   207.0
    chronic   207.1
  thrombocytic   207.9
    acute   207.0
    chronic   207.1
  undifferentiated cell (acute)   207.0
    chronic   207.1
Leukemoid reaction   289.9
Leukocythemia (*see also* Leukemia)
    207.9
Leukocytosis   289.9
Leukoderma   709.9
  syphilitic   091.2
    late   095
Leukodermia (*see also* Leukoderma)
    709.9
Leukodystrophy (cerebral)
    (metachromatic) (progressive)
    333.1
Leuko-edema, mouth   528.7
Leuko-encephalitis
  acute hemorrhagic   323
    late effects   324
  subacute sclerosing   065
    late effects   066
  van Bogaert's   065
    late effects   066
Leuko-encephalopathy (metachromatic)
    (multifocal) (progressive)   333.1
Leuko-erythroblastosis   207.9
Leuko-erythrosis   207.9
Leukokeratosis   702
  nicotina palati   528.7
Leukokraurosis
  vulva(e)   629.2
Leukolymphosarcoma   202.2
Leukoma (cornea) (adherent) - *see*
    Opacity, cornea
Leukonychia (punctata) (striata)   703.9
  congenital   757.4
Leukopathia
  unguium   703.9
    congenital   757.4
Leukopenia (malignant)   288
Leukopenic - *see* condition
Leukoplakia   702
  anus   569.2

Leukoplakia—*continued*
  bladder (postinfectional) 596.9
  buccal 528.6
  cervix (uterus) 621.0
  esophagus 530.9
  gingiva 528.6
  kidney (pelvis) (*see also* Lesion, kidney) 593.2
  larynx 508.3
  lip 528.6
  mouth 528.6
  oral (mucosa) (soft tissue) 528.6
  pelvis (kidney) (*see also* Lesion, kidney) 593.2
  penis (infectional) 607.0
  rectum 569.2
  syphilitic 095
  tongue 529.7
  ureter (postinfectional) 593.5
  urethra (postinfectional) 599.9
  uterus 625.9
  vagina 629.0
  vocal cords 508.3
  vulva 629.2
Leukopolioencephalopathy 333.1
Leukorrhea 629.3
  due to Trichomonas (vaginalis) 131
  trichomonal 131
Leukosarcoma 202.2
Leukosis (*see also* Leukemia) 207.9
Levocardia 746.8
  with situs inversus 759.0
Levulosuria 271.3
Lewandowsky's disease (primary) 017.0
  late effect or sequela 019.9
Leyden-Moebius dystrophy 330.3
Leydig cell carcinoma 186
  female 183.0
Liar, pathologic 301.7
Libman-Sacks disease 734.1
Lice (infestation) (body) (head) 132
  pubic 134.1
Lichen 697.9
  albus 701.0
  annularis 695.9
  myxedematosus 701.9
  nitidus 697.1
  obtusus corneus 697.9
  pilaris 757.2
    acquired 701.1
  planus (chronicus) 697.0
    sclerosus (et atrophicus) 701.0
  ruber 696.4
    acuminatus 696.4
    moniliforme 697.9
    of Wilson 697.0
    planus 697.0

Lichen—*continued*
  sclerosus (et atrophicus) 701.0
  scrofulosus (primary) 017.0
    late effect or sequela 019.9
  simplex
    chronicus 698.3
    circumscriptus 698.3
  spinulosus 757.2
    mycotic 117.9
  striata 697.9
  urticatus 698.2
Lichenification 698.3
  psychogenic 305.0
Lichenoides tuberculosis (primary) 017.0
  late effect or sequela 019.9
Lichtheim's disease or syndrome 281.0
Lien migrans 289.5
Lientery - *see* Diarrhea
Ligament - *see* condition
Lightning (burn) (effects) (incineration) (shock) (stroke) (struck by) 994.0
Lightwood's disease 273.8
Lignac-de Toni-Fanconi-Debre syndrome 270.3
Lignac-Fanconi syndrome 270.3
Lignac's disease 270.3
Ligneous thyroiditis 245.1
Limb - *see* condition
Limitation motion, sacro-iliac 726
Limited cardiac reserve - *see* Disease, heart
Lindau(-von Hippel) disease 759.8
Linea corneae senilis 378.4
Lines
  Beau's 703.9
  Harris' 723.9
Lingua
  geographica 529.1
  nigra (villosa) 529.3
  plicata 529.5
    congenital 750.0
  tylosis 529.7
Lingual - *see* condition
Linitis (gastric) 535
  plastica 151.9
  suppurative 535
Liomyoma (*see also* Neoplasm, connective tissue, benign) 215
  prostate 600
  skin (*see also* Dermatofibroma) 216.8
  uterus 218
Lip - *see* condition
Lipedema - *see* Edema
Lipemia (retinal) 279
  essential 272.0
  familial 272.0
  hereditary 272.0

Lipidosis 272.9
  cerebral (infantile) (juvenile) (late)
    333.0
  cerebroside 272.2
  cerebrospinal 272.9
  cholesterol 272.9
  diabetic - see category 250
  glycolipid 272.2
  hereditary, dystopic 272.2
Lipochondrodystrophy 273.8
Lipodystrophia progressiva 279
Lipodystrophy (progressive) 279
  insulin 962.3
  intestinal 039.9
Lipofibroma - see Lipoma
Lipoglycoproteinosis 279
Lipogranuloma, sclerosing 686.9
Lipogranulomatosis 279
  kidney 279
Lipoid - see also condition
  histiocytosis 272.2
    essential 272.2
  nephrosis (see also Nephrosis) 581
  proteinosis of Urbach 279
Lipoidemia (see also Lipemia) 279
Lipoidosis - see also Lipidosis
Lipoma (embryonal) 214.9
  skin 214.0
  specified site NEC 214.9
  spermatic cord 214.1
  subcutaneous tissue 214.0
Lipomatosis 279
  embryonal - see Lipoma
Lipomyohemangioma - see Lipoma
Lipomyoma - see Lipoma
Lipomyosarcoma (see also Neoplasm,
    connective tissue, malignant)
    171.9
Lipomyxoma - see Lipoma
Lipomyxosarcoma (see also Neoplasm,
    connective tissue, malignant)
    171.9
Liposarcoma (see also Neoplasm,
    connective tissue, malignant)
    171.9
Lipping
  cervix 621.9
  spine 713.1
  vertebra 713.1
Lipschutz ulcer 629.9
Lipuria 789.2
  bilharziasis 120.0
Lisping 306.0
Lissauer's paralysis 094.1
Lissencephalia, lissencephaly 743.2
Listerellose 027.0

Listeriose 027.0
Listeriosis 027.0
  fetal 027.0
Lithemia 274
Lithiasis - see also Calculus
  hepatic (see also Cholelithiasis) 574.9
  urinary 594
Lithopedion 779.9
  mother 634.2
Lithosis 515.0
  with tuberculosis 010
Lithuria 789.9
Little league elbow 724.3
Little's disease (see also Palsy, cerebral,
    spastic) 343.1
Littre's
  gland - see condition
  hernia - see Hernia, Littre's
Littritis (see also Urethritis) 597
Livedo 782.3
  annulares 782.3
  racemosa 782.3
  reticularis 782.3
Liver - see condition
Lloyd's syndrome 258.1
Loa loa 125.2
Loasis 125.2
Lobar - see condition
Lobo's disease or blastomycosis 116.9
Lobstein's disease 756.6
Lobster-claw hand 755.5
Lobulation (congenital) - see also
    Anomaly, specified type NEC
  kidney, fetal 753.3
  liver, abnormal 751.6
  spleen 758.0
Lobule, lobular - see condition
Local, localized - see condition
Locked bowel or intestine (see also
    Obstruction, intestine) 560.9
Locking
  joint (see also Derangement, joint)
    724.9
  knee 724.5
Lockjaw (see also Tetanus) 037
Loeffler's
  endocarditis 421.0
  pneumonia 519.2
  syndrome 519.2
Loiasis 125.2
Lone Star fever 082.9
Long flap, hymen 752.6
Longitudinal stripes or grooves, nails
    703.9
  congenital 757.4
Loop
  intestine (see also Volvulus) 560.2

Loop — *continued*
  intrascleral nerve   378.6
  vascular on papilla (optic)   744.8
Loose - *see also* condition
  bodies in joint   729.9
    elbow   729.3
    hip   729.5
    knee   729.6
    shoulder   729.2
    specified joint NEC   729.9
    spine   729.1
  body sheath, tendon   733.9
  cartilage (joint) - *see* Loose bodies in
      joint
  sesamoid, joint - *see* Loose bodies in
      joint
  tooth, teeth   525.9
Loosening, epiphysis   723.9
Looser-Milkman syndrome   265.2
Lop ear (deformity)   745.2
Lorain-Levi syndrome   253.1
Lorain's disease or syndrome   253.1
Lordosis (acquired)   735.9
  congenital   756.2
  due to posture (incorrect)   735.9
  late effect
    acute poliomyelitis   044
    rickets   265.1
  rachitic   265.1
  tuberculous   015.0
    late effect or sequela   019.3
Loss
  appetite   784.0
    hysterical   300.1
    psychogenic   305.5
  blood - *see* Hemorrhage
  control, sphincter, rectum   785.6
    nonorganic origin   306.7
  extremity or member, traumatic, current
      - *see* Amputation, traumatic
  fluid (acute)   788.0
    fetus or newborn   778.9
  hearing - *see* Deafness
  memory (*see also* Amnesia)   780.7
  mind (*see also* Psychosis)   299
  organ or part - *see* Absence, by site,
      acquired
  sense, smell, taste or touch (*see also*
      Disturbance, sensation)   781.6
  sight (acquired) (complete) (congenital)
      - *see* Blindness
  spinal fluid
    headache   997.0
  substance of
    bone   723.9
    cartilage (joint) (*see also* Disease,
        joint)   729.9

Loss — *continued*
  substance of — *continued*
    cartilage (joint) — *continued*
      ear   387.9
      vitreous (humor)   378.9
    voice (*see also* Aphonia)   783.5
    weight (cause unknown)   788.4
Louis-Bar syndrome   275.0
Louping ill   063.1
  late effects   066
Lousiness   132
  pubic   134.1
Low
  basal metabolic rate   788.9
  birth weight   777
    with multiple births   769.4
    for classification of births in hospital
        - *see* Newborn
  blood pressure   458.0
  cardiac reserve - *see* Disease, heart
  frequency deafness - *see* Deafness
  function - *see also* Hypofunction
    kidney (*see also* Lesion, kidney)
        593.2
    liver   573.9
  hemoglobin   285.9
  implantation, placenta - *see* Placenta,
      previa
  insertion, placenta - *see* Placenta,
      previa
  lying
    kidney (*see also* Lesion, kidney)
        593.2
    organ or site, congenital - *see*
        Malposition, congenital
    placenta - *see* Placenta, previa
  platelets (blood) (*see also*
      Thrombocytopenia)   287.1
  reserve kidney (*see also* Lesion, kidney)
      593.2
  salt syndrome   788.0
Lowe's syndrome   270.8
Lower extremity - *see* condition
L-shaped kidney   753.3
Ludwig's
  angina   528.3
  disease   528.3
Lues (venerea), luetic - *see* Syphilis
Lumbago   717.0
Lumbalgia   728.7
Lumbar - *see* condition
Lumbarization, vertebra   756.1
Lump kidney   753.3
Lunacy (*see also* Psychosis)   299
Lung - *see* condition
Lupoid (miliary) of Boeck   135

Lupus (exedens) (Hilliard's) (miliaris
disseminatus faciei) (vulgaris)
017.0
Cazenave's 695.4
discoid (local) 695.4
disseminated 734.1
erythematodes (discoid) (local) 695.4
erythematosus (discoid) (local) 695.4
disseminated 734.1
systemic 734.1
hydralazine 973.5
late effect or sequela 019.9
nephritis 734.1
nontuberculous, not disseminated
695.4
pernio (Besnier) 135
tuberculous 017.0
late effect or sequela 019.9
Lusung - see Dermatophytosis
Lutembacher's disease or syndrome
746.4
Luteoma (ovary) 256.0
Lutz-Splendore-Almeida disease 116.2
Luxatio bulbi due to birth injury (see also
Birth injury NEC 772.9
Luxation - see also Dislocation
eyeball due to birth injury (see also
Birth injury NEC) 772.9
genital organs (external) NEC - see
Wound, open, genital organs
lachrymal, lacrimal gland
(postinfectional) 378.3
lens (old) (partial) (spontaneous) 378.8
congenital 744.8
penis - see Wound, open, penis
scrotum - see Wound, open, scrotum
testis - see Wound, open, testis
L-xyloketosuria 271.8
Lycanthropy (see also Psychosis) 299
Lyell's syndrome 695.1
due to drug (see also Table of adverse
effects) 977.9
Lymph
gland or node - see condition
scrotum (see also Infestation, filarial)
125.9
Lymph hemangioma - see Hemangioma
Lymphadenia, aleukemic 204.9
acute 204.0
chronic 204.1
Lymphadenitis 289.3
with
abortion - see Abortion, by type, with
sepsis

Lymphadenitis — continued
with — continued
ectopic gestation - see categories
631.0-631.3
acute, unspecified site 683
aleukemic or leukemic 204.9
acute 204.0
chronic 204.1
any site, except mesenteric 289.3
acute 683
chronic 289.1
subacute 289.1
breast, puerperal, postpartum 678
chancroidal (congenital) 099.0
chronic 289.1
mesenteric 289.2
dermatopathic 695.9
due to
anthracosis 515.1
with tuberculosis 010
diphtheria (toxin) 032
lymphogranuloma venereum 099.1
gonorrheal 098.8
infectional 683
mesenteric (acute) (chronic)
(nonspecific) (subacute) 289.2
due to Bacillus typhi- 001
tuberculous 014
late effect or sequela 019.9
puerperal, postpartum, childbirth 670
purulent 683
pyogenic 683
regional 079.3
septic 683
streptococcal 683
subacute, unspecified site 289.1
suppurative 683
syphilitic (early) 091.8
late 095
tuberculous - see Tuberculosis, lymph
gland
venereal 099.1
Lymphadenoid goiter 245.1
Lymphadenoma 202.9
malignant 202.2
multiple 202.2
spleen 202.9
Lymphadenopathy (general) 782.7
due to toxoplasmosis (acquired) 130.0
congenital (active) 130.1
late effects 130.2
Lymphadenosis 782.7
Lymphangiectasis 457
conjunctiva 457
postinfectional 457
scrotum 457

Lymphangio-endothelioma 227.2
  malignant - *see* Neoplasm, connective
    tissue, malignant
Lymphangiofibroma 227.2
Lymphangioma (any site) (capillary)
    (cavernous) (circumscriptum)
    (congenital) (simple) 227.2
  malignant - *see* Neoplasm, connective
    tissue, malignant
Lymphangiosarcoma - *see* Neoplasm,
    connective tissue, malignant
Lymphangitis 457
  with
    abortion - *see* Abortion, by type, with
      sepsis
    abscess - *code by* site under Abscess
    cellulitis - *code by* site under
      Cellulitis
    ectopic gestation - *see* categories
      631.0-631.3
  acute (with abscess or cellulitis) 682.9
    specified site - *code by* site under
      Abscess
  breast, puerperal, postpartum 678
  chancroidal 099.0
  chronic (any site) 457
  gangrenous 457
  penis
    acute 607.5
    gonococcal (acute) 098.0
      chronic or duration of 2 months or
        over 098.1
  puerperal, postpartum, childbirth 670
  strumous, tuberculous 017.1
    late effect or sequela 019.9
  subacute (any site) 457
  tuberculous - *see* Tuberculosis, lymph
    gland
Lymphatic (vessel) - *see* condition
Lymphatism 254
  scrofulous 017.1
    late effect or sequela 019.9
Lymphatocele 227.2
Lymphectasia 457
Lymphedema (*see also* Elephantiasis)
    457
  praecox 457
  secondary 457
  surgical NEC 998.9
    postmastectomy (syndrome) 997.3
Lymphendothelioma 227.2
  malignant - *see* Neoplasm, connective
    tissue, malignant
Lymphepithelioma - *see* Neoplasm,
    malignant
Lymphoblastic - *see* condition

Lymphoblastoma 200.1
  giant cell 200.0
  giant follicular 202.0
  Hodgkin's 201
  macrofollicular 202.0
  malignant 200.1
Lymphoblastosis NEC 204.9
  acute 204.0
  chronic 204.1
Lymphocele 457
Lymphochloroma 202.2
Lymphocythemia (aleukemic) 204.9
  acute 204.0
  chronic 204.1
Lymphocytic
  chorio-encephalitis (acute) (serous)
    079.2
  choriomeningitis (acute) (serous) 079.2
  leukemia 204.9
    acute 204.0
    chronic 204.1
Lymphocytoma 200.1
Lymphocytomatosis 200.1
Lymphocytosis 289.9
  infectious (acute) 075
Lymphoepithelioma - *see* Neoplasm,
    malignant
Lymphogranuloma (malignant) 201
  inguinale 099.1
  venereal (any site) 099.1
    with stricture of rectum 099.1
  venereum 099.1
Lymphogranulomatosis 201
  benign (Boeck's sarcoid) (Schaumann's)
    135
  Hodgkin's 201
  malignant 201
  pernicious 201
Lymphoid - *see* condition
Lympholeukoblastoma 202.2
Lymphoma (any site) NEC 202.2
  benign 202.9
  compound 202.2
  follicular 200.1
  generalized 202.2
  giant cell 200.0
  giant follicular 202.0
  histiocytic 200.0
  Hodgkin's 201
  lymphoblastic 200.1
  macrofollicular 202.0
  malignant 202.2
  multiple 202.2
  ocular 202.9
  reticulum cell 200.0
  single 202.2

Lymphomatosis - *see* Lymphoma
Lymphopathia
  venereum 099.1
  veneris 099.1
Lymphopenia 289.9
  familial 275.0
Lymphoreticulosis
  benign (of inoculation) 079.3
Lymphorrhea 457

Lymphosarcoma (generalized),
    lymphosarcomatosis 200.1
  Hodgkin's 201
  lymphoblastic 200.1
  lymphocytic 200.1
  reticulum cell 200.0
Lymphostasis 457
Lypemania (*see also* Melancholia) 296.2
Lyssa 071

M

Macacus ear 745.2
Maceration
  fetus (cause not stated) 779.0
  wet feet, tropical (syndrome) 991.4
Macrocephalia, macrocephaly 756.0
Macrocheilia (congenital) 745.8
Macrochilia (congenital) 745.8'
Macrocolon 751.2
Macrocornea 744.2
Macrocytic - see condition
Macrocytosis 289.9
Macrodactylia, macrodactylism (fingers)
    (thumbs) 755.5
  toes 755.7
Macrodontia 520.2
Macrogenitosomia (praecox) (male)
    273.6
Macroglobulinemia (idiopathic) (primary)
    275.5
  Waldenstrom's 275.5
Macroglossia (congenital) 750.0
  acquired 529.9
Macrognathia, macrognathism (congenital)
    (mandibular) (maxillary) 524.0
Macrogyria (congenital) 743.2
Macrohydrocephalus (see also
    Hydrocephalus) 347.9
Macromastia (see also Hypertrophy,
    breast) 611.1
Macropsia 377.4
Macrosigmoid 569.9
  congenital 751.2
Macrostomia (congenital) 745.8
Macrotia (external ear) (congenital)
    745.2
Macula
  cornea, corneal - see also Opacity,
    cornea
    due to infection 371.9
  degeneration 377.1
    cerebral 333.0
Maculae ceruleae 132
Madarosis 704
Madelung's
  deformity 755.5
  disease 279
  radius deformity 755.5
Madness (see also Psychosis) 299
Madura
  disease 117.4
  foot 117.4
Maduromycosis 117.4

Maffucchi's syndrome 756.5
Main en griffe (acquired) 738.2
  congenital 755.5
Majocchi's disease 709.9
Major - see condition
Mal cerebral (idiopathic) (see also
    Epilepsy) 345.9
Mal comitial (see also Epilepsy) 345.9
Mal de los pintos (see also Pinta) 103.9
Mal de Meleda 757.2
Mal de mer 994.6
Mal lie
  complicating delivery - see
    Presentation, abnormal,
    complicating delivery
  during pregnancy (undelivered) 634.9
  fetus or newborn - see categories 766.0-
    766.9
Malabar itch - see Dermatophytosis
Malabsorption 269.1
  calcium 269.9
  carbohydrate 269.0
  fat 269.0
  galactose 271.2
  glucose 271.8
  isomaltose 271.8
  lactose (hereditary) 271.8
  monosaccharide 271.8
  protein 269.0
  sucrose 271.8
  syndrome 269.1
    postgastrectomy 998.9
Malacia, bone 265.2
  juvenile (see also Rickets) 265.0
Malacoplakia
  bladder 596.9
  pelvis (kidney) (see also Lesion, kidney)
    593.2
  ureter 593.5
  urethra 599.9
Malacosteon 265.2
  juvenile (see also Rickets) 265.0
Maladaptation - see Maladjustment
Maladie de Roger 746.3
Maladie du cri du chat 759.4
Maladie du sommeil 087.8
Maladjustment
  nutritional 269.9
  simple, adult 307
  situational acute 307
  social, without manifest psychiatric
    disorder Y13

Malaise 796.0
Malakoplakia
bladder 596.9
pelvis (kidney) (see also Lesion, kidney) 593.2
ureter 593.5
urethra 599.9
Malaria, malarial (fever) 084.9
cardiac 084.9
cerebral 084.9
continued 084.0
estivo-autumnal 084.0
falciparum 084.0
hemorrhagic 084.9
liver 084.9
malariae 084.2
malignant 084.0
tertian 084.0
mixed infections 084.8
ovale 084.3
pernicious, acute 084.0
Plasmodium, P.
falciparum 084.0
malariae 084.2
ovale 084.3
vivax 084.1
quartan 084.2
quotidian 084.0
recurrent 084.9
induced (therapeutically) 084.5
remittent 084.9
spleen 084.9
subtertian 084.0
tertian 084.1
benign 084.1
malignant 084.0
tropical 084.0
typhoid 084.9
vivax 084.1
Malassez's disease (cystic) 607.9
Malassimilation 269.1
Maldescent, testicle 752.1
Maldevelopment - see also Anomaly
brain 743.9
colon 751.4
fetus or newborn 778.9
hip 755.7
congenital dislocation 755.6
mastoid process 756.0
middle ear 745.0
spine 756.2
toe 755.7
Male type pelvis
complicating delivery - see Android pelvis, complicating delivery

Male type pelvis — continued
noted during pregnancy (undelivered) 634.9
Malformation (congenital) - see also Anomaly
bone 756.9
bursa 756.9
circulatory system NEC 747.9
digestive system NEC 751.9
lower 751.4
upper 750.9
eye 744.9
gum 750.9
heart NEC 746.9
valve 746.6
internal ear 745.0
joint NEC 755.9
muscle 756.9
nervous system (central) 743.9
pelvic organs or tissues
complicating delivery 657.9
fetus or newborn - see categories 764.0-764.9
noted during pregnancy (undelivered) 634.9
placenta - see Placenta, abnormal
respiratory organ NEC 748.9
sense organs NEC 743.9
skin NEC 757.9
spinal cord 743.9
tendon 756.9
throat 750.9
tooth, teeth NEC 520.9
umbilical cord - see Complications, umbilical cord
umbilicus 758.9
urinary system NEC 753.9
Malfunction - see also Dysfunction
catheter device (in dialysis) 997.4
colostomy 998.7
enteric stoma 998.7
enterostomy 998.7
gastro-enteric 536.9
pacemaker 997.5
prosthetic device, internal 997.5
artery replacement 997.5
heart valve 997.5
Malgaigne's fracture - see Fracture, pelvis
Malherbe's tumor (see also Trichoepithelioma) 216.1
Malibu disease 918.0
Malignancy - see also Neoplasm, malignant
generalized 199.0
Malignant - see condition
Malingerer (idiopathic) 796.1

Malingering 796.1
  without sickness 796.1
Mallet finger (intrinsic) (acquired) 738.3
  congenital 755.5
  late effect of rickets 265.1
Malleus 024
Mallory-Weiss syndrome 530.9
Mallory's bodies 034.1
Malnutrition 269.9
  intrauterine 778.9
  lack of care, or neglect (child) (infant)
      994.9
  malignant 267
  protein 267
Malocclusion (teeth) 524.4
  due to
    abnormal swallowing 524.5
    missing teeth 524.3
    mouth breathing 524.5
    tongue, lip or finger habits 524.5
  temporomandibular (joint) 524.1
Malposition
  cervix - *see* Malposition, uterus
  congenital
    adrenal (gland) 758.1
    alimentary tract 751.8
      lower 751.4
      upper 750.8
    aorta 747.2
    appendix 751.4
    arterial trunk 747.2
    artery (peripheral) 747.6
      coronary 746.8
      pulmonary 747.6
    auditory canal 745.2
      causing impairment of hearing
          745.0
    auricle (ear) 745.2
      causing impairment of hearing
          745.0
      cervical 745.4
    biliary duct or passage 751.6
    bladder (mucosa) 753.8
      exteriorized or extroverted 753.5
    brachial plexus 743.8
    brain tissue 743.2
    breast 757.2
    bronchus 748.3
    cecum 751.4
    clavicle 755.5
    colon 751.4
    digestive organ or tract NEC 751.8
      lower 751.4
      upper 750.8
    ear (auricle) (external) 745.2
      ossicles 745.0

Malposition—*continued*
  congenital—*continued*
    endocrine (gland) NEC 758.3
    epiglottis 748.3
    eustachian tube 745.2
    eye 744.8
    facial features 745.8
    fallopian tube 752.5
    finger(s) 755.5
      supernumerary 755.0
    foot 755.7
    gallbladder 751.6
    gastrointestinal tract 751.8
    genitalia, genital organ(s) or tract
      female 752.8
        external 752.6
        internal NEC 752.5
      male 752.8
    glottis 748.3
    hand 755.5
    heart 746.8
      dextrocardia 746.8
        with complete transposition of
            viscera 759.0
    hepatic duct 751.6
    hip (joint) 755.6
    intestine (large) (small) 751.4
      with anomalous adhesions, fixation
          or malrotation 751.1
    joint NEC 755.9
    kidney 753.3
    larynx 748.3
    limb 755.9
      lower 755.7
      upper 755.5
    liver 751.6
    lung (lobe) 748.6
    nail(s) 757.4
    nerve 743.8
    nervous system NEC 743.8
    nose, nasal (septum) 748.1
    organ or site not listed - *see*
          Anomaly, specified type NEC
    ovary 752.5
    pancreas 751.7
    parathyroid (gland) 758.3
    patella 755.7
    peripheral vascular system (any
          vessel) 747.6
    pituitary (gland) 758.3
    respiratory organ or system NEC
      748.9
    rib (cage) 756.4
      supernumerary in cervical region
          756.3
    scapula 755.5

Malposition — *continued*
  congenital — *continued*
    shoulder 755.5
    spinal cord 743.3
    spine 756.2
    spleen 758.0
    sternum 756.4
    stomach 750.8
    symphysis pubis 755.7
    testicle, testis (undescended) 752.1
    thymus (gland) 758.3
    thyroid (gland) (tissue) 758.2
      cartilage 748.3
    toe(s) 755.7
      supernumerary 755.0
    tongue 750.0
    trachea 748.3
    uterus 752.5
    vein(s) (peripheral) 747.6
      great 747.4
      portal 747.4
      pulmonary 747.4
    vena cava (inferior) (superior) 747.4
  fetus
    complicating delivery (*see also*
      Presentation, abnormal,
      complicating delivery) 656.9
      fetus or newborn - *see* categories
        766.0-766.9
    noted before delivery 634.9
  gallbladder (*see also* Disease,
    gallbladder) 576.9
  gastro-intestinal tract 569.9
  intestine 569.9
  pelvic organs or tissues
    complicating delivery 657.9
      fetus or newborn - *see* categories
        764.0-764.9
    noted during pregnancy 634.9
  placenta - *see* Placenta previa
  stomach 537.9
  uterus or cervix (acute) (acquired)
    (adherent) (any degree)
    (asymptomatic) (postinfectional)
    (postpartal, old) 624.9
    anteflexion or anteversion (*see also*
      Anteversion, uterus) 624.1
    complicating
      delivery 657.9
        fetus or newborn - *see* categories
          764.0-764.9
      pregnancy (undelivered) 634.9
    flexion 624.9
      lateral (*see also* Lateroversion,
        uterus) 624.1
    inversion 624.9

Malposition — *continued*
  uterus or cervix — *continued*
    lateral (flexion) (version) (*see also*
      Lateroversion, uterus) 624.1
    pregnant or gravid (undelivered)
      634.9
    retroflexion or retroversion (*see also*
      Retroversion, uterus) 624.0
    specified type NEC 624.1
Malposture 733.9
Malpresentation - *see* Presentation,
  abnormal
Malrotation
  cecum 751.1
  colon 751.1
  intestine 751.1
  kidney 753.3
  spine or vertebra 729.1
Malum coxae senilis 713.0
Malunion, fracture - code as Fracture,
  late effect
  current - *see* Fracture
Mammillitis (*see also* Mastitis) 611.0
  puerperal, postpartum 678
Mammitis (*see also* Mastitis) 611.0
  puerperal, postpartum 678
Mammoplasia 611.9
Mangled NEC (*see also* nature and site of
  injury) 996.9
Mania 296.1
  alcoholic (acute) (chronic) 291.9
  Bell's 296.1
  chronic 296.1
  compulsive 300.3
  delirious (acute) 296.1
  hysterical 300.1
  puerperal 296.1
  recurrent 296.1
  senile 296.1
  unproductive 296.8
  uremic - *see* Uremia
Manic-depressive insanity, psychosis, or
  reaction 296.9
  agitated 296.0
  alternating 296.3
  circular 296.3
  depressed (type), depressive 296.2
  manic 296.1
  mixed NEC 296.8
  perplexed 296.8
  stuporous 296.8
Manson's
  disease 120.1
  pyosis 684
  schistosomiasis 120.1
Mansonellosis 125.5

Manual - *see* condition
Maple syrup (urine) disease 270.4
Marasmus 268
  brain 347.1
  due to malnutrition 268
  intestinal 569.9
  nutritional 268
  senile 794
  tuberculous NEC (*see also*
      Tuberculosis) 011.9
Marble
  bones 756.7
  skin 782.3
March
  foot 825.0
  hemoglobinuria 283.9
Marchand multiple nodular hyperplasia
      (liver) - *see* Cirrhosis, postnecrotic
Marchiafava-Bignami syndrome or disease
      341
Marchiafava-Micheli syndrome 283.9
Marchiafava's disease 341
Marcus Gunn sydrome 743.8
Marfan's
  congenital syphilis 090.4
  disease 090.4
  syndrome 759.8
    meaning congenital syphilis 090.4
Marginal
  implantation, placenta - *see* Placenta
      previa
  placenta - *see* Placenta, abnormal
  sinus (hemorrhage) (rupture)
        (complicating delivery) 651.1
      fetus or newborn 770.1
      undelivered 632.2
Marie-Bamberger disease 723.1
Marie-Charcot-Tooth neuropathic atrophy
      muscle 330.0
Marie-Strumpell
  arthritis 712.4
  disease 712.4
Marie's
  cerebellar ataxia 332.1
  syndrome 253.0
Marion's disease 596.9
Mark
  port wine (*see also* Hemangioma)
      227.0
  raspberry (*see also* Hemangioma)
      227.0
  strawberry (*see also* Hemangioma)
      227.0
  tattoo 709.1
Maroteaux-Lamy syndrome 273.8
Marrow (bone)
  arrest 284

Marrow (bone) — *continued*
  poor function 289.9
Martin's disease 717.9
Masculinization female with adrenal
      hyperplasia or tumor 255.0
Masochism 302.7
Masons' lung 515.0
  with tuberculosis 010
Mass
  abdominal 796.0
  benign - *see* Neoplasm, benign
  cystic - *see* Cyst
  kidney (*see also* Lesion, kidney) 593.2
  malignant - *see* Neoplasm, malignant
  pelvic 796.0
  specified organ or site NEC - *see*
      Disease of specific organ or site
  substernal thyroid 240.9
Massive - *see* condition
Mast cell disease 757.2
Mastalgia 786.7
  psychogenic 305.6
Masters-Allen syndrome 616.9
Mastitis (acute) (adolescent) (comedo)
        (diffuse) (infantile) (interstitial)
        (lobular) (neonatorum)
        (nonsuppurative) (parenchymatous)
        (phlegmonous) (plasma cell) (simple)
        (suppurative) 611.0
  chronic (cystic) 610
  cystic (Schimmelbusch's type) 610
  lactational 678
  puerperal, postpartum 678
Mastocytosis 757.2
  systemic 757.2
Mastodynia 786.7
  psychogenic 305.6
Mastoid - *see* condition
Mastoidalgia 387.9
Mastoiditis (coalescent) (hemorrhagic)
        (pneumococcal) (streptococcal)
        (suppurative) 383.9
  with
    abscess, ear (middle) acute 382.0
    catarrh, middle ear, chronic 382.1
    myringitis, acute 382.0
    otitis (media) 382.9
      acute 382.0
      chronic 382.1
    otorrhea 382.9
      acute 382.0
      chronic 382.1
    panotitis, acute 382.0
    suppuration, ear, acute 382.0
    tympanitis, acute 382.0

Mastoiditis, etc. — *continued*
  acute, subacute   383.0
    with
      abscess, ear (middle), acute   382.0
      myringitis, acute   382.0
      otitis (media) (acute)   382.0
      panotitis, acute   382.0
      suppuration, ear, acute   382.0
      tympanitis, acute   382.0
  chronic (necrotic) (recurrent)   383.1
    with
      catarrh, middle ear (chronic)
        382.1
      otitis (media) (chronic)   382.1
      otorrhea (chronic)   382.1
  tuberculous   015.8
    late effect or sequela   019.6
Mastopathy, mastopathia   611.9
  chronica cystica   610
  estrogenic, oestrogenica   610
  ovarian origin   610
Mastoplasia   611.9
Masturbation (adult)   305.6
  childhood   308
Maternal condition, affecting fetus or
    newborn
  acute yellow atrophy of liver   762.5
  albuminuria   762.0
  chorio-amnionitis   763.9
  congenital heart disease (conditions in
      746)   760.1
  cortical necrosis of kidney (acute)
      (bilateral)   762.9
  death NEC   769.5
  diabetes mellitus (conditions in 250)
      761.1
    manifest diabetes in the infant - *see*
      category 250
  disease NEC   761.9
    circulatory system, chronic
        (conditions in 410-458, 747)
        760.3
    genitourinary system, chronic
        (conditions in 590-599, 610-
        629)   760.5
  eclampsia   762.2
  hepatitis acute, malignant, or subacute
      762.5
  hyperemesis (with neuritis)   762.4
  hypertension (arising during pregnancy)
      (with pre-eclampsia)   762.1
    with eclampsia   762.2
    chronic (conditions in 400-404)
        760.2
  infection (antepartum) (intrapartum)
      NEC   763.9
    amniotic fluid   763.9

Maternal condition, etc. — *continued*
  infection, etc. — *continued*
    genitourinary tract (conditions in 595,
        612-614, 616.0, 620, 622,
        629.4)   763.1
    urinary tract NEC   763.1
  influenza (conditions in 470-474)
      761.2
    manifest influenza in the infant - *see*
        Influenza
  injury (conditions in 800-999, E800-
      E999)   761.5
  necrosis of liver (acute) (subacute)
      762.5
  nephritis (acute) (subacute) (conditions
      in 580, 581, 583, 593.2)   762.0
    chronic (conditions in 582)   760.4
  nephrosis (conditions in 581, 593.1)
      762.0
  neuritis   762.9
    with hyperemesis or vomiting   762.4
    chronic   761.9
  operation unrelated to current delivery
      761.6
  phlebitis   763.9
    chronic   760.3
  phlegmasia alba dolens   763.9
  pre-eclampsia   762.1
  pyelitis or pyelonephritis, arising during
      pregnancy (conditions in 590.1)
      763.0
    chronic   760.5
  renal disease or failure (acute)   762.0
    chronic   760.5
  rheumatic heart disease (chronic)
      (conditions in 393-398)   760.0
  rubella (conditions in 056)   761.3
    manifest rubella in the infant or fetus
        056
  syphilis (conditions in 090-097)   761.0
    manifest syphilis in the infant or fetus
        090.0
  thrombophlebitis   763.9
    chronic   760.3
  toxemia (of pregnancy)   762.3
    eclamptic   762.2
    nephritic   762.0
    not of pregnancy   761.9
    pre-eclamptic   762.1
    uremic   762.0
  toxoplasmosis (conditions in 130)
      761.4
    manifest toxoplasmosis in the infant
        or fetus   130.1
  transmission of chemical substance
      through the placenta   761.7
  uremia   762.0

Maternal condition, etc. — *continued*
  vomiting (pernicious) (persistent)
      (vicious) (with neuritis)   762.4
Maternity - *see* Delivery
Mauriac's syndrome - *see* category 250
Maxilla, maxillary - *see* condition
Mazoplasia   610
McArdle(-Schmid)(-Pearson) disease
      (glycogen storage)   271.1
McQuarrie's syndrome   251
Measles (black) (hemorrhagic)
      (suppressed)   055
  German, French, or liberty   056
Meatitis, urethral (*see also* Urethritis)
      597
Meatus, meatal - *see* condition
Meckel's
  diverticulitis   751.0
  diverticulum (displaced) (hypertrophic)
      751.0
Meconium
  ileus   273.0
  peritonitis NEC   778.9
  plug syndrome (newborn) NEC   778.9
Median - *see also* condition
  bar (prostate)   600
  vesical orifice   600
Mediastinitis (acute) (chronic)   519.9
  actinomycotic   113
  syphilitic   095
  tuberculous   012.9
    with pneumoconiosis (conditions in
        515)   010
    late effect or sequela   019.0
Mediastinopericarditis (*see also*
      Pericarditis)   423
Mediastinum, mediastinal - *see* condition
Medicine poisoning (by overdose)   977.9
  specified drug or substance - *see* Table
      of adverse effects
Mediterranean
  disease or syndrome (hemipathic) (*see
      also* Thalassemia)   282.4
  fever (*see also* Brucellosis)   023.9
    familial   276
    kala-azar   085.0
    leishmaniasis   085.0
Medulla - *see* condition
Medullated, fibers, fibres
  optic (nerve)   377.6
  retina   377.4
Medulloblastoma (*see also* Neoplasm,
      nervous system, malignant)   192.9
  brain   191
  posterior fossa (cranii)   191
  spinal cord   192.2
  vermis (cerebelii)   191

Medullo-epithelioma (*see also* Neoplasm,
      nervous system, malignant)   192.9
Megacaryocytic - *see* Megakaryocytic
Megacolon (acquired) (functional)
      (idiopathic) (not Hirschsprung's
      disease)   569.9
  aganglionic   751.2
  congenital, congenitum   751.2
  Hirschsprung's (disease)   751.2
  psychogenic   305.5
Mega-esophagus   530.0
  congenital   750.8
Megakaryocytic
  leukemia - *see* Leukemia,
      megakaryocytic
  myeloid metaplasia, spleen   209
Megalencephaly   743.2
Megalerythema   057.0
Megalo-appendix   751.4
Megalocephalus, megalocephaly NEC
      756.0
Megalocornea   744.8
Megalodactylia (fingers) (thumbs)   755.5
  toes   755.7
Megaloduodenum   751.4
Megalo-esophagus   530.0
  congenital   750.8
Megalogastria (congenital)   750.8
Megalomania   306.9
Megalophthalmos   744.8
Megalopsia   377.4
Megalosplenia - *see* Splenomegaly
Megalo-ureter   593.5
  congenital   753.2
Megarectum   569.2
Megasigmoid   569.9
  congenital   751.2
Mega-ureter   593.5
  congenital   753.2
Megrim   346
Meibomian
  cyst infected   362
  gland - *see* condition
  infarction (eyelid)   378.2
  sty, stye   362
Meibomitis   362
Meige's disease   757.0
Meigs' syndrome   220.9
Meischer's disease   704
Melancholia   296.2
  agitated   296.0
  climacteric   296.0
  hypochondriac   300.7
  intermittent   296.2
  involutional   296.0
  menopausal   296.0

Melanosis — *continued*
addisonian 255.1
tuberculous 017.9
late effect or sequela 019.9
adrenal 255.1
colon 569.9
conjunctiva 378.3
congenital 744.8
cornea (presenile) (senile) 378.4
congenital 744.8
prenatal 744.8
diabetic - *see* category 250
eye 378.9
congenital 744.8
lenticularis progressiva 757.2
liver 573.9
Riehl 709.9
sclera 378.6
congenital 744.8
suprarenal 255.1
tar 709.9
toxic 709.9
Melanotic sarcoma or tumor - *see*
Melanoma
Melanuria 789.9
Melasma 709.9
adrenal (gland) 255.1
suprarenal (gland) 255.1
Melena 785.7
with ulcer (*see also* Ulcer, by site)
533.9
newborn 778.2
Meleney's
gangrene (cutaneous) 686.0
ulcer (chronic undermining) 686.0
Melioidosis 025
Melitensis, febris 023.0
Melitococcosis 023.0
Melkersson's syndrome 350
Mellitus, diabetes - *see* Diabetes
Melorheostosis (bone) (leri) 723.9
Melotia 745.2
Membrana
capsularis lentis posterior 744.8
epipapillaris 744.8
Membranacea placenta - *see* Placenta,
abnormal
Membranaceous uterus 625.9
Membrane, membranous - *see also*
condition
folds, congenital - *see also* Web,
congenital
Jackson's 751.1
over face (causing asphyxia) (*see also*
Asphyxia, newborn) 776.9
premature rupture - *see* Rupture,
membranes

Membrane, etc. — *continued*
pupillary persistent 744.8
retained (with hemorrhage)
(complicating delivery) 652
causing delayed hemorrhage (during
puerperium) 677.1
secondary (eye) 374.1
unruptured (causing asphyxia) (*see also*
Asphyxia, newborn) 776.9
Memory disturbance, lack, or loss (*see
also* Amnesia) 780.7
Mendacity pathologic 301.7
Menetriere's disease 269.9
Meniere's
disease 385
syndrome 385
vertigo 385
Meninges, meningeal - *see* condition
Meningioma (angioblastic) (benign) 225.9
brain 225.2
malignant 192.9
brain 192.1
spinal cord 192.3
skin 216.8
spinal cord 225.4
Meningismus 780.8
due to serum or vaccine 999.1
infectional 780.8
influenzal NEC 474
pneumococcal 780.8
Meningitis (basal) (basic) (basilar) (brain)
(catarrhal) (cerebral) (cervical)
(chronic) (congenital) (congestive)
(diffuse) (fibrinopurulent)
(hemorrhagic) (infantile) (infectious)
(membranous) (metastatic)
(nonmeningococcal) (nonspecific)
(pontine) (postinfectious)
(progressive) (purulent) (septic)
(serosa circumscripta) (simple)
(spinal) (subacute) (suppurative)
(sympathica) (toxic) 320.9
abacterial NEC (*see also* Meningitis,
aseptic) 045.9
alcoholic 303.2
aseptic (acute) 045.9
Coxsackie virus 045.0
due to
arbovirus - *see* categories 060-068
poliovirus 042
ECHO virus 045.1
enterovirus 045.9
herpes simplex 054
herpes zoster 053.9
leptospiral 100.8
lymphocytic choriomeningitis 079.2
mumps 072

Meningitis—*continued*
 bacterial NEC 320.9
  gram-negative 320.9
   late effects 324
 cancerous 198.4
 carcinomatous 198.4
 caseous 013.0
  late effect or sequela 019.1
 cerebrospinal (acute) (chronic)
     (diplococcal) (endemic) (epidemic)
     (fulminant) (infectious)
     (malignant) (meningococcal)
     (sporadic) 036.0
  H. influenzae 320.0
   late effects 324
  influenzal 320.0
   late effects 324
  nonmeningococcal (endemic)
     (fulminant) (purulent) 320.9
   late effects 324
  nonspecific 320.9
   late effects 324
  pneumococcal 320.1
   late effects 324
  purulent 320.9
   H. influenzae 320.0
    late effects 324
   influenzal 320.0
    late effects 324
   late effects 324
   pneumococcal 320.1
    late effects 324
   specified organism NEC 320.8
    late effects 324
  septic or suppurative 320.9
   H. influenzae 320.0
    late effects 324
   influenzal 320.0
    late effects 324
   late effects 324
   pneumococcal 320.1
    late effects 324
   specified organism NEC 320.8
    late effects 324
  streptococcal 320.8
   late effects 324
  tuberculous 013.0
   late effect or sequela 019.1
 cryptococcic 116.0
 diplococcal 036.0
 due to
  actinomycosis 113
  mumps 072
  oidiomycosis 112
  preventive immunization, inoculation
     or vaccination 999.1
  sporotrichosis 117.1

Meningitis—*continued*
 E. coli 320.8
 epidemic 036.0
 Friedlander (bacillus) 320.8
  late effects 324
 gonococcal 098.8
 gram-negative cocci 036.0
 gram-positive cocci 320.8
  late effects 324
 H. influenzae 320.0
  late effects 324
 influenzal 320.0
  late effects 324
 late effects 324
 leptospiral (aseptic) 100.8
 Listerella (monocytogenes) 027.0
 Listeria monocytogenes 027.0
 lymphocytic (acute) (benign) (serous)
     079.2
 meningococcal 036.0
 miliary 013.0
  late effect or sequela 019.1
 Mima polymorpha 320.8
 mycotic 117.9
 Neisseria 036.0
 nonbacterial NEC (*see also* Meningitis,
     aseptic) 045.9
 ossificans 347.9
 pneumococcal 320.1
  late effects 324
 Salmonella 003.9
 serous NEC (*see also* Meningitis,
     aseptic) 045.9
  lymphocytic 079.2
 specified organism NEC 320.8
  late effects 324
 staphylococcal 320.8
  late effects 324
 sterile 320.9
  late effects 324
 streptococcal (acute) 320.8
  late effects 324
 syphilitic 094.9
  congenital 090.4
 torula 116.0
 traumatic (complication of injury)
     995.9
 tuberculous 013.0
  late effect or sequela 019.1
 typhoid 001
 viral, virus (*see also* Meningitis, aseptic)
     045.9
 Wallgren's (*see also* Meningitis, aseptic)
     045.9
Meningocele (spinal) 741.9
 with hydrocephalus 741.0
 cerebral 743.0

Meningocerebritis - *see* Meningitis
Meningococcemia (acute)　036.1
　with meningitis　036.0
　chronic　036.1
Meningococcus, meningococcal (*see also*
　　condition)　036.9
Meningo-encephalitis (*see also* Meningitis)
　　320.9
　acute　046
　chronic　094.1
　diffuse　094.1
　diphasic　063.2
　　late effects　066
　due to
　　blastomycosis NEC (*see also*
　　　Blastomycosis)　116.9
　　mumps　072
　　toxoplasmosis　130.9
　　　acquired　130.0
　　　congenital (active)　130.1
　　　　late effects　130.2
　epidemic　036.0
　infectious (acute)　046
　influenzal　320.0
　　late effects　324
　late effects　324
　lymphocytic (serous)　079.2
　parasitic NEC　123.9
　serous　046
　　lymphocytic　079.2
　specific　094.1
　syphilitic　094.1
　toxic　320.9
　tuberculous　013.0
　　late effect or sequela　019.1
　virus NEC　046
Meningo-encephalocele　743.0
　syphilitic　094.9
　　congenital　090.4
Meningo-encephalomyelitis (*see also*
　　Meningitis)　320.9
　acute　046
　congenital　320.9
　disseminated　320.9
　　H. influenzae　320.0
　　　late effects　324
　　influenzal　320.0
　　　late effects　324
　　late effects　324
　　pneumococcal　320.1
　　　late effects　324
　　specified organism NEC　320.8
　　　late effects　324
　due to
　　actinomycosis　113

Meningo-encephalomyelitis — *continued*
　due to — *continued*
　　Torula　116.0
　　Toxoplasma or toxoplasmosis　130.9
　　　acquired　130.0
　　　congenital (active)　130.1
　　　　late effects　130.2
　　influenzal　320.0
　　　late effects　324
　　late effects　324
Meningo-encephalomyelopathy　781.7
Meningo-encephalopathy　781.7
Meningo-encephalopoliomyelitis　040
　late effects　044
Meningomyelitis (*see also* Meningitis)
　　320.9
　blastomycotic NEC (*see also*
　　　Blastomycosis)　116.9
　due to
　　Torula　116.0
　　H. influenzae　320.0
　　　late effects　324
　late effects　324
　lethargic　065
　　late effects　066
　meningococcal　036.0
　pneumococcal　320.1
　　late effects　324
　specified organism NEC　320.8
　　late effects　324
　syphilitic　094.9
　tuberculous　013.0
　　late effect or sequela　019.1
Meningomyelocele　741.9
　with hydrocephalus　741.0
　syphilitic　094.9
Meningomyeloneuritis - *see* Meningitis
Meningoradiculitis - *see* Meningitis
Meningovascular - *see* condition
Menometrorrhagia　626.6
Menopause, menopausal (symptoms)
　　(syndrome)　627
　arthritis (any site) NEC　714.9
　artificial　627
　crisis　627
　depression　296.0
　　agitated　296.0
　　psychotic　296.0
　insanity　296.0
　melancholia　296.0
　paranoid state　297.1
　paraphrenia　297.1
　premature　627
　psychoneurosis, unspecified　627
　psychosis NEC　299
　surgical　627
　toxic polyarthritis NEC　714.9

Menorrhagia (primary) 626.2
  menopausal 627
  postclimacteric 626.7
  postmenopausal 626.7
  preclimacteric 626.2
  puberty (menses retained) 626.2
Menses, retention 626.9
Menstrual
  disorders NEC 626.9
  period, normal 793.8
Menstruation
  absent 626.0
  delayed 626.9
  disorder NEC 626.9
    psychogenic 305.6
  during pregnancy 634.9
  excessive 626.2
  frequent 626.4
  infrequent 626.9
  irregular 626.5
  latent 626.9
  membranous 626.9
  painful (primary) (secondary) 626.3
    psychogenic 305.6
  precocious 626.9
  protracted 626.9
  retained 626.9
  retrograde 626.9
  scanty 626.1
  suppression 626.9
  vicarious (nasal) 626.9
Mentagra (see also Sycosis) 704
Mental - see also condition
  deficiency - see Retardation, mental
  deterioration (see also Psychosis) 299
  disorder (see also Disorder, mental)
    300.9
  exhaustion 300.5
  insufficiency (congenital) (see also
    Retardation, mental) 315.9
  observation without need for further
    medical care 793.0
  retardation - see Retardation, mental
  subnormality - see Retardation, mental
  upset (see also Disorder, mental)
    300.9
Meralgia paraesthetica 355.1
Mercurial - see condition
Mercurialism NEC 985.0
Merergasia 300.9
Merocele 551.0
  gangrenous, incarcerated, irreducible,
    strangulated or with obstruction
    (intestinal) 553.0
Merycism (see also Rumination) 784.7
Merzbacher-Pelizaeus disease 333.1

Mesaortitis (nonsyphilitic) 446.9
Mesarteritis - see Arteritis
Mesencephalitis (see also Encephalitis)
  323
  late effects 324
Mesenchymoma - see also Neoplasm,
  connective tissue, malignant
  liver 155.0
Mesentery, mesenteric - see condition
Mesiodens, mesiodentes 520.1
  causing crowding 524.3
Mesioocclusion 524.2
Mesocolon - see condition
Mesonephroma 184.9
  of Schiller 183.0
  ovary 183.0
Mesophlebitis - see Phlebitis
Mesostromal dysgenesis 744.8
Mesothelioma (fibrous) (see also
  Neoplasm, benign) 228
  malignant - see Neoplasm, malignant
  peritoneum 158.9
    fibrous 211.7
  pleura 163.0
    fibrous 212.4
Metabolism disorders NEC 279
Metagonimiasis 121.9
Metagonimus infestation (small intestine)
  121.9
Metal
  pigmentation 709.9
  polishers' disease 515.0
    tuberculous 010
Metalliferous miners' lung 516.0
Metamorphopsia 377.4
Metamorphosis, fatty 279
  localized - see Degeneration by site,
    fatty
Metaplasia
  cervix (squamous) 621.9
  endometrium (squamous) 625.9
  kidney (pelvis) (squamous) (see also
    Lesion, kidney) 593.2
  myeloid (agnogenic) 209
  spleen 289.5
    megakaryocytic myeloid 209
    myelogenous 209
  squamous cell, bladder 596.9
Metastasis, metastatic
  abscess - see Abscess
  calcification 279
  neoplasm
    from specified site - see Neoplasm,
      malignant, by site
    to specified site - see Secondary
      neoplasm, by site

Metatarsalgia 787.1
  Morton's 357.9
Metatarsus, metatarsal - *see also*
    condition
  adductus, valgus or varus (congenital)
    754.8
Meteorism 785.4
Methemoglobinemia 289.9
  acquired 289.9
  congenital 289.9
  enzymatic 289.9
  Hb M disease 289.9
  hereditary 289.9
Methemoglobinuria (*see also*
    Hemoglobinuria) 789.4
Methioninemia 270.8
Metritis (acute) (catarrhal) (chronic)
    (septic) (subacute) (suppurative) (*see*
    also Endometritis) 622.0
  cervical (*see also* Cervicitis) 620.9
  hemorrhagic 625.9
Metropathia hemorrhagica 625.9
Metroperitonitis (*see also* Disease, pelvis,
    inflammatory) 616.0
Metrorrhagia 626.6
  arising during pregnancy - *see*
    Hemorrhage, pregnancy
  postpartum (complicating delivery)
    653
  primary 626.6
  psychogenic 305.6
Metrorrhexis, complicating delivery - *see*
    Rupture, uterus, complicating
    delivery
Metrosalpingitis (*see also* Salpingo-
    oophoritis) 614
Metrostaxis 626.6
Metrovaginitis (*see also* Endometritis)
    622.0
Mibelli's disease 757.2
Mice, joint - *see* Loose bodies in joint
Micrencephalon 743.1
Microangiopathy
  thrombotic 446.5
Microcephalus, microcephalic,
    microcephaly 743.1
  due to toxoplasmosis (congenital)
    130.1
Microcolon (congenital) 751.4
Microcornea (congenital) 744.8
Microcytic - *see* condition
Microdontia 520.2
Microdrepanocytosis (*see also*
    Thalassemia) 282.4
Microgastria (congenital) 750.8
Microgenia 524.0

Microgenitalia (congenital) 752.8
Microglossia (congenital) 750.0
Micrognathia, micrognathism (congenital)
    (mandibular) (maxillary) 524.0
Microgyria (congenital) 743.2
Micro-infarct of heart (*see also*
    Insufficiency, coronary) 411.9
Microlithiasis, alveolar, lung 519.2
Micromyelia (congenital) 743.3
Microphakia (congenital) 744.8
Microphthalmia (congenital) 744.1
Microphthalmos (congenital) 744.1
  due to toxoplasmosis (congenital)
    130.1
Micropsia 377.4
Microsporon furfur infestation 111.0
Microsporosis - *see also* Dermatophytosis
    nigra 111.1
Microstomia (congenital) 745.8
Microtia (external ear) (congenital) 745.2
Micturition
  disorder - *see* category 786
    psychogenic 305.6
  frequency (nocturnal) 786.3
    psychogenic 305.6
  painful 786.0
    psychogenic 305.6
Mid plane - *see* condition
Middle
  ear - *see* condition
  lobe syndrome 519.0
Migraine (any type or site) (idiopathic)
    346
Migratory, migrating - *see* condition
Mikulicz's
  disease 527.8
  syndrome 527.8
Miliaria 705.1
  crystallina 705.1
  rubra (tropicalis) 705.1
Miliary - *see* condition
Milium (*see also* Cyst, sebaceous) 706.2
  colloid 709.9
  eyelid 706.2
Milk
  crust 691
  excess secretion 678
  fever, female 678
  poisoning 988.9
  retention 678
  sickness 988.9
Milk-leg
  complicating pregnancy 634.9
    fetus or newborn 763.9
  nonpuerperal 451.0

Milk-leg—*continued*
  puerperal, postpartum, childbirth
      671.0
Milkman's disease or syndrome 265.2
Milky urine - *see* Chyluria
Mill's disease 348.0
Millar's asthma 508.3
Millard-Gubler syndrome 344.1
Millard-Gubler-Foville paralysis 344.1
Millstone makers'
  asthma - *see* Millstone makers', lung
  lung 515.0
    with tuberculosis 010
Milroy's disease 757.0
Miners'
  asthma - *see* Miners', lung
  elbow 731.2
  lung 515.1
    with tuberculosis 010
  nystagmus 300.8
  phthisis 010
  tuberculosis 010
Minkowski-Chauffard syndrome (*see also*
      Spherocytosis) 282.0
Minor - *see* condition
Minor's disease 349.9
Minot-von Willebrand-Jurgen disease
      286.3
Minot's disease 778.2
Minus (and plus) hand (intrinsic) 738.2
Miosis (pupil) 378.6
Mirror writing 306.1
Misadventure (prophylactic) (therapeutic)
      (*see also* Complications) 999.9
  administration of insulin 962.3
  infusion - *see* Complications, infusion
  local applications NEC (of
        fomentations, plasters, etc.)
        999.9
    burn or scald - *see* Burn
  medical care NEC (early) (late) 999.9
    adverse effect of drugs or chemicals
      - *see* Table of adverse effects
    burn or scald - *see* Burn
  radiation - *see* Effect, adverse, radiation
  radiotherapy - *see* Effect, adverse,
        radiotherapy
  surgical procedure (early) (late) - *see*
        Complications, surgical
        procedure
  transfusion - *see* Complications,
        transfusion
  vaccination or other immunilogical
        procedure - *see* Complications,
        vaccination
Misanthropy 301.7
Miscarriage - *see* Abortion, spontaneous

Misplaced, misplacement
  kidney (*see also* Lesion, kidney) 593.2
    congenital 753.3
  organ or site, congenital NEC - *see*
        Malposition, congenital
Missed
  abortion (undelivered) 634.2
  delivery (at or near term) 634.2
  labor (at or near term) (undelivered)
      634.2
Missing - *see also* Absence
  incus (ear) 387.9
  vertebrae (congenital) 756.2
Mitchell's disease 443.8
Mite(s)
  diarrhea 133.9
  grain (itch) 133.9
  hair follicle (itch) 133.9
  in sputum 133.9
Mitral - *see* condition
Mittelschmerz 626.3
Mixed - *see* condition
Mljet disease 757.2
Mobile, mobility
  cecum 751.4
  excessive - *see* Hypermobility
  gallbladder 751.0
  organ or site, congenital NEC - *see*
        Malposition, congenital
Moebius
  disease 346
  syndrome 350
Moeller's
  disease 264
  glossitis 529.4
Molar pregnancy (abortion) (*see also*
        Abortion, other) 645.9
  undelivered 634.9
Molarisation, molarization
  premolars 520.2
Mold(s) in vitreous 117.9
Molding
  head (during birth) (*see also* Birth
        injury, bone or nerve) 772.2
Mole (pigmented) (nonpigmented) 757.1
  benign 757.1
  blood (abortion) (*see also* Abortion,
        other) 645.9
    undelivered 634.9
  Breus' (abortion) (*see also* Abortion,
        other) 645.9
    undelivered 634.9
  cancerous - *see* Melanoma
  carneous (abortion) (*see also* Abortion,
        other) 645.9
    undelivered 634.9

Mole — *continued*
destructive 181
ectopic - *see* Pregnancy, ectopic
fleshy (abortion) (*see also* Abortion,
other) 645.9
undelivered 634.9
hairy 757.1
hemorrhagic (abortion) (*see also*
Abortion, other) 645.9
undelivered 634.9
hydatid, hydatidiform (benign)
(complicating pregnancy)
(delivered) (undelivered) 634.0
malignant (change) 181
infected 757.1
invasive 181
malignant - *see* Melanoma
pregnancy (abortion) (*see also* Abortion,
other) 645.9
undelivered 634.9
tubal - *see* Pregnancy, tubal
vesicular - *see* Mole, hydatid,
hydatidiform
Mollities - *see also* Softening
ossium 265.2
Molluscum
contagiosum 079.0
epitheliale 079.0
fibrosum (*see also* Dermatofibroma)
216.8
pendulum (*see also* Dermatofibroma)
216.8
Monckeberg's arteriosclerosis,
degeneration, disease, or sclerosis
(*see also* Arteriosclerosis,
peripheral) 440.2
Mondor's disease (*see also* Phlebitis)
451.9
Mongolian, mongolianism, mongolism,
mongoloid 759.3
spot 757.1
Monilethrix (congenital) 757.3
Monilia infestation 112
Moniliasis (any site) (generalized) 112
Monoblastic - *see* condition
Monocytic - *see* condition
Monocytosis 289.9
Monomania (*see also* Psychosis) 299
Mononeuritis 355.9
Mononucleosis, infectious 075
Monoplegia 344.0
brain (current episode) (*see also*
Disease, cerebrovascular NEC)
438.9
fetus or newborn (*see also* Birth
injury, brain) 772.0

Monoplegia — *continued*
brain, etc. — *continued*
late effect or residual NEC 344.0
due to specified lesion - *see*
Monoplegia, late effect of
cerebral - *see* Monoplegia, brain
congenital (cerebral) (spastic) (spinal) -
see Monoplegia, infantile
cortical - *see* Monoplegia, brain
embolic (current episode) (*see also*
Embolism, brain) 434.9
late effect or residual 344.0
hysterical (transient) 300.1
infantile (cerebral) (spastic) (spinal)
343.1
with other types of motor disturbance
(e.g., ataxic, athetoid, atonic,
rigidity, or tremor) 343.9
athetoid 343.2
with other types of motor
disturbance (e.g., ataxic,
atonic, rigidity, spastic or
tremor) 343.9
specified type NEC 343.9
late effect or residual of
acute poliomyelitis (conditions in 040-
043) 044
birth injury, intracranial or spinal
(conditions in 764-768 or 772
with fourth digit .0 or .1) - *see*
Monoplegia, infantile
cerebral laceration or contusion
(conditions in 851.0, 851.1)
851.9
fracture or fracture dislocation of
vertebral column with spinal
cord lesion (conditions in
806.0-806.7) 806.9
intracranial
abscess or pyogenic infection
(conditions in 320-323) 324
hemorrhage following injury
(conditions in 853.0, 853.1)
853.9
vascular lesion (conditions in 430-
438) 344.0
spinal cord lesion (nontraumatic)
349.1
traumatic (conditions in 958.0-
958.7) 958.9
subarachnoid, subdural or extradural
hemorrhage, following injury
(conditions in 852.0, 852.1)
852.9
viral encephalitis (conditions in 062-
065) 066

Monoplegia — *continued*
  old or longstanding NEC   344.0
    due to specified lesion - *see*
      Monoplegia, late effect of
  psychogenic   305.1
    specified as conversion reaction
      300.1
  residual NEC   344.0
    due to specified lesion - *see*
      Monoplegia, late effect of
  spastic (cerebral) (infantile) (spinal)
      343.1
    with other types of motor disturbance
      (e.g., ataxic, athetoid, atonic,
      rigidity, or tremor)   343.9
    not infantile or congenital (cerebral)
      344.0
      late effect or residual NEC   344.0
        due to specified lesion - *see*
          Monoplegia, late effect of
    spinal   349.1
      late effect or residual NEC
        349.1
        due to specified lesion - *see*
          Monoplegia, late effect
          of
  spinal (cord)   349.1
    late effect or residual NEC   349.1
      due to specified lesion - *see*
        Monoplegia, late effect of
  thrombotic (current episode) (*see also*
      Thrombosis, brain)   433.9
    late effect or residual   344.0
  transient   787.0
Monorchism, monorchidism   752.1
Monster, monstrosity   759.2
  acephalic   740
  composite   759.1
  compound   759.1
  double   759.1
  twin   759.1
Monteggia's fracture - *see* Fracture, ulna,
    upper end
Moore's syndrome   345.9
Mooren's ulcer (cornea)   363.0
Mooser's bodies   081.0
Moral
  deficiency   301.7
  imbecility   301.7
Morax-Axenfeld conjunctivitis   360
Morbilli   055
Morbus
  Beigel   111.2
  caducus (*see also* Epilepsy)   345.9
  caeruleus   746.8
  comitialis (*see also* Epilepsy)   345.9

Morbus — *continued*
  cordis - *see also* Disease, heart
    valvulorum - *see* Endocarditis
  coxae   729.5
    tuberculous - *see* Tuberculosis, hip
  hemorrhagicus neonatorum   778.2
  maculosus neonatorum   778.2
  regius (*see also* Jaundice)   785.2
  renum (*see also* Lesion, kidney)   593.2
  senilis   713.0
Morel-Kraepelin disease (*see also*
    Schizophrenia)   295.9
Morel-Moore syndrome   723.4
Morel-Morgagni syndrome   723.4
Morgagni
  cyst, organ, hydatid, or appendage
    752.8
  syndrome   723.4
Morgagni-Stokes-Adams syndrome (*see
    also* Block, heart)   427.3
Moria (*see also* Psychosis)   299
Moron - *see* Retardation, mental, mild
Morphea   701.0
Morphinism   304.0
Morphinomania   304.0
Morquio-Brailsford (type)
  disease   273.8
  kyphosis   273.8
Morquio-Ullrich disease   273.8
Morquio's disease or syndrome   273.8
Morsus humanus (open wound) - *see*
    Wound, open
  skin surface intact - *see* Contusion
Mortification (dry) (moist) (*see also*
    Gangrene)   445.9
Morton's
  disease   357.9
  foot   357.9
  metatarsalgia   357.9
  neuralgia   357.9
  neuroma   357.9
  toe   357.9
Morvan's disease   349.0
Mosaicism, mosaic (autosomal)
    (chromosomal)   759.4
  sex   759.5
Motion sickness (from travel, any vehicle)
    (from roundabouts or swings)
    994.6
Motor neurone disease (manifestations)
    NEC   348.9
Mottled (enamel) teeth   520.3
Mottling enamel (teeth) (endemic) (non-
    endemic)   520.3
Mouchet's disease   722.2
Mould(s) (in vitreous)   117.9

Moulders'
  bronchitis 515.0
    with tuberculosis 010
    tuberculosis 010
Mountain
  sickness 993.2
Mouse, joint - *see* Loose bodies in joint
Mouth - *see* condition
Movable
  coccyx 723.9
  kidney (*see also* Lesion, kidney) 593.2
    congenital 753.3
  organ or site, congenital NEC - *see*
      Malposition, congenital
  spleen 289.5
Movements, dystonic 780.3
Mucinosis
  cutaneous 701.9
  papular 701.9
Mucocele
  appendix 543
  buccal cavity 528.9
  gallbladder (*see also* Disease,
      gallbladder) 576.9
  lachrymal, lacrimal sac 378.3
  salivary gland (any) 527.6
  sinus (accessory) (nasal) 505
  turbinate (bone) (middle) (nasal) 505
Muco-enteritis 564.1
Mucoperiostitis
  tympanic
    osteoclastic 387.9
Mucopolysaccharidosis (types 1-6) 273.8
Mucormycosis 117.8
  lung 117.8
Mucositis
  necroticans agranulocytica 288
  tympanic
    sclerosing 387.9
Mucous - *see also* condition
  patches (syphilitic) 091.2
    congenital 090.0
Mucoviscidosis 273.0
Mucus
  asphyxia or suffocation (*see also*
      Asphyxia, mucus) 933
    newborn (*see also* Aspiration, content
        of birth canal) 776.0
  plug 933
    newborn (*see also* Aspiration, content
        of birth canal) 776.0
    tracheobronchial 934
      newborn (*see also* Aspiration,
          content of birth canal)
          776.0
Muguet 112

Mulberry molars 090.5
Mule-spinners' cancer - *see* Neoplasm,
    skin, malignant
Multipartita placenta - *see* Placenta,
    abnormal
Multiple, multiplex - *see also* condition
  birth
    fetus or newborn 769.4
      low birthweight 769.4
    for classification of births in hospital
        - *see* Newborn
  digits (congenital) 755.0
  organ or site not listed - *see* Accessory
Multisclerosis 796.0
Mumps 072
  with oophoritis 072
  encephalitis 072
  meningitis (aseptic) 072
  meningo-encephalitis 072
  orchitis 072
  pancreatitis 072
Mumu (*see also* Infestation, filarial)
    125.9
Munchausen syndrome 306.9
Munchmeyer's disease 733.2
Mural - *see* condition
Murdock's syndrome 273.8
Murmur (cardiac) (heart) (organic) (*see
    also* Endocarditis) 424.9
  aortic (valve) (*see also* Endocarditis,
      aortic) 395.9
  benign - *see* Action, heart, irregular
  diastolic - *see* Endocarditis
  Flint (*see also* Endocarditis, aortic)
      395.9
  functional (*see also* Action, heart,
      irregular) 427.9
  Graham Steell (*see also* Endocarditis,
      pulmonary) 424.9
  mitral (valve) - *see* Endocarditis, mitral
  nonorganic (*see also* Action, heart,
      irregular) 427.9
  organic nonvalvular - *see* Disease, heart
  presystolic, mitral - *see* Endocarditis,
      mitral
  pulmonic (valve) (*see also* Endocarditis,
      pulmonary) 424.9
  systolic (valvular) - *see* Endocarditis
  tricuspid (valve) - *see* Endocarditis,
      tricuspid
  valvular - *see* Endocarditis
Murri's disease 283.9
Muscle, muscular - *see* condition
Musculoneuralgia 717.9
Mushrooming hip 729.5
Musical knee 729.8

Mutism (*see also* Aphasia) 781.5
    deaf (acquired) (congenital) 388
    hysterical 300.1
Myalgia (intercostal) (lumbar) 717.9
    epidemic 074.1
    psychogenic 305.1
    traumatic NEC 996.9
Myasthenia, myasthenic 733.9
    cordis - *see* Failure, heart
    gravis 733.0
    stomach 536.9
        psychogenic 305.5
    syndrome, residual of viral encephalitis
        066
Mycelium infection NEC 117.9
Mycetismus 988.1
Mycetoma 117.4
    bone 117.4
    foot 117.4
    madurae 117.4
    maduromycotic 117.4
    nocardial 117.8
Mycobacteriosis - *see* Mycobacterium
Mycobacterium, mycobacterial (infection)
        031.9
    acid-fast (bacilli) (pulmonary) 031.0
        nonpulmonary 031.9
    anonymous (pulmonary) 031.0
        nonpulmonary 031.9
    atypical (acid-fast bacilli) (pulmonary)
        031.0
        nonpulmonary 031.9
    balnei 031.9
    Battey (pulmonary) 031.0
    chromogenic (acid-fast bacilli) 031.9
        pulmonary 031.0
    fortuitum 031.9
        pulmonary 031.0
    kakerifu 031.9
    kansasii (pulmonary) 031.0
        nonpulmonary 031.9
    kasongo 031.9
    leprae - *see* Leprosy
    luciflavum (pulmonary) 031.0
        nonpulmonary 031.9
    nonphotochromogenic (acid-fast bacilli)
        (pulmonary) 031.0
        nonpulmonary 031.9
    photochromogenic (acid-fast bacilli)
        (pulmonary) 031.0
        nonpulmonary 031.9
    rapid growers 031.9
    scotochromogenic (acid-fast bacilli)
        031.9
    tuberculosis (human, bovine) - *see*
        Tuberculosis

Mycobacterium, etc. — *continued*
    tuberculosis — *continued*
        avian type (pulmonary) 031.0
            nonpulmonary 031.9
        ulcerans 031.9
Mycosis, mycotic 117.9
    cutaneous NEC 111.9
    ear 111.9
    fungoides 202.1
    mouth 112
    pharynx 117.9
    skin NEC 111.9
    stomatitis 112
    systemic NEC 117.9
    tonsil 117.9
    vagina, vaginitis 112
Mydriasis (pupil) 378.6
Myelatelia 743.3
Myelemia 205.9
    acute 205.0
    chronic 205.1
Myelinoclasis, perivascular, acute 323
    late effects 324
Myelitic syndrome, residual of viral
        encephalitis 066
Myelitis (acute) (ascending) (cerebellar)
        (childhood) (chronic) (descending)
        (diffuse) (disseminated)
        (postinfectious) (pressure)
        (progressive) (spinal cord)
        (streptococcal) (subacute)
        (transverse) 323
    late effects 324
    malignant 192.2
    optic neuritis in 341
    postvaccinal 999.1
    syphilitic (transverse) 094.9
    tuberculous 013.9
        late effect or sequela 019.1
    virus 079.9
Myeloblastic - *see* condition
Myeloblastoma (*see also* Leukemia,
        myeloid) 205.9
Myelocele 741.9
    with hydrocephalus 741.0
Myelochloroma 202.2
Myelocystocele 741.9
    with hydrocephalus 741.0
Myelocythemia 205.9
    acute 205.0
    chronic 205.1
Myelocytic - *see* condition
Myelocytoma 203
Myelodysplasia (spinal cord) 743.3
Myelo-encephalitis - *see* Encephalitis
Myelofibrosis (osteosclerosis) 209

Myelogenous - *see* condition
Myeloid - *see* condition
Myeloleukodystrophy   333.1
Myeloma (hemic) (malignant) (multiple)
    (plasma cell)   203
  benign   202.9
  endothelial - *see* Neoplasm, bone,
    malignant
Myelomalacia   349.9
Myelomata, multiple   203
Myelomatosis   203
Myelomeningitis - *see* Meningitis
Myelomeningocele (spinal cord)   741.9
  with hydrocephalus   741.0
Myelopathic - *see* condition
Myelopathy (spinal cord) (toxic)   349.9
  with pernicious anemia   281.0
  cervical   728.4
  lumbar   728.8
  necrotic   323
  thoracic   728.6
  transverse   349.9
Myelophthisis   289.9
Myeloradiculitis   354
Myeloradiculodysplasia (spinal)   743.3
Myelosarcoma   203
Myelosclerosis   209
  disseminated, of nervous system   340
Myelosis (aleukemic) (leukopenic) (*see*
    also Leukemia, myeloid)   205.9
  erythremic (acute)   207.2
  megakaryocytic   209
  multiple   209
  non-leukemic   209
Myiasis   134.0
  cavernous   134.0
Myo-adenoma, prostate   600
Myoblastoma (*see also* Neoplasm,
    connective tissue, malignant)   171.9
  granular cell (*see also* Neoplasm,
    connective tissue, benign)   215
Myocardial - *see* condition
Myocardiopathy   425
Myocarditis (chronic) (degenerative) (fatty)
    (fibroid) (interstitial) (old)
    (progressive) (senile)   428
  with
    arteriosclerosis (conditions in 440)
      (*see also* Ischemia, heart)
      412.9
    hypertension (benign) (conditions in
      401) (*see also* Hypertension,
      heart)   402
    malignant (*see also* Hypertension,
      malignant with heart
      involvement)   400.1

Myocarditis — *continued*
  with — *continued*
    rheumatic fever (conditions in 390)
      active (*see also* Myocarditis, acute,
        rheumatic)   391.2
      inactive or quiescent (with chorea)
        398
  active   422
    rheumatic   391.2
      with chorea (acute) (rheumatic)
        (Sydenham's)   392.0
  acute or subacute (interstitial)   422
    rheumatic   391.2
      with chorea (acute) (rheumatic)
        (Sydenham's)   392.0
  arteriolar - *see* Ischemia, heart
  arteriosclerotic (*see also* Ischemia,
    heart)   412.9
  aseptic of newborn   074.2
  bacterial (acute)   422
  congenital   746.8
  Coxsackie (virus)   074.2
  epidemic of newborn   074.2
  Fiedler's (acute) (isolated)   422
  hypertensive (*see also* Hypertension,
    heart)   402
  malignant (*see also* Hypertension,
    malignant with heart
    involvement)   400.1
  idiopathic   422
  infective   422
  isolated   422
  malignant   422
  rheumatic (chronic) (inactive) (with
    chorea)   398
    active or acute   391.2
      with chorea (acute) (rheumatic)
        (Sydenham's)   392.0
  septic   422
  syphilitic   093.9
    chronic   093.9
  toxic   422
    rheumatic (*see also* Myocarditis,
      acute, rheumatic)   391.2
  tuberculous   017.9
    late effect or sequela   019.9
  typhoid   001
  valvular - *see* Endocarditis
  virus, viral (except Coxsackie)   422
    of newborn (Coxsackie)   074.2
Myocardium, myocardial - *see* condition
Myocardosis   425
Myoclonia
  essential   347.9
  massive   780.3
Myoclonic jerks   780.3

Myoclonus 780.3
  facial 350
  pharyngeal 508.9
  simplex 780.3
Myodiastasis 733.9
Myo-endocarditis - *see* Endocarditis
Myoepithelioma (clear-cell) (*see also*
      Adenoma, sweat glands) 216.2
Myofasciitis (acute) 717.9
  low back 717.9
Myofibroma (*see also* Neoplasm,
      connective tissue, benign) 215
  uterus 218
Myofibrosis 717.9
  heart (*see also* Insufficiency,
      myocardial) 428
  humeroscapular region 717.1
  scapulohumeral 717.1
Myofibrositis 717.9
  scapulohumeral 717.1
Myogelosis (occupational) 733.9
Myoglobinuria 273.8
Myoglobulinuria, primary 273.8
Myokymia - *see* Myoclonus
Myolipoma (*see also* Lipoma) 214.9
Myoma 218
  cervix 218
  complicating delivery 657.9
    fetus or newborn - *see* categories
      764.0-764.9
  malignant - *see* Neoplasm, uterus,
      malignant
  not of uterus - *see also* Neoplasm,
      connective tissue, benign
    malignant - *see* Neoplasm, connective
      tissue, malignant
  noted during pregnancy 634.9
  prostate 600
Myomalacia 733.9
  cordis, heart (*see also* Insufficiency,
      myocardial) 428
Myometritis (*see also* Endometritis) 622.0
Myometrium - *see* condition
Myopathy 733.9
  facioscapulohumeral 330.3
  nemaline 273.8
  primary 733.9
  progressive NEC 733.9
  scapulohumeral 330.3
Myopericarditis (*see also* Pericarditis)
      423
Myopia (axial) (congenital) (increased
      curvature or refraction, nucleus of
      lens) (malignant) (progressive) 370.0
Myosarcoma (*see also* Neoplasm,
      connective tissue, malignant) 171.9

Myosis 378.6
Myositis 717.9
  clostridial 039.0
  due to posture 717.9
  epidemic 074.1
  fibrosa or fibrous (chronic) 733.2
    Volkmann (complicating trauma) 995.7
  infective 732
  multiple - *see* Polymyositis
  occupational 717.9
  orbital, chronic 369.9
  ossificans or ossifying (circumscribed)
      (progressive) (traumatic) 733.2
  purulent 732
  rheumatic 717.9
  rheumatoid 717.9
  suppurative 732
  traumatic (old) 717.9
Myotonia (acquisita) (intermittens) 733.9
  atrophica 330.4
  congenita 330.9
  dystrophica 330.4
Myotonic pupil 378.6
Myriapodiasis 134.2
Myringitis - *see* Otitis media
Mysophobia 300.2
Mytilotoxism 988.0
Myxadenitis
  labialis 528.5
Myxedema (infantile) 244
  circumscribed 242.2
  congenital 243
  cutis 701.9
  localized (pretibial) 242.2
  papular 701.9
  pituitary 244
  postpartum 244
  pretibial 242.2
  thyroid (gland) 244
Myxochondroma (*see also* Chondroma)
      213.2
Myxochondrosarcoma - *see* Neoplasm,
      cartilage, malignant
Myxofibrochondroma (*see also*
      Chondroma) 213.2
Myxofibroma (*see also* Neoplasm,
      connective tissue, benign) 215
Myxofibrosarcoma - *see* Neoplasm,
      connective tissue, malignant
Myxolipoma (*see also* Lipoma) 214.9
Myxoma (*see also* Neoplasm, connective
      tissue, benign) 215
Myxosarcoma (*see also* Neoplasm,
      connective tissue, malignant) 171.9
  breast 217
  malignant 174

N

Naegeli's
  disease 287.3
  leukemia, monocytic 205.1
Naevoxantho-endothelioma 272.0
Naffziger's syndrome 357.0
Naga sore (*see also* Ulcer, skin) 707.9
Nagele's pelvis 738.8
  complicating delivery - *see* Deformity,
    pelvis, complicating delivery
  noted during pregnancy (undelivered)
    634.9
Nail - *see also* condition
  biting, child 308
Nanism, nanosomia (*see also* Dwarfism)
  258.9
  pituitary 253.1
  renis, renalis 593.0
Nanukayami 100.8
Napkin rash 692.9
Narcissism 302.8
Narcolepsy 347.0
  late effect, viral encephalitis 066
Narcosis
  carbon dioxide (respiratory) 783.2
  due to drug - *see* Table of adverse
    effects ,
Narcotism (chronic) (*see also* listing under
  Dependence) 304.9
  acute NEC 967.9
    specified drug - *see* Table of adverse
      effects
Narrow
  anterior chamber angle 378.6
  pelvis (inlet) (outlet)
    complicating delivery - *see*
      Deformity, pelvis, complicating
      delivery
    noted during pregnancy (undelivered)
      634.9
Narrowing
  artery NEC 447
  auditory canal (external) 387.9
  cerebral arteries (*see also* Ischemia,
    cerebral) 437.9
  cicatricial - *see* Cicatrix
  coronary artery (*see also* Ischemia,
    heart) 412.9
    due to syphilis 093.9
      congenital 090.5
  ear, middle 387.9

Narrowing—*continued*
  eustachian tube 387.9
  eyelid 378.2
  intervertebral
    disc or space NEC - *see*
      Displacement, intervertebral
      disc
  joint space, hip 729.5
  larynx 508.9
  mesenteric artery (with gangrene)
    444.2
  palate 524.9
  palpebral fissure 378.2
  retinal artery 377.0
  ureter 593.3
  urethra (*see also* Stricture, urethra)
    598
Narrowness, abnormal, eyelid 744.8
Nasal - *see* condition
Nasolachrymal, nasolacrimal - *see*
  condition
Nasopharyngeal - *see also* condition
  pituitary gland 758.3
Nasopharyngioma - *see* Neoplasm,
  pharynx
Nasopharyngitis (acute) (infective)
  (subacute) 460
  chronic 502.1
  septic 034.0
  streptococcal 034.0
  suppurative (chronic) 502.1
  ulcerative (chronic) 502.1
Nasopharynx, nasopharyngeal - *see*
  condition
Natal
  tooth, teeth 520.6
Nausea (*see also* Vomiting) 784.1
  epidemic 079.8
  gravidarum - *see* Hyperemesis,
    gravidarum
  marina 994.6
Navel - *see* condition
Nearsightedness 370.0
Nebula, cornea - *see* Opacity, cornea
Necator americanus infestation 126.1
Necatoriasis 126.1
Neck - *see* condition
Necrencephalus (*see also* Softening, brain)
  438.9
Necrobacillosis 039.9

Necrobiosis 796.0
  brain or cerebral (*see also* Disease,
      cerebrovascular NEC) 438.9
  lipoidica 709.9
    diabeticorum - *see* category 250
Necrolysis, toxic epidermal 695.1
  due to drug (*see also* Table of adverse
      effects) 977.9
Necrophilia 302.8
Necrosis, necrotic (ischemic) (*see also*
      Gangrene) 445.9
  adrenal (capsule) (gland) 255.9
  antrum 508.9
  aorta (hyaline) (*see also* Aneurysm,
      aorta) 441.9
    cystic medial 441.0
  bladder (aseptic) (sphincter) 596.9
  bone 720.1
    acute 720.0
    aseptic or avascular 723.5
    ethmoid 508.9
    jaw 526.4
    tuberculous - *see* Tuberculosis, bone
  brain (softening) (*see also* Softening,
      brain) 438.9
  breast (aseptic) (fat) 611.0
  bronchi 519.9
  central nervous system NEC (*see also*
      Softening, brain) 438.9
  cerebellar (*see also* Softening, brain)
      438.9
  cerebral (softening) (*see also* Softening,
      brain) 438.9
  cornea (*see also* Keratitis) 363.9
  cystic medial (aorta) 441.0
  dental (*see also* Caries, dental) 521.0
  ear (aseptic) (ossicle) 387.9
  esophagus 530.9
  ethmoid (bone) 508.9
  eyelid 378.2
  fat (generalized) 279
    localized - *see* Degeneration by site,
        fatty
  gallbladder (*see also* Cholecystitis)
      575
  gastric 537.9
  heart - *see* Infarct, myocardium
  hepatic (*see also* Necrosis, liver) 570
  hip (aseptic) (avascular) 723.5
  intestine (any part) - *see* Gangrene,
      intestine
  jaw 526.4
  kidney (acute) (bilateral) (*see also*
      Lesion, kidney) 593.2
    cortical 593.2
      with abortion - *see* Abortion, by
          type, with toxemia

Necrosis, necrotic—*continued*
  kidney—*continued*
    cortical—*continued*
      arising during pregnancy 639.9
        fetus or newborn 762.9
      puerperal, postpartum 639.9
    papillary (*see also* Pyelitis) 590.1
  larynx 508.3
  liver (acute) (congenital) (massive)
      (subacute) 570
    with abortion - *see* Abortion, by type,
        with toxemia
    arising during pregnancy 639.0
      fetus or newborn 762.5
    puerperal, postpartum 639.0
  lung 513
  lymphatic gland 683
  mammary gland 611.0
  mastoid (chronic) - *see* Mastoiditis,
      chronic
  mesentery (fat) - *see* Gangrene,
      mesentery
  mitral valve - *see* Endocarditis, mitral
  myocardium, myocardial - *see* Infarct,
      myocardium
  nose 508.9
  omentum (fat) - *see* Gangrene,
      mesentery
  orbit, orbital 378.9
  ovary (*see also* Salpingo-oophoritis)
      614
  pancreas (aseptic) (duct) (fat) 577.9
    acute 577.0
    infective 577.0
  peritoneum (fat) - *see* Gangrene,
      mesentery
  pharynx 462
    in granulocytopenia 288
  phosphorus - *see* Table of adverse
      effects
  pituitary (gland) (Sheehan) 253.1
  placenta - *see* Placenta, abnormal
  pneumonia 513
  pulmonary 513
  pulp (dental) 522.1
  pylorus 537.9
  radiation - *see* Effect, adverse, radiation
  radium - *see* Effect, adverse,
      radioactive substance
  renal - *see* Necrosis, kidney
  sclera 378.6
  scrotum 607.9
  skin or subcutaneous tissue NEC
      445.9
  spine, spinal (column) 720.1
    acute 720.0

Necrosis, necrotic — *continued*
  spine, spinal — *continued*
    cord 349.9
  spleen 289.5
  stomach 537.9
  stomatitis 528.1
  subcutaneous fat
    fetus or newborn 778.9
  subendocardial - *see* Infarct,
    myocardium
  suprarenal (capsule) (gland) 255.9
  testis 607.9
  thymus (gland) 254
  tonsil 500
  tooth, teeth (*see also* Caries, dental)
    521.0
  trachea 519.9
  tuberculous NEC - *see* Tuberculosis
  tubular (acute) (anoxic) (toxic) (*see also*
    Nephrosis, tubular) 593.1

Necrosis, necrotic — *continued*
  umbilical cord - *see* Complications,
    umbilical cord
  vagina 629.9
  vertebra 720.1
    acute 720.0
    tuberculous - *see* Tuberculosis, spine
    x-ray - *see* Effect, adverse, x-rays
Necrospermia 606
Negativism 301.7
Neglect (newborn) 994.9
  after or at birth 994.9
Neisserian infection NEC - *see*
  Gonococcus
Nelaton's tumor - *see* Teratoma
Nematodiasis NEC 127.9
  ancylostoma (*see also* Ancylostomiasis)
    126.9
Neonatal - *see also* condition
  tooth, teeth 520.6
Neonatorum - *see* condition

	Malignant	Benign	Unspecified
Neoplasm, neoplastic..	199.1	228	239.9

Note — Secondary malignant neoplasms are classified differently from primary neoplasms of the same sites. The code numbers given in the following list apply to primary malignant neoplasms and to malignant neoplasms unspecified as to whether primary or secondary. For the code numbers for secondary neoplasms, *see* Secondary neoplasm.

For most benign neoplasms classifiable to category 216, a dash (. —) appears in the fourth digit code position. Where a dash appears one of the following fourth digits should be used:

    .0 *Epidermis*
    .1 *Hair follicles and sebaceous glands*
    .2 *Sweat glands and sweat ducts*
    .8 *Other*
    .9 *Unspecified*

	Malignant	Benign	Unspecified
abdomen, abdominal..	195.0	228	239.9
organ..	195.0	228	239.9
viscera..	195.0	228	239.9
wall..	173.6	216.–	232.2
abdominopelvic..	195.0	228	239.9
accessory sinus — *see* Neoplasm, sinus			
acromion (process)...	170.4	213.9	232.0
adenoid (tissue) (pharynx)..	147	210.7	239.0
adrenal gland..	194.0	226.0	239.1
functionally active NEC..	194.0	255.0	255.0
ala nasi (external)...	173.3	216.–	232.2
alimentary canal or tract NEC..	159	211.9	230.9
alveolus (process or ridge)..	143.9	210.4	239.0
lower..	143.1	210.4	239.0
upper..	143.0	210.4	239.0
ampulla of Vater...	156.2	211.5	230.5

	Malignant	Benign	Unspecified

Neoplasm, neoplastic — *continued*

	Malignant	Benign	Unspecified
ankle NEC	195.9	228	239.9
anorectal	154.2	211.4	230.4
antrum (Highmore) (maxillary)	160.2	212.0	231.0
anus, anal (skin)	173.6	216.-	232.2
canal	154.2	211.4	230.4
sphincter	154.2	211.4	230.4
aorta	171.1	227.1	232.1
aortic body	194.8	226.8	239.1
appendix	153.0	211.3	230.3
areola (female) (male)	174	217	233
arm NEC	195.9	228	239.9
artery — *see also* Neoplasm, connective tissue			
benign — *see* Hemangioma			
arytenoid (cartilage)	161.8	212.1	231.1
auditory			
canal (external)	173.2	216.-	232.2
internal	160.1	212.0	231.0
nerve	192.0	225.1	238.2
auricle, ear	195.9	228	239.9
cartilage	171.0	215	232.1
auricular canal (external)	173.2	216.-	232.2
internal	160.1	212.0	231.0
auris, ear	195.9	228	239.9
autonomic nerve or nervous system	192.5	225.6	238.7
ganglion — *see* Neoplasm, nervous system, ganglion			
axilla, axillary	195.9	228	239.9
fold	173.6	216.-	232.2
lymph			
channel or vessel	171.1	227.2	232.1
gland or node (*see also* Neoplasm, lymph gland)	196.3	228	239.9
back NEC	195.9	228	239.9
Bartholin's gland	184.1	221.2	236.2
basilar	191	225.0	238.1
Bichat's fat pad	145.0	210.4	239.0
bile or biliary (tract)	156.9	211.5	230.5
canals, interlobular	155.1	211.5	230.5
duct or passage (common) (extrahepatic)	156.1	211.5	230.5
intrahepatic	155.1	211.5	230.5
interlobular	155.1	211.5	230.5
bladder (urinary) (sphincter) (orifice)	188	223.3	237.6
blood vessel — *see also* Neoplasm, connective tissue			
benign — *see* Hemangioma			
bone (periosteum)	170.9	213.9	232.0
acromion (process)	170.4	213.9	232.0
ankle	170.8	213.9	232.0
arm NEC	170.4	213.9	232.0
astragalus	170.8	213.9	232.0
back NEC	170.2	213.9	232.0
calcaneus	170.8	213.9	232.0
carpus (any)	170.5	213.9	232.0
cartilage NEC	170.9	213.9	232.0
costal	170.3	213.9	232.0
rib	170.3	213.9	232.0

Neoplasm, neoplastic — *continued*
  bone — *continued*
    cartilage NEC — *continued*

	Malignant	Benign	Unspecified
semilunar	170.8	213.9	232.0
chest wall	170.3	213.9	232.0
clavicle	170.3	213.9	232.0
coccygeal vertebra	170.6	213.9	232.0
coccyx	170.6	213.9	232.0
costal cartilage	170.3	213.9	232.0
cuboid	170.8	213.9	232.0
cuneiform	170.9	213.9	232.0
ankle	170.8	213.9	232.0
wrist	170.5	213.9	232.0
digital	170.9	213.9	232.0
finger	170.5	213.9	232.0
toe	170.8	213.9	232.0
ear (meatus)	170.0	213.9	232.0
elbow	170.4	213.9	232.0
ethmoid (labyrinth)	170.0	213.9	232.0
face	170.0	213.9	232.0
lower jaw	170.1	213.9	232.0
femur (any part)	170.7	213.9	232.0
fibula (any part)	170.7	213.9	232.0
finger (any)	170.5	213.9	232.0
foot	170.8	213.9	232.0
forearm	170.4	213.9	232.0
frontal	170.0	213.9	232.0
hand	170.5	213.9	232.0
heel	170.8	213.9	232.0
hip	170.6	213.9	232.0
humerus (any part)	170.4	213.9	232.0
ilium	170.6	213.9	232.0
inferior maxilla	170.1	213.9	232.0
innominate	170.6	213.9	232.0
intervertebral cartilage or disc	170.2	213.9	232.0
intraorbital	170.0	213.9	232.0
ischium	170.6	213.9	232.0
jaw (upper)	170.0	213.9	232.0
lower	170.1	213.9	232.0
knee	170.8	213.9	232.0
leg NEC	170.7	213.9	232.0
long	170.9	213.9	232.0
lower limbs NEC	170.7	213.9	232.0
upper limbs NEC	170.4	213.9	232.0
lower jaw	170.1	213.9	232.0
lower limb (long bones) NEC	170.7	213.9	232.0
short bones	170.8	213.9	232.0
lunate	170.5	213.9	232.0
malar	170.0	213.9	232.0
mandible	170.1	213.9	232.0
marrow	202.2	202.9	202.9
maxilla, maxillary (superior)	170.0	213.9	232.0
inferior	170.1	213.9	232.0
meatus (ear)	170.0	213.9	232.0

	Malignant	Benign	Unspecified
Neoplasm, neoplastic — *continued*			
bone — *continued*			
metacarpus (any)	170.5	213.9	232.0
metatarsus (any)	170.8	213.9	232.0
navicular	170.8	213.9	232.0
nose, nasal	170.0	213.9	232.0
occipital	170.0	213.9	232.0
olefactory groove	170.0	213.9	232.0
orbit	170.0	213.9	232.0
os magnum	170.5	213.9	232.0
osseous meatus	170.0	213.9	232.0
parietal	170.0	213.9	232.0
patella	170.8	213.9	232.0
pelvic	170.6	213.9	232.0
phalanges	170.9	213.9	232.0
foot	170.8	213.9	232.0
hand	170.5	213.9	232.0
pisiform	170.5	213.9	232.0
pubic	170.6	213.9	232.0
radius (any part)	170.4	213.9	232.0
rib	170.3	213.9	232.0
sacral vertebra	170.6	213.9	232.0
sacrum	170.6	213.9	232.0
scaphoid	170.5	213.9	232.0
scapula (any part)	170.4	213.9	232.0
sella turcica	170.0	213.9	232.0
semilunar	170.5	213.9	232.0
short	170.9	213.9	232.0
lower limbs	170.8	213.9	232.0
upper limbs	170.5	213.9	232.0
shoulder	170.4	213.9	232.0
skeleton, skeletal NEC	170.9	213.9	232.0
skull	170.0	213.9	232.0
sphenoid	170.0	213.9	232.0
spine, spinal (column)	170.2	213.9	232.0
coccyx	170.6	213.9	232.0
sacrum	170.6	213.9	232.0
sternum	170.3	213.9	232.0
superior maxilla	170.0	213.9	232.0
tarsus (any)	170.8	213.9	232.0
temporal	170.0	213.9	232.0
thumb	170.5	213.9	232.0
tibia (any part)	170.7	213.9	232.0
toe (any)	170.8	213.9	232.0
trapezium	170.5	213.9	232.0
trapezoid	170.5	213.9	232.0
turbinate	170.0	213.9	232.0
ulna (any part)	170.4	213.9	232.0
unciform	170.5	213.9	232.0
upper			
jaw	170.0	213.9	232.0
limb (long bones) NEC	170.4	213.9	232.0
short bones	170.5	213.9	232.0
vertebra (column)	170.2	213.9	232.0

	Malignant	Benign	Unspecified
Neoplasm, neoplastic — *continued*			
bone — *continued*			
vertebra (column) — *continued*			
coccyx	170.6	213.9	232.0
sacrum	170.6	213.9	232.0
vomer	170.0	213.9	232.0
wrist	170.5	213.9	232.0
xiphoid process	170.3	213.9	232.0
book leaf (mouth)	144	210.3	239.0
bowel — *see* Neoplasm, intestine			
brachial plexus	192.4	225.5	238.6
brain (lobe) (ventricle)	191	225.0	238.1
membrane	192.1	225.2	238.3
meninges	192.1	225.2	238.3
branchial (cleft) (vestiges)	146.8	210.6	239.0
breast (female) (male) (connective tissue) (glandular tissue) (skin) (soft parts)	174	217	233
Brenner	183.0	220.9	220.9
broad ligament	183.1	221.0	236.0
bronchiogenic, bronchogenic (lung)	162.1	212.3	231.3
bronchus	162.1	212.3	231.3
brow	173.3	216.–	232.2
buccal (cavity) NEC	145.9	210.4	239.0
commissure	145.0	210.4	239.0
groove (lower) (upper)	145.0	210.4	239.0
mucosa	145.0	210.4	239.0
bulbo-urethral gland	189.9	223.8	237.9
bursa — *see also* Neoplasm, connective tissue			
pharyngeal	147	210.7	239.0
buttock NEC	173.6	216.–	232.2
canal of Nuck	184.1	221.2	236.2
canaliculi			
biliferi	155.1	211.5	230.5
intrahepatic	155.1	211.5	230.5
canthus (eye)	173.1	216.–	232.2
capillary — *see also* Neoplasm, connective tissue			
benign — *see* Hemangioma			
caput coli	153.0	211.3	230.3
cardia	151.0	211.1	230.1
cardiac orifice (stomach)	151.0	211.1	230.1
cardio-esophagus	151.0	211.1	230.1
carina (tracheal)	162.0	212.2	231.2
carotid (artery)	171.0	227.1	232.1
body	194.8	226.4	239.1
carpus (any bone)	170.5	213.9	232.0
cartilage (articular) (joint) NEC (*see also* Neoplasm, bone)	170.9	213.9	232.0
arytenoid	161.8	212.1	231.1
auricular	171.0	215	232.1
bronchi	162.1	212.3	231.3
costal	170.3	213.9	232.0
cricoid	161.8	212.1	231.1
cuneiform	161.8	212.1	231.1
ear (external)	171.0	215	232.1
ensiform	170.3	213.9	232.0
epiglottis	161.8	212.1	231.1

	Malignant	Benign	Unspeci- fied
Neoplasm, neoplastic *— continued*			
cartilage (articular) *— continued*			
eyelid	171.0	215	232.1
larynx, laryngeal	161.8	212.1	231.1
nose, nasal	160.0	212.0	231.0
pinna	171.0	215	232.1
rib	170.3	213.9	232.0
semilunar (knee)	170.8	213.9	232.0
thyroid	161.8	212.1	231.1
trachea	162.0	212.2	231.2
cauda equina	192.2	225.3	238.4
cavum septi pellucidi	191	225.0	238.1
cecum	153.0	211.3	230.3
central nervous system *— see* Neoplasm, nervous system			
cerebellopontine	191	225.0	238.1
cerebellum, cerebellar	191	225.0	238.1
cerebrum, cerebral	191	225.0	238.1
cervical lymph			
channel or vessel	171.0	227.2	232.1
gland or node (*see also* Neoplasm, lymph gland)	196.0	228	239.9
cervicofacial	173.3	216.–	232.2
cervix (stump) (uteri) (uterus)	180	219.9	234.1
cheek (external)	173.3	216.–	232.2
internal	145.0	210.4	239.0
chest wall NEC	195.9	228	239.9
chiasma opticum	192.0	225.1	238.2
chin	173.3	216.–	232.2
cholangiolitic	155.1	211.5	230.5
choroid	190	224	238.0
plexus	191	225.0	238.1
chromaffin tissue	194.8	226.8	239.1
adrenal, suprarenal	194.0	226.0	239.1
carotid body	194.8	226.4	239.1
ciliary			
body	190	224	238.0
nerve	192.0	225.1	238.2
clavicle	170.3	213.9	232.0
clitoris	184.1	221.2	236.2
coccygeal			
body or glomus	194.8	226.8	239.1
vertebra	170.6	213.9	232.0
coccyx	170.6	213.9	232.0
colon *— see* Neoplasm, intestine, large			
common duct	156.1	211.5	230.5
conjunctiva	190	224	238.0
connective tissue NEC	171.9	215	232.1

Note — Neoplasms of connective tissue (bursa, fascia, ligament, muscle, soft parts, synovial membranes, tendon, etc.) or of types that indicate connective tissue, are to be coded as for neoplasms of the stated site except for those sites listed below or sites otherwise classifiable to 195, 228 or 239 (171.0–171.9, 215, 232.1).

Neoplasms of the types coded to 214 and 227 remain at these categories for all sites, except for angioma and hemangioma of nervous system and retina (225, 224).

The following are common types of neoplasm of connective tissue:

Malignant: angiosarcoma, fibrosarcoma, hemangiosarcoma, leiomyosarcoma, liposarcoma, lymphangiosarcoma, myosarcoma, myxosarcoma, perithelioma, rhabdomyosarcoma, and rhabdosarcoma.

Benign: angioma, desmoid tumor, endothelioma, fibroma, leiomyoma, lymphangioma, myoma, myxoma and rhabdomyoma.

	Malignant	Benign	Unspecified
Neoplasm, neoplastic — *continued*			
connective tissue — *continued*			
abdominal wall	171.1	215	232.1
ankle	171.3	215	232.1
arm	171.2	215	232.1
auricle (ear)	171.0	215	232.1
axilla	171.1	215	232.1
back	171.1	215	232.1
breast (female) (male)	174	217	233
buttock	171.1	215	232.1
cheek	171.0	215	232.1
chest wall	171.1	215	232.1
chin	171.0	215	232.1
coccygeal body or glomus	194.8	226.8	239.1
diaphragm	171.1	215	232.1
ear (external)	171.0	215	232.1
elbow	171.2	215	232.1
eyelid	171.0	215	232.1
face	171.0	215	232.1
finger	171.2	215	232.1
foot	171.3	215	232.1
forearm	171.2	215	232.1
groin	171.1	215	232.1
hand	171.2	215	232.1
head	171.0	215	232.1
heart	171.1	215	232.1
heel	171.3	215	232.1
hip	171.3	215	232.1
hypochondrium	171.1	215	232.1
iliopsoas muscle	171.3	215	232.1
jaw	143.9	210.4	239.0
knee	171.3	215	232.1
leg	171.3	215	232.1
lower limb	171.3	215	232.1
myocardium	171.1	215	232.1
nates	171.1	215	232.1
neck	171.0	215	232.1
orbit	171.0	215	232.1
pelvis	171.1	215	232.1
perineum	171.1	215	232.1
popliteal space	171.3	215	232.1
psoas muscle	171.1	215	232.1

	Malignant	Benign	Unspeci-fied
Neoplasm, neoplastic — *continued*			
connective tissue — *continued*			
shoulder	171.2	215	232.1
skin (dermis) NEC	173.9	216.8	232.2
thigh	171.3	215	232.1
thorax	171.1	215	232.1
thoracic duct	171.1	227.2	232.1
thumb	171.2	215	232.1
toe	171.3	215	232.1
trunk	171.1	215	232.1
upper limb	171.2	215	232.1
wrist	171.2	215	232.1
cornea	190	224	238.0
corpora			
cavernosa			
female	184.1	221.2	236.2
male	187.0	222.1	237.1
quadrigemina	191	225.0	238.1
corpus			
albicans	183.0	220.9	220.9
lutem	183.0	220.9	220.9
uteri	182.0	219.9	234.9
costal cartilage	170.3	213.9	232.0
Cowper's gland	189.9	223.8	237.9
cranial nerve	192.0	225.1	238.2
optic	192.0	225.1	238.2
craniobuccal pouch	194.3	226.2	226.2
craniopharyngeal (duct or pouch)	194.3	226.2	226.2
cricoid cartilage	161.8	212.1	231.1
cutaneous — *see* Neoplasm, skin			
cutis — *see* Neoplasm, skin			
cystic duct (common)	156.1	211.5	230.5
diaphragm	171.1	215	232.1
digestive organs, system, tube, or tract NEC	159	211.9	230.9
disease, generalized	199.0	228	199.0
disseminated	199.0	228	199.0
Douglas' cul-de-sac or pouch	158.9	211.7	230.7
duodenojejunal junction	152.0	211.2	230.2
duodenum	152.0	211.2	230.2
dura (mater)	192.9	225.9	238.9
cerebral	192.1	225.2	238.3
spinal	192.3	225.4	238.5
ear (external)	195.9	228	239.9
auricle or auris	195.9	228	239.9
canal external	173.2	216.-	232.2
cartilage	171.0	215	232.1
external meatus	173.2	216.-	232.2
inner	160.1	212.0	231.0
middle	160.1	212.0	231.0
skin	173.2	216.-	232.2
ejaculatory duct	187.8	222.8	237.2
elbow NEC	195.9	228	239.9
en cuirasse	174	—	—

	Malignant	Benign	Unspecified
Neoplasm, neoplastic—*continued*			
endocervix	180	219.9	234.1
endocrine gland NEC	194.9	226.9	239.1
adrenal	194.0	226.0	239.1
functionally active NEC	194.0	255.0	255.0
aortic body	194.8	226.8	239.1
carotid body	194.8	226.4	239.1
chromaffin tissue	194.8	226.8	239.1
adrenal, suprarenal	194.0	226.0	239.1
carotid body	194.8	226.4	239.1
craniobuccal pouch	194.3	226.2	226.2
craniopharyngeal duct or pouch	194.3	226.2	226.2
hypophyseal duct	194.3	226.2	226.2
intrasellar	194.3	226.2	226.2
ovary	183.0	220.9	235
functionally active	183.0	256.0	256.0
pancreas—*see* Neoplasm, pancreas			
parathyroid	194.1	226.8	239.1
pineal	194.4	226.3	239.1
pituitary	194.3	226.2	226.2
functionally active	194.3	253.0	253.0
Rathke's pouch	194.3	226.2	226.2
sella turcica	194.3	226.2	226.2
suprarenal	194.0	226.0	239.1
functionally active	194.0	255.0	255.0
testis	186	222.0	237.0
functionally active	186	257.0	257.0
thymus	194.2	226.1	239.1
thyroid	193	226.8	239.1
endometrium (stroma)	182.0	219.9	234.9
ensiform cartilage	170.3	213.9	232.0
enteric—*see* Neoplasm, intestine			
epididymis	187.8	222.8	237.2
epidural	192.9	225.9	238.9
epiglottis (cartilage)	161.8	212.1	231.1
anterior surface	146.8	210.6	239.0
epipleural	163.0	212.4	231.4
epoophoron	183.1	221.0	236.0
esophagus	150	211.0	230.0
ethmoid (sinus)	160.8	212.0	231.0
bone or labyrinth	170.0	213.9	232.0
Eustachian tube	160.1	212.0	231.0
Ewing's—*see* Neoplasm, bone, malignant			
external			
meatus (ear)	173.2	216.–	232.2
os uteri	180	219.9	234.1
extradural	192.9	225.9	238.9
extrarectal	195.1	228	239.9
extremity (upper) (lower) NEC	195.9	228	239.9
eye	190	224	238.0
glioma	190	224	190
eyebrow	173.3	216.–	232.2
eyelid (lower) (upper) (skin)	173.1	216.–	232.2
cartilage	171.0	215	232.1

	Malignant	Benign	Unspecified
Neoplasm, neoplastic — *continued*			
face NEC	173.3	216.-	232.2
fallopian tube (accessory)	183.1	221.0	236.0
fascia — *see* Neoplasm, connective tissue			
fauces, faucial NEC	146.9	210.6	239.0
pillars	146.8	210.6	239.0
femur (any part)	170.7	213.9	232.0
fibula (any part)	170.7	213.9	232.0
finger NEC	195.9	228	239.9
flank NEC	195.9	228	239.9
follicle, Nabothian	180	219.9	234.1
foot NEC	195.9	228	239.9
foramen cecum of tongue	141.1	210.1	239.0
forearm NEC	195.9	228	239.9
forehead	173.3	216.-	232.2
frenulum			
labii — *see* Neoplasm, lip			
linguae	141.3	210.1	239.0
frontal			
bone	170.0	213.9	232.0
meninges	192.1	225.2	238.3
sinus	160.8	212.0	231.0
fundus			
stomach	151.8	211.1	230.1
uterus	182.0	219.9	234.9
gall duct (extrahepatic)	156.1	211.5	230.5
intrahepatic	155.1	211.5	230.5
gallbladder	156.0	211.5	230.5
ganglion (sympathetic) — *see* Neoplasm, nervous system, ganglion			
Gartner's duct	183.1	221.0	236.0
gastric — *see* Neoplasm, stomach			
gastrocolic	159	211.9	230.9
gastro-intestinal (tract)	159	211.9	230.9
generalized	199.0	228	199.0
genital organ			
female NEC	184.9	221.9	236.9
specified site NEC	184.8	221.8	236.8
male NEC	187.9	222.9	237.2
specified site NEC	187.8	222.8	237.2
genito-urinary			
female	184.9	221.9	236.9
male	187.9	222.9	237.2
gingiva (alveolar) (marginal)	143.9	210.4	239.0
lower	143.1	210.4	239.0
upper	143.0	210.4	239.0
glabella	173.3	216.-	232.2
gland, glandular (lymphatic) (system) — *see also* Neoplasm, lymph gland			
endocrine — *see* Neoplasm, endocrine gland			
salivary — *see* Neoplasm, salivary gland			
glans penis	187.0	222.1	237.1
glossopharyngeal sulcus	146.8	210.6	239.0
glottis	161.0	212.1	231.1

	Malignant	Benign	Unspecified

Neoplasm, neoplastic — *continued*
  intestine, intestinal — *continued*
    large — *continued*

	Malignant	Benign	Unspecified
hepatic flexure	153.1	211.3	230.3
ileocecum	153.0	211.3	230.3
sigmoid flexure (lower) (upper)	153.3	211.3	230.3
splenic flexure	153.1	211.3	230.3
lymph			
channel or vessel	——	227.2	——
malignant or unspecified — *code as* Neoplasm, intestine			
gland or node (*see also* Neoplasm, lymph gland)	196.2	228	239.9
small	152.9	211.2	230.2
duodenum	152.0	211.2	230.2
ileum	152.2	211.2	230.2
jejunum	152.1	211.2	230.2
tract NEC	153.9	211.3	230.3
intra-abdominal	195.0	228	239.9
intracranial	191	225.0	238.1
intra-ocular	190	224	238.0
intra-orbital	190	224	238.0
bone	170.0	213.9	232.0
eye	190	224	238.0
glioma	190	224	190
intrasellar	194.3	226.2	226.2
bone	170.0	213.9	232.0
intrathoracic (cavity) (organs NEC)	163.9	212.9	231.9
iris	190	224	238.0
ischiorectal fossa	195.1	228	239.9
ischium	170.6	213.9	232.0
islands of Langerhans	157.9	251	251
jaw (bone) (upper)	170.0	213.9	232.0
lower	170.1	213.9	232.0
soft tissues	143.9	210.4	239.0
lower	143.1	210.4	239.0
upper	143.0	210.4	239.0
jejunum	152.1	211.2	230.2
joint NEC (*see also* Neoplasm, bone)	170.9	213.9	232.0
bursa or synovial membrane — *see* Neoplasm, connective tissue			
kidney	189.0	223.0	237.3
calyx	189.1	223.1	237.4
embryonal (adults)	189.0	223.0	189.0
hilus	189.1	223.1	237.4
pelvis	189.1	223.1	237.4
knee NEC	195.9	228	239.9
Krukenberg's (malignant) (secondary)	198.9	——	198.9
labia (majora) (minora)	184.1	221.2	236.2
labial fold	184.1	221.2	236.2
labium (majus) (minus)	184.1	221.2	236.2
lachrymal, lacrimal (apparatus) (caruncle) (gland) (sac)	190	224	238.0
laryngopharynx	148.9	210.8	239.0
larynx NEC	161.9	212.1	231.1
cartilage	161.8	212.1	231.1
extrinsic NEC	161.8	212.1	231.1

	Malignant	Benign	Unspeci-fied
Neoplasm, neoplastic — *continued*			
larynx NEC — *continued*			
intrinsic	161.0	212.1	231.1
ventricle	161.8	212.1	231.1
leg NEC	195.9	228	239.9
ligament — *see also* Neoplasm, connective tissue			
broad	183.1	221.0	236.0
Mackenrodt's	183.1	221.0	236.0
round	183.1	221.0	236.0
sacro-uterine	183.1	221.0	236.0
uterine	183.1	221.0	236.0
utero-ovarian	183.1	221.0	236.0
uterosacral	183.1	221.0	236.0
lingual NEC (*see also* Neoplasm, tongue)	141.9	210.1	239.0
lip (mucous membrane)	140.9	210.0	239.0
both lips	140.2	210.0	239.0
skin	173.0	216.–	232.2
commissure	140.9	210.0	239.0
lower	140.1	210.0	239.0
skin	173.0	216.–	232.2
upper	140.0	210.0	239.0
liver	197.8	211.5	230.5
primary	155.0	———	———
lumbrosacral plexus	192.4	225.5	238.6
lung	162.1	212.3	231.3
lymph, lymphatic			
channel NEC (*see also* Neoplasm, connective tissue)	171.9	227.2	232.1
gland	196.9	228	239.9
axilla, axillary	196.3	228	239.9
brachial	196.3	228	239.9
bronchopulmonary	196.1	228	239.9
cervical	196.0	228	239.9
epitrochlear	196.3	228	239.9
face	196.0	228	239.9
groin	196.4	228	239.9
head	196.0	228	239.9
iliac	196.4	228	239.9
inguina, inguinal	196.4	228	239.9
intestinal	196.2	228	239.9
intra-abdominal	196.2	228	239.9
intrathoracic	196.1	228	239.9
limb			
lower	196.4	228	239.9
upper	196.3	228	239.9
lower limb	196.4	228	239.9
mediastinal	196.1	228	239.9
mesenteric	196.2	228	239.9
multiple sites in categories 196.0–196.7	196.8	228	239.9
neck	196.0	228	239.9
popliteal	196.4	228	239.9
primary (any site)	202.2	202.9	202.9
retroperitoneal	196.2	228	239.9
specified site not classifiable to 196.0–196.4	196.7	228	239.9
splenic	196.2	228	239.9

	Malignant	Benign	Unspecified
Neoplasm, neoplastic — *continued*			
lymph, lymphatic — *continued*			
gland — *continued*			
supraclavicular	196.0	228	239.9
tibial	196.4	228	239.9
tracheobronchial	196.1	228	239.9
upper limb	196.3	228	239.9
Virchow's	196.0	228	239.9
node — *see also* Neoplasm, lymph gland			
primary	202.2	202.9	202.9
vessel (*see also* Neoplasm, connective tissue)	171.9	227.2	232.1
lymphadenoid tissue, pharynx	147	210.7	239.0
Mackenrodt's ligament	183.1	221.0	236.0
malar	170.0	213.9	232.2
region — *see* Neoplasm, cheek			
mammary gland (female) (male)	174	217	233
mandible	170.1	213.9	232.0
alveolar process or ridge	143.1	210.4	239.0
marrow (bone)	202.2	202.9	202.9
mastoid (antrum) (cavity)	160.1	212.0	231.0
bone or process	170.0	213.9	232.0
maxilla, maxillary (superior)	170.0	213.9	232.0
alveolar process or ridge	143.0	210.4	239.0
inferior — *see* Neoplasm, mandible			
sinus	160.2	212.0	231.0
meatus			
external (ear)	173.2	216.-	232.2
osseous	170.0	213.9	232.0
mediastinum, mediastinal	163.1	212.5	231.5
lymph			
channel or vessel	163.1	227.2	231.5
gland or node (*see also* Neoplasm, lymph gland)	196.1	228	239.9
medulla oblongata	191	225.0	238.1
meibomian gland	173.1	216.1	232.2
melanotic — *see* Melanoma			
meninges	192.9	225.9	238.9
brain	192.1	225.2	238.3
spinal cord	192.3	225.4	238.5
mesentery, mesenteric	158.9	211.7	230.7
lymph			
channel or vessel	158.9	227.2	230.7
gland or node (*see also* Neoplasm, lymph gland)	196.2	228	239.9
meso-appendix	158.9	211.7	230.7
mesocolon	158.9	211.7	230.7
mesopharynx (oral)	146.9	210.6	239.0
peritonsillar	146.8	210.6	239.0
pillars of fauces	146.8	210.6	239.0
specified part NEC	146.8	210.6	239.0
tonsil	146.0	210.5	239.0
vallecula (epiglottis)	146.8	210.6	239.0
mesosalpinx	183.1	221.0	236.0
mesovarium	183.1	221.0	236.0
metacarpus (any bone)	170.5	213.9	232.0
metastatic NEC (*see also* Metastasis neoplasm)	199.0	——	199.0

	Malignant	Benign	Unspeci-fied
Neoplasm, neoplastic — *continued*			
metatarsus (any bone)	170.8	213.9	232.0
milk duct	174	217	233
mixed NEC (*see also* Tumor, mixed)	199.1	228	228
mons veneris	184.1	221.2	236.2
motor tract	192.9	225.9	238.9
brain	191	225.0	238.1
spinal	192.2	225.3	238.4
mouth NEC	145.9	210.4	239.0
floor	144	210.3	239.0
and ventral surface tongue	144	210.3	239.0
roof	145.1	210.4	239.0
specified site NEC	145.8	210.4	239.0
vestibule	145.0	210.4	239.0
mucous membrane of lip (exposed) (internal) — *see* Neoplasm, lip			
mullerian duct			
female	184.9	221.9	236.9
male	186	222.0	237.0
multiple NEC	199.0	228	199.0
muscle — *see* Neoplasm, connective tissue			
mycardium	171.1	215	232.1
myometrium	182.0	219.9	234.9
Nabothian gland (follicle)	180	219.9	234.1
nail	173.9	216.8	232.2
finger	173.7	216.8	232.2
toe	173.8	216.8	232.2
nares, naris (anterior) (posterior)	160.0	212.0	231.0
nasal — *see* Neoplasm, nose			
nasolabial groove	173.3	216.–	232.2
nasopharynx	147	210.7	239.0
nates	173.6	216.–	232.2
neck NEC	195.9	228	239.9
nervous system (central) NEC	192.9	225.9	238.9
auditory nerve	192.0	225.1	238.2
antonomic	192.5	225.6	238.7
brachial plexus	192.4	225.5	238.6
brain (lobe) (ventricle)	191	225.0	238.1
membrane or meninges	192.1	225.2	238.3
cauda equina	192.2	225.3	238.4
cavum septi pellucidi	191	225.0	238.1
cerebellopontine	191	225.0	238.1
cerebellum, cerebellar	191	225.0	238.1
cerebrum, cerebral	191	225.0	238.1
choroid plexus	191	225.0	238.1
ciliary nerve	192.0	225.1	238.2
corpora quadrigemina	191	225.0	238.1
cranial	191	225.0	238.1
meninges	192.1	225.2	238.3
nerve (any)	192.0	225.1	238.2
dura (mater)	192.9	225.9	238.9
cerebral	192.1	225.2	238.3
spinal	192.3	225.4	238.5
extradural	192.9	225.9	238.9

	Malignant	Benign	Unspecified

Neoplasm, neoplastic — *continued*

nervous system, etc. — *continued*

	Malignant	Benign	Unspecified
ganglion, ganglionic (parasympathetic) (sympathetic)......	192.5	225.6	238.7
cranial nerve, except ciliary....................................	192.0	225.1	238.2
ciliary...............	192.5	225.6	238.7
gasserian..........	192.5	225.6	238.7
insular tissue, brain.............	191	225.0	238.1
intracranial..........	191	225.0	238.1
lumbosacral plexus...............	192.4	225.5	238.6
medulla (oblongata).............	191	225.0	238.1
meninges............	192.9	225.9	238.9
brain..........	192.1	225.2	238.3
spinal cord...........	192.3	225.4	238.5
motor tract.........	192.9	225.9	238.9
brain....	191	225.0	238.1
spinal.................	192.2	225.3	238.4
nerve (peripheral)............	192.4	225.5	238.6
acoustic..............	192.0	225.1	238.2
auditory...............	192.0	225.1	238.2
autonomic..........	192.5	225.6	238.7
ciliary..........	192.0	225.1	238.2
cranial (any)...........	192.0	225.1	238.2
ganglion (parasympathetic) (sympathetic)...................	192.5	225.6	238.7
cranial nerve, except ciliary...............	192.0	225.1	238.2
ciliary......	192.5	225.6	238.7
parasympathetic or sympathetic........................	192.5	225.6	238.7
optic...........................	192.0	225.1	238.2
sciatic.......	192.4	225.5	238.6
spinal (root)........	192.4	225.5	238.6
parasympathetic..........	192.5	225.6	238.7
ganglion — *see* Neoplasm, nervous system, ganglion			
peripheral nerve...........	192.4	225.5	238.6
pons (angle) (varolii)...............	191	225.0	238.1
sciatic nerve........	192.4	225.5	238.6
spinal			
bulb........	191	225.0	238.1
cord........	192.2	225.3	238.4
membrane or meninges...............	192.3	225.4	238.5
nerve (root)............	192.4	225.5	238.6
subdural.........	192.9	225.9	238.9
sympathetic...........	192.5	225.6	238.7
thalamus.........	191	225.0	238.1
nipple (female) (male)...........	174	217	233
nose, nasal...........	160.0	212.0	231.0
ala (external)...........	173.3	216.–	232.2
bone........	170.0	213.9	232.0
cartilage........	160.0	212.0	231.0
cavity........	160.0	212.0	231.0
external (skin)........	173.3	216.–	232.2
fossa........	160.0	212.0	231.0
internal........	160.0	212.0	231.0
mucosa........	160.0	212.0	231.0
posterior space........	160.0	212.0	231.0

	Malignant	Benign	Unspecified
Neoplasm, neoplastic—*continued*			
nose, nasal—*continued*			
septum	160.0	212.0	231.0
sinus—*see* Neoplasm, sinus			
turbinate	170.0	213.9	232.0
nostril	160.0	212.0	231.0
olfactory groove	170.0	213.9	232.0
omentum	158.9	211.7	230.7
optic nerve or chiasm	192.0	225.1	238.2
oral cavity NEC	145.9	210.4	239.0
orbit	190	224	238.0
bone	170.0	213.9	232.0
eye	190	224	238.0
glioma	190	224	190
soft parts	171.0	215	232.1
oro-lingual	145.9	210.4	239.0
oropharynx—*see* Neoplasm, mesopharynx			
osseous meatus	170.0	213.9	232.0
ovary	183.0	220.9	235
functionally active	183.0	256.0	256.0
oviduct	183.1	221.0	236.0
palate (hard) (soft)	145.1	210.4	239.0
palpebra	173.1	216.–	232.2
pancreas	157.9	211.6	230.6
body	157.8	211.6	230.6
duct of Wirsung	157.0	211.6	230.6
functionally active	157.9	251	251
head	157.0	211.6	230.6
islet cells	157.9	251	251
neck	157.8	211.6	230.6
tail	157.8	211.6	230.6
papillae			
filiform (lingual) (tongue)	141.1	210.1	239.0
foliate (lingual) (tongue)	141.2	210.1	239.0
fungiform (lingual) (tongue)	141.2	210.1	239.0
lenticular (lingual) (tongue)	141.2	210.1	239.0
lingual NEC	141.1	210.1	239.0
vallate (lingual) (tongue)	141.1	210.1	239.0
parametrium	183.1	221.0	236.0
paranephric	158.0	211.7	230.7
pararectal	195.1	228	239.9
parasagittal (region)	195.9	228	239.9
parathyroid (gland)	194.1	226.8	239.1
paratubal	183.1	221.0	236.0
para-urethral	195.1	228	239.9
paravaginal	195.1	228	239.9
paroophoron	183.1	221.0	236.0
parotid gland	142.0	210.2	239.0
parovarium	183.1	221.0	236.0
patella	170.8	213.9	232.0
pelvis, pelvic	195.1	228	239.9
bone	170.6	213.9	232.0
floor	195.1	228	239.9
renal	189.1	223.1	237.4

	Malignant	Benign	Unspecified
Neoplasm, neoplastic — *continued*			
pelvis, pelvic — *continued*			
viscera	195.1	228	239.9
pelvo-abdominal	195.1	228	239.9
penis	187.0	222.1	237.1
peri-anal	173.6	216.-	232.2
pericardium	171.1	215	232.1
perinephric	158.0	211.7	230.7
perineum	195.1	228	239.9
periosteum — *see* Neoplasm, bone			
peripheral nerve	192.4	225.5	238.6
perirectal (tissue)	195.1	228	239.9
perirenal (tissue)	158.0	211.7	230.7
peritoneum, peritoneal (cavity)	158.9	211.7	230.7
peritonsillar tissue	146.8	210.6	239.0
peri urethral tissue	195.1	228	239.9
phalanges	170.9	213.9	232.0
foot	170.8	213.9	232.0
hand	170.5	213.9	232.0
pharynx, pharyngeal	149	210.9	239.0
bursa	147	210.7	239.0
region	149	210.9	239.0
tonsil	146.0	210.5	239.0
pillars of fauces	146.8	210.6	239.0
pineal (body) (gland) (of brain)	194.4	226.3	239.1
pinna (ear) NEC	195.9	228	239.9
cartilage	171.0	215	232.1
piriform fossa or sinus	148.1	210.8	239.0
pituitary (body) (gland) (lobe) (of brain)	194.3	226.2	226.2
functionally active NEC	194.3	253.0	253.0
placenta	181	219.9	234.9
pleura, pleural (cavity)	163.0	212.4	231.4
plexus			
brachial	192.4	225.5	238.6
choroid	191	225.0	238.1
lumbosacral	192.4	225.5	238.6
pons (varolii) (angle)	191	225.0	238.1
popliteal space	173.8	216.-	232.2
postcricoid region	148.0	210.8	239.0
prechiasmal	192.0	225.1	238.2
prepuce	187.0	222.1	237.1
presacral	195.1	228	239.9
prostate (gland)	185	600	600
pubes	173.6	216.-	232.2
pubic bone	170.6	213.9	232.0
pudenda, pudendum (female)	184.1	221.2	236.2
pulmonary	162.1	212.3	231.3
pylorus	151.1	211.1	230.1
pyriform fossa or sinus	148.1	210.8	239.0
radius (any part)	170.4	213.9	232.0
Rathke's pouch	194.3	226.2	226.2
rectosigmoid (junction)	154.0	211.4	230.4
rectovaginal septum or wall	195.1	228	239.9
rectum	154.1	211.4	230.4

	Malignant	Benign	Unspecified
Neoplasm, neoplastic — *continued*			
renal..	189.0	223.0	237.3
calyx..	189.1	223.1	237.4
hilus..	189.1	223.1	237.4
pelvis...	189.1	223.1	237.4
respiratory organs or system (upper) NEC..........................	163.9	212.9	231.9
retina..	190	224	238.0
retrobulbar...	191	225.0	238.1
retrocecal..	158.0	211.7	230.7
retrohepatic..	158.0	211.7	230.7
retromolar area...	145.0	210.4	239.0
retro-orbital...	191	225.0	238.1
retroperitoneal (space) (tissue)...................................	158.0	211.7	230.7
lymph			
channel or vessel...	158.0	227.2	230.7
gland or node (*see also* Neoplasm, lymph gland)...........	196.2	228	239.9
retropharyngeal...	149	210.9	239.0
retrovesical..	195.1	228	239.9
rib...	170.3	213.9	232.0
round ligament..	183.1	221.0	236.0
sacro-uterine ligament..	183.1	221.0	236.0
sacrum, sacral (vertebra)...	170.6	213.9	232.0
salivary gland or duct..	142.9	210.2	239.0
mixed, gland unspecified......................................	142.9	210.2	210.2
parotid..	142.0	210.2	239.0
mixed...	142.0	210.2	210.2
sublingual...	142.8	210.2	239.0
mixed...	142.8	210.2	210.2
submaxillary...	142.8	210.2	239.0
mixed...	142.8	210.2	210.2
salpinx (uterina)...	183.1	221.0	236.0
scalp...	173.4	216.–	232.2
scapula (any part)..	170.4	213.9	232.0
scar NEC (*see also* Neoplasm, skin)..............................	173.9	216.–	232.2
sclera..	190	224	238.0
scrotum...	173.5	216.–	232.2
sebaceous gland, unspecified site.................................	173.9	216.1	232.2
specified site — *see* Neoplasm, skin			
sella turcica...	194.3	226.2	226.2
bone...	170.0	213.9	232.0
seminal vesicle...	187.8	222.8	237.2
shoulder NEC..	195.9	228	239.9
sigmoid flexure (lower) (upper)...................................	153.3	211.3	230.3
sinus (accessory)...	160.9	212.0	231.0
bone (any)...	170.0	213.9	232.0
ethmoidal..	160.8	212.0	231.0
frontal..	160.8	212.0	231.0
maxillary..	160.2	212.0	231.0
nasal..	160.9	212.0	231.0
pyriform...	148.1	210.8	239.0
sphenoidal...	160.8	212.0	231.0
skeleton, skeletal NEC..	170.9	213.9	232.0
Skene's gland...	189.9	223.8	237.9
skin NEC..	173.9	216.–	232.2

	Malignant	Benign	Unspecified

Neoplasm, neoplastic — *continued*
  skin NEC — *continued*

	Malignant	Benign	Unspecified
abdominal wall	173.6	216.-	232.2
ankle	173.8	216.-	232.2
anus	173.6	216.-	232.2
arm	173.7	216.-	232.2
auricle (ear)	173.2	216.-	232.2
auricular canal (external)	173.2	216.-	232.2
axilla, axillary fold	173.6	216.-	232.2
back	173.6	216.-	232.2
breast	174	217	233
brow	173.3	216.-	232.2
buttock	173.6	216.-	232.2
canthus (eye)	173.1	216.-	232.2
cheek	173.3	216.-	232.2
chest wall	173.6	216.-	232.2
chin	173.3	216.-	232.2
clavicular area	173.6	216.-	232.2
clitoris	184.1	221.2	236.2
ear (external)	173.2	216.-	232.2
eyebrow	173.3	216.-	232.2
eyelid	173.1	216.-	232.2
face NEC	173.3	216.-	232.2
female genital organ	184.1	221.2	236.2
clitoris	184.1	221.2	236.2
labium	184.1	221.2	236.2
vulva	184.1	221.2	236.2
finger	173.7	216.-	232.2
foot	173.8	216.-	232.2
forearm	173.7	216.-	232.2
forehead	173.3	216.-	232.2
glabella	173.3	216.-	232.2
groin	173.6	216.-	232.2
hand	173.7	216.-	232.2
head NEC	173.4	216.-	232.2
heel	173.8	216.-	232.2
hip	173.8	216.-	232.2
hypochondrium	173.6	216.-	232.2
jaw	173.3	216.-	232.2
knee	173.8	216.-	232.2
leg	173.8	216.-	232.2
lip (lower) (upper)	173.0	216.-	232.2
lower limb	173.8	216.-	232.2
male genital organ	187.9	222.9	237.2
penis	187.0	222.1	237.1
prepuce	187.0	222.1	237.1
scrotum	173.5	216.-	232.2
nates	173.6	216.-	232.2
neck	173.4	216.-	232.2
nose (external)	173.3	216.-	232.2
penis	187.0	222.1	237.1
perineum	173.6	216.-	232.2
pinna	173.2	216.-	232.2
popliteal space	173.8	216.-	232.2

	Malignant	Benign	Unspeci-fied
Neoplasm, neoplastic *— continued*			
skin NEC *— continued*			
prepuce..	187.0	222.1	237.1
pubes...	173.6	216.–	232.2
scalp..	173.4	216.–	232.2
scapular region.....................................	173.6	216.–	232.2
scrotum...	173.5	216.–	232.2
shoulder..	173.7	216.–	232.2
supraclavicular fossa...............................	173.4	216.–	232.2
temple..	173.3	216.–	232.2
thigh..	173.8	216.–	232.2
thumb...	173.7	216.–	232.2
toe...	173.8	216.–	232.2
trunk..	173.6	216.–	232.2
umbilicus...	173.6	216.–	232.2
upper limb...	173.7	216.–	232.2
vulva..	184.1	221.2	236.2
wrist..	173.7	216.–	232.2
skull...	170.0	213.9	232.0
soft parts or tissues *— see* Neoplasm, connective tissue			
spermatic cord..	187.8	222.8	237.2
sphenoid..	160.8	212.0	231.0
bone	170.0	213.9	232.0
sinus	160.8	212.0	231.0
spine, spinal (column)................................	170.2	213.9	232.0
bulb	191	225.0	238.1
coccyx..	170.6	213.9	232.0
cord..	192.2	225.3	238.4
lower..	170.2	213.9	232.0
lumbosacral..	170.2	213.9	232.0
membrane...	192.3	225.4	238.5
meninges	192.3	225.4	238.5
nerve (root)..	192.4	225.5	238.6
root	192.4	225.5	238.6
sacrum..	170.6	213.9	232.0
spleen, splenic..	202.2	227.1	232.1
flexure (colon).......................................	153.1	211.3	230.3
lymph			
channel or vessel................................	202.2	227.2	232.1
gland or node (*see also* Neoplasm, lymph gland)........	196.2	228	239.9
sternum...	170.3	213.9	232.0
stomach...	151.9	211.1	230.1
antrum..	151.8	211.1	230.1
body...	151.8	211.1	230.1
cardiac orifice.......................................	151.0	211.1	230.1
curvature (greater) (lesser)	151.8	211.1	230.1
fundus...	151.8	211.1	230.1
pylorus..	151.1	211.1	230.1
subcutaneous (nodule) (tissue) N EC *— see* Neoplasm, con-nective tissue			
subdural..	192.9	225.9	238.9
subglottic	161.8	212.1	231.1
sublingual	144	210.3	239.0
gland or duct..	142.8	210.2	239.0
mixed	142.8	210.2	210.2

	Malignant	Benign	Unspecified
Neoplasm, neoplastic — *continued*			
submandibular gland	142.8	210.2	239.0
mixed	142.8	210.2	210.2
submaxillary gland or duct	142.8	210.2	239.0
mixed	142.8	210.2	210.2
submental	195.9	228	239.9
subpleural	162.1	212.3	231.3
substernal	163.1	212.5	231.5
sudoriferous, sudoriparous gland, site unspecified	173.9	216.2	232.2
specified site — *see* Neoplasm, skin			
suprarenal (capsule) (gland)	194.0	226.0	239.1
functionally active	194.0	255.0	255.0
suprasellar (region)	191	225.0	238.1
bone	170.0	213.9	232.0
sweat gland (apocrine) (eccrine), site unspecified	173.9	216.2	232.2
specified site — *see* Neoplasm, skin			
sympathetic nerve or nervous system	192.5	225.6	238.7
ganglion — *see* Neoplasm, nervous system, ganglion			
synovial membrane — *see* Neoplasm, connective tissue			
tarsus (any bone)	170.8	213.9	232.0
temple	173.3	216.-	232.2
temporal region	195.9	228	239.9
tendon — *see* Neoplasm, connective tissue			
testicle, testis, testes	186	222.0	237.0
thalamus	191	225.0	238.1
thigh NEC	195.9	228	239.9
thorax, thoracic (cavity) (organs NEC)	163.9	212.9	231.9
duct	171.1	227.2	232.1
wall NEC	195.9	228	239.9
throat	149	210.9	239.0
thumb NEC	195.9	228	239.9
thymus (gland)	194.2	226.1	239.1
thyroglossal duct	193	226.8	239.1
thyroid (gland)	193	226.8	239.1
cartilage	161.8	212.1	231.1
tibia (any part)	170.7	213.9	232.0
toe NEC	195.9	228	239.9
tongue	141.9	210.1	239.0
base	141.0	210.1	239.0
borders	141.2	210.1	239.0
foramen cecum	141.1	210.1	239.0
frenulum	141.3	210.1	239.0
papillae NEC (*see also* Neoplasm, papillae)	141.1	210.1	239.0
posterior angle	141.0	210.1	239.0
surface	141.9	210.1	239.0
dorsal	141.1	210.1	239.0
ventral	141.3	210.1	239.0
and floor of mouth	144	210.3	239.0
tip	141.2	210.1	239.0
tonsil	146.0	210.5	239.0
tonsil	146.0	210.5	239.0
fauces, faucial	146.0	210.5	239.0
lingual	146.0	210.5	239.0
pharyngeal	146.0	210.5	239.0

	Malignant	Benign	Unspeci-fied
Neoplasm, neoplastic — *continued*			
tonsil — *continued*			
pillars...:	146.8	210.6	239.0
tonsillar area or fossa	146.0	210.5	239.0
trachea (cartilage) (mucosa)	162.0	212.2	231.2
tracheobronchial	162.0	212.2	231.2
lymph			
channel or vessel	162.0	227.2	231.2
gland or node (*see also* Neoplasm, lymph gland)	196.1	228	239.9
tubo-ovarian	183.1	221.0	236.0
tunica vaginalis	187.8	222.8	237.2
turbinate (bone)	170.0	213.9	232.0
ulna (any part)	170.4	213.9	232.0
umbilicus, umbilical	173.6	216.–	232.2
urachus	189.9	223.8	237.9
ureter	189.2	223.2	237.5
ureter-bladder junction	189.9	223.8	237.9
urethra, urethral (gland)	189.9	223.8	237.9
urinary organ NEC	189.9	223.9	237.9
bladder	188	223.3	237.6
utero-ovarian ligament	183.1	221.0	236.0
uterosacral ligament	183.1	221.0	236.0
uterus, uteri, uterine	182.9	219.9	234.9
adnexa NEC	183.9	221.9	236.9
body	182.0	219.9	234.9
cervix	180	219.9	234.1
external os	180	219.9	234.1
fundus	182.0	219.9	234.9
ligament	183.1	221.0	236.0
uveal tract	190	224	238.0
uvula	145.8	210.4	239.0
vagina, vaginal (vault) (wall)	184.0	221.1	236.1
vaginovesical :	184.0	221.1	236.1
septum	195.1	228	239.9
vallecula (epiglottis)	146.8	210.6	239.0
vas deferens	187.8	222.8	237.2
vascular — *see also* Neoplasm, connective tissue			
benign — *see* Hemangioma			
Vater's ampulla	156.2	211.5	230.5
vein, venous — *see also* Neoplasm, connective tissue			
benign — *see* Hemangioma			
ventriculus — *see* Neoplasm, stomach			
vertebra (column)	170.2	213.9	232.0
coccyx	170.6	213.9	232.0
sacrum	170.6	213.9	232.0
vesical (orifice)	188	223.3	237.6
vesicle, seminal	187.8	222.8	237.2
vesicorectal	188	223.3	237.6
vesicovaginal	188	223.3	237.6
septum	195.1	228	239.9
vestibule of mouth	145.0	210.4	239.0
Virchow's gland	196.0	228	239.9
viscera NEC	195.0	228	239.9
vitreous (humor)	190	224	238.0

	Malignant	Benign	Unspeci-fied
Neoplasm, neoplastic — *continued*			
vocal cords (true)	161.0	212.1	231.1
false	161.8	212.1	231.1
vulva	184.1	221.2	236.2
vulvovaginal gland	184.1	221.2	236.2
Wilms'	189.0	——	189.0
windpipe	162.0	212.2	231.2
Wolffian (body) (duct)			
female	184.9	221.9	236.9
male	187.8	222.8	237.2
womb — *see* Neoplasm, uterus			
wrist NEC	195.9	228	239.9
xiphoid process	170.3	213.9	232.0

Nephralgia 786.0

Nephritis, nephritic (albuminuric)
(azotemic) (catarrhal) (congenital)
(degenerative) (diffuse)
(disseminated) (Ellis, type I)
(epithelial) (exudative) (familial)
(focal) (glomerular) (granular)
(granulomatous) (hemorrhagic)
(infantile) (interstitial)
(nonsuppurative excretory) (type I)
(uremic) 583
with
abortion - *see* Abortion, by type, with
toxemia
edema - *see* Nephritis, subacute
hypertension, malignant (*see also*
Hypertension, malignant with
renal involvement) 400.3
acute 580
with
abortion - *see* Abortion, by type,
with toxemia
hypertension, malignant (*see also*
Hypertension, malignant
with renal involvement)
400.3
arising during pregnancy 636
fetus or newborn 762.0
puerperal, postpartum 636
alcoholic 303.2
arising during pregnancy 636
fetus or newborn 762.0
arteriolar (*see also* Hypertension,
kidney) 403
arteriosclerotic (*see also* Hypertension,
kidney) 403
ascending (*see also* Pyelitis) 590.1
calculous, calculus 592
cardiac (*see also* Hypertension,
cardiorenal) 404

Nephritis, nephritic — *continued*
cardiovascular (*see also* Hypertension,
cardiorenal) 404
chronic 582
with hypertension, malignant (*see*
also Hypertension, malignant
with renal involvement) 400.3
arteriosclerotic (*see also*
Hypertension, kidney) 403
maternal, affecting fetus or newborn
760.4
cirrhotic (*see also* Sclerosis, renal) 584
croupous - *see* Nephritis, acute
desquamative - *see* Nephritis, subacute
gonococcal (acute) 098.0
chronic or duration of 2 months or
over 098.1
gouty 274
gravidarum - *see* Nephritis, arising
during pregnancy
hereditary 759.8
hydremic - *see* Nephritis, subacute
infective (*see also* Pyelitis) 590.1
latent or quiescent - *see* Nephritis,
chronic
lead 984
lupus 734.1
necrotic, necrotizing (*see also*
Nephrosis, tubular) 593.1
nephrotic - *see* Nephritis, subacute
old - *see* Nephritis, chronic
parenchymatous (acute) (chronic) - *see*
Nephritis, subacute
polycystic 753.1
pregnancy - *see* Nephritis, arising
during pregnancy
puerperal, postpartum 636
purulent (*see also* Pyelitis) 590.1

Nephritis, nephritic—*continued*

salt losing (*see also* Lesion, kidney) 593.2

salt wasting (*see also* Lesion, kidney) 593.2

saturnine 984

septic (*see also* Pyelitis) 590.1

staphylococcus (*see also* Pyelitis) 590.1

streptotrichosis 113

subacute 581

  with

    abortion - *see* Abortion, by type, with toxemia

    hypertension, malignant (*see also* Hypertension, malignant with renal involvement) 400.3

  arising during pregnancy 636

    fetus or newborn 762.0

  puerperal, postpartum 636

suppurative (acute) (*see also* Pyelitis) 590.1

syphilitic (late) 095

  congenital 090.5

  early 091.8

toxic - *see* Nephritis, acute

trench - *see* Nephritis, acute

tubal, tubular (acute) (chronic) - *see* Nephritis, subacute

tuberculous 016.0

  late effect or sequela 019.2

type II (Ellis) - *see* Nephritis, subacute

vascular - *see* Hypertension, kidney

Nephroblastoma 189.0

Nephrocalcinosis 279

Nephrocystitis, pustular (*see also* Pyelitis) 590.1

Nephrolithiasis (congenital) (pelvis) (recurrent) 592

Nephroma (malignant) 189.0

benign 223.0

Nephronephritis (*see also* Nephrosis) 581

Nephropathy (*see also* Disease, renal) 593.2

analgesic 593.2

diabetic - *see* category 250

obstructive (*see also* Lesion, kidney) 593.2

  congenital 753.2

sickle cell (*see also* Disease, sickle cell) 282.5

Nephroptosis (*see also* Lesion, kidney) 593.2

congenital 753.3

Nephropyosis (*see also* Abscess, kidney) 590.2

Nephrorrhagia (*see also* Lesion, kidney) 593.2

Nephrosclerosis (arteriolar) (arteriosclerotic) (benign) (chronic) (hyaline) (*see also* Hypertension, kidney) 403

gouty 274

hyperplastic - *see* Nephrosclerosis, malignant

malignant (*see also* Hypertension, malignant with renal involvement) 400.3

senile (*see also* Sclerosis, renal) 584

Nephrosis, nephrotic (Epstein's) (lipid) (lipoid) (syndrome) 581

with

  abortion - *see* Abortion, by type, with toxemia

  hypertension, malignant (*see also* Hypertension, malignant with renal involvement) 400.3

acute - *see* Nephrosis, tubular

anoxic - *see* Nephrosis, tubular

arising during pregnancy 636

  fetus or newborn 762.0

bile (*see also* Disease, gallbladder) 576.9

chemical - *see* Nephrosis, tubular

cholemic (*see also* Disease, gallbladder) 576.9

diabetic - *see* category 250

hemoglobinuric - *see* Nephrosis, tubular

ischemic - *see* Nephrosis, tubular

lower nephron - *see* Nephrosis, tubular

necrotizing - *see* Nephrosis, tubular

puerperal, postpartum 636

radiation - *see* Effect, adverse, radiotherapy

syphilitic 095

toxic - *see* Nephrosis, tubular

tubular (acute) 593.1

  with abortion - *see* Abortion, by type, with toxemia

  arising during pregnancy 636

    fetus or newborn 762.0

  puerperal, postpartum 636

  radiation - *see* Effect, adverse, radiotherapy

Nephroso-nephritis hemorrhagic (endemic) 067.5

Nerve - *see* condition

Nerves 790.0

Nervous (*see also* condition) 790.0

heart 305.3

Nervous—*continued*
  stomach 305.5
  tension 790.0
Nervousness 790.0
Nettle rash (*see also* Urticaria) 708.9
Nettleship's disease 757.2
Neumann's disease 694
Neuralgia, neuralgic (acute) (*see also*
      Neuritis) 355.9
  ankle 355.1
  axilla 355.1
  brain 355.0
  breast 355.1
  cerebral 355.0
  cheek 355.0
  chin 355.0
  ear 384.9
    middle 355.0
  finger 355.1
  flank 355.1
  foot 355.1
  forearm 355.1
  forehead 355.0
  groin 355.1
  hand 355.1
  head 355.0
  heel 355.1
  hip 355.1
  Hunt's 053.1
  iliac region 355.1
  infra-orbital 351
  inguinal 355.1
  jaw 355.0
  knee 355.1
  larynx 355.9
  loin 355.1
  lumbar 355.1
  malarial (*see also* Malaria) 084.9
  mastoid 387.9
  maxilla 355.0
  middle ear 355.0
  Morton's 357.9
  mouth 355.0
  nasopharynx 355.0
  nose 355.0
  occipital 355.0
  ophthalmic 377.6
  orbital region 355.0
  perineum 355.1
  pharynx 355.9
  pleura 511.0
  postauricular 355.0
  pre-auricular 355.0
  pubic region 355.1
  sacro-iliac joint 353
  scalp 355.0

Neuralgia, neuralgic—*continued*
  shoulder 355.1
  Sluder's 355.0
  sphenopalatine (ganglion) 355.0
  supra-orbital (functional) 355.0
  sympathetic 355.1
  temporomandibular 355.0
  temporomaxillary 355.0
  thigh 355.1
  throat 355.9
  thumb 355.1
  tongue 355.0
  wrist 355.1
  writer's 300.8
Neurapraxia - *see* Injury, nerve, by site
Neurasthenia 300.5
  cardiac 305.3
  gastric 305.5
  heart 305.3
  postfebrile NEC 309.1
    due to specified condition - *see* listing
        under Disorder, mental
Neurilemmoma (peripheral nerve) 225.5
  acoustic 225.1
    malignant 192.0
  cranial nerve 225.1
    malignant 192.0
  ganglion (parasympathetic)
        (sympathetic) 225.6
    ciliary 225.6
      malignant 192.5
    cranial nerve, except ciliary 225.1
      malignant 192.0
    malignant 192.5
  malignant 192.4
  parasympathetic, sympathetic (nerve)
        225.6
    malignant 192.5
  sympathetic 225.6
Neurilemoma - *see* Neurilemmoma
Neurinoma - *see also* Neurilemmoma
  multiple 743.4
Neuritis (acute) (degenerative) (pressure)
        (*see also* Neuralgia) 355.9
  with
    abortion - *see* Abortion, by type, with
        toxemia
    hyperemesis gravidarum 638.0
      fetus or newborn 762.4
  abducens (nerve) 369.9
  accessory nerve 355.9
  acoustic (nerve) 384.9
    syphilitic 094.9
  alcoholic 303.2
  amyloid, any site 276
  anterior crural 355.1

Neuritis—*continued*
  arising during pregnancy 639.9
    with hyperemesis (gravidarum)
        638.0
      fetus or newborn 762.4
    fetus or newborn 762.9
  arm 352
  ascending 355.1
  auditory (nerve) 384.9
  back 355.1
  brachial (nerve) 352
  cancerous (*see also* Neoplasm,
        malignant) 199.1
  cardiac - *see* Disease, heart
  cervical 355.1
  chest 355.1
    wall 355.1
  costal region 355.1
  cranial nerve 355.0
    eighth or acoustic 384.9
    eleventh or accessory 355.0
    fifth or trigeminal 351
    first or olfactory 355.0
    fourth or trochlear 369.9
    ninth or glossopharyngeal 355.0
    second or optic 367
    seventh or facial 350
      newborn (*see also* Birth injury,
          bone or nerve) 772.2
    sixth or abducens 369.9
    tenth or vagus 355.0
    third or oculomotor 369.9
    twelfth or hypoglossal 355.0
  Dejerine-Sottas 355.9
  diabetic - *see* category 250
  diphtheritic 032
  due to
    beriberi 261
    displacement, prolapse, protrusion or
        rupture, intervertebral disc
        725.9
      cervical, cervicodorsal,
          cervicothoracic 725.0
      lumbar, lumbosacral 725.1
      specified site NEC 725.8
    herniation, nucleus pulposus 725.9
      cervical, cervicodorsal,
          cervicothoracic 725.0
      lumbar, lumbosacral 725.1
      specified site NEC 725.8
  endemic 261
  facial 350
    newborn (*see also* Birth injury, bone
        or nerve) 772.2
  general 354
  geniculate ganglion 350

Neuritis—*continued*
  geniculate ganglion—*continued*
    due to herpes 053.1
  glossopharyngeal (nerve) 355.0
  gouty 274
  hypoglossal (nerve) 355.0
  ileo-inguinal nerve 355.1
  infectious (multiple) 354
  intercostal (nerve) 355.1
  interstitial 355.9
    hypertrophic progressive 355.9
  leg 355.1
  median nerve 352
  multiple (acute) (infective) 354
    endemic 261
  multiplex endemica 261
  neck 355.1
  nerve NEC 355.9
    root (*see also* Radiculitis) 728.9
  oculomotor (nerve) 369.9
  olfactory nerve 355.0
  optic (nerve) 367
    hereditary 367
    meningococcal 036.8
    sympathetic 367
  pelvic 355.1
  peripheral (nerve) 355.9
  pneumogastric nerve 355.0
  post-herpetic 053.9
  progressive 355.9
    hypertrophic interstitial 355.9
  puerperal, postpartum 639.9
  radial nerve 352
  retrobulbar 367
  rheumatic (chronic) 717.9
  sacral region 355.1
  sciatic (nerve) 353
    due to displacement of intervertebral
        disc - *see* Displacement,
        intervertebral disc
  serum 999.5
  spinal (nerve) 355.1
    root (*see also* Radiculitis) 728.9
  subscapular (nerve) 352
  suprascapular (nerve) 352
  syphilitic 095
  thoracic 355.1
  toxic 355.9
    with abortion - *see* Abortion, by type,
        with toxemia
    arising during pregnancy (*see also*
        Neuritis arising during
        pregnancy) 639.9
    due to unspecified poison 355.9
    puerperal, postpartum 639.9
  trifacial 351

Neuritis — *continued*
  trigeminal   351
  trochlear (nerve)   369.9
  typanic plexus   384.9
  ulnar nerve   352
  vagus (nerve)   355.0
Neuro-avitaminosis   266.9
Neuroblastoma   192.5
  adrenal   192.5
  central nervous system - *see* Neoplasm,
    nervous system, malignant
  eye   190
  retinal   190
  suprarenal (medulla)   192.5
  sympatheticum   192.5
Neurochorioretinitis   367
Neurocirculatory asthenia   305.3
Neurocytoma   238.7
  adrenal gland   238.7
  central nervous system - *see* Neoplasm,
    nervous system
Neurodermatitis (circumscribed)
    (circumscripta) (local)   698.3
  atopic   691
  diffuse (Brocq)   691
  disseminated   691
  psychogenic   305.0
Neurodermatosis, psychogenic   305.0
Neuro-encephalomyelopathy, optic   341
Neuro-epithelioma - *see also* Neoplasm,
    nervous system, malignant
  adrenal gland   192.5
  choroid   190
  eye   190
  eyelid   192.4
  optic nerve   192.0
  retina   190
Neurofibroma (*see also* Neurilemmoma)
    225.5
  multiple   743.4
Neurofibromatosis   743.4
  malignant   192.4
  skin   743.4
Neurofibrosarcoma (peripheral nerve)
    192.4
  acoustic nerve   192.0
  central nervous system - *see* Neoplasm,
    nervous system, malignant
  cranial nerve   192.0
  ganglion (parasympathetic)
    (sympathetic)   192.5
  ciliary   192.5
  cranial nerve, except ciliary   192.0
  parasympathetic, sympathetic (nerve)
    192.5

Neurogenic - *see also* condition
  bladder NEC   596.9
  heart   305.3
Neuroglioma - *see also* Neoplasm,
    nervous system, malignant
  choroid   190
  eye   190
  nose   212.0
  optic nerve   192.0
  retina   190
Neurolathyrism   988.2
Neuroleprosy   030.1
Neuroma (plexiform) (*see also*
    Neurilemmoma)   225.5
  acoustic   225.1
  adrenal gland   225.6
  amputation (traumatic) - *see also* Injury,
    nerve, by site
  surgical complication (late)   997.2
  appendix   543
  auditory nerve   225.1
  digital   357.9
  interdigital   357.9
  intermetatarsal   357.9
  Morton's   357.9
  multiple   743.4
  optic   225.1
  traumatic (with open wound) - *see*
    Injury nerve, by site
Neuromatosis   743.4
Neuromyalgia   717.9
Neuromyasthenia (epidemic)   065
  late effects   066
Neuromyelitis   355.1
  ascending   354
  optica   341
Neuromyopathy   348.9
Neuromyositis   733.9
Neuromyxoma (*see also* Neurilemmoma)
    225.5
Neuronitis   355.9
  ascending (acute)   355.1
Neuroparalytic - *see* condition
Neuropathy, neuropathic   357.9
  with pernicious anemia   281.0
  alcoholic   303.2
  axillary nerve   357.1
  brachial plexus   357.0
  cervical plexus   357.0
  Djerine-Sottas   355.9
  diabetic - *see* category 250
  entrapment - *see* Compression, nerve
  facial nerve   350
  hypertropic
    interstitial   355.9
  intercostal nerve   357.9

Neuropathy, neuropathic — *continued*
  ischemic 357.9
  median nerve 357.2
  multiple (acute) (chronic) 357.9
  peripheral nerve NEC 357.9
    with pernicious anemia 281.0
    autonomic 358.9
    radicular 728.9
      brachial 728.3
      cervical 728.4
      hereditary sensory 349.0
      lumbar 728.8
      lumbosacral 728.8
      thoracic 728.6
    sciatic 353
    spinal nerve NEC 357.9
    toxic 357.9
    ulnar nerve 357.3
    vitamin B12 281.0
Neurophthisis 357.9
  peripheral (*see also* Neuropathy)
    357.9
    diabetic - *see* category 250
Neuroretinitis 367
Neurosarcoma - *see* Neurofibrosarcoma
Neurosclerosis (*see also* Neuropathy)
  357.9
Neurosis, neurotic 300.9
  anancastic 300.3
  anankastic 300.3
  anxiety (state) 300.0
  asthenic 300.5
  bladder 305.6
  cardiac (reflex) 305.3
  cardiovascular 305.3
  climacteric, unspecified type 627
  colon 305.5
  compensation 300.1
  compulsive, compulsion 300.3
  conversion 300.1
  craft 300.8
  cutaneous 305.0
  depressive (reaction) (type) 300.4
  due to or associated with physical
    condition - *see* listing under
    Disorder, mental
  environmental 300.9
  fatigue 300.5
  functional (*see also* Disorder,
    psychosomatic) 305.9
  gastric 305.5
  gastro-intestinal 305.5
  heart 305.3
  hypochondriacal 300.7
  hysterical 300.1
  impulsive 300.3

Neurosis, neurotic — *continued*
  inco-ordination 305.2
    larynx 305.2
    vocal cord 305.2
  intestine 305.5
  larynx 305.2
    hysterical 300.1
    sensory 305.2
  menopause, unspecified type 627
  mixed NEC 300.8
  musculoskeletal 305.1
  obsessional 300.3
    phobia 300.3
  obsessive-compulsive 300.3
  occupational 300.8
  ocular 305.8
  organ (*see also* Disorder,
    psychosomatic) 305.9
  pharynx 305.2
  phobic 300.2
  psychasthenic (type) 300.8
  railroad 300.1
  rectum 305.5
  respiratory 305.2
  rumination 305.5
  senile 300.9
  sexual 305.6
  situational 300.8
  specified type NEC 300.8
  state 300.9
    with depersonalization episode
      300.6
  stomach 305.5
  vasomotor 305.3
  visceral 305.5
  war 300.1
Neurosyphilis (arrested) (early) (late)
    (latent) (inactive) (recurrent) 094.9
  with ataxia (cerebellar) (locomotor)
    (spastic) (spinal) 094.0
  acute meningitis 094.9
  aneurysm 094.9
  arachnoid (adhesive) 094.9
  arteritis (any artery) 094.9
  asymptomatic 094.9
  congenital 090.4
  dura (mater) 094.9
  general paresis 094.1
  gumma 094.9
  hemorrhagic 094.9
  juvenile (asymptomatic) (meningeal)
    090.4
  leptomeninges (aseptic) 094.9
  meningeal 094.9
  meninges (adhesive) 094.9
  meningovascular (diffuse) 094.9

Neurosyphilis, etc. — *continued*
  optic atrophy 094.9
  parenchymatous (degenerative) .094.1
  paresis (*see also* Paresis, general)
    094.1
  paretic 094.1
  relapse 094.9
  remission in (sustained) 094.9
  serological 094.9
  tabes (dorsalis) 094.0
    juvenile 090.4
  tabetic 094.0
  taboparesis 094.1
    juvenile 090.4
  thrombosis 094.9
  vascular 094.9
Neurotic (*see also* Neurosis) 300.9
  excoriation 698.4
    psychogenic 305.0
Neurotmesis - *see* Injury, nerve, by site
Neurotoxemia - *see* Toxemia
Neutropenia, neutropenic (chronic)
    (cyclical) (genetic) (infantile)
    (periodic) (pernicious) 288
  malignant 288
  splenomegaly 288
Nevocarcinoma - *see* Melanoma
Nevolipoma 757.1
Nevoxantho-endothelioma 272.0
Nevus (angiomatous) (capillary)
    (cavernous) (cutaneous NEC)
    (flammeus) (hemangiomatous) (port
    wine) (sanguineous) (strawberry)
    (Unna's) (vascular) (vasculosus) (*see
    also* Hemangioma) 227.0
  acanthotic (*see also* Keratosis,
    seborrheic) 216.0
  amelanotic 757.1
  anemic, anemicus 709.9
  araneus 448
  avasculosus 709.9
  blue 757.1
  cellular 757.1
  comedonicus 757.2
  compound 757.1
  conjunctiva 224
  dermoepidermal 757.1
  elasticus 757.1
  fibrosus 757.1
  hairy 757.1
  intradermal 757.1
  Jadassohn-Tieche 757.1
  junctional 757.1
  linear 757.1
  lipomatodes 757.1
  lipomatosus 757.1

Nevus, etc. — *continued*
  lymphatic 227.2
  lymphaticus 227.2
  malignant - *see* Melanoma
  marginal 757.1
  nonpigmented 757.1
  nonvascular 757.1
  oral mucosa
    white sponge 528.7
  osteohypertrophic, flammeus 759.8
  papillaris 757.1
  papillomatosus 757.1
  pigmented, pigmentosus (papillomatous)
    (verrucous) 757.1
    vulva 757.1
  pilosus 757.1
  sebaceous (senile) (*see also*
    Trichoepithelioma) 216.1
  spider 448
  spilus 757.1
  stellar 448
  syringocystadenomatous papilliferus
    (*see also* Adenoma, sweat glands)
    216.2
  unius lateris 757.1
  verrucous 757.1
New
  growth - *see* Neoplasm
  tissue - *see* Neoplasm
Newborn (infant) (born in hospital)
    (liveborn) (single) Y20

Note — The following fourth-digit subdivisions are for use with categories Y20–
Y29 to indicate method of delivery:
  .0 Spontaneous delivery
  .1 Low forceps delivery
  .2 Mid or high forceps delivery
  .3 Cesarean section
  .9 Other (including breech extraction, with or without forceps)

---

  admitted after birth (not sick) Y00.5
    immature or premature - *see*
      Immaturity
  immature or premature Y21
  multiple born (three or more infants) (all
    liveborn) Y26
    immature or premature Y28
    one or more mates not liveborn Y27
      immature or premature Y29
  not liveborn - *see* Death, fetus
  twin (mate liveborn) Y22
    immature or premature Y24
    mate not liveborn Y23
      immature or premature Y25

Newcastle's disease 078.8
Niacin (amide) deficiency 262
Nicolas-Durand-Favre disease 099.1
Nicolas-Favre disease 099.1
Nicotinic acid (amide) deficiency 262
Niemann-Pick disease or splenomegaly
    272.2
Night
  blindness 378.9
    congenital 378.9
    vitamin A deficiency 260.0
  sweats 788.1
  terrors, child 308
Nightmare 306.4
Nipple - see condition
Nisbet's chancre 099.0
Nitritoid
  crisis or reaction 961.1
Nitrogen retention, extrarenal 788.9
Nitrosohemoglobinemia 289.9
Njovera 104.0
No diagnosis 796.9
No disease (found) 793.9
Nocardiosis 117.8
  lung 113
Nocturia 786.3
  psychogenic 305.6
Nocturnal
  dyspnea (paroxysmal) 783.2
  emissions 607.9
  enuresis 786.2
    psychogenic 306.6
  frequency (micturition) 786.3
    psychogenic 305.6
Nodal rhythm, auriculoventricular - see
    Action, heart, irregular
Node(s)
  Heberden's 713.0
  larynx 508.3
  lymph - see condition
  milkers' 051
  Osler's 421.0
  rheumatic 718
  Schmorl's - see Displacement,
      intervertebral disc
  singers' 508.3
  tuberculous - see Tuberculosis, lymph
      gland
  vocal cords 508.3
Nodosities, Haygarth's 713.0
Nodule(s), nodular
  actinomycotic 113
  arthritic - see Arthritis, nodosa
  cutaneous 788.3
  inflammatory - see Inflammation

Nodule(s), nodular—continued
  juxta-articular 102.7
    syphilitic 095
    yaws 102.7
  larynx 508.3
  milkers' 051
  prostate 600
  rheumatoid - see Arthritis, rheumatoid
  scrotum (inflammatory) 607.5
  singers' 508.3
  solitary
    lung 519.2
  subcutaneous 788.3
  thyroid (gland) (see also Goiter,
      nodular) 241.9
  vocal cords 508.3
Noli-me-tangere - see Neoplasm, skin,
    malignant
Noma (gangrenous) (hospital) (infective)
    528.1
  auricle (see also Gangrene) 445.9
  mouth 528.1
  pudendi (see also Vulvitis) 622.1
  vulvae (see also Vulvitis) 622.1
Nomadism 301.7
Nonclosure - see also Imperfect closure
  ductus
    arteriosus 747.0
    botalli 747.0
  eustachian valve 746.8
  foramen
    botalli 746.4
    ovale 746.4
Nondescent (congenital) - see also
    Malposition, congenital
  cecum 751.1
  colon 751.1
  testicle 752.1
Nondevelopment (newborn) 778.9
  brain 743.1
    specified part 743.2
  heart 746.8
  organ or site, congenital NEC - see
      Hypoplasia
Nonengagement
  head NEC
    complicating delivery 655
      fetus or newborn - see categories
        765.0-765.9
Nonexpansion lung (newborn) (see also
    Asphyxia, newborn) 776.9
Nonfilarial - see condition
Nonfunctioning
  gallbladder (see also Disease,
      gallbladder) 576.9
  kidney (see also Lesion, kidney) 593.2

Nonfunctioning—*continued*
  labyrinth 387.9
Nonhealing stump (surgical) 997.2
  traumatic - code as Amputation,
    traumatic, by site, complicated
Noninsufflation, fallopian tube 615.9
Nonmalignant neoplasm - *see* Neoplasm,
  benign
Non-ovulation 615.9
Nonpatent fallopian tube 615.9
Nonpneumatization, lung (*see also*
  Asphyxia, newborn) 776.9
Nonreflex bladder 596.9
Nonretention food 784.1
Nonrotation - *see* Malrotation
Nonsecretion urine 786.5
  newborn 753.3
Nontraumatic - *see* condition
Nonunion
  fracture - code as Fracture, late effect
    current - *see* Fracture
  organ or site, congenital NEC - *see*
    Imperfect closure
  symphysis pubis, congenital 755.7
  top sacrum, congenital 756.1
Nonviability 777
Nonvisualization gallbladder (*see also*
  Disease, gallbladder) 576.9
Nonvitalized tooth 522.9
Normal
  delivery 650
    anesthetic death 662
  pregnancy examination Y06

North American blastomycosis 116.1
Nose, nasal - *see* condition
Nosebleed 783.0
Nosomania 299
Nosophobia 300.2
Nostalgia 307
Notch of iris 744.4
Notching nose, congenital (tip) 748.1
Nothnagel's
  syndrome 373.9
  vasomotor acroparesthesia 443.8
Novy's relapsing fever (American) 088.1
Nuchal hitch (arm) - *see* Malposition,
  fetus
Nucleus pulposus - *see* condition
Numbness (*see also* Disturbance,
  sensation) 781.6
Nuns' knee 731.6
Nutmeg liver 573.9
Nutrition deficient or insufficient
  (particular kind of food) 269.9
  due to
    insufficient food 994.2
    lack of
      care 994.9
      food 994.2
Nyctalopia 378.9
  vitamin A deficiency 260.0
Nycturia 786.3
  psychogenic 305.6
Nymphomania 302.8
Nystagmus 781.1
  congenital 744.8
  miner's 300.8

O

Oat cell carcinoma (lung) 162.1

Obermeyer's relapsing fever (European) 088.0

Obesity (simple) 277
  adrenal 255.9
  constitutional 277
  endocrine 258.9
  endogenous 258.9
  exogenous 277
  familial 277
  glandular 258.9
  hypothyroid (see also Hypothyroidism) 244
  nutritional 277
  pituitary 253.1
  thyroid (deficiency) (see also Hypothyroidism) 244

Oblique - see condition

Obliteration
  abdominal aorta 446.9
  appendix (lumen) 543
  artery 447
  ascending aorta 446.9
  bile ducts (see also Disease, gallbladder) 576.9
    congenital 751.5
  common duct (see also Disease, gallbladder) 576.9
    congenital 751.5
  endometrium 625.9
  eye, anterior chamber 378.6
  fallopian tube 615.9
  lymphatic vessel 457
  organ or site, congenital NEC - see Atresia
  placental blood vessels - see Placenta, abnormal
  ureter 593.5
  urethra 599.9
  vein 458.9

Observation
  following operation or treatment - see Follow-up
  postpartum Y07
  routine check-up only - see Examination
  without need for further medical care (with complaints or symptoms) 793.9

Observation—continued
  without need for, etc. — continued
    for
      disease 793.9
        digestive 793.8
        heart 793.8
        mental 793.0
        specified NEC 793.8
        unspecified 793.9
      injuries (accidental) 793.8
      neoplasm 793.8
        malignant 793.1
      tuberculosis 793.8

Obsession, obsessional 300.3
  ideas and mental images 306.9
  impulses 300.3
  neurosis 300.3
  phobia 300.3
  psychasthenia 300.3
  ruminations 306.9
  state 300.3
  syndrome 300.3

Obsessive-compulsive
  neurosis 300.3
  reaction 300.3

Obstetric - see also condition
  procedure - see Delivery
  shock
    with abortion - see Abortion, by type
    complicating delivery 661.8

Obstetrical trauma NEC (complicating delivery) 660.9
  fetus or newborn - see categories 768.0-768.9

Obstipation (see also Constipation) 564.0

Obstruction, obstructed, obstructive
  airway 519.9
  alimentary canal (see also Obstruction, intestine) 560.9
  aortic (heart) (valve) (see also Endocarditis, aortic) 395.9
  aqueduct of Sylvius 347.9
    congenital 742
      with spina bifida 741.0
    Arnold-Chairi 741.0
  artery (see also Embolism, artery) 444.9
    retinal (central) 377.0
  bile duct or passage (see also Obstruction, gallbladder) 576.0

Obstruction, etc. — *continued*
bile duct, etc. — *continued*
congenital 751.5
biliary duct or passage (*see also*
Obstruction, gallbladder) 576.0
congenital 751.5
birth canal (by cancer, cyst, or tumor)
complicating delivery 657.9
fetus or newborn - *see* categories
764.0-764.9
noted during pregnancy (undelivered)
634.9
bladder neck 596.2
congenital 753.6
bowel (*see also* Obstruction, intestine)
560.9
bronchus 519.9
bubonocele 552
canal, ear 387.9
cardia 537.9
caval veins (inferior) (superior) 458.1
cecum (*see also* Obstruction, intestine)
560.9
circulatory 458.9
colon (*see also* Obstruction, intestine)
560.9
common duct (*see also* Obstruction,
gallbladder) 576.0
congenital 751.5
coronary (artery) (heart) (*see also*
Ischemia, heart) 412.9
cystic duct (*see also* Obstruction,
gallbladder) 576.0
congenital 751.5
duodenum 537.9
ejaculatory duct 607.9
enterocele 553.9
epigastrocele 553.2
epiplocele 553.9
esophagus 530.3
eustachian tube (complete) (partial)
387.9
exomphalos 553.1
fallopian tube (bilateral) 615.9
fecal 560.3
with hernia - *see* Hernia, by site, with
obstruction
foramen of Monro (congenital) 742
with spina bifida 741.0
foreign body - *see* Foreign body
gallbladder 576.0
with calculus, cholelithiasis, stones
574.9
congenital 751.6
gastric outlet - *see* Obstruction, pylorus

Obstruction, etc. — *continued*
gastro-intestinal (*see also* Obstruction,
intestine) 560.9
hepatic 573.9
duct (*see also* Obstruction,
gallbladder) 576.0
congenital 751.5
hernia (*see also* Hernia, by site, with
obstruction) 553.9
icterus (*see also* Obstruction,
gallbladder) 576.0
ileocecal coil (*see also* Obstruction,
intestine) 560.9
ileum (*see also* Obstruction, intestine)
560.9
intestine (mechanical) (neurogenic)
(paroxysmal) (postinfectional)
(reflex) (with gangrene) 560.9
with
adhesions (intestinal) (peritoneal)
560.4
hernia - *see* Hernia, by site, with
obstruction
adynamic (*see also* Ileus) 560.1
by gallstone 560.3
with hernia - *see* Hernia, by site,
with obstruction
congenital (large) (small) 751.4
malignant - *see* Neoplasm, intestine,
malignant
volvulus 560.2
jaundice (*see also* Obstruction,
gallbladder) 576.0
jejunum (*see also* Obstruction, intestine)
560.9
kidney (*see also* Lesion, kidney) 593.2
labor, complicating delivery 657.9
fetus or newborn - *see* categories
768.0-768.9
lachrymal, lacrimal (apparatus) (duct)
368
congenital 744.8
lachrymonasal, lacrimonasal duct 368
lacteal with steatorrhea 269.0
larynx 508.3
congenital 748.3
liver 573.9
cirrhotic - *see* Cirrhosis, liver
lung 519.2
lymphatic 457
mediastinum 519.9
merocele 553.0
mitral - *see* Endocarditis, mitral
nasal 508.9
duct 368
nasolachrymal, nasolacrimal duct 368

Obstruction, etc. — *continued*
  nasopharynx 508.9
  nose 508.9
  omentocele 553.9
  omphalocele 553.1
  organ or site, congenital NEC - *see*
      Atresia
  pancreatic duct 577.9
  parotid gland 527.9
  pelvo-ureteral junction (*see also*
      Obstruction, ureter) 593.3
  pharynx 508.9
  portal (circulation) (vein) 452
  prostate 600
  pulmonary valve (heart) (*see also*
      Endocarditis, pulmonary) 424.9
  pyemic - *see* Septicemia
  pylorus 537.0
    congenital 750.1
    infantile 750.1
  rectosigmoid (*see also* Obstruction,
      intestine) 560.9
  rectum 569.2
  respiratory 519.9
  retinal (artery) (central) (vein) 377.0
  rupture (nontraumatic) 553.9
  salivary duct (any) 527.9
  sarco-epiplocele 553.9
  sarco-epiplomphalocele 553.1
  sigmoid (*see also* Obstruction, intestine)
    560.9
  sinus - *see* Sinusitis
  Stensen's duct 527.9
  stomach 537.9
    congenital 750.8
  submaxillary gland 527.9
  thoracic duct 457
  thrombotic - *see* Thrombosis
  trachea 519.9
  tricuspid - *see* Endocarditis, tricuspid
  upper respiratory, congenital 748.8
  ureter (pelvic juncture) (functional)
    593.3
    congenital 753.2
    due to calculus 592
  urethra 599.9
    congenital 753.6
  urinary (moderate) 596.2
    organ or tract (lower) 599.9
    prostatic valve 599.9
  uropathy 599.9
  uterus 625.9
  vagina 629.7
  valvular - *see* Endocarditis
  vein, venous 458.9
    caval (inferior) (superior) 458.1

Obstruction, etc. — *continued*
  vein, etc. — *continued*
    thrombotic - *see* Thrombosis
  vena cava (inferior) (superior) 458.1
  vesical 596.2
  vesico-urethral orifice 596.2
  vessel NEC 458.9
Obturator - *see* condition
Occlusio pupillae 378.6
Occlusion
  anus 569.2
    congenital 751.3
    infantile 751.3
  aqueduct of Sylvius 347.9
    congenital 742
      with spina bifida 741.0
  arteries of extremities 444.4
  artery - *see also* Embolism, artery
    basilar, carotid, cerebellar, choroidal,
      hypophyseal, pontine,
      precerebral, or vertebral - *see*
      Occlusion, precerebral artery
    brain or cerebral (*see also*
      Thrombosis, brain) 433.9
  basilar (artery) (*see also* Occlusion,
    precerebral artery) 432.9
  bile duct (*see also* Obstruction,
    gallbladder) 576.0
    congenital 751.5
  bowel (*see also* Obstruction, intestine)
    560.9
  brain (artery) (vascular) (*see also*
    Thrombosis, brain) 433.9
  carotid (artery) (common) (internal) (*see*
    also Occlusion, precerebral
    artery) 432.9
  cerebellar (artery) (*see also* Occlusion,
    precerebral artery) 432.9
  cerebral (artery) (*see also* Thrombosis,
    brain) 433.9
  cerebrovascualr (*see also* Thrombosis,
    brain) 433.9
    diffuse (*see also* Ischemia, cerebral)
      437.9
  cervical canal (*see also* Stricture,
    cervix) 621.5
    by falciparum malaria 084.0
  cervix (uteri) (*see also* Stricture, cervix)
    621.5
  colon (*see also* Obstruction, intestine)
    560.9
  coronary (artery) (thrombotic) (*see also*
    Infarct, myocardium) 410.9
  embolic - *see* Embolism
  fallopian tube 615.9
    congenital 752.5

Occlusion—*continued*
  gallbladder (*see also* Obstruction,
      gallbladder)   576.0
    congenital   751.6
  gingiva, traumatic   523.9
  hymen   629.7
    congenital   752.6
  intestine (*see also* Obstruction,
      intestine)   560.9
  kidney (*see also* Lesion, kidney)   593.2
  lachrymal, lacrimal apparatus   378.3
  lung   519.2
  lymph or lymphatic channel   457
  mammary duct   611.9
  mesenteric artery (embolic) (thrombotic)
      (with gangrene)   444.2
  nose   508.9
    congenital   748.0
  organ or site, congenital NEC - *see*
      Atresia
  oviduct   615.9
    congenital   752.5
  periodontal, traumatic   523.9
  peripheral arteries   444.4
  posterior lingual, of mandibular teeth
      524.2
  precerebral artery   432.9
    with hypertension (benign) (conditions
        in 401)   432.0
      malignant (*see also* Hypertension,
          malignant with
          cerebrovascular
          involvement)   400.2
    puerperal, postpartum, childbirth
        674
  puncta lacrimalia   378.3
  pupil   378.6
  pylorus (*see also* Stricture, pylorus)
      537.0
  renal artery   444.3
  retinal (artery) (vein)   377.0
  thoracic duct   457
  ureter (complete) (partial) (*see also*
      Stricture, ureter)   593.3
    congenital   753.2
  urethra (*see also* Stricture, urethra)
      598
    congenital   753.6
  uterus   625.9
  vagina   629.7
  vascular NEC   458.9
  vein - *see* Thrombosis
  vena cava   453
  ventricle (brain) NEC   347.9

Occlusion—*continued*
  vertebral (artery) (left) (right) (*see also*
      Occlusion, precerebral artery)
      432.9
  vessel (blood)   458.9
  vulva   629.7
Occupational - *see* condition
Ochlophobia   300.2
Ochronosis (endogenous)   270.6
  with chloasma of eyelid   270.6
Ocular muscle - *see* condition
Oculogyric
  crisis or disturbance   781.1
    late effect, viral encephalitis   066
    psychogenic   305.8
Oculomotor syndrome   781.1
  residual of viral encephalitis   066
Odontalgia   525.9
Odontoclasis - *see* Wound, open, face
Odontogenesis
  imperfecta   520.5
Odontoma   210.4
  follicular   526.0
Odontomyelitis (closed) (open)   522.0
Odontonecrosis   521.0
Odontorrhagia   525.9
Oestriasis   134.0
Offences, sex, in children   308
Oguchi's disease (retina)   378.9
Ohara's disease   021
Oidiomycosis   112
Old age   794
  dementia   290.0
Olfactory - *see* condition
Oligemia   285.9
Oligergasia (*see also* Retardation, mental)
      315.9
Oligocythemia   285.9
Oligodendroblastoma (*see also* Neoplasm,
      nervous system, malignant)   192.9
Oligodendroglioma (*see also* Neoplasm,
      nervous system, malignant)   192.9
Oligodendroma (*see also* Neoplasm,
      nervous system, malignant)   192.9
Oligodontia (*see also* Anodontia)   520.0
Oligohydramnios (complicating pregnancy)
      634.9
  complicating delivery   661.8
  fetus or newborn   769.9
Oligohydrosis   705.0
Oligomenorrhea   626.1
Oligophrenia (*see also* Retardation,
      mental)   315.9
  phenylpyruvic   270.0
Oligospermia   606

Oligotrichia 704
  congenita 757.3
Oliguria 786.5
Ollier's disease 756.5
Omentitis (*see also* Peritonitis) 567.9
Omentocele 551.9
  gangrenous, incarcerated, irreducible,
      strangulated or with obstruction
      (intestinal) 553.9
Omentum, omental - *see* condition
Omphalitis 686.9
Omphalocele 551.1
  gangrenous, incarcerated, irreducible,
      strangulated or with obstruction
      (intestinal) 553.1
Omphalomesenteric duct persistent
      751.0
Omphalorrhagia, newborn 778.9
Onanism 305.6
Onchocerciasis 125.3
Onchocercosis 125.3
Oncocytoma (salivary gland) 210.2
  jaw 210.4
  specified site NEC - *see* Neoplasm,
      benign
Oneirophrenia 295.4
Onychauxis 703.9
  congenital 757.4
Onychia (with lymphangitis) 681
Onychitis (with lymphangitis) 681
Onychocryptosis 703.0
Onychodystrophy 703.9
  congenital 757.4
Onychogryphosis 703.9
Onycholysis 703.9
Onychomadesis 703.9
Onychomalacia 703.9
Onychomycosis - *see* Dermatophytosis
Onychophagy 788.9
  child problem 308
Onychoptosis 703.9
Onychorrhexis 703.9
  congenital 757.4
Onychoschizia 703.9
Onychotrophia (*see also* Atrophy, nail)
      703.9
Onyxis - *see* Ingrowing nail
Onyxitis (with lymphangitis) 681
Oophoritis (cystic) (infectional)
      (interstitial) (*see also* Salpingo-
      oophoritis) 614
  fetal (acute) 752.5
Opacities enamel (teeth) (fluoride)
      (nonfluoride) 520.3
Opacity
  cornea 371.9

Opacity—*continued*
  cornea—*continued*
    congenital 744.8
    degenerative 371.9
    inflammatory 371.9
    late effect of trachoma (healed) 077
    postoperative 371.0
    subendothelial (striped) 371.9
    subepithelial (striped) 371.9
  lens (*see also* Cataract) 374.9
  optic nerve fibers, fibres 377.6
  snowball 378.9
  vitreous (humor) 377.4
    congenital 744.8
Opalescent dentin 520.5
Open, opening
  abnormal, organ or site, congenital - *see*
      Imperfect closure
  false - *see* Imperfect closure
  wound - *see* Wound, open
Openbite (anterior) (posterior) 524.2
Operation NEC 796.9
  causing multilation of fetus 773
  exploratory 796.9
  for delivery
    fetus or newborn (*see also* Birth
        injury NEC) 772.9
  maternal, unrelated to current delivery,
      affecting fetus or newborn 761.6
Operational fatigue 300.8
Operative - *see* condition
Ophthalmia (catarrhal) (purulent) 360
  actinic rays 360
  allergic 360
    with hay fever 507
  blennorrhagic (neonatorum) 098.2
  diphtheritic 032
  due to
    dust 360
    lagophthalmos 360
  Egyptian 076
  electrica 360
  gonococcal (neonatorum) 098.2
  metastatic 366
  migraine 346
  neonatorum, newborn 360
    gonococcal 098.2
  nodosa 360
  sympathetic 366
Ophthalmitis - *see* Ophthalmia
Ophthalmoneuromyelitis 341
Ophthalmoplegia (*see also* Strabismus)
      373.9
  bilateral 373.9
  diabetic - *see* category 250

Ophthalmoplegia—*continued*
  exophthalmic 242.0
  interna 373.0
  migraine 346
  Parinaud's 373.9
  unilateral 373.9
Opisthognathism 524.0
Opisthorchiasis 121.0
Opitz's disease 289.5
Opiumism 304.0
Oppenheim-Urbach disease - *see* category
  250
Oppenheim's disease 330.2
Opthalmocele (congenital) 744.8
Optic nerve - *see* condition
Orbit - *see* condition
Orchitis (gangrenous) (nonspecific) (septic)
  (suppurative) 604
  blennorrhagic (acute) 098.0
    chronic or duration of 2 months or
      over 098.1
  gonococcal (acute) 098.0
    chronic or duration of 2 months or
      over 098.1
  mumps 072
  parotidea 072
  syphilitic 095
  tuberculous 016.2
    late effect or sequela 019.2
Orf 057.8
Organ of Morgagni 752.8
Organic - *see also* condition
  heart - *see* Disease, heart
  insufficiency 796.0
Orifice - *see* condition
Ormond's disease 593.3
Ornithosis 073
Orotaciduria, oroticaciduria (congenital)
  (hereditary) (pyrimidine deficiency)
  281.4
Orthopnea 783.2
Os, uterus - *see* condition
Osgood-Schlatter
  disease 722.2
  osteochondrosis 722.2
Osler-Rendu disease 448
Osler-Vaquez disease 208
Osler's
  disease 208
  nodes 421.0
Osmidrosis 705.9
Osseous - *see* condition
Ossification
  artery - *see* Arteriosclerosis
  auricle (ear) 387.9
  bronchi 519.9

Ossification—*continued*
  cardiac (*see also* Insufficiency,
    myocardial) 428
  cartilage (senile) 729.9
  coronary (artery) (*see also* Ischemia,
    heart) 412.9
  diaphragm 733.9
  ear 387.9
  falx cerebri 347.9
  fascia 733.9
  fontanel
    defective or delayed 756.0
    premature 756.0
  heart (*see also* Insufficiency,
    myocardial) 428
    valve - *see* Endocarditis
  larynx 508.3
  meninges (cerebral) 347.9
    spinal 349.9
  multiple, eccentric centers 723.9
  muscle 733.9
  myocardium, myocardial (*see also*
    Insufficiency, myocardial) 428
  penis 607.9
  periarticular 729.9
  sclera 378.6
  tendon 733.3
  trachea 519.9
  tympanic membrane 387.9
  vitreous (humor) 378.9
Osteitis (*see also* Osteomyelitis) 720.2
  alveolar 526.5
  condensans (ilii) 720.1
  deformans 721
  due to yaws 102.6
  fibrosa NEC 723.9
    cystica (generalisata) 252.0
    disseminata 756.7
    osteoplastica 252.0
  fragilitans 756.6
  Garre's (sclerosing) 720.1
  jaw (acute) (chronic) (lower)
    (suppurative) (upper) 526.4
  parathyroid 252.0
  petrous bone, acute - *see* Mastoiditis,
    acute
  sclerotic, nonsuppurative 720.1
  tuberculosa
    cystica (of Jungling) 135
    multiplex cystoides 135
Osteo-arthritis (degenerative)
    (hypertrophic) (polyarticular)
    (rheumatoid) 713.0
  distal interphalangeal 713.0
  spine, spinal (any part) (cervical)
    (lumbar) 713.1

Osteo-arthropathy 723.9
  hypertrophic pulmonary 723.1
  secondary, hypertrophic 723.1
Osteo-arthrosis - *see also* Osteo-arthritis
  deformans alkaptonurica 270.6
Osteoblastoma - *see* Neoplasm, bone,
    malignant
Osteocarcinoma - *see* Neoplasm, bone,
    malignant
Osteochondritis (*see also*
      Osteochondrosis) 722.9
  dissecans 722.5
  multiple 756.7
  syphilitic (congenital) 090.0
Osteochondrocarcinoma - *see* Neoplasm,
    bone, malignant
Osteochondrocarcinosarcoma - *see*
    Neoplasm, bone, malignant
Osteochondrodermodysplasia 756.7
Osteochondrodystrophy 273.8
  deformans 273.8
  familial 273.8
  fetalis 756.5
Osteochondroma (*see also* Exostosis)
      213.0
  bursa 215
  multiple, congenital 756.5
Osteochondromatosis (*see also* Exostosis)
      213.0
  synovial 215
Osteochondromyxoma 213.9
Osteochondromyxosarcoma - *see*
    Neoplasm, bone, malignant
Osteochondrosarcoma - *see* Neoplasm,
    bone, malignant
Osteochondrosis 722.9
  adult spine 722.9
  calcaneus 722.2
  capitular epiphysis (femur) 722.1
  carpal scaphoid 722.2
  coxae juvenilis 722.1
  deformans juvenilis (coxae) 722.1
  dissecans (knee) (shoulder) 722.5
  femoral capital epiphysis 722.1
  femur 722.1
  Freiberg's 722.2
  ilium 722.2
  juvenile, juvenilis 722.2
    capitular epiphysis 722.1
    clavicle, sternal epiphysis 722.2
    coxae 722.1
    deformans 722.1
    hip 722.1
    medial cuneiform bone 722.2
    specified site NEC 722.2
    spine 722.0

Osteochondrosis — *continued*
  juvenile, juvenilis — *continued*
    vertebra (body) 722.0
      epiphyseal plates 722.0
    Kienbock's 722.2
    Kohler's 722.2
    Legg-Perthes(-Calve) 722.1
    lunate bone 722.2
    metatarsal (head) 722.2
    navicular 722.2
    os calcis 722.2
    Osgood-Schlatter 722.2
    Scheuermann's 722.0
    spine (juvenile) 722.0
      adult 722.9
    syphilitic (congenital) 090.0
    tarsal scaphoid 722.2
    tibia (tuberosity) 722.2
    tuberculous - *see* Tuberculosis, bone
    vertebral (juvenile) 722.0
      adult 722.9
Osteoclastic tumor 213.9
  malignant - *see* Neoplasm, bone,
      malignant
Osteoclastoma 213.9
  malignant - *see* Neoplasm, bone,
      malignant
Osteoclastosis 213.9
Osteocopic pain 723.9
Osteodynia 723.9
Osteodystrophy
  parathyroid 252.0
  renal 593.0
Osteofibrochondroma 213.9
Osteofibroma 213.9
Osteofibrosarcoma - *see* Neoplasm, bone,
    malignant
Osteogenesis imperfecta 756.6
Osteogenic - *see* condition
Osteoma (any bone) 213.1
  nasal sinus 212.0
  osteoid 213.9
  tongue 210.1
Osteomalacia 265.2
  infantile (*see also* Rickets) 265.0
  juvenile (*see also* Rickets) 265.0
  pelvis 265.2
  vitamin D-resistant 273.4
Osteomalacosis 265.2
Osteomyelitis (general) (infective)
      (localized) (purulent) (pyogenic)
      (septic) (staphylococcal)
      (streptococcal) (suppurative) (with
      periostitis) 720.2
  acute or subacute 720.0
  chronic or old 720.1

Osteomyelitis, etc. — *continued*
   Garre's 720.1
   jaw (acute) (chronic) (lower)
      (suppurative) (upper) 526.4
   nonsuppurating 720.1
   petrous bone - *see* Mastoiditis
   sclerosing
      nonsuppurative 720.1
   syphilitic 095
      congenital 090.0
   tuberculous - *see* Tuberculosis, bone
   typhoid 001
Osteomyelofibrosis 209
Osteomyelosclerosis 209
Osteomyxochondroma 213.9
Osteonecrosis 720.1
Osteopathia
   condensans disseminata 756.7
   hyperostotica multiplex infantilis
      756.7
Osteopecilia 756.7
Osteoperiostitis (*see also* Osteomyelitis)
   720.2
Osteopetrosis (familial) 756.7
Osteophyte - *see* Exostosis
Osteoplastic tumor 213.9
   malignant - *see* Neoplasm, bone,
      malignant
Osteopoikilosis 756.7
Osteoporosis 723.0
   post-traumatic 723.0
   senilis 723.0
Osteopsathyrosis 756.6
Osteosarcoma - *see* Neoplasm, bone,
   malignant
Osteosclerosis 756.7
   fragilis (generalisata) 756.7
   myelofibrosis 209
Osteosclerotic anemia 209
Osteosis cutis 709.9
Ostium
   atrioventriculare commune 746.5
   primum or secundum (arteriosum)
      (defect) (persistent) 746.4
Ostrum-Furst syndrome 756.7
Otalgia (reflex) 384.9
Othematoma 387.9
Otitis 381.9
   with abscess, caries, disease, empyema
      or necrosis of mastoid,
      endomastoiditis, mastoiditis,
      osteitis of petrous bone or
      petrositis - *see* Otitis media with
      these conditions
   acute 381.0
   chronic 381.1

Otitis — *continued*
   diffuse parasitic 136
   externa (acute) 380
      tropical 111.9
   insidiosa 386
   interna 384.0
   media (hemorrhagic) (purulent)
      (staphylococcal) (streptococcal)
      (suppurative) 381.9
   with
      abscess of mastoid, acute 382.0
      caries of mastoid process, chronic
         382.1
      empyema of mastoid, acute 382.0
      endomastoiditis, acute 382.0
      mastoid
         disease 382.9
            acute 382.0
            chronic 382.1
         necrosis, chronic 382.1
      mastoiditis 382.9
         acute 382.0
         chronic 382.1
      osteitis, petrous bone, acute 382.0
      petrositis, acute 382.0
   acute (serous) 381.0
      with
         abscess of mastoid (acute)
            382.0
         empyema of mastoid (acute)
            382.0
         endomastoiditis (acute) 382.0
         mastoid disease (acute) 382.0
         mastoiditis (acute) 382.0
         osteitis, petrous bone (acute)
            382.0
         petrositis (acute) 382.0
   chronic (secretory) (serous) (with
      effusion) 381.1
      with
         caries of mastoid process
            (chronic) 382.1
         mastoid disease or necrosis
            (chronic) 382.1
         mastoiditis (chronic) 382.1
   tuberculous 017.3
      late effect or sequela 019.9
Otolith syndrome 387.9
Otomycosis (diffuse) 111.9
Otopathy 387.9
Otoporosis 386
Otorrhagia 387.9
   traumatic - *see* nature of injury
Otorrhea (*see also* Otitis, media) 381.9
   cerebrospinal 387.9
Otosclerosis (general) 386

Otospongiosis 386
Otto's disease or pelvis 713.0
  complicating delivery - *see* Deformity,
    pelvis, complicating delivery
  noted during pregnancy (undelivered)
    634.9
Outburst, aggressive 306.9
Outlet - *see* condition
Outstanding ears (bilateral) 745.2
Ovalocytosis (hereditary) (*see also*
    Elliptocytosis) 282.1
Ovaritis (cystic) (*see also* Salpingo-
    oophoritis) 614
Ovary, ovarian - *see* condition
Overactive
  hypothalmus 253.9
  thyroid (*see also* Hyperthyroidism)
    242.2
Overbite (deep) (excessive) (horizontal)
    (vertical) 524.2
Overbreathing (*see also* Hyperventilation)
    783.2
Overdevelopment - *see also* Hypertrophy
  breast 611.1
  congenital, prostate 752.8
  nasal bones 738.0
Overdistension - *see* Distension
Overdose, overdosage (drug) 977.9
  specified drug or substance - *see* Table
    of adverse effects
Overeating 278.9
Overexertion (effects) (exhaustion) 994.5
Overexposure (effects) (exhaustion)
    994.4
Overfeeding 278.9
Overgrowth, bone NEC 723.9
Overheated (places) (effects) - *see* Heat

Overjet 524.2
Overlaid, overlying (suffocation) 994.7
Overlapping
  toe (acquired) 729.9
    congenital (fifth toe) 755.7
Overnutrition (*see also*
    Hyperalimentation) 278.9
Overriding
  aorta 747.2
  finger 729.9
    congenital 755.5
  toe 729.9
    congenital 755.7
Oversize
  fetus
    complicating delivery 655
    fetus or newborn - *see* categories
      765.0-765.9
Overstrained 790.1
  heart - *see* Disease, heart
Overweight 277
Overwork 790.1
Oviduct - *see* condition
Ovotestis 752.0
Ovulation (cycle)
  failure or lack of 615.9
  pain 626.3
Owren's disease (*see also* Defect,
    coagulation) 286.9
Ox heart - *see* Hypertrophy, cardiac
Oxalosis 271.8
Oxaluria 271.8
Oxycephaly, oxycephalic 756.0
  syphilitic, congenital 090.0
Oxyuriasis 127.3
Oxyuris vermicularis (infestation) 127.3
Ozena 502.1

P

Pachyderma, pachydermia 701.9
  cachexia 244
  laryngitis 508.3
  larynx (verrucosa) 508.3

Pachydermatocele (congenital) 757.2
  acquired 701.9

Pachydermatosis 701.9
Pachymeningitis (adhesive) (basal) (brain)
  (cerebral) (cervical) (chronic)
  (circumscribed) (external) (fibrous)
  (hemorrhagic) (hypertrophic)
  (internal) (purulent) (spinal)
  (suppurative) (*see also* Meningitis)
  320.9

Pachyonychia (congenital) 757.4
Packing after onset of labor
  fetus or newborn (*see also* Birth injury
    NEC) 772.9

Paget's disease 721
  bone 721
  breast 174
  malignant 174
  nipple 174
  osteitis deformans 721
  scrotum 173.5
  skin - *see* Neoplasm, skin, malignant

Pain(s)
  abdominal 785.5
  anginoid (*see also* Pain, precordial)
    782.0
  anus 569.2
  arch 787.1
  arm 787.1
  back (postural) 728.9
    low 728.7
    psychogenic 305.1
  bile duct (*see also* Disease, gallbladder)
    576.9
  bladder 786.0
  bone 723.9
  breast 786.7
    psychogenic 305.6
  cecum 785.5
  cervicobrachial 728.2
  chest 783.7
  coccyx 728.9
  colon 785.5
  common duct (*see also* Disease,
    gallbladder) 576.9
  coronary - *see* Angina
  ear 384.9

Pain(s) — *continued*
  epigastrium 785.5
  extremity (lower) (upper) 787.1
  eye 378.9
  facial 351
    nerve 350
  false (labor) (undelivered) 634.7
  finger 787.1
  flank 785.5
  foot 787.1

  gas (intestinal) 785.4
  gastric 536.9
  genital organ (female) (male) 786.7
    psychogenic 305.6
  groin 785.5

  hand 787.1
  head (*see also* Headache) 791
  heart (*see also* Pain, precordial) 782.0

  infra-orbital 351
  insufficient, poor, weak
    complicating delivery 657.9
      fetus or newborn - *see* categories
        767.0-767.9
  intermenstrual 626.3

  jaw 526.9
  joint 787.3
    psychogenic 305.1

  kidney 786.0

  labor, spurious (undelivered) 634.7
  leg 787.1
  limb 787.1
  low back 728.7
  lumbar region 728.7

  mastoid 384.9
  maxilla 526.9
  metacarpophalangeal 787.1
  metatarsophalangeal 787.1
  mouth 528.9
  muscle 717.9

  nasal 508.9
  nasopharynx 508.9
  neck NEC 728.0
    psychogenic 305.1
  nerve - *see* Neuralgia
  neuromuscular 717.9
  nose 508.9

  ophthalmic 378.9
  orbital region 378.9
  osteocopic 723.9
  ovary 786.7

Pain(s) — *continued*
  ovary — *continued*
    psychogenic 305.6
  over heart (*see also* Pain, precordial)
    782.0
  ovulation 626.3
  penis 786.7
    psychogenic 305.6
  pericardial (*see also* Pain, precordial)
    782.0
  pharynx 508.9
  pleura, pleural, pleuritic 783.7
  preauricular 387.9
  precordial (region) 782.0
    psychogenic 305.3
  psychogenic 305.9
    cardiovascular system 305.3
    gastrointestinal system 305.5
    genitourinary system 305.6
    heart 305.3
    musculo-skeletal system 305.1
    respiratory system 305.2
    skin 305.0
  radicular (spinal) (*see also* Radiculitis)
    728.9
  rectum 569.2
  rheumatic, muscular 717.9
  rib 783.7
  root (spinal) (*see also* Radiculitis)
    728.9
  sacro-iliac 728.7
  sciatic 353
  scrotum 786.7
    psychogenic 305.6
  seminal vesicle 786.7
  spermatic cord 786.7
  spinal root (*see also* Radiculitis) 728.9
  stomach 536.9
  temporomandibular (joint) 787.3
  temporomaxillary joint 787.3
  testicle 786.7
    psychogenic 305.6
  thoracic spine 728.5
    with radicular and visceral pain
      728.5
  tibia 787.1
  toe 787.1
  tongue 529.6
  tooth 525.9
  trigeminal 351
  ureter 786.0
  urinary (organ) (system) 786.0
  uterus 786.7
    psychogenic 305.6
  vertebrogenic (syndrome) (*see also*
    Radiculitis) 728.9

Pain(s) — *continued*
  very frequent, very strong
    complicating delivery 661.1
    fetus or newborn - *see* categories
      767.0-767.9
  vesical 786.0
Painful - *see also* Pain
  coitus (female) (male) 786.7
    psychogenic 305.6
  ejaculation (semen) 786.7
  erection 786.6
  menstruation 626.3
    psychogenic 305.6
  scar 709.0
  wire sutures 998.9
Painter's colic 984
Palate - *see* condition
Palatoplegia 528.9
Palatoschisis 749.0
  with cleft lip 749.2
Palilalia 781.5
Pallor 782.3
Palmar - *see* condition
  fascia - *see* condition
Palpable
  cecum 569.9
  kidney (*see also* Lesion, kidney) 593.2
  liver 573.9
  ovary 615.9
  spleen - *see* Splenomegaly
Palpitation (heart) 782.1
  psychogenic 305.3
Palsy (*see also* Paralysis) 344.9
  atrophic diffuse 348.9
  Bell's 350
  brachial plexus 357.0
    due to or with birth injury (*see also*
      Birth injury, bone or nerve)
      772.2
  brain NEC - *see also* Palsy, cerebral
    not congenital or infantile (*see also*
      Disease, cerebrovascular
      NEC) 438.9
    syphilitic 094.9
      congenital 090.4
  bulbar (progressive) (chronic) 348.1
    pseudo NEC 344.9
    supranuclear NEC 344.9
  cerebral (congenital) (infantile) 343.9
    with mixed types of motor
      disturbance (types classifiable
      under more than one of the
      titles 343.0-343.9) 343.9
    ataxic (type of motor disturbance)
      343.9

Palsy—*continued*
  cerebral, etc. —*continued*
    athetoid (type of motor disturbance)
      343.2
    atonic (type of motor disturbance)
      343.9
    late effect of birth injury 343.9
      specified type of motor disturbance
        - *code by* type under Palsy,
        cerebral
    not congenital or infantile - *see*
      Paralysis, brain
    rigidity (type of motor disturbance)
      343.9
    spastic (type of motor disturbance)
      343.1
      hemiplegia 343.0
    specified type of motor disturbance
      NEC 343.9
    tremor (type of motor disturbance)
      343.9
  congenital (cerebral) (spinal) - *see* Palsy,
    cerebral
  creeping 348.2
  divers' 993.3
  glossopharyngeal 356
  infantile - *see* Palsy, cerebral
  lead 984
  pseudobulbar NEC 344.9
  seventh nerve 350
  shaking (*see also* Parkinsonism) 342
  spastic (cerebral) (spinal) - *see* Palsy,
    cerebral, spastic
  tardy median 357.2
  wasting 348.2
Paltauf-Sternberg disease 201
Paludism - *see* Malaria
Panaris (with lymphangitis) 681
Panaritium (with lymphangitis) 681
Panarteritis (nodosa) 446.0
  brain or cerebral (*see also* Disease,
    cerebrovascular NEC) 438.9
Pancarditis (acute) (chronic) (*see also*
  Disease, heart) 429.9

Pancoast's syndrome or tumor 162.1
  benign 212.3

Pancreas, pancreatic - *see* condition
Pancreatitis 577.0
  acute (edematous) (hemorrhagic) 577.0
  annular 577.0
  apoplectic 577.0
  chronic (infectious) (relapsing) 577.1
  cystic 577.9
  fibrous 577.9
  gangrenous 577.0
  hemorrhagic (acute) 577.0

Pancreatitis—*continued*
  interstitial (chronic) 577.1
  acute 577.0
  malignant 577.0
  mumps 072
  suppurative 577.0
  syphilitic 095
Pancreolithiasis 577.9
Pancytolysis 289.9
Pancytopenia (congenital) 284
Panhematopenia 284
  splenic
    primary 289.4
Panhemocytopenia 284
Panhypogonadism 257.1
Panhypopituitarism 253.1
  prepubertal 253.1
Panic (attack) (state) 300.0
Panmyelophthisis 284
Panmyelosis 207.9
Panner's disease 722.2
Panneuritis endemica 261
Panniculitis 686.9
  nodular, nonsuppurative 686.9
Panniculus adiposus (abdominal) 277
Pannus 378.4
  allergic eczematous (*see also* Keratitis)
    363.9
  degenerativus 378.4
  keratic 378.4
  trachomatosus, trachomatous (active)
    076
    late effect 077
Panophthalmitis 366
Panotitis - *see* Otitis media
Pansinusitis (chronic) (hyperplastic)
    (nonpurulent) (purulent) (*see also*
    Sinusitis) 503.9
  due to fungus NEC 117.9
  tuberculous 012.9
    with pneumoconiosis (conditions in
      515) 010
    late effect or sequela 019.0

Panvalvular disease - *see* Endocarditis,
  mitral
Papageienkrankheit 073
Papilledema 377.5
  choked disc 377.5
  infectional 367
Papillitis 367
  anus 569.2
  necrotizing
    kidney (*see also* Pyelitis) 590.1
  optic 367
  rectum 569.0

Papillitis—*continued*
  renal
    necrotizing (*see also* Pyelitis) 590.1
    tongue 529.0
Papillo-adenocarcinoma - *see* Neoplasm,
    malignant
Papillo-adenocystoma - *see also*
    Neoplasm, benign
  ovary 220.1
Papillocarcinoma - *see* Epithelioma,
    malignant
Papilloma (epidermoid) (squamous cell) -
    see also Epithelioma, benign
  acuminatum (female) (male) 099.9
  auditory canal 216.0
  bladder 223.3
  breast (intracystic) (intraductal) (skin of)
    217
  choroid plexus 225.0
  colon (villous) 211.3
  conjunctiva 224
  epitheliomatous - *see* Epithelioma
  kidney 223.0
    pelvis 223.1
  larynx 212.1
    congenital 748.3
    juvenile 212.1
  malignant - *see* Epithelioma, malignant
  nose 212.0
    skin of 216.0
  thyroid 246
  uterus 219.0
  yaws, plantar or palmar 102.1
Papillomata, multiple, of yaws 102.1
Papillomatosis, ductal, breast 610
Papule 709.9
  carate (primary) 103.0
  pinta (primary) 103.0
Papulosis, malignant 446.9
Papyraceus fetus NEC 779.9
Paracephalus 759.2
Paracoccidioidomycosis 116.2
Paradentosis 523.5
Paraffinoma 999.9
Paraganglioma (chromaffin) (non-
    chromaffin) 226.8
  adrenal (gland) 255.2
  aortic body 226.8
  carotid body 226.4
  coccygeal body or glomus 226.8
  glomus jugulare 226.8
  malignant 194.8
    adrenal (gland) 194.0
  specified site NEC 226.8
Parageusia 781.4
  psychogenic 305.8

Paragonimiasis 121.2
Paragranuloma, Hodgkin's 201
Parahemophilia (*see also* Defect,
    coagulation) 286.9
Parakeratosis 701.1
  variegata 696.2
Paralysis, paralytic 344.9
  with
    broken
      back - *code by* region under
        Fracture, vertebra, with
        spinal cord lesion
      neck (closed) 806.0
        late effect 806.9
        open 806.1
    fracture, vertebra, (conditions in 805)
      - *code by* region under
      Fracture, vertebra, with spinal
      cord lesion
    syphilis 094.9
  abdomen and back muscles 357.9
  abdominal muscles 357.9
  abducens (nerve) 373.9
  abductor 357.9
  accessory nerve 356
  accommodation 370.9
    hysterical 300.1
  acoustic nerve 387.9
  agitans 342
    arteriosclerotic 342
    juvenile, with pallidal degeneration
      342
    late effect, viral encephalitis 066
    postencephalitic 066
  alcoholic 303.2
  alternating 344.1
    oculomotor 344.1
  amyotrophic 348.0
  ankle 357.9
  anterior serratus 357.9
  anus (sphincter) 569.2
  apoplectic (current episode) (*see also*
    Disease, cerebrovascular, acute)
    436.9
    late effect or residual 344.9
  arm 357.9
    due to old CVA 436.9
    hysterical 300.1
    psychogenic 305.1
    transient 787.0
    traumatic NEC (*see also* Injury,
      nerve, by site) 959.2
  arteriosclerotic (current episode) (*see*
    also Disease, cerebrovascular
    NEC) 438.9
    late effect or residual 344.9

Paralysis, etc. — *continued*
  ascending (spinal) 349.5
    acute 354
    general 349.5
  associated, nuclear 344.9
  ataxic NEC 344.9
    general 094.1
  atrophic 357.9
    infantile, acute 041
      late effect or residual 044
    muscle 357.9
    progressive 348.2
    spinal (acute) 041
      late effect 044
  attack (*see also* Disease,
      cerebrovascular, acute) 436.9
  axillar, axillary (nerve) 357.1
  Bell's 350
    newborn (*see also* Birth injury, bone
      or nerve) 772.2
  Benedikt's 344.9
  bilateral NEC 344.9
    late effect or residual NEC 344.9
    due to specified lesion - *see*
      Paralysis, late effect of
  birth (injury) (*see also* Birth injury, bone
      or nerve) 772.2
    brain (*see also* Birth injury, brain)
      772.0
      late effect or residual - *see* Palsy,
        cerebral
    intracranial (*see also* Birth injury,
      brain) 772.0
      late effect or residual - *see* Palsy,
        cerebral
    spinal cord (*see also* Birth injury,
      spinal cord) 772.1
      late effect or residual - *see* Palsy,
        cerebral
  bladder (sphincter) 596.3
    flaccid 596.3
    puerperal, postpartum, childbirth
      677.9
    sensory 596.3
    spastic 596.3
  bowel, colon or intestine (*see also* Ileus)
    560.1
  brachial plexus 357.0
    due to or with birth injury (*see also*
      Birth injury, bone or nerve)
      772.2
    newborn (*see also* Birth injury, bone
      or nerve) 772.2
  brain (current episode) (*see also*
    Disease, cerebrovascular NEC)
    438.9

Paralysis, etc. — *continued*
  brain, etc. — *continued*
    congenital - *see* Palsy, cerebral
    fetus or newborn (*see also* Birth
      injury, brain) 772.0
    infantile - *see* Palsy, cerebral
    late effect or residual NEC 344.9
      due to specified lesion - *see*
        Paralysis, late effect of
    spastic (infantile) 343.1
      with other types of motor
        disturbance (e.g., ataxic,
        athetoid, atonic, rigidity, or
        tremor) 343.9
      not infantile or congenital 344.9
    syphilitic, congenital 090.4
  bronchi 519.9
  Brown-Sequard 349.5
  bulbar (progressive) (chronic) 348.1
    infantile (*see also* Poliomyelitis,
      bulbar) 040
    poliomyelitic (*see also* Poliomyelitis,
      bulbar) 040
    pseudo 344.9
    supranuclear 344.9
  cardiac (*see also* Failure, heart) 782.4
  cerebral (current episode) - *see*
    Paralysis, brain
  cerebrocerebellar (*see also* Paralysis,
    brain) 438.9
    diplegic infantile - *see* Diplegia,
      infantile
  cerebrospinal NEC 344.9
  cervical
    plexus 357.0
    sympathetic 358.0
  Cestan-Chenais 344.1
  Charcot-Marie-Tooth type 330.0
  childhood - *see* Palsy, cerebral
  Clark's - *see* Palsy, cerebral
  compressed air 993.3
  compression (*see also* Compression,
    nerve) 357.9
  congenital (cerebral) (spinal) - *see* Palsy,
    cerebral
  conjugate movement (of eye) 781.1
    cortical (nuclear) (supranuclear)
      373.9
  convergence 373.1
  cordis (*see also* Failure, heart) 782.4
  cortical (*see also* Paralysis, brain)
    438.9
  cranial or cerebral nerve 356
    eighth or acoustic 387.9
    eleventh or accessory 356
    fifth or trigeminal 356

Paralysis, etc. — *continued*
  infantile — *continued*
    paralytic 041
      late effects 044
    progressive acute 043
      late effects 044
    spastic 343.1
      with other types of motor
        disturbance (e.g., ataxic,
        athetoid, atonic, rigidity, or
        tremor) 343.9
    spinal 043
      late effects 044
  infective 043
    late effects 044
  inferior nuclear 344.9
  insane, general or progressive 094.1
  internuclear 373.9
  interosseous 357.9
  intracranial (current episode) (*see also*
    Disease, cerebrovascular NEC)
    438.9
    due to birth injury (*see also* Birth
      injury, brain) 772.0
      late effect - *see* Palsy, cerebral
  iris 378.6
    due to diphtheria (toxin) 032
  ischemic, Volkmann's (complicating
    trauma) 995.7
  Jackson's 344.9
  jake 989.9
  Jamaica ginger 989.9
  juvenile general 090.4
  Klumpke(-Dejerine) (birth) (newborn)
    (*see also* Birth injury, bone or
    nerve) 772.2
  labioglossal (laryngeal) (pharyngeal)
    348.1
  Landry's 354
  laryngeal nerve (bilateral) (recurrent)
    (superior) (unilateral) 508.0
  larynx 508.0
    due to diphtheria (toxin) 032
  late effect or residual of
    acute poliomyelitis (conditions in 040-
      043) 044
    birth injury, intracranial or spinal
      (conditions in 764-768 or 772
      with fourth digit .0 or .1) - *see*
      Palsy, cerebral
    cerebral laceration or contusion
      (conditions in 851.0, 851.1)
      851.9
    fracture or fracture dislocation of
      vertebral column with spinal cord
      lesion (conditions in 806.0-
      806.7) 806.9

Paralysis, etc. — *continued*
  late effect, etc. — *continued*
    intracranial
      abscess or pyogenic infection
        (conditions in 320-323) 324
      hemorrhage following injury
        (conditions in 853.0, 853.1)
        853.9
      vascular lesion (conditions in 430-
        438) 344.9
      spinal cord lesion (nontraumatic)
        NEC 349.5
      traumatic (conditions in 958.0-
        958.7) 958.9
      subarachnoid, subdural or extradural
        hemorrhage, following injury
        (conditions in 852.0, 852.1)
        852.9
      viral encephalitis (conditions in 062-
        065) 066
  lateral 348.0
  lead 984
  left side - *see* Hemiplegia
  leg 357.9
    both - *see* Paraplegia
    crossed 344.9
    hysterical 300.1
    psychogenic 305.1
    transient or transitory 787.0
      traumatic NEC (*see also* Injury,
        nerve, peroneal) 959.2
  levator palpebrae superioris 378.2
  lip 781.4
  Lissauer's 094.1
  local 357.9
  longstanding NEC 344.9
    due to specified lesion - *see* Paralysis,
      late effect of
  lung 519.2
    newborn (*see also* Asphyxia,
      newborn) 776.9
  median nerve 357.2
  medullary (tegmental) 344.9
  mesencephalic NEC 344.9
    tegmental 344.9
  middle alternating 344.1
  Millard-Gubler-Foville 344.1
  motor NEC 344.9
  multiple NEC 344.9
  muscle (flaccid) 357.9
    due to lesion
      central nervous system NEC
        344.9
      nerve (*see also* Neuropathy)
        357.9
    eye (extrinsic) (*see also* Strabismus)
      373.9

Paralysis, etc. — *continued*
  muscle (flaccid) — *continued*
    eye (extrinsic) — *continued*
      intrinsic 378.9
      oblique 373.9
    ischemic (Volkmann's) (complicating
        trauma) 995.7
    postpoliomyelitic 044
    pseudohypertrophic 330.3
    spastic 343.1
      with other types of motor
        disturbance (e.g., ataxic,
        athetoid, atonic, rigidity, or
        tremor) 343.9
      not infantile or congenital 344.9
  muscular 357.9
    atrophic 357.9
    progressive 348.2
  musculocutaneous nerve 357.9
  musculospiral 357.9
  nerve 357.9
    at birth (facial) (radial) (*see also* Birth
      injury, bone or nerve) 772.2
    auditory 387.9
    cranial or cerebral - *see* Paralysis,
      cranial or cerebral nerve
    due to or with birth injury (*see also*
      Birth injury, bone or nerve)
      772.2
    facial 350
      due to or with birth injury (*see also*
        Birth injury, bone or nerve)
        772.2
      newborn (*see also* Birth injury,
        bone or nerve) 772.2
      newborn (*see also* Birth injury, bone
        or nerve) 772.2
    radial 357.9
      due to or with birth injury (*see also*
        Birth injury, bone or nerve)
        772.2
      newborn (*see also* Birth injury,
        bone or nerve) 772.2
    specified NEC - *see* nerve involved
      under Paralysis
    traumatic NEC (*see also* Injury,
      nerve) 959.2
    ulnar 357.3
  obstetrical
    newborn (*see also* Birth injury, bone
      or nerve) 772.2
  ocular 781.1
  oculomotor (nerve) (*see also*
    Strabismus) 373.9
    alternating 344.1
    external bilateral 373.1

Paralysis, etc. — *continued*
  old 344.9
    age 344.9
    due to specified lesion - *see* Paralysis,
      late effect of
  olfactory nerve 356
  optic nerve 377.6
  palate 528.9
  periodic (familial) (hypokalemic)
    (hyperkalemic) 273.4
  peripheral
    autonomic nervous system 358.9
    nerve NEC 357.9
  peroneal (nerve) 357.9
  pharynx 508.9
  phrenic (nerve) 357.9
  pneumogastric nerve 356
  poliomyelitis (current) 041
    old 044
  popliteal nerve 357.9
  postdiphtheritic 032
  postencephalitic 066
  pressure (*see also* Compression, nerve)
    357.9
  progressive 348.2
    atrophic 348.2
    general 094.1
    infantile acute 043
      late effects 044
    multiple 348.2
  pseudobulbar 344.9
  pseudohypertrophic 330.3
    muscle 330.3
  psoas 357.9
  psychogenic 305.1
  quadriceps 357.9
  radial nerve 357.9
    due to or with birth injury (*see also*
      Birth injury, bone or nerve)
      772.2
  rectus muscle (eye) (*see also*
    Strabismus) 373.9
  residual NEC 344.9
    due to specified lesion - *see* Paralysis,
      late effect of
  respiratory (muscle) (system) (tract)
    796.0
    center NEC 344.9
      fetus or newborn (*see also* Birth
        injury, brain) 772.0
      late effect or residual NEC 344.9
      due to specified lesion - *see*
        Paralysis, late effect of
    congenital (*see also* Asphyxia,
      newborn) 776.9
    newborn (*see also* Asphyxia,
      newborn) 776.9

Paralysis, etc. — *continued*
retrobulbar 378.9
right side - *see* Hemiplegia
saturnine 984
sciatic nerve 357.9
seizure (current episode) (*see also*
Disease, cerebrovascular, acute)
436.9
late effect or residual 344.9
senile 344.9
serratus magnus 357.9
shaking (*see also* Parkinsonism) 342
shoulder 357.0
soft palate 528.9
spastic (cerebral) (spinal) (cord) 343.1
with other types of motor disturbance
(e.g., ataxic, athetoid, atonic,
rigidity, or tremor) 343.9
congenital 343.1
familial 333.9
infantile 343.1
muscle 343.1
not infantile or congenital (cerebral)
344.9
late effect or residual NEC 344.9
due to specified lesion - *see*
Paralysis, late effect of
spinal 349.3
late effect or residual NEC
349.5
due to specified lesion - *see*
Paralysis, late effect of
syphilitic 094.0
sphincter, bladder - *see* Paralysis,
bladder
spinal (cord) 349.5
accessory nerve 357.9
acute 043
late effects 044
ascending acute 354
atrophic (acute) 041
late effects 044
chronic 349.5
congenital - *see* Palsy, cerebral
hereditary 333.9
infantile 043
late effects 044
late effect or residual NEC 349.5
due to specified lesion - *see*
Paralysis, late effect of
nerve NEC 357.9
progressive 348.2
spastic (congenital) (infantile) 343.1
with other types of motor
disturbance (e.g., ataxic,
athetoid, atonic, rigidity, or
tremor) 343.9

Paralysis, etc. — *continued*
spinal cord — *continued*
spastic, etc. — *continued*
with other, etc. — *continued*
not infantile or congenital 349.5
sternomastoid 356
stomach 537.9
nerve 356
stroke (current episode) (*see also*
Disease, cerebrovascular, acute)
436.9
late effect or residual 344.9
subscapularis 357.9
superior nuclear 344.9
supranuclear 350
sympathetic
cervical 358.0
nerve NEC 358.9
nervous system 358.9
syphilitic spastic spinal (Erb's) 094.9
tabetic general 094.1
thigh 357.9
throat 508.9
diphtheritic 032
muscle 508.9
thrombotic (current episode) (*see also*
Thrombosis, brain) 433.9
late effect or residual 344.9
thumb 357.9
Todd's 345.5
toe 357.9
tongue 781.4
transient
arm or leg NEC 787.0
traumatic NEC (*see also* Injury,
nerve) 959.2
trapezius 356
traumatic, transient NEC (*see also*
Injury, nerve) 959.2
trembling (*see also* Parkinsonism) 342
triceps brachii 357.9
trigeminal nerve 356
trochlear (nerve) 373.9
uremic - *see* Uremia
uveoparotitic 135
uvula 528.9
hysterical 300.1
postdiphtheritic 032
vagus nerve 356
vasomotor 358.9
velum palati 528.9
vesical - *see* Paralysis, bladder
vestibular nerve 387.9
vocal cords 508.0
Volkmann's (complicating trauma) 995.7
wasting 348.2
Weber's 344.1

Paralysis, etc. — *continued*
  wrist 357.9
Paramedial orifice urethrovesical 753.8
Paramenia 626.9
Parametritis (*see also* Disease, pelvis,
    inflammatory) 616.0
Parametrium, parametric - *see* condition
Paramnesia (*see also* Amnesia) 780.7
Paramolar 520.1
  causing crowding 524.3
Paramyloidosis 276
Paramyoclonus multiplex 347.9
Paramyotonia 330.9
  congenita 330.9
Parangi (*see also* Yaws) 102.9
Paranoia 297.0
  alcoholic 291.3
Paranoid
  dementia 295.3
    praecox (acute) 295.3
    senile 290.0
  personality 301.0
  psychosis 297.9
    alcoholic 291.3
    climacteric 297.1
    involutional 297.1
    menopausal 297.1
    senile 297.9
  reaction (chronic) 297.9
    acute 298.3
  schizophrenia (acute) 295.3
  state 297.9
    climacteric 297.1
    involution 297.1
    menopausal 297.1
    senile 297.9
  tendencies 301.0
  traits 301.0
  trends 301.0
  type, psychopathic personality 301.0
Paraparesis (*see also* Paralysis) 344.9
Paraphasia 781.5
Paraphimosis (congenital) 605
  chancroidal 099.0
Paraphrenia, paraphrenic (late) 297.9
  climacteric 297.1
  dementia 295.3
  involutional 297.1
  menopausal 297.1
  schizophrenia (acute) 295.3
Paraplegia 344.2
  with
    broken
      back - *code by* region under
        Fracture, vertebra, with
        spinal cord lesion

Paraplegia —*continued*
  with — *continued*
    fracture, vertebra (conditions in 805)
      - *code by* region under
      Fracture, vertebra, with spinal
      cord lesion
  ataxic 281.0
  brain (current episode) (*see also*
      Disease, cerebrovascular NEC)
      438.9
    late effect or residual NEC 344.2
    due to specified lesion - *see*
        Paraplegia, late effect of
    spastic (infantile) - *see* Paraplegia,
      spastic
  cerebral - *see* Paraplegia, brain
  congenital (cerebral) (spastic) (spinal) -
    see Paraplegia, infantile
  cortical - *see* Paraplegia, brain
  functional (hysterical) 300.1
  hysterical 300.1
  infantile (cerebral) (spastic) (spinal)
    343.1
    with other types of motor disturbance
      (e.g., ataxic, athetoid, atonic,
      rigidity, or tremor) 343.9
    athetoid 343.2
      with other types of motor
        disturbance (e.g., ataxic,
        atonic, rigidity, spastic, or
        tremor) 343.9
    specified type NEC 343.9
  late effect or residual of
    acute poliomyelitis (conditions in 040-
      043) 044
    birth injury, intracranial or spinal
      (conditions in 764-768 or 772
      with fourth digit .0 or .1) - *see*
      Paraplegia, infantile
    cerebral laceration or contusion
      (conditions in 851.0, 851.1)
      851.9
    fracture or fracture dislocation of
      vertebral column with spinal
      cord lesion (conditions in
      806.0-806.7) 806.9
    intracranial
      abscess or pyogenic infection
        (conditions in 320-323) 324
      hemorrhage following injury
        (conditions in 853.0, 853.1)
        853.9
      vascular lesion (conditions in 430-
        438) 344.2
    spinal cord lesion (nontraumatic)
      NEC 349.3

Paraplegia—*continued*
  late effect, etc.—*continued*
    spinal cord lesion—*continued*
      traumatic (conditions in 958.0-
          958.7) 958.9
      subarachnoid, subdural or extradural
          hemorrhage, following injury
          (conditions in 852.0, 852.1)
          852.9
      viral encephalitis (conditions in 062-
          065) 066
  old or longstanding NEC 344.2
    due to specified lesion - *see*
        Paraplegia, late effect of
  Pott's 015.0
    late effect or sequela 019.3
  psychogenic 305.1
  residual NEC 344.2
    due to specified lesion - *see*
        Paraplegia, late effect of
  senile NEC 344.2
  spastic (cerebral) (spinal) 343.1
    with other types of motor disturbance
        (e.g., ataxic, athetoid, atonic,
        rigidity, or tremor) 343.9
    congenital 343.1
    due to birth injury 343.1
    Erb's spinal 094.9
    hereditary 333.9
    not infantile or congenital (cerebral)
        344.2
      late effect or residual NEC 344.2
        due to specified lesion - *see*
            Paraplegia, late effect of
      spinal 349.3
        late effect or residual NEC
            349.3
          due to specified lesion - *see*
              Paraplegia, late effect of
    primary 343.1
    secondary 343.1
    spinal (cord) 349.3
      late effect or residual NEC 349.3
        due to specified lesion - *see*
            Paraplegia, late effect of
      traumatic - *see* Injury, spinal, by
          region
    syphilitic (spastic) 094.9
    traumatic NEC - *see* Injury, spinal, by
        region
Paraproteinemia 275.9
Parapsoriasis 696.2
  en plaques 696.2
  guttata 696.2
  retiformis 696.2
  varioliformis (acuta) 696.2

Parascarlatina 057.8
Parasitic - *see also* condition
  disease NEC (*see also* Infestation)
      136
    intestinal NEC 129
    skin NEC 134.9
  stomatitis 112
  sycosis (beard) (scalp) 110.0
  twin 759.1
Parasitism NEC 136
  intestinal NEC 129
  skin NEC 134.9
  specified - *see* Infestation
Parasitophobia 300.2
Paraspadias 752.8
Paraspasm facialis 350
Parathyroid gland - *see* condition
Parathyroprivic tetany 252.1
Paratrachoma 078.0
Paratrophy 279
Paratyphlitis (*see also* Appendicitis) 541
Paratyphoid (fever) - *see* Fever,
      paratyphoid
Paratyphus - *see* Fever, paratyphoid
Para-urethral duct 753.8
Para-urethritis 599.9
  gonococcal (acute) 098.0
    chronic or duration of 2 months or
        over 098.1
Paravaginitis (*see also* Vaginitis) 622.1
Parencephalitis (*see also* Encephalitis)
      323
Parergasia 299
Paresis (*see also* Paralysis) 344.9
  bladder (sphincter) 596.3
    tabetic 094.0
  bowel, colon or intestine (*see also* Ileus)
      560.1
  extrinsic muscle, eye (*see also*
      Strabismus) 373.9
  general 094.1
    arrested 094.1
    brain 094.1
    cerebral 094.1
    insane 094.1
    juvenile 090.4
      remission 090.4
    progressive 094.1
    remission (sustained) 094.1
    tabetic 094.1
  heart (*see also* Failure, heart) 782.4
  insane 094.1
  juvenile 090.4
  peripheral progressive 357.9
  pseudohypertrophic 330.3
  senile NEC 344.9

Paresis—*continued*
  stomach 537.9
  syphilitic (general) 094.1
    congenital 090.4
  vesical NEC 596.3
Paresthesia (*see also* Disturbance,
    sensation) 781.6
  Berger's 781.6
  Bernhardt 355.1
Paretic
  convulsions 094.1
  dementia 094.1
Parinaud's
  conjunctivitis 360
  oculoglandular syndrome 360
  ophthalmoplegia 373.9
  syndrome 781.1
Parkinson's disease or syndrome - *see*
    Parkinsonism
Parkinsonian epilepsy 342
  postencephalitic or late effect of viral
      encephalitis 066
Parkinsonism 342
  arteriosclerotic 342
  late effect of viral encephalitis 066
  postencephalitic 066
  syphilitic 094.9
Parodontitis 523.4
Parodontosis 523.5
Paronychia (with lymphangitis) 681
  chronic 681
    candidal 112
  tuberculous (primary) 017.0
    late effect or sequela 019.9
Parorexia NEC 306.5
  hysterical 300.1
Parosmia 781.4
  psychogenic 305.8
Parotid gland - *see* condition
Parotiditis (*see also* Parotitis) 527.2
Parotitis 527.2
  chronic 527.2
  epidemic 072
  infectious 072
  nonspecific toxic 527.2
  not mumps 527.2
  post operative 527.2
  purulent 527.2
  septic 527.2
  suppurative (acute) 527.2
  surgical 527.2
Parrot's disease 090.0
Parry-Romberg syndrome 356
Parry's disease 242.0
Parson's disease 242.0
Particolored infant 757.2

Parturition - *see* Delivery
Passage false, urethra 599.9
Passive - *see* condition
Pasteurella septica 027.9
Patches
  mucous (syphilitic) 091.2
    congenital 090.0
  smokers' (mouth) 528.6
Patellar - *see* condition
Patent - *see also* Imperfect closure
  atrioventricular ostium 746.5
  canal of Nuck 752.8
  cervix 621.9
    causing abortion - *see* Abortion,
        spontaneous
    complicating pregnancy 634.9
      fetus or newborn 769.0
  ductus arteriosus or botalli 747.0
  eustachian valve 746.8
  foramen
    botalli 746.4
    ovale 746.4
  interauricular septum 746.4
  interventricular septum 746.3
  omphalomesenteric duct 751.0
  os (uteri) - *see* Patent, cervix
  urachus 753.8
  vitelline duct 751.0
Paterson(-Brown)-Kelly syndrome 280
Pathologic, pathological - *see also*
    condition
  asphyxia 796.0
  emotionality 306.9
  liar 301.7
  mendacity 301.7
  personality 301.9
  sexuality (*see also* Deviation, sexual)
      302.9
Pathology (of) - *see* Disease
Patulous - *see also* Patent
  anus 569.2
Pavy's disease (*see also* Lesion, kidney)
      593.2
Paxton's disease 111.2
Pearl-worker's disease 720.1
Pectenosis 569.2
Pectoral - *see* condition
Pectus
  carinatum (congenital) 756.4
    acquired 738.8
    rachitic - *see* Rickets
  excavatum (congenital) 756.4
    acquired 738.8
    rachitic - *see* Rickets
Pedatrophia 268
Pederosis 302.2

Pediculosis (infective) 132
  capitis 132
  corporis 132
  pubis 134.1
  vulvae 134.1
Pedophilia 302.2
Peg shaped teeth 520.2
Pel-Ebstein disease 201
Pel's crisis 094.0
Pelade (see also Alopecia) 704
Pelger-Huet anomaly or syndrome 289.9
Peliosis (rheumatica) 287.0
Pelizaeus-Merzbacher
  disease 333.1
  sclerosis diffuse cerebral 333.1
Pellagra 262
  alcoholic or with alcoholism 262
Pellegrini-Stieda disease or syndrome
  729.8
Pellizzi's syndrome 258.9
Pelvic - see also condition
  kidney 753.3
Pelvioectasis (see also Lesion, kidney)
  593.2
Pelviolithiasis 592
Pelviperitonitis
  female (see also Disease, pelvis,
    inflammatory) 616.0
  male (see also Peritonitis) 567.9
Pelvis - see condition or type
Pemphigoid, bullous 694
Pemphigus 694
  benign 694
    chronic familial 757.2
  Brazilian 694
  congenital
    traumatic 757.2
  conjunctiva 694
  erythematosus 694
  foliaceous 694
  gangrenous (see also Gangrene) 445.9
  malignant 694
  neonatorum 684
  syphilitic (congenital) 090.0
  vegetans 694
  vulgaris 694
  wildfire 694
Pendred's syndrome 243
Pendulous breast 611.1
Penetrating wound - see also Wound,
  open
  with internal injury - see Injury,
    internal, by site, with open
    wound

Penetration, pregnant uterus by
  instrument, complicating delivery
  - see Obstetrical trauma
Penicilliosis of lung 117.3
Penis - see condition
Penitis 607.5
Pentalogy (of Fallot) 746.2
Pentosuria (essential) 271.8
Pepper's syndrome 194.0
Perforated - see Perforation
Perforation (nontraumatic)
  appendix 540.0
  atrial septum, multiple 746.4
  bile duct (see also Disease, gallbladder)
    576.9
  bladder (urinary) - see also Injury,
    internal, bladder
    complicating delivery - see
      Obstetrical trauma
  bowel 569.4
  cecum 540.0
  cervix (uteri) - see also Injury, internal,
    uterus
    complicating delivery - see
      Laceration cervix,
      complicating delivery
  colon 569.4
  common duct (bile) (see also Disease,
    gallbladder) 576.9
  cornea 378.4
    due to ulceration 363.0
  diverticulum (see also Diverticula)
    562.1
  duodenum, duodenal (ulcer) - see Ulcer,
    duodenum, with perforation
  ear drum - see Perforation, tympanum
  esophagus 530.4
  foreign body (external site) - see
    Wound, open, complicated
    internal site, by ingested object - see
      Foreign body
  gallbladder or duct (see also Disease,
    gallbladder) 576.9
  gastric (ulcer) - see Ulcer, stomach,
    with perforation
  heart valve - see Endocarditis
  ileum 569.4
  instrumental, surgical (any site) 998.2
  intestine 569.4
    ulcerative NEC 569.4
  jejunum, jejunal 569.4
    ulcer - see Ulcer, gastrojejunal, with
      perforation
  mastoid (antrum) (cell) 387.9
  membrana tympani - see Perforation,
    tympanum

Perforation (nontraumatic) — *continued*
nasal
  septum 508.9
    congenital 748.1
    syphilitic 095
  sinus (*see also* Sinusitis) 503.9
    congenital 748.1
palate (hard) 526.9
  soft 528.9
    syphilitic 095
  syphilitic 095
palatine vault 526.9
  syphilitic 095
  congenital 090.5
pelvic
  floor
    complicating delivery - *see*
      Laceration, perineum,
      complicating delivery
  organ, complicating delivery - *see*
    Obstetrical trauma
perineum
  complicating delivery - *see*
    Laceration, perineum,
    complicating delivery
pharynx 508.9
rectum 569.2
sigmoid 569.4
sinus - *see* Sinusitis
stomach (due to ulcer) - *see* Ulcer,
    stomach, with perforatiom
surgical (accidental) (any site) (by
    instrument) 998.2
traumatic
  external - *see* Wound, open
  internal organ - *see* Injury, internal,
    by site
tympanum (membrane) (nontraumatic)
    387.2
  traumatic - *see* Wound, open, ear
typhoid, gastro-intestinal 001
ulcer - *see* Ulcer, by site, with
    perforation
ureter 593.5
urethra
  complicating delivery - *see*
    Laceration, urethra,
    complicating delivery
uterus - *see also* Injury, internal, uterus
  complicating delivery - *see*
    Obstetrical trauma
uvula 528.9
  syphilitic 095
vagina
  complicating delivery - *see*
    Laceration, perineum,
    complicating delivery

Perforation (nontraumatic) — *continued*
viscus NEC 796.0
vulva
  complicating delivery - *see*
    Laceration, perineum,
    complicating delivery
Peri-adenitis mucosa necrotica recurrens
    528.2
Peri-appendicitis (*see also* Appendicitis)
    541
Peri-arteritis (nodosa) (infectious) 446.0
Peri-arthritis (joint) 717.9
  Duplay's 717.1
  gonococcal 098.3
  humeroscapularis 717.1
  scapulohumeral 717.1
  shoulder 717.1
Peri-arthrosis (angioneural) - *see* Peri-
    arthritis
Peribronchitis 491
  tuberculous (*see also* Tuberculosis,
    pulmonary) 011.9
Pericapsulitis, adhesive (shoulder) 717.1
Pericarditis (calcareous) (constrictive)
    (fibrous) (granular) (hemorrhagic)
    (plastic) (with decompensation)
    (with effusion) 423
  with
    rheumatic fever (conditions in 390)
      active (*see also* Pericarditis,
        rheumatic) 391.0
      inactive or quiescent (*see also*
        Pericarditis, chronic) 393
  acute (rheumatic) 391.0
    with chorea (acute) (rheumatic)
      (Sydenham's) 392.0
    benign 420
    nonrheumatic 420
    nonspecific 420
  adhesive or adherent (rheumatic) (with
    chorea) (*see also* Pericarditis,
    chronic) 393
  acute - *see* Pericarditis, acute
    nonrheumatic 423
  bacterial (acute) (subacute) (with serous
    or seropurulent effusion) 420
  chronic (rheumatic) (with chorea) 393
    nonrheumatic 423
  Coxsackie 074.2
  fibrinocaseous 017.9
    late effect or sequela 019.9
  fibrinopurulent 420
  fibrinous - *see* Pericarditis, rheumatic
  idiopathic 420
  infective 420
  pneumococcal 420

Pericarditis, etc. — *continued*
  purulent 420
  rheumatic (active) (acute) (with effusion)
      (with pneumonia) 391.0
    with chorea (acute) (rheumatic)
        (Sydenham's) 392.0
    chronic or inactive (with chorea)
        393
  septic 420
  serofibrinous - *see* Pericarditis,
    rheumatic
  suppurative 420
  syphilitic 093.9
  tuberculous 017.9
    late effect or sequela 019.9
  uremic - *see* Nephritis, chronic
  viral 420
Pericardium, pericardial - *see* condition
Pericellulitis (*see also* Cellulitis) 682.9
Pericementitis 523.4
Pericholecystitis (*see also* Cholecystitis)
  575
Perichondritis
  auricle 387.9
  bronchus 491
  ear (external) 387.9
  larynx 508.3
    syphilitic 095
    typhoid 001
  nose 508.9
  trachea 508.9
Periclasia 523.5
Pericolitis 569.9
Pericoronitis 523.4
Pericystitis (acute) (*see also* Cystitis)
  595
Pericytoma (*see also* Neoplasm,
    connective tissue, malignant)
    171.9
  benign - *see* Hemangioma
Peridiverticulitis (*see also* Diverticula)
  562.1
Periduodenitis 535
Peri-endocarditis - *see* Endocarditis
Peri-endothelioma - *see* Neoplasm,
  connective tissue, malignant
Peri-epididymitis (*see also* Epididymitis)
  604
Perifolliculitis (abscedens) 704
  capitis, abscedens et suffodiens 704
  scalp 704
  superficial pustular 684
Perigastritis (acute) 535
Perigastrojejunitis 535
Perihepatitis (acute) 573.0
  gonococcal 098.8

Peri-ileitis (subacute) 569.9
Perilabyrinthitis (acute) 384.0
Perimeningitis - *see* Meningitis
Perimetritis (*see also* Disease, pelvis,
  inflammatory) 616.0
Perimetrosalpingitis (*see also* Salpingo-
  oophoritis) 614
Perinephric - *see* condition
Perinephritic - *see* condition
Perinephritis (acute) (*see also* Infection,
  kidney) 590.9
  purulent (*see also* Abscess, kidney)
    590.2
Perineum, perineal - *see* condition
Perineuritis 355.9
Periodic - *see also* condition
  disease (familial) 276
  edema 708.0
  fever 276
  paralysis (familial) 273.4
  peritonitis 276
  polyserositis 276
  somnolence 347.9
Periodontal cyst 522.8
Periodontitis (chronic) (complex) (local)
    (simplex) 523.4
  acute 523.3
  apical 522.6
    acute 522.4
Periodontoclasia 523.5
Periodontosis 523.5
Perionychia (with lymphangitis) 681
Peri-oophoritis (*see also* Salpingo-
  oophoritis) 614
Peri-orchitis (*see also* Orchitis) 604
Periosteum, periosteal - *see* condition
Periostitis (acute) (chronic) (circumscribed)
    (diffuse) (infective) (purulent)
    (streptococcal) (suppurative) 720.3
  with osteomyelitis 720.2
    acute or subacute 720.0
    chronic or old 720.1
  alveolar 526.5
  alveolodental 526.5
  dental 526.5
  gonorrheal 098.8
  jaw (lower) (upper) 526.4
  monomelic 723.9
  orbital 369.9
  syphilitic 095
    congenital 090.0
  tuberculous - *see* Tuberculosis, bone
  yaws (hypertrophic) (early) (late) 102.6
Periostosis 720.3
  with osteomyelitis 720.2
    acute or subacute 720.0

Periostosis—*continued*
  with osteomyelitis—*continued*
    chronic or old   720.1
    hyperplastic   723.1
Periphlebitis (*see also* Phlebitis)   451.9
  retina   377.0
  tuberculous   017.9
    late effect or sequela   019.9
    retina   017.2
      late effect or sequela   019.9
Peripneumonia - *see* Pneumonia
Periproctitis   569.0
Periprostatitis (*see also* Prostatitis)   601
Perirectal - *see* condition
Perirenal - *see* condition
Perisalpingitis (*see also* Salpingo-
    oophoritis)   614
Perisigmoiditis   569.9
Perisplenitis (infectional)   289.5
Perispondylitis - *see* Spondylitis
Peristalsis visible or reversed   785.8
Peritendinitis - *see also* Tenosynovitis
  adhesive (shoulder)   717.1
Perithelioma - *see* Neoplasm, connective
    tissue, malignant
Peritoneum, peritoneal - *see* condition
Peritonitis (acute) (adhesive) (B. coli)
      (congenital) (diaphragmatic) (diffuse)
      (disseminated) (fibrinopurulent)
      (fibrinous) (fibropurulent) (fibrous)
      (focal) (generalized) (hemorrhagic)
      (idiopathic) (localized) (perforative)
      (phlegmonous) (pneumococcal)
      (primary) (purulent) (septic)
      (serofibrinous) (staphylococcal)
      (streptococcal) (subdiaphragmatic)
      (subphrenic) (suppurative) (with
      adhesions) (with effusion)   567.9
  with or following
    abortion - *see* Abortion, by type, with
        sepsis
    abscess   567.0
    appendicitis   540.0
    ectopic gestation - *see* categories
        631.0-631.3
  bile, biliary (*see also* Disease,
      gallbladder)   576.9
  cancerous   197.6
  diphtheritic   032
  fibrocaseous   014
    late effect or sequela   019.9
  gonococcal   098.8
  malignant   197.6
  meconium (newborn) NEC   778.9
  pancreatic   577.9
  paroxysmal, benign   276

Peritonitis, etc. — *continued*
  pelvic
    female (*see also* Disease, pelvis,
        inflammatory)   616.0
    male NEC   567.9
  periodic   276
  puerperal, postpartum, childbirth   670
  syphilitic   095
    congenital   090.0
  tuberculous   014
    late effect or sequela   019.9
Peritonsillar - *see* condition
Peritonsillitis   501
Perityphlitis (*see also* Appendicitis)   541
Peri-ureteritis   593.5
Peri-urethral - *see* condition
Peri-urethritis (gangrenous)   599.9
Peri-uterine - *see* condition
Perivaginitis (*see also* Vaginitis)   622.1
Perivasitis (chronic)   607.5
Perivesiculitis (seminal) (*see also*
        Vesiculitis)   607.4
Perleche   686.9
  due to
    moniliasis   112
    riboflavin deficiency   263.0
Pernicious - *see* condition
Pernio   443.2
Persecution delusion   306.9
Perseveration (tonic)   781.5
Persistence, persistent (congenital)   758.8
  anal membrane   751.3
  arteria stapedia   745.0
  atrioventricular canal   746.5
  branchial cleft   745.4
  bulbus cordis in left ventricle   746.8
  canal of Cloquet   744.8
  capsule (opaque)   744.8
  cilioretinal artery or vein   744.8
  cloaca   751.4
  communication - *see* Fistula, congenital
  convolutions
    aortic arch   747.2
    fallopian tube   752.5
    oviduct   752.5
    uterine tube   752.5
  double aortic arch   747.2
  ductus
    arteriosus   747.0
    botalli   747.0
  fetal
    circulation   747.9
    form of cervix (uteri)   752.5
  foramen
    botalli   746.4
    ovale   746.4

Persistence, etc. — *continued*
 Gartner's duct   752.8
 hyaloid
  artery (generally incomplete)   744.8
  system   744.8
 lanugo   757.3
 left
  posterior cardinal vein   747.4
  root with right arch of aorta   747.2
  superior vena cava   747.4
 Meckel's diverticulum   751.0
 nail(s), anomalous   757.4
 occiput posterior
  complicating delivery   656.8
   fetus or newborn - *see* categories
    766.0 766.9
 omphalomesenteric duct   751.0
 organ or site not listed - *see* Anomaly,
   specified type NEC
 ostium arteriosum primum or secundum
   746.4
 ostium atrioventriculare commune
   746.5
 ovarian rests in fallopian tube   752.5
 pancreatic tissue in intestinal tract
   751.4
 primary
  teeth   520.6
  vitreous hyperplasia   744.8
 pupillary membrane   744.8
  iris   744.8
 right aortic arch   747.2
 sinus
  urogenitalis   752.8
  venosus with imperfect incorporation
    in right auricle   747.4
 thymus (gland)   254
 thyroglossal duct   758.2
 thyrolingual duct   758.2
 truncus arteriosus or communis   746.0
 tunica vasculosa lentis   744.8
 urachus   753.8
 vitelline duct   751.0
Personality
 affective   301.1
 aggressive   301.3
 amoral   301.7
 anancastic   301.4
 anankastic   301.4
 antisocial   301.7
 asocial   301.7
 asthenic   301.6
 change, disorder, disturbance NEC
   301.9
  with
   sociopathic disturbance   301.7

Personality — *continued*
 change, disorder, etc. — *continued*
  due to or associated with physical
    condition - *see* listing under
    Disorder, mental
  transient, following acute or special
    stress   307
 compulsive   301.4
 cyclothymic   301.1
 dual   301.8
 dyssocial   301.7
 eccentric   301.8
 emotionally unstable   301.5
 explosive   301.3
 histrionic   301.5
 hyperthymic   301.1
 hypothymic   301.1
 hysterical   301.5
 immature   301.8
 inadequate   301.6
 labile   301.5
 morally defective   301.7
 multiple   301.8
 obsessional   301.4
 obsessive(-compulsive)   301.4
 paranoid   301.0
 passive-aggressive   301.8
 passive(-dependent)   301.6
 pathologic NEC   301.9
 pattern
  defect NEC   301.9
  disturbance NEC   301.9
 pseudosocial   301.7
 psychoneurotic NEC   300.9
 psychopathic   301.9
  with
   amoral trend   301.7
   antisocial trend   301.7
   asocial trend   301.7
   mixed types   301.7
 schizoid   301.2
 sociopathic   301.7
  antisocial   301.7
  dyssocial   301.7
 unstable (emotional)   301.5
Perthes' disease   722.1
Pertussis (*see also* Whooping cough)
   033.9
Perversion, perverted
 appetite   306.5
  hysterical   300.1
 function
  anterior lobe, pituitary (gland)   253.9
  pineal gland   258.9
  placental hormones - *see* Placenta,
    abnormal

Perversion, perverted—*continued*
  function—*continued*
    posterior lobe, pituitary (gland)
      253.9
    sense of smell or taste 781.4
      psychogenic 305.8
    sexual (*see also* Deviation, sexual)
      302.9
Pervious, congenital - *see also* Imperfect
  closure
  ductus arteriosus 747.0
Pes (congenital) (*see also* Talipes) 754.9
  acquired (any type except planus)
    738.6
  adductus 754.9
  cavus 754.0
  planus (acquired) (any degree) 736
    congenital 755.7
    rachitic 265.1
  valgus 754.8
Pest (*see also* Plague) 020.9
Pestis (*see also* Plague) 020.9
  bubonica 020.0
  fulminans 020.0
  pneumonica 020.1
Petechia, petechiae 287.0
Petges-Clejat or Petges-Clegat syndrome
  716.0
Petit mal (idiopathic) 345.0
Petit's disease (*see also* Hernia,
  diaphragm) 551.3
Petrositis - *see* Mastoiditis
Peutz-Jeghers disease or syndrome
  211.9
Peyronie's disease 607.9
Pfeiffer's disease 075
Phacentocele 378.8
  traumatic 921
Phacocele (old) 378.8
  traumatic 921
Phagedena (dry) (moist) (*see also*
    Gangrene) 445.9
  geometric 686.0
  penis 607.9
  tropical (*see also* Ulcer, skin) 707.9
  vulva (*see also* Vulvitis) 622.1
Phagedenic - *see* condition
Phakoma 378.8
Phantom limb (syndrome) 781.6
Pharyngitis (acute) (catarrhal) (gangrenous)
    (infective) (malignant)
    (membranous) (phlegmonous)
    (pneumococcal)
    (pseudomembranous) (simple)
    (staphylococcal) (subacute)
    (suppurative) (ulcerative) (viral)
    462

Pharyngitis, etc.—*continued*
  with influenza, flu, or grippe 472
  aphthous 074.0
  chronic 502.0
  Coxsackie virus 074.0
  diphtheritic 032
  follicular 502.0
  granular (chronic) 502.0
  herpetic 054
  influenzal 472
  septic 034.0
  streptococcal 034.0
  tuberculous 012.9
    with pneumoconiosis (conditions in
      515) 010
    late effect or sequela 019.0
  vesicular 074.0
Pharyngoconjunctivitis, viral 078.2
Pharyngolaryngitis (acute) 465
  chronic 508.9
  septic 034.0
Pharyngoplegia 508.9
Pharyngotracheitis (acute) 465
  chronic 508.9
Pharynx, pharyngeal - *see* condition
Phenomenon
  Arthus' 999.4
  jaw-winking 743.8
  L. E. cell 734.1
  lupus erythematosus cell 734.1
  Raynaud's (secondary) 443.0
  vasomotor 782.5
  vasospastic 443.9
  vasovagal 782.5
  Wenckebach's (*see also* Block, heart)
    427.3
Phenylketonuria 270.0
Pheochromoblastoma 194.8
  adrenal (gland) 194.0
Pheochromocytoma (adrenal gland)
    255.2
  adrenalin producing 255.2
  ectopic 255.2
  malignant 194.0
    specified site, except of adrenal gland
      194.8
  noradrenalin producing 255.2
  specified site, except of adrenal gland
    - *see* Paraganglioma
Phimosis (congenital) 605
  chancroidal 099.0
  due to infection 605
Phlebectasia (*see also* Varicose vein)
    454.9
  congenital 747.6
Phlebitis (infective) (pyemic) (septic)
    (suppurative) 451.9

Phlebitis, etc. — *continued*
  with
    abortion - *see* Abortion, by type, with
        sepsis
    ectopic gestation - *see* categories
        631.0-631.3
  breast
    superficial 451.9
  cavernous (venous) sinus - *see* Phlebitis,
      intracranial (venous) sinus
  cerebral (venous) sinus - *see* Phlebitis,
      intracranial (venous) sinus
  chest wall, superficial 451.9
  complicating pregnancy 634.9
    fetus or newborn 763.9
  cranial (venous) sinus - *see* Phlebitis,
      intracranial (venous) sinus
  femoral 451.0
  gouty 274
  hepatic veins 451.9
  ilio-femoral 451.0
  intracranial (venous) sinus (any) 321
    late effects 324
    nonpyogenic (*see also* Disease,
        cerebrovascular NEC) 438.9
  lateral (venous) sinus - *see* Phlebitis,
      intracranial (venous) sinus
  leg 451.0
  longitudinal sinus - *see* Phlebitis,
      intracranial (venous) sinus
  lower extremity 451.0
  migrans, migrating (superficial) 453
  portal 572
  puerperal, postpartum, childbirth
      671.9
    intracranial venous sinus 674
    lower extremities 671.0
    pelvis 671.9
    specified site NEC 677.9
  retina 377.0
  saphenous 451.0
  sarcomatous - *see* Neoplasm, malignant
  sinus (meninges) - *see* Phlebitis,
      intracranial (venous) sinus
  specified site NEC 451.9
  syphilitic 093.9
  ulcerative 451.9
    leg 451.0
    lower extremity 451.0
  umbilicus 451.9
  uterus (septic) (*see also* Endometritis)
      622.0
  varicose (leg) (lower extremity) (*see also*
      Varicose vein) 454.9
Phleboliths 458.9

Phlebosclerosis 458.9
Phlebothrombosis - *see* Thrombosis
Phlegmasia
  alba dolens 451.0
    complicating pregnancy 634.9
      fetus or newborn 763.9
    nonpuerperal 451.0
    puerperal, postpartum, childbirth
        671.0
  cerulea dolens 451.0
Phlegmon (*see also* Abscess) 682.9
  broad ligament (*see also* Disease,
      pelvis, inflammatory) 616.0
  diffuse (with lymphangitis) NEC 682.9
  erysipelatous (*see also* Erysiplas) 035
  femoral (with lymphangitis) 682.4
  iliac (fossa) 540.0
  pelvic (female) (*see also* Disease, pelvis,
      inflammatory) 616.0
  pelvis, male (cellular tissue) (with
      lymphangitis) 682.1
  perimetric (*see also* Disease, pelvis,
      inflammatory) 616.0
  perinephric (*see also* Abscess, kidney)
      590.2
  peri-urethral (*see also* Infection,
      urinary) 599.0
  peri-uterine (*see also* Disease, pelvis,
      inflammatory) 616.0
  retro-uterine (*see also* Disease, pelvis,
      inflammatory) 616.0
  skin (with lymphangitis) NEC 682.9
  thigh (with lymphangitis) 682.4
  throat 508.9
Phlegmonous - *see* condition
Phlyctenulosis (conjunctiva) 360
  allergic (nontuberculous) 360
  cornea 363.9
  tuberculous 017.2
    late effect or sequela 019.9
Phobia, phobic 300.2
  obsessional 300.3
  reaction 300.2
Phocas' disease 610
Phocomelia 755.4
  lower limb 755.3
  upper limb 755.2
Phoria (*see also* Strabismus) 373.9
Phosphatemia 788.9
Phosphaturia 279
Photodermatitis 692.9
  contactant - *see* Dermatitis, due to
Photophobia 781.2
Photophthalmia 360
Photopsia 377.4
Photoretinitis 377.4

Photosensitiveness   692.9
  contactant - *see* Dermatitis, due to
Photosensitization, skin   692.9
  contactant - *see* Dermatitis, due to
Phrenitis   323
  late effects   324
Phrynoderma   260.8
Phthiriasis (pubis)   134.1
Phthirus infestation   134.1
Phthisis (*see also* Tuberculosis)   011.9
  bulbi (infectional)   378.9
  colliers'   010
  eyeball (due to infection)   378.9
  millstone makers'   010
  miners'   010
  potters'   010
  sandblasters'   010
  stonemasons'   010
Phycomycosis   117.8
Physalopteriasis   127.1
Physiological cup, large, optic papilla
    377.6
Phytobezoar   938
  intestine   936
  stomach   935
Pian (*see also* Yaws)   102.9
Pianoma   102.1
Piarhemia   279
  bilharziasis   120.9
Pica   306.5
  hysterical   300.1
Pick-Niemann disease   272.2
Pick's
  disease (lipoid histiocytosis) 272.2
    brain   290.1
    liver   423
  syndrome
    heart   423
    liver   423
  tubular adenoma   256.0
Pickwickian syndrome   277
Piebaldism, classic   270.8
Piedra   111.2
  beard   111.2
    black   111.8
    white   111.2
  black   111.8
  scalp   111.8
    black   111.8
    white   111.2
  white   111.2
Pierre Robin syndrome   756.0
Pigeon
  breast or chest (acquired)   738.8
    congenital   756.4
    rachitic - *see* Rickets

Pigeon—*continued*
  breeder's lung   114
  toe   738.6
Pigmentation (abnormal)   709.9
  anomalies NEC   709.9
  arsenical   709.9
  conjunctiva   378.3
  cornea   378.4
  lids, congenital   757.2
  limbus corneae   378.4
  metals   709.9
  optic papilla, congenital   744.8
  retina (congenital) (grouped) (nevoid)
    744.6
  scrotum, congenital   757.2
Pigmented
  mole   757.1
  nevus (papillomatous) (verrucous)
    757.1
Piles (bleeding) (external) (internal)
    (prolapsed) (rectum) (strangulated)
    (thrombosed) (ulcerated)   455
Pili annulati or torti (congenital)   757.3
Pill roller hand (intrinsic)   738.2
Pilonidal cyst, fistula, or sinus (infected)
    (rectum)   685
Pimple   709.9
Pinched nerve - *see* Compression, nerve
Pineal body or gland - *see* condition
Pinealoblastoma   194.4
Pinealoma   226.3
  malignant   194.4
Pinguecula   378.3
Pinhole meatus (*see also* Stricture,
    urethra)   598
Pink
  disease   985.0
  eye   360
Pinkus' disease   697.1
Pinpoint
  meatus (*see also* Stricture, urethra)
    598
  os (uteri) (*see also* Stricture, cervix)
    621.5
Pinselhaare (congenital)   757.3
Pinta   103.9
  cardiovascular lesions   103.2
  chancre (primary)   103.0
  erythematous plaques   103.1
  hyperchromic lesions   103.1
  hyperkeratosis   103.1
  lesions   103.9
    cardiovascular   103.2
    hyperchromic   103.1
    intermediate   103.1
    late   103.2
    mixed   103.3

Pinta — *continued*
  lesions — *continued*
    primary 103.0
    skin (achromic) (cicatricial)
        (dyschromic) 103.2
      mixed (achromic and hyperchromic)
        103.3
    papule (primary) 103.0
    skin lesions (achromic) (cicatricial)
        (dyschromic) 103.2
      mixed (achromic and hyperchromic)
        103.3
    vitiligo 103.2
Pintid 103.0
Pinworms (disease) (infection) (infestation)
    127.3
Pistol wound - *see* Gunshot wound
Pita - *see* Dermatophytosis
Pitch cancer - *see* Neoplasm, skin,
    malignant
Pithecoid pelvis - *see* Anthropoid pelvis
Pithiatism 300.1
Pitted
  teeth 520.4
Pitting (in the sense of edema) (*see also*
    Edema) 782.6
  lip 782.6
  nail 703.9
    congenital 757.4
Pituitary gland - *see* condition
Pityriasis 696.5
  alba 696.5
  capitis 690
  circinata (et maculata) 696.3
  Hebra's 695.9
  lichenoides et varioliformis 696.2
  maculata (et circinata) 696.3
  pilaris 757.2
    acquired 701.1
  rosea 696.3
  rubra (Hebra's) 695.9
    pilaris 696.4
  simplex 690
  streptogenes 696.5
  versicolor 111.0
    scrotal 111.0
Placenta, placental
  ablatio (complicating delivery) 651.1
    with abortion - *see* Abortion, by type
    fetus or newborn 770.1
    undelivered 632.1
  abnormal, abnormality (complicating
      pregnancy) (delivered)
      (undelivered) 634.1
    causing complicated delivery 661.8
    fetus or newborn 770.8

Placenta, placental — *continued*
  abruptio (complicating delivery) 651.1
    with abortion - *see* Abortion, by type
    fetus or newborn 770.1
    undelivered 632.1
  accreta (complicating delivery) (with
      hemorrhage) 652
  adherent (complicating delivery) (with
      hemorrhage) 652
  apoplexy - *see* Placenta, separation
  battledore - *see* Placenta, abnormal
  bipartita - *see* Placenta, abnormal
  centralis - *see* Placenta, previa
  circumvallata - *see* Placenta, abnormal
  cyst (amniotic) - *see* Placenta, abnormal
  deficiency - *see* Placenta, insufficiency
  degeneration - *see* Placenta, abnormal
  detachment (complicating delivery)
      (partial) (premature) (with
      hemorrhage) 651.1
    fetus or newborn 770.1
    undelivered 632.1
  dimidiata - *see* Placenta, abnormal
  disease (complicating pregnancy)
      (delivered) (undelivered) 634.1
    causing complicated delivery 661.8
    fetus or newborn 770.8
  duplex - *see* Placenta, abnormal
  dysfunction - *see* Placenta, insufficiency
  fenestrata - *see* Placenta, abnormal
  fibrosis - *see* Placenta, abnormal
  hematoma - *see* Placenta, abnormal
  hemorrhage NEC - *see also* Placenta,
      separation
    fetus or newborn 770.1
  hyperplasia - *see* Placenta, abnormal
  increta (complicating delivery) (with
      hemorrhage) 652
  infarction (complicating pregnancy)
      (delivered) (undelivered) 634.1
    causing complicated delivery 661.8
    fetus or newborn 770.2
  insertion, vicious - *see* Placenta, previa
  insufficiency
    causing complicated delivery 661.8
    fetus or newborn 770.9
  lateral - *see* Placenta, previa
  low implantation or insertion - *see*
      Placenta, previa
  malformation - *see* Placenta, abnormal
  malposition - *see* Placenta, previa
  marginal sinus (complicating delivery)
      (hemorrhage) (rupture) 651.1
    fetus or newborn 770.1
    undelivered 632.2

Placenta, placental—*continued*
  marginalis, marginata - *see* Placenta,
      abnormal
  membranacea - *see* Placenta, abnormal
  multilobed - *see* Placenta, abnormal
  multipartita - *see* Placenta, abnormal
  necrosis - *see* Placenta, abnormal
  percreta (complicating delivery) (with
      hemorrhage) 652
  perverted hormone function - *see*
      Placenta, abnormal
  polyp (puerperal, postpartum) 677.9
    with abortion (*see also* Abortion,
        other) 645.9
  previa (central) (centralis) (complete)
      (complicating delivery) (lateral)
      (marginal) (marginalis) (partial)
      (partialis) 651.0
    with abortion - *see* Abortion, by type
    fetus or newborn 770.0
    undelivered 632.0
  retention (complicating delivery) (with
      hemorrhage) 652
    fragments, complicating puerperium
        (delayed hemorrhage) 677.1
  separation (complicating delivery)
      (normally implanted) (partial)
      (premature) (with hemorrhage)
      651.1
    with abortion - *see* Abortion, by type
    fetus or newborn 770.1
    undelivered 632.1
  septuplex - *see* Placenta, abnormal
  small - *see* Placenta, abnormal
  softening (premature) - *see* Placenta,
      abnormal
  spuria - *see* Placenta, abnormal
  succenturiata - *see* Placenta, abnormal
  syphilitic 095
  transmission of chemical substance
      affecting fetus or newborn
      761.7
  tripartita - *see* Placenta, abnormal
  triplex - *see* Placenta, abnormal
  varicose vessel - *see* Placenta, abnormal
  vicious insertion - *see* Placenta, previa
Placentitis
  causing complicated delivery 661.8
  complicating pregnancy (delivered)
      (undelivered) 634.9
  fetus or newborn 763.9
Plagiocephaly (skull) 756.0
Plague 020.9
  bubonic 020.0
  lymphatic gland 020.0
  pneumonic 020.1

Plague—*continued*
  pulmonary 020.1
  pulmonic 020.1
  septicemic 020.9
  tonsillar (septicemic) 020.9
Plaque
  artery, arterial - *see* Arteriosclerosis
  calcareous - *see* Calcification
  cervix (uteri) (calcified) 621.9
  tongue 529.9
Plasma cell myeloma 203
Plasmacytosis 289.9
Plasmocytoma 203
Plaster ulcer (*see also* Decubitus) 707.0
Plastic surgery (cosmetic) Y11.9
  for prominent
    ear Y11.1
    nose Y11.0
Platybasia 756.0
Platyonychia (congenital) 757.4
  acquired 703.9
Platypelloid pelvis - *see* Flat pelvis
Pleura, pleural - *see* condition
Pleuralgia 783.7
Pleurisy (acute) (adhesive) (chronic)
      (costal) (diaphragmatic) (double)
      (dry) (fetid) (fibrinous) (fibrous)
      (interlobar) (latent) (lung) (old)
      (plastic) (residual) (sicca) (sterile)
      (subacute) (unresolved) (with
      adherent pleura) 511.0
  with
    effusion (without mention of cause)
        012.2
      with pneumoconiosis (conditions in
          515) 010
      late effect or sequela 019.0
      nontuberculous 511.2
        bacterial 511.1
      pneumococcal 511.1
      staphylococcal 511.1
      streptococcal 511.1
      tuberculous 012.1
        with pneumoconiosis (conditions
            in 515) 010
        late effect or sequela 019.0
    influenza, flu, or grippe 472
    tuberculosis - *see* Pleurisy,
        tuberculous
  encysted 511.2
  exudative (*see also* Pleurisy with
      effusion) 012.2
  fibrinopurulent 510
  fibropurulent 510
  hemorrhagic 511.1
  influenzal 472

Pleurisy etc. — *continued*
  pneumococcal 511.0
    with effusion 511.1
  purulent 510
  septic 510
  serofibrinous (*see also* Pleurisy with
    effusion) 012.2
  seropurulent 510
  serous (*see also* Pleurisy with effusion)
    012.2
  staphylococcal 511.0
    with effusion 511.1
  streptococcal 511.0
    with effusion 511.1
  suppurative 510
  traumatic (post) (current) - *see* Injury,
    internal, pleura
  tuberculous (with effusion) 012.1
    with pneumoconiosis (conditions in
      515) 010
    late effect or sequela 019.0
Pleuritis sicca - *see* Pleurisy
Pleurobronchopneumonia - *see*
  Pneumonia, broncho
Pleurodynia 783.7
  epidemic 074.1
Pleurohepatitis 573.0
Pleuropericarditis (*see also* Pericarditis)
  423
Pleuropneumonia (acute) (bilateral)
  (double) (septic) (*see also*
  Pneumonia) 486
  chronic (*see also* Fibrosis, lung) 517
Pleurorrhea (*see also* Hydrothorax)
  511.2
Plica
  polonica 132
  tonsil 500
Plicated tongue 529.5
  congenital 750.0
Plug
  bronchus NEC 519.9
  meconium (newborn) NEC 778.9
  mucus - *see* Mucus, plug
Plumbism 984
Plummer-Vinson syndrome 280
Plummer's disease 242.1
Pluricarential syndrome of infancy 267
Plus (and minus) hand (intrinsic) 738.2
Pneumathemia (*see also* Air embolism)
  995.0
Pneumatic drill disease 443.0
Pneumatocele 519.2
  intracranial 347.9
Pneumatosis
  cystoides intestinalis 569.9

Pneumatosis — *continued*
  peritonei 569.9
Pneumaturia 596.9
Pneumocephalus 347.9
Pneumococcemia 038.2
  with pneumonia - *see* Pneumonia,
    pneumococcal
Pneumococcus, pneumococcal - *see*
  condition
Pneumoconiosis (due to) (inhalation of)
  515.9
  with tuberculosis 010
  aluminum 516.0
  asbestos 515.2
    with tuberculosis 010
  bagasse 516.1
  bauxite 516.0
  beryllium 516.0
  coal miner (simple) 515.1
    with tuberculosis 010
  cotton dust 516.1
  diatomite fibrosis 515.0
    with tuberculosis 010
  dust NEC 516.1
    inorganic 516.0
    lime 515.0
      with tuberculosis 010
    marble 515.0
      with tuberculosis 010
  fumes (from silo) 516.2
  graphite 516.0
  mica 515.9
    with tuberculosis 010
  moldy hay 516.1
  rheumatoid 515.9
    with tuberculosis 010
  silica 515.0
    with tuberculosis 010
    and carbon 515.1
      with tuberculosis 010
  silicate NEC 515.9
    with tuberculosis 010
  talc 515.9
    with tuberculosis 010
Pneumocystosis 136
Pneumoenteritis 025
Pneumohemopericardium (*see also*
  Pericarditis) 423
Pneumohemothorax (*see also*
  Hemothorax) 511.2
Pneumohydropericardium (*see also*
  Pericarditis) 423
Pneumohydrothorax (*see also*
  Hydrothorax) 511.2
Pneumomediastinum 492
Pneumomycosis 117.8

Pneumonia, etc. — *continued*
  interstitial, etc. — *continued*
    Friedlander's bacillus 482.0
    Hemophilus influenzae 482.1
    hypostatic 514
    influenzal 471
    Klebsiella 482.0
    plasma cell 136
    pneumococcal 481
    specified organism NEC 483
    staphylococcal 482.3
    streptococcal 482.2
    viral, virus 480
  Klebsiella 482.0
  lipid 519.2
  lipoid 519.2
  lobar (bacterial NEC) (diplococcal)
    (disseminated) (interstitial)
    (pneumococcal, any type or
    mixed) 481
    with influenza 471
    chronic (*see also* Fibrosis, lung) 517
    Friedlander's bacillus 482.0
    Hemophilus influenzae 482.1
    hypostatic 514
    influenzal 471
    Klebsiella 482.0
    specified organism NEC 483
    staphylococcal 482.3
    streptococcal 482.2
    viral, virus 480
  lobe - *see* Pneumonia, lobar
  lobular (confluent) - *see* Pneumonia,
    broncho
  Loeffler's 519.2
  massive - *see* Pneumonia, lobar
  measles 055
  meconium (*see also* Aspiration, content
    of birth canal) 776.0
  metastatic NEC 482.9
  Mycoplasma 483
  necrotic 513
  orthostatic 514
  parenchymatous (*see also* Fibrosis,
    lung) 517
  passive 514
  patchy - *see* Pneumonia, broncho
  plasma cell 136
  pleurolobar - *see* Pneumonia, lobar
  pleuropneumonia-like organism 483
  pneumococcal (broncho) (lobar) 481
  Pneumocystis (carinii) 136
  postinfectional NEC 482.9
  Proteus 482.9
  psittacosis 073
  specified organism NEC 483

Pneumonia, etc. — *continued*
  spirochetal 104.9
  staphylococcal (broncho) (lobar) 482.3
  static, stasis 514
  streptococcal (broncho) (lobar) 482.2
  traumatic (complication) (early)
    (secondary) 995.9
  tuberculous (any) (*see also*
    Tuberculosis, pulmonary) 011.9
  tularemic 021
  viral, virus (adenovirus) (broncho)
    (interstitial) (lobar) (respiratory
    syncytial) (parainfluenza) (variety
    X) 480
    with influenza, flu, or grippe 471
  white (congenital) 090.0
Pneumonic - *see* condition
Pneumonitis (acute) (primary) (*see also*
  Pneumonia) 486
  cholesterol 519.2
  due to toxoplasmosis 130.9
    acquired 130.0
    congenital (active) 130.1
    late effects 130.2
  eosinophilic 519.2
Pneumonoconiosis - *see* Pneumoconiosis
Pneumopathy NEC 519.2
Pneumopericarditis (*see also* Pericarditis)
  423
Pneumopericardium - *see also* Pericarditis
  traumatic (post) 860.0
    with open wound into thorax 860.1
    late effect 860.9
Pneumopericardium (*see also* Pericarditis)
  423
Pneumophagia (psychogenic) 305.5
Pneumopleurisy, pneumopleuritis (*see*
  also Pneumonia) 486
Pneumopyopericardium 420
Pneumopyothorax (*see also*
  Pyopneumothorax) 510
Pneumorrhagia 783.1
  newborn 778.2
  tuberculous (*see also* Tuberculosis,
    pulmonary) 011.9
Pneumosiderosis 516.0
Pneumothorax 512
  congenital (*see also* Syndrome,
    respiratory distress) 776.2
  due to operative injury of chest wall or
    lung 998.9
  fetus or newborn (*see also* Syndrome,
    respiratory distress) 776.2
  spontaneous 512
    fetus or newborn (*see also* Syndrome,
    respiratory distress) 776.2

Pneumothorax — *continued*
  sucking 512
  tense valvular, infectional 512
  tension 512
  traumatic 860.0
    with open wound into thorax 860.1
    late effect 860.9
  tuberculous (*see also* Tuberculosis,
      pulmonary) 011.9
Podagra 274
Podencephalus 759.2
Poikiloderma 709.9
  Civatte's 709.9
  congenital 757.2
  vasculare atrophicans 709.9
Poikilodermatomyositis 716.0

Pointed ear 745.2

Poise imperfect 733.9

Poison ivy, oak, sumac or other vine
    dermatitis 692.6

Poisoning (acute) - *see also* Table of
    adverse effects
  Bacillus, B.
    aertrycke 003.9
      due to food 003.0
    botulinus 005.1
    choleraesuis 003.9
      due to food 003.0
    paratyphosus 003.9
      due to food 003.0
    suipestifer 003.9
      due to food 003.0
  bacterial toxins NEC 005.9
  blood (general) - *see* Septicemia
  botulism 005.1
  bread, moldy, mouldy - *see* Poisoning,
    food
  chronic, specified substance - *see* listing
      under Dependence, if not listed,
      see Table of adverse effects
  damaged meat - *see* Poisoning, food
  decomposed food - *see* Poisoning, food
  diseased food - *see* Poisoning, food
  epidemic, fish, meat, or other food - *see*
    Poisoning, food
  fava bean 282.2
  fish (bacterial) - *see also* Poisoning,
    food
    noxious 988.9
  food (acute) (bacterial) (diseased)
    (infected) NEC 005.9
    due to
      Bacillus
        aertrycke 003.0
        botulinus 005.1
        cereus 005.8

Poisoning, etc. — *continued*
  food, etc. — *continued*
    due to — *continued*
      Bacillus — *continued*
        choleraesuis 003.0
        paratyphosus 003.0
        suipestifer 003.0
      Clostridium (perfringens) (welchii)
        005.2
        botulinum 005.1
      Salmonella (aertrycke)
        (choleraesuis) (enteritidis)
        (typhimurium) 003.0
      specified bacteria NEC 005.8
      Staphylococcus 005.0
      Streptococcus 005.8
      Vibrio parahaemolyticus 005.8
    noxious or naturally toxic 988.9
  ice cream - *see* Poisoning, food
  malarial - *see* Malaria
  meat - *see* Poisoning, food
  mushroom (noxious) 988.1
  mussel - *see also* Poisoning, food
    noxious 988.0
  noxious foodstuffs NEC 988.9
  pork - *see also* Poisoning, food
    trichinosis 124
  ptomaine - *see* Poisoning, food
  putrefaction, food - *see* Poisoning, food
  Salmonella (aertryke) (choleraesuis)
    (enteritidis) (typhimurium) 003.9
    due to food 003.0
  sausage - *see also* Poisoning, food
    trichinosis 124
  shellfish - *see also* Poisoning, food
    noxious 988.0
  Staphylococcus, food 005.0
  toxic, from disease NEC 796.0
  truffles - *see* Poisoning, food
  uremic - *see* Uremia
  uric acid 274

Poker spine 712.4

Policemen's disease 355.1

Polio-encephalitis (acute) (bulbar) 040
  chronic 044
  inferior 348.1
  influenzal 474
  late effects 044
  noncontagious 323
  superior hemorrhagic (acute)
    (Wernicke's) 263.9
  Wernicke's 263.9

Polio-encephalomyelitis (acute) (anterior)
    (bulbar) 040
  late effects 044

Polio-encephalopathy, superior
  hemorrhagic, due to lack of vitamin
  B complex 263.9
  with
    beriberi 261
    pellagra 262
Poliomeningo-encephalitis (see also
  Meningitis) 320.9
Poliomyelitis (acute) (anterior) (epidemic)
  043
  with
    paralysis 041
      bulbar 040
    abortive 042
    ascending 043
      progressive 043
    bulbar 040
    chronic 348.2
    deformities 044
    infancy 043
    late effects 044
    lateral, acute 323
      late effect 324
    nonepidemic 043
    nonparalytic 042
    old with deformity 044
    posterior, acute 054
    residual 044
    sequelae 044
    spinal, acute 043
    syphilitic (chronic) 094.9
Poliosis (eyebrow) (eyelashes) (see also
  Canities) 704
  circumscripta (congenital) 757.3
    acquired 704
Pollakiuria 786.3
  psychogenic 305.6
Pollinosis 507
Pollitzer's disease 705.9
Polyadenitis (see also Adenitis) 289.3
  malignant 020.0
Polyangiitis (essential) 446.0
Polyarteritis (nodosa) (renal) 446.0
Polyarthralgia 787.3
  psychogenic 305.1
Polyarthritis - see also Arthritis
  migratory - see Fever, rheumatic
  rheumatic 714.9
    fever (acute) - see Fever, rheumatic
Polycarential syndrome of infancy 267
Polychondritis (atrophic) (chronic)
  (relapsing) 729.9
Polycoria 744.8
Polycystic (disease) (congenital) 758.8
  degeneration, kidney 753.1
  kidney 753.1

Polycystic — continued
  liver 751.6
  lung 748.4
  ovary, ovaries 256.9
  spleen 758.0
Polycythemia 208
  acquired 289.0
  chronic 208
  due to high altitude 289.0
  emotional 289.0
  hypertonica 289.0
  hypoxemic 289.0
  myelopathic 208
  primary 208
  rubra 208
  secondary 289.0
  splenomegalic 208
  stress 289.0
  vera 208
Polycytosis cryptogenica 289.0
Polydactylism 755.0
Polyglandular
  deficiency 258.1
  dyscrasia 258.1
  dysfunction 258.1
Polyhydramnios (complicating pregnancy)
  (see also Hydramnios) 634.3
Polymastia 757.2
Polymenorrhea 626.4
Polymyalgia 717.9
  arteritica 446.4
  rheumatica 717.9
Polymyositis (acute) (chronic)
  (hemorrhagic) 716.1
  with skin involvement 716.0
  ossificans (generalisata) (progressiva)
    733.2
Polyneuritis, polyneuritic 354
  acute
    idiopathic 354
  alcoholic 303.9
  due to lack of vitamin NEC 263.9
  endemic 261
  erythredema 985.0
  febrile 354
  infective (acute) 354
  nutritional 269.9
Polyneuropathy
  arsenical (see also Table of adverse
    effects) 985.1
  lead 984
  peripheral 357.9
Polyopia 781.1
Polyorchism, polyorchidism 752.8
Polyorrhomenitis (peritoneal) 569.9
  pleural - see Pleurisy

Polyostotic fibrous dysplasia 756.7

Polyotia 745.1

Polyp, polypus (adenomatous) - *see also* Neoplasm, benign
accessory sinus 505
adenoid tissue 505
antrum 505
anus, anal (canal) 211.4
Bartholin's gland 221.2
broad ligament 221.0
cervix (mucous) (uteri) 219.0
complicating delivery 657.9
fetus or newborn - *see* categories 764.0-764.9
non-neoplastic 621.9
choanal 505
clitoris 221.2
colon 211.3
dental 522.0
ear (middle) 387.9
endometrium 219.0
epoophoron 221.0
ethmoidal (sinus) 505
fallopian tube 221.0
frontal (sinus) 505
gum 523.9
labia 221.2
larynx (mucous) 508.1
lymphoid (benign) 202.9
malignant - *see* Neoplasm, malignant
maxillary
sinus 505
middle ear 387.9
myometrium 219.0
nares (posterior) 505
nasal cavity, septum or sinus 505
nose (mucous) 505
ovary 220.9
oviduct 221.0
paratubal 221.0
paroophoron 221.0
pharynx 210.9
congenital 750.8
placental (puerperal, postpartum) 677.9
with abortion (*see also* Abortion, other) 645.9
pudenda 221.2
pulpal 522.0
rectum 211.4
sinus (accessory) (ethmoidal) (frontal) (maxillary) (nasal) (sphenoidal) 505
sphenoidal (sinus) 505
stomach (epithelial) 211.1
turbinate, mucous membrane 505

Polyp, polypus, etc. — *continued*
ureter 223.2
uterine ligament 221.0
uterus (body) (cervix) (corpus) (mucous) 219.0
complicating delivery 657.9
fetus or newborn - *see* categories 764.0-764.9
vagina 221.1
vocal cord (mucous) 508.1
vulva 221.2

Polyphagia 278.9

Polypoid - *see* condition

Polyposis - *see also* Polyp
coli 211.3
familial (coli) 211.9
intestinal adenomatous 211.3

Polyradiculitis 354

Polysarcia 277

Polyserositis (peritoneal) 569.9
periodic 276
pleural - *see* Pleurisy
tuberculous 018.9
with
lung (*see also* Tuberculosis, pulmonary) 011.9

Polytrichia (*see also* Hypertrichosis) 704

Polyunguia 757.4
acquired 703.9

Polyuria (nocturnal) 786.4

Pompe's disease (glycogen storage) 271.1

Pompholyx 705.9

Poncet's disease 015.9
late effect or sequela 019.6

Pond fracture - *see* Fracture, skull, vault

Ponos 085.0

Pons, pontine - *see* condition

Poor vision NEC 370.9

Poradenitis, nostras 099.1

Porencephaly (congenital) (developmental) 743.2
acquired 347.9
nondevelopmental 347.9
traumatic (post) 850.9

Porocephaliasis 134.2

Porokeratosis 757.2

Poroma, eccrine (*see also* Adenoma, sweat glands) 216.2

Porphyria (acute) (congenital) (erythropoietic) (familial) (hepatic) (intermittent) (latent) (Swedish) (South African) 273.1
acquired 279
cutanea tarda
hereditaria 273.1
symptomatica 279

Porphyria, etc. — *continued*
  due to drugs - *see* Table of adverse
    effects
  secondary 279
  toxic NEC 279
  variegata 273.1
Porphyrinuria (congenital) 273.1
  acquired 279
Porphyruria (congenital) 273.1
  acquired 279
Port wine nevus, mark, or stain (*see also*
    Hemangioma) 227.0
Portal - *see* condition
Position
  fetus, abnormal - *see* Malposition, fetus
  teeth, faulty 524.3
Positive
  serology 097.1
  VDRL 097.1
Postcardiotomy syndrome 997.1
Postcaval
  ureter 753.4
Postcholecystectomy syndrome 998.9
Postclimacteric bleeding 626.7
Postcommissurotomy syndrome 997.1
Postcricoid region - *see* condition
Postencephalitic - *see* condition
Posterior - *see* condition
Posterolateral sclerosis (spinal cord)
  281.0
Postexanthematous - *see* condition
Postfebrile - *see* condition
Postgastrectomy dumping syndrome
  997.9
Posthemiplegic chorea 344.1
Postherpetic neuralgia (zoster) 053.9
Posthitis 607.5
Postimmunization complication or
    reaction - *see* Complications,
    vaccination
Postinfectious - *see* condition
Postmastectomy lymphedema (syndrome)
  997.3
Postmaturity, postmature (fetus or
    newborn) 778.1
  causing complicated delivery 661.8
  pregnancy (undelivered) (with failure of
    induction) 634.9
Postmenopausal endometrium (atrophic)
  625.0
  suppurative (*see also* Endometritis)
    622.0
Postnatal - *see* condition
Postoperative NEC 796.9
Postpartum - *see also* condition
  observation Y07

Postpoliomyelitic - *see* condition
Post-term infant (*see also* Postmaturity)
  778.1
Postures, hysterical 300.1
Postvaccinal reaction or complication -
  see Complications, vaccination
Postvalvulotomy syndrome 997.1
Potatorium, chronic 303.1
Pott's
  curvature (spinal) 015.0
    late effect or sequela 019.3
  disease 015.0
    late effect or sequela 019.3
  fracture - *see* Fracture, ankle
  spinal curvature 015.0
    late effect or sequela 019.3
  tumor, puffy (*see also* Osteomyelitis)
    720.2
Potter's
  asthma 515.0
    tuberculous 010
  lung 515.0
    tuberculous 010
  syndrome (with renal agenesis) 753.0
Pouch
  bronchus 748.3
  Douglas' - *see* condition
  esophagus, esophageal 750.8
    acquired 530.2
  gastric 537.9
  pharynx 750.8
Poulet's disease 712.3
Poultrymen's itch 133.9
Preacher's voice 783.5
Pre-auricular appendage 745.1
Prebetalipidproteinemia
  familial 272.0
Precancerous dermatosis 702
Precipitate labor
  complicating delivery 661.1
  fetus or newborn - *see* categories
    767.0-767.9
Preclimacteric bleeding 626.2
Precocious
  menstruation 626.9
  puberty 258.9
Precocity sexual (female) (male) NEC
  258.9
  with
    adrenal hyperplasia or tumor 255.0
    ovarian hyperfunction or tumor
      256.0
Precordial pain 782.0
  psychogenic 305.3
Prediabetes, prediabetic 789.5

Pre-eclampsia, pre-eclamptic (albuminuria)
(nephritic) (toxemia) (uremic)
with abortion - *see* Abortion, by type,
with toxemia
arising during pregnancy 637.0
fetus or newborn 762.1
puerperal, postpartum 637.0
Pregnancy (single) (uterine)
abdominal 631.4
with sepsis (conditions in categories
635, 670, 671 or 673.9) 631.0
fetus or newborn 769.3
abnormal NEC 634.9
ampullar - *see* Pregnancy, tubal
broad ligament - *see* Pregnancy, ectopic
cervical - *see* Pregnancy, ectopic
complicated by
abnormal, abnormality 634.9
cord (umbilical) 634.9
pelvis (bony) 634.9
placenta, placental (vessel) 634.1
position
cervix 634.9
fetus or fetuses (undelivered)
634.9
placenta 632.0
uterus 634.9
uterus (congenital) 634.9
abscess or cellulitis
bladder 635.1
genital organ or tract (conditions in
categories 612-614, 616.0,
620, 622 and 629.4) 630
kidney 635.0
urinary tract NEC 635.9
air embolism (any site) 634.8
albuminuria (acute) (subacute) 636
eclamptic 637.1
pre-eclamptic 637.0
amnionitis 634.9
anemia (arising during pregnancy, not
secondary to hemorrhage)
633.9
iron deficiency (conditions in
category 280) 633.1
macrocytic (conditions in category
281) 633.0
atrophy, yellow (acute) (liver)
(subacute) 639.0
auto-intoxication NEC 637.9
bicornis or bicornuate uterus 634.9
cervicitis (conditions in category 620)
630
chloasma (gravidarum) 634.9
chorea (gravidarum) 637.1
convulsions (eclamptic) (uremic)
637.1

Pregnancy, etc. — *continued*
complicated by — *continued*
cystitis (any type) 635.1
death of fetus (in utero) (near term)
634.2
deciduitis 634.9
displacement, any, uterus or cervix
634.9
eclampsia, eclamptic (albuminuria)
(coma) (convulsions) (delirium)
(nephritis) (uremia) 637.1
embolism (any site) 634.9
air 634.8
emesis (gravidarum) 638.9
with neuritis 638.0
endometritis (conditions in category
622.0) 630
decidual 634.9
enuresis 634.9
excessive weight gain NEC 634.9
false labor (pains) (without delivery)
634.7
fatigue 634.9
gangrene
bladder 635.1
genital organ or tract 630
hematoma (vulva) 634.9
hemorrhage (before onset of labor)
(concealed) (undelivered)
632.9
accidental 632.1
due to
afibrinogenemia or other
coagulation defect
(conditions in category
286) 632.4
marginal sinus (rupture) 632.2
placenta previa 632.0
premature separation, placenta
632.1
threatened abortion 632.3
unavoidable 632.0
hepatitis acute, subacute, or
malignant 639.0
herniation of uterus 634.9
hydatidiform mole (delivered)
(undelivered) 634.0
hydramnios 634.3
hydrops amnii 634.3
hydrorrhea 634.9
hyperemesis (gravidarum) 638.9
with neuritis 638.0
hypertension (arising during) (with
pre-eclampsia) 637.0
hysteralgia 634.9
icterus gravis 639.0

Pregnancy, etc. — *continued*
  complicated by — *continued*
    infection   634.9
      amniotic fluid   634.9
      bladder   635.1
      genital organ or tract (conditions in
         categories 612-614, 616.0,
         620, 622 and 629.4)   630
      kidney (conditions in category 590)
         635.0
      urinary (tract)   635.9
    inflammation
      bladder   635.1
      genital organ or tract (conditions in
         categories 612-614, 616.0,
         620, 622 and 629.4)   630
      kidney (conditions in categories
         580, 581, and 583)   636
      urinary tract NEC   635.9
    mal lie (fetus or fetuses) (undelivered)
      634.9
    malformation, uterus (congenital)
      634.9
    malposition
      fetus or fetuses (in uterus)
      ·   (undelivered)   634.9
      uterus or cervix (undelivered)
        634.9
    menstruation   634.9
    missed
      abortion   634.2
      delivery (at or near term)   634.2
      labor (at or near term)   634.2
    necrosis
      genital organ or tract   630
      kidney or renal   636
        cortex, cortical   639.9
      liver (conditions in category 670)
        639.0
    nephritis (conditions in categories
      580, 581 and 583)   636
    nephrosis (acute) (tubular) (conditions
      in categories 581 and 593.1)
      636
    neuritis (toxic)   639.9
      with hyperemesis (conditions in
        category 638.9)   638.0
    oligohydramnios   634.9
    pelvic inflammatory disease
      (conditions in category 616.0)
      630
    placenta, placental
      abnormality   634.1
      abruptio or ablatio (undelivered)
        632.1
      detachment (undelivered)   632.1
      disease   634.1

Pregnancy, etc. — *continued*
  complicated by — *continued*
    placenta, etc. — *continued*
      low implantation (undelivered)
        632.0
      malformation   634.1
      malposition (undelivered)   632.0
      previa (undelivered)   632.0
      separation (premature) (undelivered)
        632.1
    placentitis   634.9
    polyhydramnios   634.3
    postmaturity   634.9
    pre-eclampsia, pre-eclamptic
      (albuminuria) (nephritis)
      (toxemia) (uremia)   637.0

    premature rupture of membranes,
      without delivery   634.4
    prolapse, uterus   634.9
    pruritis (neurogenic)   634.9
    ptyalism   634.9
    pyelitis (conditions in category 590)
      635.0
    renal disease or failure   636
    retention, retained
      dead ovum   634.9

    Rh immunization, incompatibility or
      sensitization   634.5
    rupture
      amnion (premature) (undelivered)
        634.4
      membranes (premature)
        (undelivered)   634.4
      uterus (undelivered)   634.9
    salivation (excessive)   634.9
    salpingo-oophoritis (conditions in
      categories 612-614)   630
    septicemia (conditions in category
      038)   634.9
    spasms, uterus (abnormal)   634.7
    spurious labor pains, without delivery
      634.7
    superfecundation   634.9
    superfetation   634.9
    threatened abortion or premature
      delivery (undelivered)   632.3
    thrombophlebitis   634.9
    thrombosis (any site)   634.9
    torsion of uterus   634.9
    toxemia   637.9
      eclamptic (nephritic) (uremic)
        637.1
      nephritic   636
      pre-eclamptic (nephritic) (uremic)
        637.0
      uremic   636

Pregnancy, etc. — *continued*
  complicated by — *continued*
    uremia 636
      eclamptic 637.1
    uremic coma, delirium, dropsy,
        intoxication, toxemia,
        poisoning 636
    vaginitis or vulvitis (conditions in
        category 622.1) 630
    varicose
      placental vessels 634.1
      veins 634.9
    varicosity
      labia or vulva 634.9
    vomiting (incoercible) (pernicious)
        (persistent) (uncontrollable)
        (vicious) 638.9
      with neuritis 638.0
  complications NEC 634.9
  cornual - *see* Pregnancy, ectopic
  death from NEC 634.9
  delivered - *see* Delivery
  ectopic NEC 631.9
    with sepsis (conditions in categories
        635, 670, 671 or 673.9) 631.3
    fetus or newborn 769.3
  examination for, unconfirmed Y00.4
  extra-uterine - *see* Pregnancy, ectopic
  fallopian - *see* Pregnancy, tubal
  false 300.1
  in double uterus 634.9
  interstitial - *see* Pregnancy, ectopic
  intraligamentous - *see* Pregnancy,
      ectopic
  intramural - *see* Pregnancy, ectopic
  intraperitoneal - *see* Pregnancy,
      abdominal
  isthmian - *see* Pregnancy, tubal
  molar (abortion) (*see also* Abortion,
      other) 645.9
    undelivered 634.9
  multiple
    undelivered 634.9
  mural - *see* Pregnancy, ectopic
  normal (prenatal care) Y06
  ovarian 631.6
    with sepsis (conditions in categories
        635, 670, 671 or 673.9) 631.2
    fetus or newborn 769.3
  spurious 300.1
  tubal (with abortion) (with rupture)
      631.5
    with sepsis (conditions in categories
        635, 670, 671 or 673.9) 631.1
    fetus or newborn 769.3
  unconfirmed (by examination) Y00.4

Pregnant uterus - *see* condition
Preiser's disease 723.0
Premature - *see also* condition
  beats, auricular or ventricular (*see also*
      Action, heart, irregular) 427.9
  birth NEC 777
  closure
    foramen ovale 746.8
  confinement, delivery, or labor - *see
      also* Delivery
    less than 28 weeks gestation
      dead fetus - *see* Abortion, by type
      liveborn infant - *see* Delivery
  contraction
    auricular (*see also* Action, heart,
        irregular) 427.9
    auriculoventricular (*see also* Action,
        heart, irregular) 427.9
    heart (extrasystole) (*see also* Action,
        heart, irregular) 427.9
    junctional (*see also* Action, heart,
        irregular) 427.9
    ventricular (*see also* Action, heart,
        irregular) 427.9
  infant NEC 777
    for classification of births in hospital
        - *see* Newborn
  lungs (*see also* Syndrome, respiratory
      distress) 776.2
  menopause 627
  puberty 258.9
    due to adenoma adrenal 255.0
  rupture membranes or amnion
    complicating delivery 661.0
    fetus or newborn 769.1
    without delivery 634.4
  senility 258.9
  separation, placenta (partial) - *see*
      Placenta, separation
  ventricular systole (*see also* Action,
      heart, irregular) 427.9
Prematurity NEC 777
  for classification of births in hospital -
      see Newborn
  physiological 777
Premenstrual
  endometrium 626.9
  tension 626.9
Premolarisation, cuspids 520.2
Prenatal care (normal pregnancy) Y06
Prenatal death, cause unknown 779.9
Prepartum - *see* condition
Preponderance left or right ventricular -
    see Disease, heart
Prepuce - *see* condition
Presbycardia 794

Presbycusis 389.9
Presbyophrenia 309.6
Presbyopia 370.2
Presenile - see also condition
  aging 258.9
  dementia 290.1
Presenility 258.9
Presentation, abnormal
  complicating delivery 656.9
    arm or hand 656.4
    breech (footling) (frank) 656.0
    brow 656.2
    chin 656.3
    compound 656.4
    extended head 656.3
    face 656.3
      to pubes 656.8
    oblique 656.4
    shoulder 656.4
    transverse 656.1
  fetus or newborn - see categories 766.0-766.9
  noted during pregnancy (undelivered) 634.9
  umbilical cord - see Prolapse, umbilical cord
Prespondylolisthesis (congenital) 756.1
Pressure
  area, skin ulcer (see also Decubitus) 707.0
  atrophy, spine 723.9
  birth
    fetus or newborn (see also Birth injury NEC) 772.9
  brachial plexus 357.0
  brain 347.9
    injury at birth (see also Birth injury, brain) 772.0
  cerebral - see Pressure, brain
  cone, tentorial 347.9
    injury at birth (see also Birth injury, brain) 772.0
  excessive, delivery
    fetus or newborn (see also Birth injury NEC) 772.9
  funis - see Compression, umbilical cord
  hyposystolic 458.0
  increased
    intracranial 347.9
      injury at birth (see also Birth injury, brain) 772.0
    intra-ocular, causing rupture of cornea 378.4
  lumbosacral plexus 357.9
  mediastinum 519.9
  necrosis (chronic) (skin) (see also Decubitus) 707.0

Pressure—continued
  nerve - see Compression, nerve
  paralysis (see also Compression, nerve) 357.9
  sore (chronic) (see also Decubitus) 707.0
  spinal cord 349.9
  ulcer (chronic) (see also Decubitus) 707.0
  venous, increased 458.9
Priapism 786.6
Prickling sensation (see also Disturbance, sensation) 781.6
Prickly heat 705.1
Primary - see condition
Primipara, old
  complicating delivery 657.9
    fetus or newborn - see categories 764.0-764.9
Primula dermatitis 692.6
Primus varus (bilateral) - see Talipes, varus
Pringle's disease (see also Trichoepithelioma) 216.1
Prizefighter ear 872.9
Problem
  child 308
  feeding (infant) (newborn) 269.9
  mental hygiene, adult 300.9
  neurological NEC 796.0
  personality (see also Disorder, personality) 301.9
  psychiatric NEC 300.9
    due to or associated with physical condition (see also listing under Disorder, mental) 309.9
Procidentia
  anus (sphincter) 569.1
  female NEC 623.9
  rectum (sphincter) 569.1
  stomach 537.9
  uteri 623.4
Proctalgia 569.2
  fugax 564.9
  spasmodic 564.9
    psychogenic 305.5
Proctitis (catarrhal) (gangrenous) (ulcerative) 569.0
  amebic 006.9
    with liver abscess 006.0
  gonococcal 098.8
  tuberculous 014
    late effect or sequela 019.9
Proctocele
  female 623.1
  male 569.1

Proctoptosis 569.1
Proctosigmoiditis 569.0
  ulcerative (chronic) 563.1
Proctospasm 564.9
  psychogenic 305.5
Profichet's syndrome 729.9
Progeria 258.9
Prognathism (mandibular) (maxillary)
    524.1
Progressive - *see* condition
Prolapse, prolapsed
  anus, anal (canal) (sphincter) 569.1
  arm or hand, complicating delivery
      656.4
    fetus or newborn - *see* categories
        766.0-766.9
  bladder (mucosa) (sphincter) (acquired)
      congenital (female) (male) 753.8
    female 623.0
    male 596.9
  cecostomy 998.7
  cecum 569.9
  cervix, cervical (stump) (hypertrophied)
      623.4
    congenital 752.5
    postpartal, old 623.4
  ciliary body 378.6
  colon (pedunculated) 569.9
  colostomy 998.7
  conjunctiva 378.3
  cord - *see* Prolapse, umbilical cord
  disc (intervertebral) - *see* Displacement,
      intervertebral disc
  eye implant 998.9
  fallopian tube 615.9
  female genital organ NEC 623.9
  fetal extremity, complicating delivery
      656.4
    fetus or newborn - *see* categories
        766.0-766.9
  funis - *see* Prolapse, umbilical cord
  gastric (mucosa) 537.9
  globe 378.9
  ileostomy bud 998.7
  intervertebral disc - *see* Displacement,
      intervertebral disc
  intestine (small) 569.9
  iris 378.6
  kidney (*see also* Lesion, kidney) 593.2
    congenital 753.3
  laryngeal muscles or ventricle 508.3
  leg, complicating delivery 656.4
    fetus or newborn - *see* categories
        766.0-766.9
  liver 573.9
  meatus urinarius 599.9

Prolapse, etc. — *continued*
  organ or site, congenital NEC - *see*
      Malposition, congenital
  ovary 615.0
  pelvic (floor), female 623.9
  perineum female 623.9
  pregnant uterus (undelivered) 634.9
  rectum (mucosa) (sphincter) 569.1
  spleen 289.5
  stomach 537.9
  umbilical cord
    complicating delivery 661.3
    fetus or newborn 771.1
      with compression 771.0
  ureter 593.5
    with obstruction 593.3
  ureterovesical orifice 593.5
  urethra (acquired) (infected) (mucosa)
      599.9
    congenital 753.8
  uterus 623.4
    congenital 752.5
    postpartal (old) 623.4
    pregnant, complicating delivery
        657.9
      fetus or newborn - *see* categories
          764.0-764.9
  uveal 378.6
  vagina (anterior) (posterior) (wall)
      623.9
  vitreous (humor) 378.9
  womb - *see* Prolapse, uterus
Prolapsus, female 623.9
Proliferative - *see* condition
Prolongation of coagulation or
      prothrombin time (*see also* Defect,
      coagulation) 286.9
Prominauris 745.2
Prominence of auricle (congenital) (ear)
    745.2
Prominent
  ischial spine or sacral promontory
    complicating delivery - *see*
        Deformity, pelvis, complicating
        delivery
    noted during pregnancy (undelivered)
        634.9
Pronation
  ankle 738.6
  foot 738.6
    congenital 755.7
Proptosis (ocular) 781.1
  thyroid 242.0
Prostate, prostatic - *see* condition
Prostatism 600

Prostatitis (acute) (chronic) (congestive)
(granulomatous) (subacute)
(suppurative) 601
due to Trichomonas (vaginalis) 131
fibrous 600
gonococcal 098.0
chronic or duration of 2 months or
over 098.1
hypertrophic 600
malignant 185
trichomonal 131
tuberculous 016.2
late effect or sequela 019.2
Prostatocystitis (see also Prostatitis) 601
Prostatorrhea 602
Prostration 790.1
fetus or newborn 778.9
heat - see Heat, exhaustion
nervous 300.5
senile 794
Protanopia (anomalous trichromat)
(complete) (incomplete) 377.3
Protein
deficiency 267
malnutrition 267
sickness (prophylactic) (therapeutic)
999.5
Proteinemia 788.9
Proteinosis
alveolar, lung or pulmonary 519.2
lipid 279
lipoid (of Urbach) 279
Proteinuria (see also Albuminuria) 789.0
Bence Jones NEC 203
Protrusion
acetabulum (into pelvis) 738.8
complicating delivery - see
Deformity, pelvis, complicating
delivery
noted in pregnancy (undelivered)
634.9
intervertebral disc - see Displacement,
intervertebral disc
nucleus pulposus - see Displacement,
intervertebral disc
Prurigo 698.2
Besnier's 691
Hebra's 698.2
mitis 698.2
nodularis 697.9
psychogenic 305.0
Pruritus, pruritic 698.9
ani 698.0
psychogenic 305.0
conditions NEC 698.9
psychogenic 305.0

Pruritus, etc. – continued
diabetic - see category 250
ear 698.9
genital organ(s) 698.1
psychogenic 305.0
gravidarum 634.9
neurogenic (any site) 305.0
psychogenic (any site) 305.0
scrotum 698.1
psychogenic 305.0
senile 698.9
Trichomonas 131
vulva, vulvae 698.1
psychogenic 305.0
Psammocarcinoma - see Neoplasm,
malignant
Psammoma (see also Neoplasm,
meninges, benign) 225.9
brain 225.0
choroid plexus 225.0
malignant (see also Neoplasm,
meninges, malignant) 192.9
brain 191
choroid plexus 191
ovary 220.1
Pseudarthrosis, pseudo-arthrosis (bone)
723.9
joint following fusion (see also Disease,
joint) 729.9
spine 729.0
Pseudo-aneurysm - see Aneurysm
Pseudo-angina (pectoris) - see Angina
Pseudo-angioma 452
Pseudo-arteriosus 747.8
Pseudocholera 025
Pseudochromhidosis 705.9
Pseudocirrhosis, liver, pericardial 423
Pseudocroup 464
Pseudocyesis 300.1
Pseudocyst
lung 519.2
pancreas 577.9
Pseudodiphtheria 464
Pseudo-erosion cervix, congenital 752.5
Pseudo-erythromelalgia 357.9
Pseudoglanders 025
Pseudoglioma 364
Pseudogoiter 246
Pseudohallucination 781.8
Pseudohemi-anesthesia (see also
Disturbance, sensation) 781.6
Pseudohemophilia (Bernuth's) (hereditary)
(type B) 286.3
A 287.9
Pseudohermaphroditism 752.7
female 752.7
with adrenocortical disorder 273.6

Psychosis—*continued*
  affective NEC—*continued*
    senile 296.9
  alcoholic 291.9
    with
      delirium tremens 291.0
      hallucinosis 291.2
    amnestic confabulatory 291.1
    Korsakoff's, Korsakov's, Korsakow's
      291.1
    paranoid type 291.3
    polyneuritic 291.1
  alternating 296.3
  anergastic (*see also* Psychosis, organic)
    294.9
  arteriosclerotic 293.0
  circular 296.3
  climacteric (*see also* Psychosis,
    involutional) 299
  confusional 299
    reactive 298.2
  depressive 296.2
    involutional 296.0
    psychogenic 298.0
    reactive (from emotional stress,
      psychological trauma) 298.0
  due to or associated with physical
    condition - *see* Psychosis,
    organic
  exhaustive 299
  hypomanic 296.1
  hysterical 299
    acute 298.1
  involutional 299
    depressive 296.0
    melancholic 296.0
    paranoid (state) 297.1
    paraphrenia 297.1
  Korsakoff's, Korsakov's, Korsakow's
    (alcoholic) 291.1
    nonalcoholic 299
  mania (phase) 296.1
  manic 296.1
  manic-depressive 296.9
    agitated 296.0
    alternating 296.3
    circular 296.3
    depressive 296.2
    manic 296.1
    mixed NEC 296.8
    perplexed 296.8
    stuporous 296.8
  menopausal (*see also* Psychosis,
    involutional) 299
  mixed schizophrenic and affective
    295.7

Psychosis—*continued*
  organic NEC 294.9
    due to or associated with
      abscess
        brain 292.9
      accident, cerebrovascular 293.1
      addiction
        alcohol (*see also* Psychosis,
          alcoholic) 291.9
        drug 294.3
      alcohol intoxication, acute 291.9
      alcoholism (conditions in 303) - *see*
        category 291
      anomaly
        brain, congenital 293.9
      anoxia (at birth) 293.5
      apoplexy 293.1
      arteriosclerosis (cerebral) 293.0
      bacteremia 294.2
      bronchopneumonia 294.2
      cerebral condition - *see* categories
        292, 293
      childbirth 294.4
      chorea, Huntington's 293.4
      concussion 293.5
      contusion, cerebral 293.5
      Cushing's syndrome 294.0
      deficiency
        nutritional 294.1
        vitamin 294.1
      degeneration
        brain 293.4
          senile 290.0
        central nervous system 293.4
      dependence
        alcohol (*see also* Psychosis,
          alcoholic) 291.9
        drug (conditions in 304) 294.3
      diabetes mellitus 294.0
      disease
        brain, cerebral 293.9
          arteriosclerotic 293.0
          degenerative 293.4
          infective NEC 292.9
          inflammatory - *see* categories
            292.2, 292.3
          neoplastic 293.3
          senile 290.0
          syphilitic - *see* categories
            292.0, 292.1
          vascular - *see* categories 293.0,
            293.1
      central nervous system
        degenerative 293.4
        encephalitis - *see* categories
          292.2, 292.3

Psychosis — *continued*
  organic NEC — *continued*
    due to or associated with — *continued*
      disease — *continued*
        central nervous, etc. — *continued*
          intracranial infection - *see*
              category 292
          syphilitic - *see* categories
              292.0, 292.1
        cerebrovascular   293.1
          arteriosclerotic   293.0
        Cushing's   294.0
        endocrine (conditions in 240-258)
            294.0
        Jakob-Creutzfeldt   290.1
        liver   294.1
          alcoholic (*see also* Psychosis,
              alcoholic)   291.9
        metabolic NEC (conditions in
            270-279)   294.1
        nutritional (conditions in 260-
            269)   294.1
        Pelizaeus-Merzbacher's   293.4
        Schilder's   293.4
        thyroid   294.0
      disorder
        endocrine (conditions in 240-258)
            294.0
          due to therapeutic use of
              endocrine substance
              294.3
        metabolic NEC (conditions in
            270-279)   294.1
        nutritional (conditions in 260-
            269)   294.1
      disturbance
        cerebrovascular NEC (conditions
            in 430-436, 438)   293.1
        electrolyte   294.1
      electrocution trauma to brain
          293.5
      embolism
        cerebral   293.1
      encephalitis (*see also* categories
          292.2, 292.3)   292.3
        acute infectious   292.2
        epidemic (conditions in 062-065)
            292.2
        following infection   292.3
        idiopathic   292.3
        specified type NEC   292.3
        traumatic   293.5
        unknown cause   292.3
        viral   292.2
      encephalomyelitis (*see also*
          categories 292.2, 292.3)
          292.3

Psychosis — *continued*
  organic NEC — *continued*
    due to or associated with — *continued*
      encephalomyelitis, etc. — *continued*
        acute disseminated   292.3
        epidemic   292.2
      encephalopathy, progressive
          subcortical   293.4
      epilepsy (conditions in 345)   293.2
      fever   294.2
        rheumatic, acute   294.2
        typhoid   294.2
        typhus   294.2
      fracture
        face bones   293.5
        skull (base) (vault)   293.5
      general paralysis, paresis (of insane)
          (conditions in 094.1)   292.0
        juvenile   292.1
      hemorrhage
        cerebral   293.1
          following injury   293.5
        extradural   293.1
          following injury   293.5
        subarachnoid   293.1
          following injury   293.5
        subdural   293.1
          following injury   293.5
      hyperthyroidism   294.0
      hypothyroidism   294.0
      hypoxia (at birth)   293.5
      infarction
        cerebral   293.1
      infection
        brain - *see* category 292
        generalized   294.2
        intracranial - *see* category 292
        systemic   294.2
          specified type NEC   294.2
      inflammation
        brain - *see* categories 292.2,
            292.3
      influenza   294.2
      injury
        brain (birth) (from electric
            current) (surgical)   293.5
        intracranial (conditions in 850-
            854)   293.5
      intoxication
        alcoholic (acute) (pathological)
            (*see also* Psychosis,
            alcoholic)   291.9
        drug (conditions in 960-979)
            294.3
        gas   294.3
        lead   294.3

Psychosis — *continued*
  organic NEC — *continued*
    due to or associated with — *continued*
      intoxication — *continued*
        metal (heavy)   294.3
        poison (conditions in 981-989)
            294.3
      ischemia
        cerebral   293.0
          transient   293.1
        cerebrovascular (generalized)
            293.0
      Jakob-Creutzfeldt's disease or
        syndrome   290.1
      laceration, cerebral   293.5
      leukodystrophy (cerebral)
        (progressive)   293.4
      malaria   294.2
      meningitis   292.9
      multiple sclerosis   293.4
      myxedema   294.0
      neoplasm (benign) (malignant)
        brain   293.3
        cerebral (meninges)   293.3
        intracranial   293.3
        pineal (gland)   293.3
        pituitary (gland)   293.3
      neurosyphilis   292.1
        juvenile   292.1
        paretic   292.0
      occlusion
        pre-cerebral artery   293.1
      pellagra   294.1
      pneumonia   294.2
      poisoning (acute) (chronic)   294.3
        blood   294.2
      postoperative period   294.9
      presenility   290.1
      puerperium   294.4
      sclerosis
        brain   293.4
        multiple   293.4
      senility   290.0
      septicemia   294.2
      space-occupying lesion, brain
        293.3
      specified physical condition NEC
        294.8
      stroke   293.1
      surgery, brain   293.5
      syphilis, central nervous system
        (conditions in 090.4, 094.0,
        094.9)   292.1
      tabes dorsalis   292.1
      taboparesis   292.0
        juvenile   292.1

Psychosis — *continued*
  organic NEC — *continued*
    due to or associated with — *continued*
      thrombosis
        cerebral   293.1
      thyrotoxicosis   294.0
      trauma   294.8
        brain (birth) (from electric
          current) (surgical)   293.5
      tuberculosis NEC   294.2
        brain   292.9
      typhoid (fever)   294.2
      typhus (fever)   294.2
      unspecified physical condition
        294.9
  paranoiac   297.0
  paranoid   297.9
    alcoholic   291.3
    climacteric   297.1
    involutional   297.1
    menopausal   297.1
    schizophrenic   295.3
    senile   297.9
  paroxysmal   299
  polyneuritic
    alcoholic   291.1
  postencephalitic NEC   292.3
  postoperative
    specified type - *see* categories 295-
      298
    unspecified type   294.9
  presbyophrenic (type)   290.0
  presenile   290.1
  puerperal
    specified type - *see* categories 295-
      298
    unspecified type   294.4
  reactive (from emotional stress,
    psychological trauma)   298.9
    confusion   298.2
    depressive   298.0
    excitation   298.1
  schizo-affective   295.7
  schizophrenia, schizophrenic (*see also*
    Schizophrenia)   295.9
  schizophreniform   295.8
  senile NEC   290.0
    paranoid type   297.9
    simple deterioration   290.0
    specified type - *see* categories 295-
      298
  situational (reactive)   298.9
  thyroid   294.0
Psychotic (*see also* condition)   299
  episode   299

Psychotic — *continued*
  episode — *continued*
    due to or associated with physical
      condition - *see* Psychosis,
      organic
Pterygium (eye) 372
  colli 745.5
Ptilosis 704
Ptomaine (poisoning) (*see also* Poisoning,
    food) 005.9
Ptosis (adiposa) 378.2
  cecum 569.9
  colon 569.9
  congenital (eyelid) 744.7
    specified site NEC - *see* Anomaly,
      specified type NEC
  eyelid (paralytic) 378.2
    congenital 744.7
  gastric 537.9
  intestine 569.9
  kidney (*see also* Lesion, kidney) 593.2
    congenital 753.3
  liver 573.9
  renal (*see also* Lesion, kidney) 593.2
    congenital 753.3
  splanchnic 569.9
  spleen 289.5
  stomach 537.9
  viscera 569.9
Ptyalism 527.7
  hysterical 300.1
  periodic 527.2
  pregnancy 634.9
  psychogenic 305.5
Pubertas praecox 258.9
Puberty
  abnormal 258.9
  bleeding 626.9
  delayed 258.9
  precocious 258.9
  premature 258.9
    due to
      adrenal
        adenoma 255.0
        cortical hyperfunction 255.0
      pineal tumor 258.9
      pituitary (anterior) hyperfunction
        253.0
Pudenda, pudendum - *see* condition
Puente's disease 528.5
Puerperal - *see also* condition
  abscess
    areola 678
    Bartholin's gland 670
    bladder 635.1
    breast 678

Puerperal — *continued*
  abscess — *continued*
    broad ligament 670
    cervix (uteri) 670
    corpus luteum (acute) (chronic) 670
    fallopian tube (acute) (chronic) 670
    genital organ 670
    kidney 635.0
    mammary 678
    mesosalpinx (acute) (chronic) 670
    nabothian 670
    nephritic 635.0
    nipple 678
    ovary, ovarian (acute) (chronic) 670
    oviduct (acute) (chronic) 670
    parametric 670
    para-uterine 670
    pelvic 670
    perimetric 670
    perinephric 635.0
    perinephritic 635.0
    perirenal 635.0
    peri-uterine 670
    pyemic 670
    renal 635.0
    retro-uterine 670
    round ligament 670
    suprapelvic 670
    tubal (acute) (chronic) (ruptured) 670
    tubo-ovarian (acute) (chronic) 670
    urinary tract NEC 635.9
    uterine 670
      ligament 670
      tube 670
    uterus 670
      neck 670
    vagina (wall) 670
    vaginorectal 670
    vulvovaginal gland 670
  accident NEC 677.9
  adnexitis 670
  afibrinogenemia, or other coagulation
    defect 675
  albuminuria (acute) (subacute) 636
    pre-eclamptic 637.0
  anemia 676
    due to childbearing (not secondary to
      hemorrhage) 676
    following hemorrhage 653
      intrapartum 653
      postpartum 653
  anuria 636
  apoplexy, apoplectic 674
    bulbar 674
    cerebral 674
    congestive 674

Puerperal—*continued*
  apoplexy—*continued*
    fit 674
    hemiplegia 674
    hemorrhagic (stroke) 674
    ingravescent 674
    pulmonary (artery) (vein) 673.9
    seizure 674
    serous 674
    stroke 674
  bacteremia 670
  bartholinitis 670
    suppurating 670
  blood dyscrasia 675
  Bright's disease (acute) (subacute) 636
  cellulitis - *see* Puerperal abscess
  cervicitis 670
  coagulopathy (any) 675
  complications NEC 677.9
  convulsions (albuminuric) (eclamptic)
      (nephritic) (nephrotic) (uremic)
      637.1
  cystitis (gangrenous) (septic)
      (suppurative) 635.1
  cystopyelitis 635.0
  deciduitis (acute) 670
  delirium NEC 677.9
  dementia NEC 294.4
  disease 677.9
    breast 678
    cerebrovascular (acute) 674
    pelvis inflammatory 670
    renal (acute) 636
    tubo-ovarian (acute) (chronic)
        (inflammatory) 670
    Valsuani's 676
  disorders, lactation 678
  eclampsia (nephritic) (uremic) 637.1
  edema, cervix 677.9
  embolism 673.9
    air 673.0
    amniotic fluid 673.1
    brain or cerebral 674
    cardiac 677.9
    pulmonary (artery) (vein) 673.9
    pyemic 670
    septic 670
  endocervicitis 670
  endometritis (purulent) (septic) 670
  endophlebitis - *see* Puerperal phlebitis
  endotrachelitis 670
  erysipelas 670
  failure, renal 636
  fever (meaning sepsis) 670
    meaning pyrexia (of unknown origin)
        672

Puerperal—*continued*
  fissure, nipple 678
  fistula
    breast 678
    mammary gland 678
    nipple 678
  galactophoritis 678
  gangrene
    bladder 635.1
    gas 670
    ovary (acute) (chronic) 670
    uterus 670
  hematoma, subdural 674
  hematosalpinx, infectional 670
  hemiplegia, cerebral 674
  hemorrhage 653
    brain 674
    bulbar 674
    cerebellar 674
    complicating delivery 653
    cortical 674
    delayed (uterine) 677.2
    due to retained placenta (fragments)
        677.1
    extradural 674
    internal capsule 674
    intracranial 674
    intrapontine 674
    meningeal 674
    pontine 674
    subarachnoid 674
    subcortical 674
    subdural 674
    ventricular 674
  hydropyonephrosis 635.0
  hypertrophy
    breast 678
    mammary gland 678
  induration breast (fibrous) 678
  infarction
    fallopian tube 670
    lung 673.9
    ovary 670
    pulmonary (artery) (vein)
        (hemorrhagic) 673.9
  infection 670
    Bartholin's gland 670
    breast 678
    cervix 670
    corpus luteum 670
    endocervix 670
    fallopian tube 670
    generalized 670
    genital tract NEC 670
    kidney (Bacillus coli) 635.0
    mammary gland 678

Puerperal—*continued*
  infection—*continued*
    nipple 678
    ovary 670
    pelvic 670
    perirenal 635.0
    peritoneum 670
    purulent 670
    renal 635.0
    tubo-ovarian 670
    urinary (tract) NEC 635.9
    uterus, uterine 670
    vagina 670
  inflammation
    areola 678
    Bartholin's gland 670
    breast 678
    broad ligament 670
    cervix (uteri) 670
    fallopian tube (acute) (chronic) 670
    genital organ NEC 670
    mammary gland 678
    nipple 678
    ovary (acute) (chronic) 670
    oviduct (acute) (chronic) 670
    pelvis 670
    peri-uterine 670
    tubal (acute) (chronic) 670
    tubo-ovarian (acute) (chronic) 670
    uterine ligament 670
    uterus 670
    vagina (catarrhal) 670
    vein - *see* Puerperal phlebitis
  insanity NEC 294.4
  ischemia, cerebral 674
  lymphangitis 670
    breast 678
  mammillitis 678
  mammitis 678
  mania 296.1
  mastitis (diffuse) (lobular) 678
  melancholia 296.2
  metritis (septic) (suppurative) 670
  metroperitonitis 670
  metrorrhagia (complicating delivery) 653
  metrosalpingitis (acute) (chronic) 670
  metrovaginitis 670
  milk leg 671.0
  monoplegia, cerebral 674
  necrosis
    kidney, cortical (acute) (bilateral) 639.9
    liver (acute) (subacute) (conditions in category 670) 639.0
    ovary 670

Puerperal—*continued*
  necrosis—*continued*
    renal cortex 639.9
  nephritis (acute or subacute) (conditions in 580, 581, 583) 636
    ascending 635.0
    infective 635.0
    septic 635.0
    suppurative 635.0
  nephrosis (acute) (tubular) 636
  neuritis (toxic) 639.9
  occlusion, pre-cerebral artery 674
  oophoritis (acute) (chronic) (infectional) (interstitial) 670
  ovaritis (acute) (chronic) 670
  paralysis
    bladder (sphincter) 677.9
    cerebral 674
    uremic 636
  paralytic stroke 674
  parametritis 670
  paravaginitis 670
  pelviperitonitis 670
  perimetritis 670
  perimetrosalpingitis (acute) (chronic) 670
  perinephritis 635.0
  peri-oophoritis (acute) (chronic) 670
  periphlebitis - *see* Puerperal phlebitis
  perisalpingitis (acute) (chronic) 670
  peritoneal infection 670
  peritonitis (pelvic) 670
  perivaginitis 670
  phlebitis 671.9
    intracranial venous sinus 674
    lower extremity 671.0
    pelvic (veins) 671.9
    specified site NEC 677.9
  phlegmasia alba dolens 671.0
  phlegmon - *see* Puerperal. abscess
  placental polyp 677.9
  pneumonia, embolic 673.9
    pyemic or septic 670
  pre-eclampsia. pre-eclamptic 637.0
    albuminuria 637.0
    toxemia (nephritic) 637.0
  psychoneurosis, unspecified type 309.9
  psychosis, unspecified or type classifiable to 299 294.4
  pus
    tube (rupture) 670
  pyelitis 635.0
  pyelocystitis 635.0
  pyelohydronephrosis 635.0
  pyelonephritis 635.0

Puerperal—*continued*
  pyelonephrosis 635.0
  pyemia 670
  pyocystitis 635.0
  pyohemia 670
  pyohydronephrosis 635.0
  pyometra 670
  pyonephritis 635.0
  pyonephrosis 635.0
  pyo-oophoritis (acute) (chronic) 670
  pyosalpingitis (acute) (chronic) 670
  pyosalpinx (acute) (chronic) 670
  pyrexia (of unknown origin) 672
  renal
    disease or failure (acute) (subacute)
      636
    dropsy 636
  retention
    decidua (fragments) (with delayed
      hemorrhage) 677.1
    placenta (fragments) (with delayed
      hemorrhage) 677.1
    secundines (fragments) (with delayed
      hemorrhage) 677.1
  rupture
    blood vessel in brain 674
    corpus luteum infected 670
    pus tube 670
    pyosalpinx 670
    tubal abscess 670
    uterus 677.9
  salpingitis (acute) (chronic) (follicular)
    (pseudofollicular) 670
  salpingo-oophoritis (acute) (chronic)
    670
  salpingo-ovaritis (acute) (chronic) 670
  salpingoperitonitis (acute) (chronic)
    670
  sapremia 670
  scarlatina 670
  scarlet fever 670
  seizure, cerebral 674
  sepsis 670
  septic kidney 635.0
  septicemia 670
  shock, complicating delivery 661.8
  stroke 674
  subdural hematoma 674
  subinvolution (uterus) 677.9
  sudden death (cause unknown) 677.0
  suppuration - *see* Puerperal, abscess
  syncope, complicating delivery 661.8
  tetanus 670
  thelitis 678
  thrombocytopenia 675

Puerperal—*continued*
  thrombophlebitis - *see* Puerperal,
    phlebitis
  thrombosis (venous) - *see* Thrombosis,
    puerperal
  toxemia 637.9
    eclamptic 637.1
    nephritic 636
    pre-eclamptic 637.0
  uremia 636
    pyelitic 635.0
  vaginitis 670
  varicose vein - *see* Varix, puerperal
  vulvitis 670
  vulvovaginitis 670
  white leg 671.0
Pulled muscle - *see* Sprain
Pulmolithiasis 519.2
Pulmonary *see* condition
Pulpitis (acute) (chronic) (hyperplastic)
    (suppurative) (ulcerative) 522.0
Pulpless tooth 522.9
Pulse
  alternating (*see also* Action, heart,
    irregular) 427.9
  bigeminal (*see also* Action, heart,
    irregular) 427.9
  feeble, rapid due to shock following
    injury 995.5
Pulseless disease 446.6
Pulsus alternans or trigeminy (*see also*
    Action, heart, irregular) 427.9
Punch drunk 850.9
Puncta lacrimalia occlusion 378.3
Punctiform hymen 752.6
Puncture - *see also* Wound, open
  accidental, complicating surgery 998.2
  bladder, nontraumatic 596.9
  fetal membrane (*see also* Birth injury
    NEC) 772.9
  internal organs, abdomen, chest, or
    pelvis - *see* Injury, internal
  kidney, nontraumatic (*see also* Lesion,
    kidney) 593.2

P U O (*see also* Pyrexia) 788.6
Pupillary membrane (persistent) 744.8
Pupillotonia 378.6
Purpura (primary) 287.0
  abdominal 287.0
  allergic 287.0
  anaphylactoid 287.0
  annularis telangiectodes 709.9
  arthritic 287.0
  bacterial 287.0
  capillary fragility, idiopathic 287.9
  cryoglobulinemic 275.4

Purpura (primary)—*continued*
  fibrinolytic (*see also* Fibrinolysis)
      286.4
  fulminans, fulminous 287.0
  gangrenous 287.0
  hemorrhagic, hemorrhagica (*see also*
      Thrombocytopenia) 287.1
    nodular 272.2
    not due to thrombocytopenia 287.0
  Henoch's 287.0
  idiopathic 287.0
  infectious 287.0
  malignant 287.0
  nervosa 287.0
  newborn 778.2
  nonthrombopenic 287.0
  primitive 287.0
  rheumatica 287.0
  Schonlein(-Henoch) 287.0
  scorbutic 264
  senile 287.0
  simplex 287.0
  symptomatica 287.0
  thrombocytopenic (congenital)
      (essential) (idiopathic) (*see also*
      Thrombocytopenia) 287.1
    thrombotic 446.5
  thrombohemolytic (*see also*
      Fibrinolysis) 286.4
  thrombopenic (congenital) (essential)
      (*see also* Thrombocytopenia)
      287.1
  thrombotic 446.5
    thrombocytopenic 446.5
  toxic 287.0
  visceral symptoms 287.0
Purulent - *see* condition
Pus
  absorption, general - *see* Septicemia
  in urine 789.1
  kidney (*see also* Pyelitis) 590.1
  tube (rupture) (*see also* Salpingo-
      oophoritis) 614
Pustular rash 788.2
Pustule 686.9
  malignant 022
  newborn NEC 686.9
  nonmalignant 686.9
Putnam-Dana syndrome 281.0
Putnam's disease 281.0
Putrefaction
  hospital, noma 528.1
  intestinal 569.9
Putrescent pulp (dental) 522.1
Pyarthritis - *see* Pyarthrosis

Pyarthrosis 710.9
  hip 710.2
  lower extremity, except hip 710.3
  specified site NEC 710.9
  spine 710.0
  tuberculous - *see* Tuberculosis, joint
  upper extremity (including shoulder)
      710.1
Pyelectasis (*see also* Lesion, kidney)
      593.2
Pyelitis (acute) (congenital) (cystica) (due
      to Escherichia coli) (gangrenous)
      (suppurative) (uremic) 590.1
  with
    abortion - *see* Abortion, by type, with
        sepsis
    calculus or stones 592
    contracted kidney 590.0
    ectopic gestation - *see* categories
        631.0-631.3
  arising during pregnancy 635.0
    fetus or newborn 763.0
  chronic 590.0
    with calculus 592
  gonococcal 098.0
    chronic or duration of 2 months or
        over 098.1
  puerperal, postpartum 635.0
  tuberculous 016.0
    late effect or sequela 019.2
Pyelocystitis (*see also* Pyelitis) 590.1
Pyelohydronephrosis 591
Pyelonephritis (*see also* Pyelitis) 590.1
  chronic 590.0
  syphilitic 095
Pyelonephrosis (*see also* Pyelitis) 590.1
  chronic 590.0
Pyelophlebitis - *see* Phlebitis
Pyemia, pyemic (purulent) (*see also*
      Septicemia) 038.9
  joint - *see* Pyarthrosis
  liver 572
  portal 572
  postvaccinal 999.3
  tuberculous - *see* Tuberculosis, miliary
Pygopagus 759.1
Pykno-epilepsy, pyknolepsy (idiopathic)
      345.0
Pylephlebitis 572
Pylethrombophlebitis 572
Pyloritis 535
Pylorospasm (reflex) 784.2
  congenital or infantile 750.1
  neurotic 305.5
  psychogenic 305.5
Pylorus, pyloric - *see* condition

Pyo-arthrosis - *see* Pyarthrosis
Pyocele
    mastoid - *see* Mastoiditis
    sinus (nasal) - *see* Sinusitis
    turbinate (bone) 50?.9
    urethra (*see also* Urethritis) 597
Pyococcal dermatitis 686.0
Pyocolpos (*see also* Vaginitis) 622.1
Pyocyaneus dermatitis 686.0
Pyocystitis (*see also* Cystitis) 595
Pyoderma, pyodermia NEC 686.0
    gangrenosum 686.0
    vegetans 686.0
Pyodermatitis 686.0
    vegetans 686.9
Pyogenic - *see* condition
Pyohemia - *see* Septicemia
Pyohydronephrosis (*see also* Pyelitis)
    590.1
Pyometra (*see also* Endometritis) 622.0
Pyometritis (*see also* Endometritis)
    622.0
Pyometrium (*see also* Endometritis)
    622.0
Pyomyositis 732
    ossificans 733.2
    tropical 117.9
Pyonephritis (*see also* Pyelitis) 590.1
Pyonephrosis (congenital) (*see also*
    Pyelitis) 590.1
Pyo-oophoritis (*see also* Salpingo-
    oophoritis) 614
Pyo-ovarium (*see also* Salpingo-
    oophoritis) 614
Pyopericardium 420
Pyophlebitis - *see* Phlebitis
Pyopneumopericardium 420

Pyopneumothorax (infectional) 510
    subphrenic (*see also* Peritonitis) 567.9
    tuberculous 012.1
        with pneumoconiosis (conditions in
            515) 010
        late effect or sequela 019.0
Pyorrhea (alveolar) (alveolaris)
        (inflammatory) 523.4
    amebic 006.9
        with liver abscess 006.0
    degenerative 523.5
Pyosalpingitis (*see also* Salpingo-
        oophoritis) 614
Pyosalpinx (*see also* Salpingo-oophoritis)
        614
Pyosepticemia - *see* Septicemia
Pyosis Corlett's or Manson's 684
Pyothorax 510
    tuberculous 012.1
        with pneumoconiosis (conditions in
            515) 010
        late effect or sequela 019.0
Pyo-ureter 593.5
    tuberculous 016.1
        late effect or sequela 019.2
Pyramidopallidonigral syndrome, residual
        of encephalitis, viral 066
Pyrexia (of unknown origin) 788.6
    atmospheric 992.0
    during labor (complicating delivery)
        661.8
    heat 992.0
    puerperal 672
Pyroglobulinemia 275.9
Pyromania 300.3
Pyrosis 784.3
Pyuria (bacterial) 789.1

Q

Quadricuspid aortic valve   746.6
Quadriplegia   344.3
  with
    fracture
      spine or vertebra (process) - *see*
          Fracture, vertebra, cervical,
          with spinal cord lesion
  brain (current episode) (*see also*
      Disease, cerebrovascular NEC)
      438.9
    fetus or newborn (*see also* Birth
        injury, brain)   772.0
    late effect or residual NEC   344.3
      due to specified lesion - *see*
          Quadriplegia, late effect of
  cerebral - *see* Quadriplegia, brain
  congenital (cerebral) (spinal) - *see* Palsy,
      cerebral
  cortical - *see* Quadriplegia, brain
  embolic (current episode) (*see also*
      Embolism, brain)   434.9
    late effect or residual   344.3
  infantile (cerebral) (spinal) - *see* Palsy,
      cerebral
  late effect or residual of
    acute poliomyelitis (conditions in 040-
        043)   044
    birth injury, intracranial or spinal
        (conditions in 764-768 or 772
        with fourth digit .0 or .1) - *see*
        Palsy, cerebral
    cerebral laceration or contusion
        (conditions in 851.0, 851.1)
        851.9
    fracture or fracture dislocation of
        vertebral column with spinal
        cord lesion (conditions in
        806.0-806.7)   806.9
    intracranial
      abscess or pyogenic infection
          (conditions in 320-323)   324
      hemorrhage following injury
          (conditions in 853.0, 853.1)
          853.9
      vascular lesion (conditions in 430-
          438)   344.4
    spinal cord lesion (nontraumatic)
        NEC   349.4
    traumatic (conditions in 958.0-
        958.7)   958.9

Quadriplegia – *continued*
  late effect, etc. – *continued*
    subarachnoid, subdural or extradural
        hemorrhage, following injury
        (conditions in 852.0, 852.1)
        852.9
    viral encephalitis (conditions in 062-
        065)   066
  old or longstanding NEC   344.3
    due to specified lesion - *see*
        Quadriplegia, late effect of
  residual NEC   344.3
    due to specified lesion - *see*
        Quadriplegia, late effect of
  spastic (cerebral) (congenital) (infantile)
      (spinal)   343.1
    with other types of motor disturbance
        (e.g., ataxic, athetoid, atonic,
        rigidity, or tremor)   343.9
    not congenital or infantile (cerebral)
        344.3
      late effect or residual NEC   344.3
        due to specified lesion - *see*
            Quadriplegia, late effect of
      spinal   349.4
        late effect or residual NEC
            349.4
          due to specified lesion - *see*
              Quadriplegia, late effect
              of
  spinal (cord)   349.4
    late effect or residual NEC   349.4
      due to specified lesion - *see*
          Quadriplegia, late effect of
  thrombotic (current episode) (*see also*
      Thrombosis, brain)   433.9
    late effect or residual   344.3
  traumatic - *see* Injury, spinal, cervical
Quarrelsomeness   301.3
Queensland fever   083.1
  seven day   100.8
Quervain's disease   731.4
Queyrat's erythroplasia   702
Quincke's disease or edema - *see* Edema,
    angioneurotic
Quinquaud's disease   704
Quinsy   501
  gangrenous   501

R

Rabbia   071

Rabia   071

Rabies   071
inoculation
reaction - *see* Complications,
vaccination

Rachischisis   741.9
with hydrocephalus   741.0

Rachitic - *see also* condition
deformities of spine   265.1
pelvis   265.1
complicating delivery - *see*
Deformity, pelvis, complicating
delivery
noted during pregnancy (undelivered)
634.9

Rachitis, rachitism - *see also* Rickets
acuta   265.0
fetalis   756.5
tarda   265.0

Radial nerve - *see* condition

Radiation effects - *see* Effect, adverse,
radiation

Radiculitis (pressure) (vertebrogenic)
728.9
accessory nerve   728.1
anterior crural   728.9
brachial   728.3
cervical NEC   728.4
due to displacement of intervertebral
disc (conditions in 725) - *see*
Displacement, intervertebral disc
lumbar NEC   728.8
lumbosacral   728.8
rheumatic   717.9
syphilitic   094.9
thoracic (with visceral pain)   728.5

Radiculomyelitis   354
toxic, due to
Clostridium tetani   037
Corynebacterium diphtheriae   032

Radiculopathy (*see also* Radiculitis)
728.9

Radioactive substances, adverse effect -
see Effect, adverse, radioactive
substance

Radiodermal burns (acute, chronic, or
occupational) - *see* Burn

Radiodermatitis   692.7

Radiological evidence suggestive of
pleural tuberculosis   012.1
with pneumoconiosis (conditions in
515)   010
late effect or sequela   019.0
pulmonary tuberculosis   011.5
with pneumoconiosis (conditions in
515)   010
late effect or sequela   019.0

Radiologist's cancer - *see* Neoplasm, skin,
malignant

Radionecrosis - *see* Effect, adverse,
radiation

Radium, adverse effect - *see* Effect
adverse, radioactive substance

Rage
child   308
meaning rabies   071

Raillietiniasis   123.9

Railroad neurosis   300.1

Railway spine   300.1

Raiva   071

Rales   783.2

Ramifying renal pelvis   753.3

Ramsay-Hunt syndrome   053.1
meaning dyssynergia cerebellaris
myoclonica   347.9

Ranke's primary infiltration (with
symptoms)   012.0
with pneumoconiosis (conditions in 515)
010
late effect or sequela   019.0

Ranula   527.6
congenital   750.8

Rape (*see also* nature and site of injury)
996.9

Rapid
feeble pulse, due to shock, following
injury   995.5
heart   782.2
psychogenic   305.3

Raquitismo (*see also* Rickets)   265.0

Rarefaction, bone   723.0

Rash   788.2
canker   034.1
diaper   692.9
drug - *see* Dermatitis, due to drug
ECHO 9 viral   079.8
enema   692.9
food (*see also* Allergy, food)   692.5
heat   705.1
napkin   692.9

Rash—*continued*
  nettle (*see also* Urticaria) 708.9
  pustular 788.2
  rose 788.2
    epidemic 056
  scarlet 034.1
  serum (prophylactic) (therapeutic)
      999.5
  wandering
    tongue 529.1
Rasmussen's aneurysm (*see also*
      Tuberculosis, pulmonary) 011.9
  with pneumoconiosis (conditions in 515)
      010
Raymond-Cestan syndrome (*see also*
      Occlusion, precerebral artery)
      432.9
Raymond's syndrome (*see also* Occlusion,
      precerebral artery) 432.9
Raynaud's
  disease or syndrome 443.0
  gangrene 443.0
  phenomenon (secondary) 443.0
Reaction
  acute situational maladjustment 307
  adjustment 307
    adolescence 307
    childhood 308
    infancy 308
    late life 307
  affective (*see also* Psychosis, affective)
      296.9
  aggressive 301.3
  allergic - *see* Allergy
  anaphylactic (generalized) (prophylactic)
      (therapeutic) - *see* Anaphylactic
      shock
  anesthesia - *see* Table of adverse
      effects
  anger, child 308
  antisocial 301.7
  antitoxin (prophylactic) (therapeutic) -
      see Complications, vaccination
  anxiety 300.0
  asthenic 300.5
  behavioral 306.9 .
    due to or associated with physical
        condition - *see* listing under
        Disorder, mental
  chemical substance - *see also* Table of
      adverse effects
  contact - *see* Dermatitis, due to
  compulsive 300.3
  conversion (anesthetic) (autonomic)
      (hyperkinetic) (mixed paralytic)
      (paresthetic) 300.1

Reaction—*continued*
  depressive 300.4
    affective 296.2
    manic (*see also* Psychosis, manic-
        depressive) 296.9
    neurotic 300.4
    psychoneurotic 300.4
    psychotic 298.0
  dissociative 300.1
  drug - *see also* Table of adverse effects
    contact 692.3
    external medicament 692.3
    withdrawal NEC 304.9
      specified drug - *see* listing under
          Dependence
  dysphoric 796.0
  dyssocial 301.7
  erysipeloid 027.1
  fear 300.2
    child 308
  fluid loss
    cerebrospinal 997.0
  foreign body NEC 733.6
  group delinquent 308
  Herxheimer's 999.4
  hypochondriacal 300.7
  hypoglycemic, due to insulin 962.3
  hypomanic 296.1
  hysterical 300.1
  immunization - *see* Complications,
      vaccination
  infusion - *see* Complications, infusion
  inoculation (immune serum) - *see*
      Complications, vaccination
  insulin 962.3
  leukemoid 289.9
  lumbar puncture 997.0
  lymphoid 796.0
  manic-depressive (*see also* Psychosis,
      manic-depressive) 296.9
  neurasthenic 300.5
  neurogenic (*see also* Neurosis) 300.9
  neurotic NEC 300.9
    due to or associated with physical
        condition (*see also* listing
        under Disorder, mental)
        309.9
  neurotic-depressive 300.4
  nitritoid 961.1
  obsessive(-compulsive) 300.3
  overanxious, child or adolescent 308
  paranoid (chronic) 297.9
    acute 298.3
    climacteric 297.1
    involutional 297.1
    menopausal 297.1

Reaction—*continued*
  peptic-ulcer-like, psychogenic   305.5
  personality (*see also* Disorder,
      personality)   301.9
    transient, following acute or special
        stress   307
  phobic   300.2
  postradiation - *see* Effect, adverse,
      radiation
  psychogenic NEC   300.9
  psychoneurotic (*see also* Neurosis)
      300.9
    compulsive   300.3
    due to or associated with physical
        condition (*see also* listing
        under Disorder, mental)
        309.9
    obsessive   300.3
  psychophysiologic (*see also* Disorder,
      psychosomatic)   305.9
  psychotic (*see also* Psychosis)   299
    due to or associated with physical
        condition - *see* Psychosis,
        organic
  pyelogramic   999.9
  radiation - *see* Effect, adverse, radiation
  runaway, child or adolescent   308
  scarlet fever toxin - *see* Complications,
      vaccination
  schizophrenic (*see also* Schizophrenia)
      295.9
  serological for syphilis - *see* Serology
      for syphilis
  serum (prophylactic) (therapeutic)
      999.5
    immediate   999.4
  situational   307
    acute   307
    adult   307
  skin immunity or sensitization tests (*see*
      also Tests)   Y01
  somatization (*see also* Disorder,
      psychosomatic)   305.9
  spinal puncture   997.0
  spite, child   308
  stress, gross   307
  surgical procedure - *see* Complications,
      surgical procedure
  tetanus antitoxin - *see* Complications,
      vaccination
  toxin-antitoxin - *see* Complications,
      vaccination
  transfusion (blood) (allergic) - *see*
      Complications, transfusion
  ultraviolet - *see* Effect, adverse,
      ultraviolet

Reaction—*continued*
  unsocialized agressive, child or
      adolescent   308
  vaccination (any) - *see* Complications,
      vaccination
  withdrawing, child or adolescent   308
  x-ray - *see* Effect, adverse, x-rays
Reactive depression   300.4
  neurotic   300.4
  psychoneurotic   300.4
  psychotic   298.0
Recanalization, thrombus - *see*
      Thrombosis
Receding chin   524.0
Recession
  gingival (generalized) (localized)   523.2
Recklinghausen's disease (nerves) (skin)
      743.4
  bones   252.0
Reclus' disease   610
  cystic   610
Rectalgia   569.2
Rectitis   569.0
Rectocele
  complicating delivery   657.9
    fetus or newborn - *see* categories
        764.0-764.9
  female   623.1
  male   569.1
  noted during pregnancy (undelivered)
      634.9
  vagina, vaginal (outlet)   623.1
Rectosigmoid junction - *see* condition
Rectosigmoiditis   569.0
  ulcerative (chronic)   563.1
Recto-urethral - *see* condition
Rectovaginal - *see* condition
Rectovesical - *see* condition
Rectum, rectal - *see* condition
Recurrent - *see* condition
Reduction function
  kidney (*see also* Lesion, kidney)   593.2
  liver   573.9
Redundant, redundancy
  anus   569.2
  cardia   537.9
  clitoris   629.9
  colon   569.9
  foreskin (congenital)   605
  intestine   569.9
  labia   629.9
  organ or site, congenital NEC - *see*
      Accessory
  panniculus (abdominal)   277
  prepuce (congenital)   605
  pylorus   537.9

Redundant, etc. — *continued*
  rectum   569.2
  scrotum   607.9
  sigmoid   569.9
  skin (of face)   701.9
    eyelids   378.2
  stomach   537.9
  uvula   528.9
  vagina   629.9

Reduplication - *see* Duplication

Reflex - *see also* condition
  hyperactive gag   508.9
  neurogenic
    bladder NEC   596.9
  vasovagal   782.5

Reflux
  esophageal   530.9
  gastro-esophageal   530.9
  mitral - *see* Endocarditis, mitral
  ureteral   593.5
  vesico-ureteral   593.5

Refractive error   370.9

Refsum's syndrome   332.9

Refusal of food NEC   306.5
  hysterical   300.1

Regaud's tumor   147
  not of nasopharynx - *see* Neoplasm,
    malignant

Regional - *see* condition

Regulation feeding (infant)   269.9
  routine   Y00.5

Regurgitation
  aortic (valve) (*see also* Endocarditis,
    aortic)   395.9
    syphilitic   093.9
  food (*see also* Vomiting)   784.1
    with reswallowing - *see* Rumination
  gastric contents (*see also* Vomiting)
    784.1
  heart - *see* Endocarditis
  mitral (valve) - *see* Endocarditis, mitral
  myocardial - *see* Endocarditis
  pulmonary (valve) (heart) (*see also*
    Endocarditis, pulmonary)   424.9
  tricuspid - *see* Endocarditis, tricuspid
  valve, valvular - *see* Endocarditis
  vesico-ureteral   593.5

Reichmann's disease   536.0

Reiter's disease, syndrome, or urethritis
  136

Rejection
  food NEC   306.5
    hysterical   300.1
  transplant, any organ   997.7

Relaxation
  anus (sphincter)   569.2
    due to hysteria   300.1
  arch (foot)   736
    congenital   755.7
  back ligaments   733.9
  bladder (sphincter)   596.9
  cardio-esophageal   530.9
  cervix   623.4
  inguinal rings   569.9
  joint (capsule) (ligament) (paralytic) (*see
    also* Disease, joint)   729.9
    congenital   755.9
    postpoliomyelitic   044
  lumbosacral (joint)   729.1
  pelvic floor   623.9
  perineum   623.9
  posture   733.9
  rectum (sphincter)   569.2
  sacro-iliac (joint)   726
  scrotum   607.9
  urethra (sphincter)   599.9
  uterus (outlet)   623.4
  vagina (outlet)   623.9
  vesical   596.9

Remains
  canal of Cloquet   744.8
  capsule (opaque)   744.8

Remnant
  fingernail   703.9
    congenital   757.4
  meniscus, knee   724.5
  thyroglossal duct   758.2
  tonsil (infected)   500
  urachus   753.8

Ren
  arcuatus   753.3
  mobile, mobilis (*see also* Lesion,
    kidney)   593.2
    congenital   753.3
  unguliformis   753.3

Renal - *see* condition

Rendu-Osler-Weber disease   448

Renon-Delille syndrome   253.9

Replacement-lipomatosis
  kidney   279

Reserve, decreased or low
  cardiac - *see* Disease, heart
  kidney (*see also* Lesion, kidney)   593.2

Residual - *see also* condition
  bladder   596.9
  state, schizophrenic   295.6
  urine   596.9

Resorption
  biliary (*see also* Disease, gallbladder)
    576.9
    purulent or putrid (*see also*
      Cholecystitis) 575
  dental (roots) 521.4
    alveoli 525.9
  septic - *see* Septicemia
  teeth (external) (internal) (roots) 521.4
Respiration
  Cheyne-Stokes 783.2
  decreased due to shock, following
    injury 995.5
  disorder of, psychogenic 305.2
  failure, insufficient, or poor 796.0
    newborn (*see also* Asphyxia,
      newborn) 776.9
  sighing, psychogenic 305.2
Respiratory - *see* condition
Restless leg syndrome 781.6
Rests, ovarian, in fallopian tube 752.5
Restzustand, schizophrenic 295.6
Retained - *see* Retention
Retardation
  developmental 796.0
    fetus or newborn 778.9
  endochondral bone growth 723.6
  intra-uterine growth 778.9
  mental (*see also* Note below) 315
    borderline, I.Q. 68-85 (*see also* Note
      below) 310
    mild, I.Q. 52-67 (*see also* Note
      below) 311
    moderate, I.Q. 36-51 (*see also* Note
      below) 312
    profound, I.Q. under 20 (*see also*
      Note below) 314
    severe, I.Q. 20-35 (*see also* Note
      below) 313

Note—The fourth-digit subdivisions
which may be used with the above mental
retardation categories can be identified
from the following alphabetical listing:
Retardation
  mental (conditions in categories 310–
    315)
    with or associated with
      abnormality
        autosomes........................ .5
        chromosomal, chromosomes
          (sex)........................ .5
      acrocephaly........................ .4
      acromicria........................ .5
      agyria................................ .4
      anencephaly........................ .4

Retardation—*continued*
  mental—*continued*
    with or associated with—*continued*
      aneuploidy........................... .5
      anomaly, congenital
        brain........................... .4
        cranial........................... .4
        skull........................... .4
      Apert's syndrome................... .4
      arachnodactyly....................... .2
      arginosuccinicaciduria............. .2
      ataxia Friedrich's.................. .3
      Bielkowsky's disease............... .2
      Bourneville's disease.............. .3
      chromosomal abnormality........ .5
        sex (XO) (XXX) (XXXY)
          (XXXXY) (XYY)...... .5
      citrullinemia....................... .2
      condition due to (unknown) pre-
        natal influence.............. .4
      craniostenosis...................... .4
      cretinism........................... .2
      cri-du-chat syndrome.............. .5
      cystathioninuria.................... .2
      cystinosis........................... .2
      defect
        anatomical...................... .4
        cerebral, congenital............. .4
      degeneration
        cerebellar...................... .3
        hepatolenticular................. .2
      deletion, chromosomal............. .5
      deprivation
        environmental................... .8
        psycho-social................... .8
      diabetes, maternal................. .2
      disease
        brain, gross (postnatal)......... .3
        cerebral storage................. .2
        due to (unknown) prenatal
          influence................... .4
        glycogen storage................. .2
      disnergia cerebellaris myoclonia .3
      disorder, disturbance
        growth........................... .2
        metabolic, metabolism.......... .2
        nutrition....................... .2
      Down's disease or syndrome... .5
      Edwards syndrome................. .5
      encephalopathy progressive sub-
        cortical....................... .3
      epilepsy familial progressive
        myoclonic...................... .2
      epiloia............................. .3
      familial progressive myoclonic
        epilepsy....................... .2

Retardation — *continued*
mental — *continued*
  cause unknown or unspecified...... .9
  cultural-familial........................ .8
  following
    abscess, brain....................... .0
    contusion, brain.................... .1
    cytomegalic inclusion body
      disease....................... .0
    disorder, psychiatric (major)..... .7
    emotional disturbance............. .8
      major.............................. .7
    encephalitis......................... .0
    encephalopathy
      bilirubin........................... .0
      post-immunization............... .0
      post-serum........................ .0
      post-vaccinal.................... .0
    hematoma, brain.................... .1
    hemorrhage, brain.................. .1
    hypoxia (at birth) (postnatal)... .1
    immunization....................... .0
    infection (maternal)
      (postnatal) (prenatal)...... .0
    injury (birth) (mechanical)
      (postnatal)................... .1
    intoxication (maternal)
      (postnatal) (prenatal)...... .0
      arsenic......... .0
      botulism exotoxin................. .0
      carbon monoxide................. .0
      ergot............................... .0
      lead................................ .0
      quinine............................. .0
      tetanus exotoxin.................. .0
    irradiation, prenatal................. .1
    kernicterus........................... .0
    laceration, brain.................... .1
    poisoning (chronic)................. .0
      lead................................ .0
    rubella (congenital)
      (maternal).................... .0
    syphilis (congenital)
      (maternal).................... .0
    toxemia (maternal)................. .0
    toxoplasmosis (congenital)
      (maternal).................... .0
    trauma (birth) (postnatal)......... .1
  idiopathic............................ .9
  specified cause NEC................. .9
  unknown cause....................... .9
  unspecified cause.................... .9

Retardation — *continued*
physical 796.0
  fetus or newborn 778.9

Retching (*see also* Vomiting) 784.1
Retention, retained
  bladder 786.1
    psychogenic 305.6
  cyst - *see* Cyst
  dead
    fetus (early pregnancy) (2 months or
      more after death) 634.2
      aborted or delivered - *see*
        Abortion, by type
      at or near term (undelivered)
        634.2
        with delivery - *see* Delivery
    ovum 634.9
  decidua (fragments) (complicating
    delivery) (with hemorrhage) 652
    with abortion - *see* Abortion, by type
    complicating puerperium (delayed
      hemorrhage) 677.1
  deciduous tooth 520.6
  dental root 525.9
  fecal (*see also* Constipation) 564.0
  foreign body - *see* Foreign body
  gastric 536.9
  membranes (complicating delivery) (with
    hemorrhage) 652
    complicating puerperium (delayed
      hemorrhage) 677.1
  menses 626.9
  milk (puerperal, postpartum) 678
  nitrogen, extrarenal 788.9
  placenta (complicating delivery) (with
    hemorrhage) 652
    with abortion - *see* Abortion, by type
    fragments, complicating puerperium
      (delayed hemorrhage) 677.1

  products of conception (with abortion)
    (*see also* Abortion, other) 645.9
  complicating
    delivery 652
    puerperium 677.1

  secundines (complicating delivery) (with
    hemorrhage) 652
    with abortion - *see* Abortion, by type
    complicating puerperium (delayed
      hemorrhage) 677.1

  smegma, clitoris 629.9
  urine 786.1
    psychogenic 305.6
  water (in tissues) (*see also* Edema)
    782.6

Reticulation, dust 515.9
  with tuberculosis 010

Reticulocytoma 200.0
Reticulo-endothelioma 200.0

Reticulo-endotheliosis 279
  leukemic 206.9
    acute 206.0
    chronic 206.1
  malignant 202.2
  nonlipid 279
  systemic 279
Reticulohistiocytoma 279
  giant-cell 279
Reticulohistiocytosis 279
  multicentric 279
Reticulosarcoma 200.0
Reticulosis (skin) 279
  fibromyeloid 209
    Robb-Smith's 201
  histiocytic medullary 209
  lipomelanotic 695.9
  lymphoid follicular 202.0
  malignant 202.2
  reticulum cell 200.0
Reticulum cell sarcoma 200.0
Retina, retinal - *see* condition
Retinitis (angiospastic) (atrophic) (central)
    (circinate) (exudative) (proliferans)
    (proliferating) (purulent) (septic)
    (suppurative) (vascular)
    (vasospastic) 367
  albuminurica (*see also* Nephritis,
    chronic) 582
  arteriosclerotic (*see also*
    Arteriosclerosis) 440.9
  diabetic - *see* category 250
  disciformis 377.1
  gravidarum 634.9
  juxtapapillaris 365
  leukemic - *see* Leukemia
  leukocythemic - *see* Leukemia
  luetic - *see* Retinitis, syphilitic
  pigmentosa 744.6
  punctata albescens 744.8
  renal (*see also* Nephritis, chronic) 582
  syphilitic (late) 095
    congenital 090.0
    early 091.8
  syphilitica, central, recurrent 095
  tuberculous 017.2
    late effect or sequela 019.9
Retinoblastoma 190
Retinochoroiditis 366
  juxtapapillaris 365
Retinopathy 377.6
  arteriosclerotic (*see also*
    Arteriosclerosis) 440.9
  central serous 377.0
  circinate 377.1
  diabetic - *see* category 250

Retinopathy — *continued*
  of prematurity 377.0
  pigmentary, congenital 744.6
Retinoschisis 376
  congenital 744.8
Retraction
  cervix (*see also* Retroversion, uterus)
    624.0
  drum (membrane) 387.9
  finger 738.3
  lung 519.2
  mediastinum 519.9
  nipple 611.9
    congenital 757.2
    puerperal, postpartum 678
  palmar fascia 733.5
  pleura (*see also* Pleurisy) 511.0
  ring, uterus, pathological
    complicating delivery 657.9
      fetus or newborn - *see* categories
      767.0-767.9
  sternum (congenital) 756.4
    acquired 738.8
  syndrome 744.8
  uterus (*see also* Retroversion, uterus)
    624.0
  valve (heart) - *see* Endocarditis
Retrobulbar - *see* condition
Retrocecal - *see also* condition
  appendix (congenital) 751.4
Retrocession - *see* Retroversion
Retrodisplacement - *see* Retroversion
Retroflection, retroflexion - *see*
    Retroversion
Retrognathia, retrognathism (mandibular)
    (maxillary) 524.1
Retrograde menstruation 626.9
Retroperineal - *see* condition
Retroperitoneal - *see* condition
Retroperitonitis (*see also* Peritonitis)
    567.9
Retropharyngeal - *see* condition
Retroplacental - *see* condition
Retroposition - *see* Retroversion
Retrosternal thyroid 758.2
Retroversion, retroverted
  cervix (*see also* Retroversion, uterus)
    624.0
  female NEC (*see also* Retroversion,
    uterus) 624.0
  iris 378.6
  testis (congenital) 752.1
  uterus, uterine (acute) (acquired)
    (adherent) (any degree)
    (asymptomatic) (cervix)
    (postinfectional) (postpartal, old)
    624.0

Retroversion, etc. — *continued*
  uterus, etc. — *continued*
    complicating
      delivery   657.9
        fetus or newborn - *see* categories
          764.0-764.9
        pregnancy (undelivered)   634.9
      congenital   752.5
      pregnant or gravid (undelivered)
        634.9
Reverse peristalsis   785.8
Reye's syndrome   347.9
Rh (factor)
  incompatibility, immunization or
    sensitization
    fetus   775.0
    newborn   775.0
      with kernicterus or nervous
        affection   774.0
    noted during pregnancy   634.5
    due to infusion or transfusion
      634.5
    transfusion reaction   999.7
  negative mother affecting
    fetus   775.0
    newborn   775.0
      with kernicterus or nervous
        affection   774.0
    transfusion reaction   999.7
Rhabdomyochondroma (*see also*
    Neoplasm, connective tissue,
    benign)   215
Rhabdomyolysis (idiopathic)   733.9
Rhabdomyoma NEC (*see also* Neoplasm,
    connective tissue, benign)   215
  heart or myocardium   215
    congenital   746.8
  prostate   600
  tongue   210.1
Rhabdomyosarcoma (*see also* Neoplasm,
    connective tissue, malignant)
    171.9
Rhabdosarcoma - *see* Neoplasm,
    connective tissue, malignant
Rhesus (factor) incompatibility - *see* Rh,
    incompatibility
Rheumaticosis - *see* Rheumatism
Rheumatism, rheumatic   718
  acute NEC   718
  articular (chronic) NEC   714.9
    acute or subacute - *see* Fever,
      rheumatic
  blennorrhagic   098.3
  cerebral - *see* Fever, rheumatic
  chronic NEC   718
  febrile - *see* Fever, rheumatic

Rheumatism, etc. — *continued*
  gonococcal   098.3
  heart (*see also* Disease, heart,
    rheumatic)   398
  inflammatory (acute) (chronic)
    (subacute) - *see* Fever, rheumatic
  intercostal   717.9
  joint (chronic) NEC   714.9
    acute - *see* Fever, rheumatic
  muscular   717.9
  neuralgic   717.9
  neuromuscular   717.9
  nodose - *see* Arthritis, nodosa
  nonarticular   717.9
  palindromic (any site)   712.2
  polyarticular NEC   714.9
  psychogenic   305.1
  sciatic   717.9
  septic - *see* Fever, rheumatic
  spine - *see* Arthritis, spine
  subacute NEC   718
  tuberculous NEC   015.9
    late effect or sequela   019.6
Rheumatoid - *see also* condition
  lung   515.9
    with tuberculosis   010
Rhinitis (atrophic) (catarrhal) (chronic)
    (croupous) (fibrinous) (hyperplastic)
    (hypertrophic) (membranous)
    (purulent) (suppurative) (ulcerative)
    502.1
  with
    hay fever   507
    sore throat - *see* Nasopharyngitis
  acute   460
  allergic (any cause)   507
    nonseasonal   507
  infective   460
  pneumococcal   460
  syphilitic   095
  tuberculous   012.9
    with pneumoconiosis (conditions in
      515)   010
    late effect or sequela   019.0
  vasomotor   507
Rhino-antritis (chronic) (*see also* Sinusitis,
    antrum)   503.0
Rhinodacryolith   368
Rhinolith   508.9
  nasal sinus (*see also* Sinusitis)   503.9
Rhinomegaly   508.9
Rhinopharyngitis (acute) (subacute) (*see*
    also Nasopharyngitis)   460
  chronic   502.1
  destructive ulcerating   102.5
  mutilans   102.5

Rhinophyma 695.3
Rhinorrhea 508.9
  cerebrospinal (fluid) 347.9
  paroxysmal 507
  spasmodic 507
Rhinosalpingitis 384.0
Rhinoscleroma 039.1
Rhinosporidiosis 117.0
Rhinovirus infection 460
Rhizomelique
  pseudopolyarthric 446.4
Rhoad and Bomford anemia 284
Rhus
  diversiloba dermatitis 692.6
  radicans dermatitis 692.6
  toxicodendron dermatitis 692.6
  venenata dermatitis 692.6
Rhythm
  atrioventricular nodal (see also Action,
    heart, irregular) 427.9
  escape (see also Action, heart, irregular)
    427.9
  heart, abnormal (see also Action, heart,
    irregular) 427.9
  idioventricular (see also Action, heart,
    irregular) 427.9
  nodal (see also Action, heart, irregular)
    427.9
  sleep, inversion 780.6
Rhytidosis facialis 701.9
Rib - see also condition
  cervical 756.3
Riboflavin deficiency 263.0
Rice bodies (joint) - see Loose bodies in
    joint
Richter's hernia - see Hernia, Richter's
Ricinism 989.9
Rickets (active) (acute) (adolescent) (adult)
    (chest wall) (congenital) (current)
    (infantile) (intestinal) 265.0
  celiac 269.0
  fetal 756.5
  hemorrhagic 264
  hypophosphatemic with nephrotic-
    glycosuric dwarfism 270.2
  kidney 593.0
  late effects, any 265.1
  renal 593.0
  scurvy 264
  vitamin D-resistant 273.4
Rickettsial disease NEC 083.9
Rickettsialpox 083.0
Rickettsiosis NEC 083.9
  tick-borne NEC 082.9
  vesicular 083.0
Ricord's chancre 091.0

Riddoch's syndrome 781.0
Riders' bone 733.3
Ridge, alveolus - see condition
Ridged ear 745.2
Riedel's
  lobe, liver 751.6
  struma 245.1
  thyroiditis 245.1
Rieder cell leukemia 207.9
  acute 207.0
  chronic 207.1
Riehl's melanosis 709.9
Rietti-Greppi-Micheli anemia (see also
    Thalassemia) 282.4
Rieux's hernia - see Hernia, Rieux's
Riga-Fede disease 529.0
Riggs' disease 523.4
Rigid, rigidity - see also condition
  articular, multiple
    congenital 755.8
  cervix (uteri)
    complicating delivery 657.2
      fetus or newborn - see categories
        764.0-764.9
  hymen 629.9
  pelvic floor, perineum, vagina or vulva
    complicating delivery 657.9
      fetus or newborn - see categories
        764.0-764.9
  spine 712.4
Rigors 788.9
Riley-Day syndrome 743.8
Ring(s)
  aorta 747.2
  Bandl's, complicating delivery 657.9
    fetus or newborn - see categories
      767.0-767.9
  contraction, complicating delivery
    657.9
    fetus or newborn - see categories
      767.0-767.9
  Fleischer's 273.3
  Kayser-Fleischer (cornea) 273.3
  retraction, uterus, pathological,
    complicating delivery 657.9
    fetus or newborn - see categories
      767.0-767.9
  Schatzki (esophagus) (lower) (congenital)
    750.3
    acquired 530.3
  trachea
    abnormal 748.3
  vascular (congenital) 747.2
  Vossius' 921
Ringed hair (congenital) 757.3

Ringworm (*see also* Dermatophytosis)
110.9
beard 110.0
Burmese 110.9
corporeal 110.9
foot 110.1
groin 110.9
honeycomb 110.9
scalp 110.0
Tokelau 110.9
Rise, venous pressure 458.9
Risk, suicidal 300.9
Ritter's disease 695.9
Robb-Smith's fibromyeloid reticulosis
201
Robert's pelvis 755.7
complicating delivery - *see* Deformity,
pelvis, complicating delivery
noted during pregnancy (undelivered)
634.9
Robin's syndrome 756.0
Robinson's disease (*see also* Adenoma,
sweat glands) 216.2
Roble's disease. 125.3
Rocky Mountain fever (spotted) 082.0
Rodent
cornea 363.0
dermatitis - *see* Neoplasm, skin,
malignant
ulcer - *see also* Neoplasm, skin,
malignant
cornea 363.0
Roentgen ray, adverse effect - *see* Effect,
adverse, x-ray
Roetheln 056
Roger's disease 746.3
Rokitansky-Aschoff sinuses (*see also*
Disease, gallbladder) 576.9
Rokitansky's
disease (*see also* Necrosis, liver) 570
tumor 615.2
Rollet's chancre 091.0
gonococcal 099.9
syphilitic 091.0
Romberg's disease 356
Roof, mouth - *see* condition
Rosacea 695.3
acne 695.3
keratitis 695.3
Rosary, rachitic (*see also* Rickets) 265.0
Rose's tamponade (*see also* Pericarditis)
423
Rosenbach's erysipelatoid or erysipeloid
027.1
Rosenthal's disease 286.2
Roseola 056
infantum 057.8

Rossbach's disease 536.0
psychogenic 305.5
Rostan's asthma (*see also* Failure,
ventricular, left) 427.1
Rot
Barcoo (*see also* Ulcer, skin) 707.9
knife-grinders' 010
Rotation
anomalous, incomplete or insufficient -
see Malrotation
manual
fetus or newborn (*see also* Birth
injury NEC) 772.9
spine, incomplete or insufficient 729.1
tooth, teeth 524.3
vertebra, incomplete or insufficient
729.1
Roteln 056
Roth's disease 355.1
Rothmund-Thomson syndrome 757.2
Rothmund's syndrome 757.2
Rotor's disease or syndrome 273.5
Rotundum ulcus - *see* Ulcer, stomach
Round
back (with wedging of vertebrae)
735.9
late effect of rickets 265.1
ulcer (stomach) - *see* Ulcer, stomach
worms (large) (infestation) NEC 127.0
Roussy-Levy syndrome 330.9
Rowland's disease 272.0
Rubella 056
maternal
affecting fetus or newborn 761.3
manifest rubella in infant 056
Rubenstein(-Taybia) syndrome 759.8
Rubeola (signifying measles) 055
not signifying measles 056
scarlatinosa 057.8
Rudimentary (congenital) - *see also*
Agenesis
arm 755.2
bone 756.9
cervix uteri 752.5
eye 744.1
lobule of ear 745.2
patella 755.7
tracheal bronchus 748.3
uterus 752.5
in male 752.7
solid or with cavity 752.5
vagina 752.6
Rumination 784.7
neurotic 306.9
obsessional 306.9
psychogenic 306.9

Rupia 091.2
  congenital 090.0
  tertiary 095
Rupture, ruptured 551.9
  abdominal viscera NEC 796.0
    complicating delivery - *see*
      Obstetrical trauma
  abscess (spontaneous) - *code by* site
    under Abscess
  amnion, premature
    complicating delivery 661.0
    fetus or newborn 769.1
    without delivery 634.4
  aneurysm - *see* Aneurysm
  aorta, aortic (*see also* Aneurysm, aorta)
    441.9
    syphilitic 093.0
    traumatic - *see* Injury, internal, aorta
    valve or cusp (*see also* Endocarditis,
      aortic) 395.9
  appendix (with peritonitis) 540.0
  artery 447
    brain (*see also* Hemorrhage, brain)
      431.9
    coronary (*see also* Infarct,
      myocardium) 410.9
    heart (*see also* Infarct, myocardium)
      410.9
    traumatic (complication) 995.3
  bile duct (*see also* Disease, gallbladder)
    576.9
  bladder (sphincter) 596.9
    complicating delivery - *see*
      Obstetrical trauma
    spontaneous 596.9
    traumatic - *see* Injury, internal,
      bladder
  blood vessel (*see also* Hemorrhage)
    458.9
    brain (*see also* Hemorrhage, brain)
      431.9
    heart (*see also* Infarct, myocardium)
      410.9
    traumatic (complication) 995.3
  bone - *see* Fracture
  bowel 569.9
  brain
    aneurysm (congenital) (*see also*
      Hemorrhage, subarachnoid)
      430.9
      syphilitic 094.9
    hemorrhagic (*see also* Hemorrhage,
      brain) 431.9
    injury at birth (*see also* Birth injury,
      brain) 772.0
    syphilitic 094.9

Rupture, etc. — *continued*
  capillaries 448
  cardiac (*see also* Infarct, myocardium)
    410.9
  cartilage (articular) (current) - *see also*
    Sprain
    with open wound - *see* Wound, open
    knee (*see also* Dislocation, knee)
      836.0
      old 724.5
    semilunar (*see also* Dislocation, knee)
      836.0
      old 724.5
  cecum (with peritonitis) 540.0
  cerebral aneurysm (congenital) (*see also*
    Hemorrhage, subarachnoid)
    430.9
  cervix (uteri)
    complicating delivery - *see*
      Laceration, cervix,
      complicating delivery
    traumatic - *see* Injury, internal, cervix
  chordae tendineae (infectional) - *see
    also* Endocarditis, bacterial
  choroid (direct) (indirect) 378.6
    traumatic - *see* Wound, open, eye
  circle of Willis (*see also* Hemorrhage,
    subarachnoid) 430.9
  colon 569.9
  cornea 378.4
    traumatic - *see* Wound, open, eye
  corpus luteum (infected) (ovary) 615.9
  cyst - *see* Cyst
  Descemet's membrane 378.4
    traumatic - *see* Wound, open, eye
  diaphragm - *see also* Hernia, diaphragm
    traumatic - *see* Injury, internal,
      diaphragm
  diverticulum (intestine) (*see also*
    Diverticula) 562.1
  duodenal stump 537.9
  duodenum (ulcer) - *see* Ulcer,
    duodenum, with perforation
  ear drum 387.2
    with otitis media - *see* Otitis media
    traumatic - *see* Wound, open, ear
  esophagus 530.4
  fallopian tube 615.9
    due to pregnancy - *see* Pregnancy,
      tubal
  fontanel (*see also* Birth injury, bone or
    nerve) 772.2
  gallbladder or duct (*see also* Disease,
    gallbladder) 576.9
  gastric - *see also* Rupture, stomach
    vessel 458.9

Rupture, etc. — *continued*
  globe (eye) 378.9
    traumatic - *see* Wound, open, eye
  graafian follicle (hematoma) 615.9
  heart (auricle) (ventricle) (*see also*
      Infarct, myocardium) 410.9
  hymen 629.9
  internal organ, traumatic - *see* Injury,
      internal, by site
  intervertebral disc - *see also*
      Displacement, intervertebral disc
    traumatic (current) - *see* Dislocation,
      vertebrae
  intestine 569.9
    traumatic - *see* Injury, internal,
      intestine
  iris 378.6
    traumatic - *see* Wound, open, eye
  kidney - *see also* Injury, internal,
      kidney
    due to
      birth injury (*see also* Birth injury
        NEC) 772.9
    nontraumatic (*see also* Lesion,
        kidney) 593.2
  lachrymal, lacrimal apparatus 378.3
    traumatic - *see* Wound, open, eye
  lens 378.8
    traumatic - *see* Wound, open, eye
  ligament - *see* Sprain
  liver - *see also* Injury, internal, liver
    due to
      birth injury (*see also* Birth injury
        NEC) 772.9
  lymphatic vessel 457
  marginal sinus (complicating delivery)
      (placental) (with hemorrhage)
      651.1
    fetus or newborn 770.1
    undelivered 632.2
  meaning hernia - *see* Hernia
  membrana tympani 387.2
    with otitis media - *see* Otitis media
    traumatic - *see* Wound, open, ear
  membranes, premature
    complicating delivery 661.0
    fetus or newborn 769.1
    undelivered 634.4
  meningeal artery (*see also* Hemorrhage,
      subarachnoid) 430.9
  meniscus (knee) (current injury) (*see
      also* Dislocation, knee) 836.0
    late effect 836.9
    old 724.5
      elbow 724.3
      shoulder 724.1

Rupture, etc. — *continued*
  meniscus, etc. — *continued*
    site other than knee - code as Sprain
  mesentery 569.9
  mitral (heart) (valve) - *see* Endocarditis,
      mitral
  muscle (traumatic) NEC - *see also*
      Sprain
    with open wound - *see* Wound, open
    nontraumatic 733.9
  mycotic aneurysm causing cerebral
      hemorrhage (*see also*
      Hemorrhage, brain) 431.9
  myocardium, myocardial (*see also*
      Infarct, myocardium) 410.9
    traumatic - *see* Injury, internal, heart
  nontraumatic (meaning hernia) (*see also*
      Hernia) 551.9
  obstructed (*see also* Hernia, by site,
      with obstruction) 553.9
  ovary, ovarian 615.9
    corpus luteum 615.9
    cyst 220.1
    follicle (graafian) 615.9
  oviduct 615.9
    due to pregnancy - *see* Pregnancy,
      tubal
  pancreas 577.9
    traumatic - *see* Injury, internal,
      pancreas
  papillary muscle (*see also* Infarct,
      myocardium) 410.9
  pelvic
    floor, complicating delivery - *see*
      Laceration, perineum,
      complicating delivery
    organ, complicating delivery - *see*
      Obstetrical trauma
  penis (traumatic) - *see* Wound, open,
      penis
  perineum 629.9
    complicating delivery - *see*
      Laceration, perineum,
      complicating delivery
  pregnant uterus (undelivered) (with
      hemorrhage) 634.9
    with delivery 659
      fetus or newborn - *see* categories
        768.0-768.9
  prostate (traumatic) - *see* Injury,
      internal, prostate
  pulmonary valve (heart) (*see also*
      Endocarditis, pulmonary) 424.9
  pus tube (*see also* Salpingo-oophoritis)
      614

Rupture, etc. — *continued*
pyosalpinx (*see also* Salpingo-
oophoritis) 614
rectum 569.2
traumatic - *see* Injury, internal,
rectum
retina, retinal 376
traumatic - *see* Wound, open, eye
sclera 378.6
semilunar cartilage, knee (current
injury) (*see also* Dislocation,
knee) 836.0
old 724.5
sigmoid 569.9
traumatic - *see* Injury, internal,
intestine
sinus Valsalva 747.2
spinal cord - *see also* Injury, spinal, by
region
due to birth injury (*see also* Birth
injury, spinal cord) 772.1
spleen (congenital) 289.5
due to or with birth injury (*see also*
Birth injury NEC) 772.9
in malarial districts (*see also* Malaria)
084.9
spontaneous 289.5
traumatic - *see* Injury, internal,
spleen
splenic vein 458.9
stomach 537.9
traumatic - *see* Injury, internal,
stomach
ulcer - *see* Ulcer, stomach, with
perforation
tendon (any) (traumatic) - *see also*
Sprain
with open wound - *see* Wound, open
nontraumatic 733.9
testicle (traumatic) - *see also* Wound,
open, testicle
due to syphilis 095
thoracic duct 457
tonsil 500
traumatic
external site - *see* Wound, open, by
site
internal organ (abdomen, chest, or
pelvis) - *see* Injury, internal, by
site
ligament, muscle, or tendon - *see*
Sprain
referring to hernia - *see* Hernia

Rupture, etc. — *continued*
tricuspid (heart) (valve) - *see*
Endocarditis, tricuspid
tube, tubal 615.9
abscess (*see also* Salpingo-oophoritis)
614
due to pregnancy - *see* Pregnancy,
tubal
tympanum, tympanic (membrane)
387.2
with otitis media - *see* Otitis media
traumatic - *see* Wound, open, ear
umbilical cord - *see* Complications,
umbilical cord
ureter (traumatic) - *see also* Injury,
internal, ureter
nontraumatic 593.5
urethra 599.9
complicating delivery - *see*
Laceration, urethra,
complicating delivery
traumatic - *see* Injury, internal,
urethra
uterosacral ligament 616.9
uterus (traumatic) - *see also* Injury,
internal, uterus
complicating delivery 659
fetus or newborn - *see* categories
768.0-768.9
nonpuerperal, nontraumatic 625.9
pregnant (undelivered) 634.9
puerperal 677.9
vagina - *see also* Wound, open, genital
organ
complicating delivery - *see*
Laceration, perineum,
complicating delivery
valve, valvular (heart) - *see*
Endocarditis
varicose vein - *see* Varicose vein
varix - *see* Varix
vena cava 458.9
viscus 796.0
vulva - *see also* Wound, open, genital
organ
complicating delivery - *see*
Laceration, perineum,
complicating delivery
Russell-Silver syndrome 759.8
Russell's dysentery 004.8
Rust's disease 015.0
late effect or sequela 019.3

S

Saber, sabre
  shin   090.5
  tibia   090.5
Sac lachrymal, lacrimal - *see* condition
Saccular - *see* condition
Sacculation
  aorta (nonsyphilitic) (*see also*
      Aneurysm, aorta)   441.9
    syphilitic   093.0
  bladder   596.9
  colon   569.9
  intralaryngeal (congenital) (ventricular)
    748.3
  larynx (congenital) (ventricular)   748.3
  organ or site, congenital - *see*
    Distortion
  pregnant uterus, complicating delivery
    657.9
    fetus or newborn - *see* categories
      764.0-764.9
  rectosigmoid   569.2
  sigmoid   569.9
  ureter   593.5
  urethra   599.9
Sachs-Tay disease   333.0
Sachs'
  amaurotic familial idiocy   333.0
  disease   333.0
Sacks-Libman disease   734.1
Sacralgia   728.8
Sacralization
  fifth lumbar vertebra   756.1
  incomplete (vertebra)   756.1
Sacrodynia   728.8
Sacro-iliac joint - *see* condition
Sacrum - *see* condition
Saddle
  back   735.9
  embolus, aorta   444.0
  nose   738.0
    due to syphilis   090.5
Sadism (sexual)   302.6
Saemisch's ulcer (cornea)   363.0
Sago spleen   276
Sailors' skin   709.9
Saint
  Anthony's fire (*see also* Erysipelas)
    035
  Guy's dance - *see* Chorea

Saint—*continued*
  triad (*see also* Hernia, diaphragm)
    551.3
  Vitus' dance - *see* Chorea
Salicylism   965.1
Salivary duct or gland - *see* condition
Salivation (excessive) (*see also* Ptyalism)
  527.7
Salmonella
  choleraesuis   003.9
    due to food   003.0
  enteritidis   003.9
    due to food   003.0
  infection   003.9
    due to food   003.0
  septicemia   003.9
    due to food   003.0
  typhimurium   003.9
    food poisoning   003.0
  typhosa   001
Salmonellosis   003.9
  due to food   003.0
Salpingitis (catarrhal) (fallopian tube)
    (follicular) (interstitial) (isthmica
    nodosa) (nodular) (pseudofollicular)
    (purulent) (septic) (*see also*
    Salpingo-oophoritis)   614
  ear   384.0
  eustachian (tube)   384.0
  gonococcal (chronic)   098.1
    acute   098.0
  specific (chronic)   098.1
    acute   098.0
  tuberculous   016.2
    late effect or sequela   019.2
  venereal (chronic)   098.1
    acute   098.0
Salpingocele   615.9
Salpingo-oophoritis (catarrhal) (purulent)
    (ruptured) (septic) (suppurative)
    614
  with
    abortion - *see* Abortion, by type, with
      sepsis
    ectopic gestation - *see* categories
      631.0-631.3
  acute   612
    with
      abortion - *see* Abortion, by type,
        with sepsis
      ectopic gestation - *see* categories
        631.0-631.3

Savill's disease 695.9
Scabies (any site) 133.0
Scald - *see* Burn
Scalp - *see* condition
Scaphocephaly 756.0
Scapulalgia 787.1
Scar, scarring (*see also* Cicatrix) 709.0
  adherent 709.0
  atrophic 709.0
  cervix, complicating delivery 657.9
    fetus or newborn - *see* categories
      764.0-764.9
  congenital 757.2
  cornea - *see* Opacity, cornea
  due to
    previous cesarean section
      complicating delivery 661.2
        fetus or newborn - *see* categories
          764.0-764.9
  duodenum (cap) 537.9
  hypertrophic 701.3
  keloid 701.3
  lung (base) 519.2
  muscle 733.9
  myocardium, myocardial (*see also*
    Ischemia, heart) 412.9
  painful 709.0
  postnecrotic (hepatic) (liver) - *see*
    Cirrhosis, liver, postnecrotic
  psychic 300.9
  trachea 508.9
  uterus 625.9
    complicating delivery 657.9
      fetus or newborn - *see* categories
        764.0-764.9
Scarlatina (*see also* Fever, scarlet) 034.1
  anginosa 034.1
  maligna 034.1
  myocarditis, old (*see also* Myocarditis)
    428
  puerperal, postpartum, childbirth 670
  ulcerosa 034.1
Scarlatinella 057.8
Schamberg's
  dermatitis 709.9
  dermatosis, pigmentary 709.9
  disease 709.9
Schatzki ring (esophagus) (lower)
  (congenital) 750.3
  acquired 530.3
Schaumann's
  benign lymphogranulomatosis 135
  disease 135
  syndrome 135
Scheie's syndrome 273.8
Schenck's disease 117.1

Scheuermann's disease or osteochondrosis
  722.0
Schilder(-Flatau) disease 341
Schiller's mesonephroma 183.0
Schimmelbusch's disease, cystic mastitis,
  or hyperplasia 610
Schistosoma infestation - *see* Infestation,
  Schistosoma
Schistosomiasis 120.9
  bladder 120.0
  colon 120.1
  cutaneous 120.3
  eastern 120.2
  genitourinary tract 120.0
  intestinal 120.1
  lung 120.2
  Manson's (intestinal) 120.1
  Oriental 120.2
  pulmonary 120.2
  vesical 120.0
Schizencephaly 743.2
Schizo-affective psychosis 295.7
Schizoid personality 301.2
Schizophrenia, schizophrenic (insanity)
    (psychosis) (reaction) 295.9
  acute (attack) (episode) NEC 295.4
  atypical form 295.8
  borderline 295.5
  catatonic (type) (acute) (excited)
    (withdrawn) 295.2
  childhood type 295.8
  chronic NEC 295.8
  hebephrenic (type) (acute) 295.1
  incipient 295.5
  latent 295.5
  paranoid (type) (acute) 295.3
  paraphrenic (acute) 295.3
  prepsychotic 295.5
  primary (acute) 295.0
  pseudoneurotic 295.5
  pseudopsychopathic 295.5
  residual (state) (type) 295.6
  restzustand 295.6
  schizo-affective (type) (depressed)
    (excited) 295.7
  simple (type) (acute) 295.0
  simplex (acute) 295.0
  specified type NEC 295.8
  undifferentiated 295.8
    acute 295.4
    chronic 295.8
Schizothymia 301.2
Schlafkrankeit 087.8
Schlatter-Osgood disease 722.2
Schlatter's tibia 722.2
Schloffer's tumor (*see also* Peritonitis)
  567.9

Sclerosis, sclerotic — *continued*
 cardiovascular — *continued*
  renal - *see* Hypertension, cardiorenal
 cerebellar - *see* Sclerosis, brain
 cerebral - *see* Sclerosis, brain
 cerebrospinal 340
  disseminated 340
  multiple 340
 cerebrovascular (*see also* Ischemia,
   cerebral) 437.9
 choroid 378.6
 combined (spinal cord) 281.0
  multiple 340
  subacute 281.0
 cornea 378.4
 coronary (artery) (*see also* Ischemia,
   heart) 412.9
 corpus cavernosum
  female 629.9
  male 607.9
 degenerative 347.9
 disease, heart (*see also* Ischemia, heart)
   412.9
 disseminated 340
 dorsal 340
  diabetic - *see* category 250
 dorsolateral (spinal cord) 281.0
 extrapyramidal 347.9
 eye, senile nuclear 374.9
 Friedreich's (spinal cord) 332.0
 funicular (spermatic cord) 607.9
  spinal cord - *see* Sclerosis, spinal
 general (vascular) - *see* Arteriosclerosis
 gland (lymphatic) 457
 hepatic - *see* Cirrhosis, liver
 hereditary 333.9
  cerebral 332.1
  spinal 332.0
 insular 340
  pancreas 251
 islands of Langerhans 251
  diabetic - *see* category 250
 kidney - *see* Sclerosis, renal
 larynx 508.3
 lateral 348.0
  amyotrophic 348.0
  descending 348.0
  primary 348.0
  spinal 348.0
 liver - *see* Cirrhosis, liver
 lobar, atrophic (of brain) 290.1
 lung (*see also* Fibrosis, lung) 517
 mastoid 387.9
 mitral - *see* Endocarditis, mitral
 Monckeberg's (*see also*
   Arteriosclerosis, peripheral)
   440.2

Sclerosis, sclerotic — *continued*
 multiple (cerebral) (spinal cord) 340
 myocardium, myocardial (*see also*
   Ischemia, heart) 412.9
 ovary 615.9
 pancreas 577.9
 penis 607.9
 peripheral arteries (*see also*
   Arteriosclerosis, peripheral)
   440.2
 plaques 340
 pluriglandular 258.1
 polyglandular 258.1
 posterior (spinal cord) (syphilitic)
   094.0
 posterolateral (spinal cord) 281.0
 prepuce 607.9
 presenile (Alzheimer's) 290.1
 primary, lateral 348.0
 progressive, systemic 734.0
 pulmonary (*see also* Fibrosis, lung)
   517
  artery 426
  valve (heart) (*see also* Endocarditis,
    pulmonary) 424.9
 renal 584
  with
   cystine storage disease 270.3
   hypertension (benign) (conditions in
     401) (*see also* Hypertension,
     kidney) 403
   heart (conditions in 402) (*see also*
     Hypertension, cardiorenal)
     404
   malignant (*see also*
     Hypertension, malignant
     with renal involvement)
     400.3
  arteriolar (hyaline) (*see also*
    Hypertension, kidney) 403
  hyperplastic (*see also*
    Hypertension, malignant
    with renal involvement)
    400.3
 retina (senile) (vascular) 377.0
 senile - *see* Arteriosclerosis
 spinal (cord) (progressive) 349.9
  ascending 349.9
  combined 281.0
   multiple 340
   subacute 281.0
   syphilitic 094.9
  disseminated 340
  dorsolateral 281.0
  general 349.9
  hereditary (mixed form) 332.0
  lateral (amyotrophic) 348.0

Sclerosis, sclerotic — *continued*
  spinal — *continued*
    multiple 340
    posterior (syphilitic) 094.0
    transverse 349.9
  stomach 537.9
  subendocardial, congenital 746.7
  symmetrical 349.9
  tricuspid (heart) (valve) - *see*
      Endocarditis, tricuspid
  tuberous (brain) 759.6
  tympanic membrane 387.9
  valve, valvular (heart) - *see*
      Endocarditis
  vascular - *see* Arteriosclerosis
  vein 458.9
Sclerotitis 369.9
Scoliosis (acquired) 735.0
  congenital 756.2
  idiopathic 735.0
  paralytic 735.0
  rachitic 265.1
  sciatic 353
  tuberculous 015.0
    late effect or sequela 019.3
Scoliotic pelvis 735.0
  complicating delivery - *see* Deformity,
      pelvis, complicating delivery
  noted during pregnancy (undelivered)
      634.9
Scorbutus, scorbutic 264
Scotoma (arcuate) (central) 781.0
Scratch - *see* Injury, superficial
Scrofula 017.1
  late effect or sequela 019.9
Scrofulide (primary) 017.0
  late effect or sequela 019.9
Scrofuloderma, scrofulodermia (any site)
    (primary) 017.0
  late effect or sequela 019.9
Scrofulosis (universal) 017.1
  late effect or sequela 019.9
Scrofulosus lichen (primary) 017.0
  late effect or sequela 019.9
Scrofulous - *see* condition
Scrotal tongue 529.5
  congenital 750.0
Scrotum - *see* condition
Scurvy, scorbutic 264
  gum 264
  infantile 264
  rickets 264
Seabright-Bantam syndrome 273.4
Seasickness 994.6
Seatworm 127.3
Sebaceous
  adenoma (*see also* Adenoma,
      sebaceous) 216.1

Sebaceous — *continued*
  cyst (*see also* Cyst, sebaceous) 706.2
  gland disease NEC 706.9
  tumor (*see also* Adenoma, sebaceous)
      216.1
Sebocystomatosis 706.2
Seborrhea, seborrheic 706.3
  capilitii 704
  corporis 706.3
  dermatitis 690
    infantile 691
  eczema 690
    infantile 691
  nigricans 705.9
  sicca 690
Seclusion pupil 378.6
Secondary neoplasm, secondaries
  appendix 197.5
  bladder (spincter) (urinary) (orifice)
      198.0
  bone (sites in 170) 198.5
  brain (sites in 191) 198.3
  bronchus (cartilage) 197.3
  carcinomatosis NEC 199.0
  digestive organs NEC (sites in 150,
      151, 155.1, 156, 157, 159)
      197.9
  duodenum 197.4
  generalized NEC 199.0
  intestines, intestinal 197.5
    large (sites in 153, 154) 197.5
    small (sites in 152) 197.4
  liver 197.7
  lung 197.0
  lymph gland or node 196.9
    axillary 196.3
    brachial 196.3
    bronchopulmonary 196.1
    cervical 196.0
    epitrochlear 196.3
    face 196.0
    groin 196.4
    head 196.0
    iliac 196.4
    inguinal 196.4
    intestinal 196.2
    intra-abdominal 196.2
    intrathoracic 196.1
    limb
      lower 196.4
      upper 196.3
    lower limb 196.4
    mediastinal 196.1
    mesenteric 196.2
    multiple sites 196.8
    neck 196.0
    popliteal 196.4

Secondary neoplasm, etc. — *continued*
  lymph gland or node — *continued*
    retroperitoneal 196.2
    specified site NEC 196.7
    splenic 196.2
    supraclavicular 196.0
    tibial 196.4
    tracheobronchial 196.1
    upper limb 196.3
    Virchow's 196.0
    mediastinum 197.1
    multiple unspecified sites 199.0
    nervous system NEC (sites in 190, 192)
      198.4
    peritoneum (sites in 158) 197.6
    pleura 197.2
    pulmonary 197.0
    rectum 197.5
    respiratory organs NEC (sites in 160,
      161, 162.0, 163.9) 197.3
    retroperitoneal tissue 197.6
    skin (sites in 172, 173) 198.2
    specified sites NEC (sites in 140-149,
      171, 174, 180-187, 193-195)
      198.9
    spleen 198.9
    urinary organs NEC (sites in 189)
      198.1
    vesical (orifice) 198.0
Secretion urinary
  excessive 786.4
  suppression 786.5
Section
  nerve, traumatic - *see* Injury, nerve, by
    site
Segmentation, incomplete (congenital) -
    see also Fusion
  bone NEC 756.9
  lumbosacral (joint) 756.1
  vertebra 756.2
    lumbosacral 756.1
Seizure 780.2
  akinetic 345.0
    idiopathic 345.0
    psychomotor 345.3
  apoplexy, apoplectic (*see also* Disease,
    cerebrovascular, acute) 436.9
  autonomic 300.1
  brain or cerebral (*see also* Disease,
    cerebrovascular, acute) 436.9
  convulsive (*see also* Convulsions)
    780.2
  cortical
    focal - *see* Epilepsy, partial
    idiopathic 345.9
  epileptic (*see also* Epilepsy) 345.9
  epileptiform, epileptoid 780.2

Seizure — *continued*
  epileptiform, etc. — *continued*
    focal - *see* Epilepsy, partial
  febrile 780.2
  heart - *see* Disease, heart
  hysterical 300.1
  jacksonian - *see* Epilepsy, jacksonian
  paralysis (*see also* Disease,
    cerebrovascular, acute) 436.9
  uncinate 345.3
Self-mutilation 300.9
Seminal
  vesicle - *see* condition
  vesiculitis (*see also* Vesiculitis) 607.4
Seminoma (testis) 186
Senear-Usher disease 694
Senecio jacoboea dermatitis 692.6
Senectus 794
Senescence 794
Senile (*see also* condition) 794
  cervix (atrophic) 621.6
  endometrium (atrophic) 625.0
  fallopian tube (atrophic) 615.9
  heart (failure) 794
  ovary (atrophic) 615.9
  wart (*see also* Keratosis, seborrheic)
    216.0
Senility 794
  with
    mental changes 309.6
    psychosis NEC (*see also* Psychosis,
      senile) 290.0
  premature 258.9
Sensation
  burning (*see also* Disturbance,
    sensation) 781.6
    tongue 529.6
  prickling (*see also* Disturbance,
    sensation) 781.6
Sense loss (smell) (taste) (touch) (*see also*
    Disturbance, sensation) 781.6
Sensibility disturbance (cortical) (deep)
    (vibratory) (*see also* Disturbance,
    sensation) 781.6
Sensitivity - *see also* Allergy
  carotid sinus 358.1
  methemoglobinemia 289.9
Sensitization, auto-erythrocytic 283.9
Separation
  apophysis, traumatic - code as Fracture,
    closed
  choroid 378.6
  costochondral - *see* Dislocation,
    costochondral
  epiphysis, epiphyseal, traumatic - code
    as Fracture, closed
  fracture - *see* Fracture

Septicemia, etc. — *continued*
streptococcal 038.0
suipestifer 003.9
due to food 003.0
umbilicus, newborn (organism
unspecified) 038.9
viral 079.9
Septum, septate (congenital) - *see also*
Anomaly, specified type NEC
anal 751.3
aqueduct of Sylvius 742
with spina bifida 741.0
hymen 752.6
uterus (*see also* Double uterus) 752.5
vagina 752.6
Sequestration
lung (congenital) 748.6
orbit 378.9
pulmonary artery (congenital) 747.6
Sequestrum
bone 720.1
dental 525.9
sinus - *see* Sinusitis
Serology for syphilis Y00.3
doubtful
with signs or symptoms - *code by* site
and stage under Syphilis
follow-up of latent syphilis - *see*
Syphilis, latent
false positive Y00.7
negative Y00.3
with signs or symptoms - *code by* site
and stage under Syphilis
follow-up of latent syphilis (not
needing further care) Y03.9
positive 097.1
with signs or symptoms - *code by* site
and stage under Syphilis
false Y00.7
follow-up of latent syphilis - *see*
Syphilis, latent
only finding - *see* Syphilis, latent
reactivated 097.1
Seroma - *see* Hematoma
Seropurulent - *see* condition
Serositis, multiple 569.9
peritoneal 569.9
pleural - *see* Pleurisy
Serous - *see* condition
Serum
allergy, allergic reaction 999.5
shock 999.4
arthritis 999.5
complication or reaction NEC (*see also*
Complications, vaccination)
999.5
disease NEC 999.5

Serum — *continued*
hepatitis 999.2
intoxication 999.5
jaundice (homologous) 999.2
neuritis 999.5
poisoning NEC 999.5
rash NEC 999.5
sickness NEC 999.5
Sesamoiditis 723.9
Sever's disease 722.2
Sex chromosome mosaics 759.5
Sexopathy (*see also* Deviation, sexual)
302.9
Sexual
anesthesia 305.6
deviation (*see also* Deviation, sexual)
302.9
frigidity (female) 305.6
function, disorder of (psychogenic)
305.6
immaturity (female) (male) 258.9
impotence (psychogenic) 305.6
organic origin NEC 607.9
precocity (female) (male) 258.9
with adrenal hyperplasia or tumor
255.0
sadism 302.6
Sexuality, pathologic (*see also* Deviation,
sexual) 302.9
Sezary syndrome 695.9
Shaking palsy or paralysis (*see also*
Parkinsonism) 342
Shallowness, acetabulum 723.9
Shaver's disease 516.0
Sheath (tendon) - *see* condition
Shedding nail 703.9
Sheehan's disease or syndrome 253.1
Shelf, rectal 569.2
Shell shock (current) 307
Shield kidney 753.3
Shiga's
bacillus 004.0
dysentery 004.0
Shigella (dysentery) (*see also* Dysentery,
bacillary) 004.9
carrier (state) Y05.9
Shigellosis (*see also* Dysentery, bacillary)
004.9
Shin splints 844
Shingles - *see* Herpes, zoster
Shipyard eye or disease 078.1
Shock 782.9
allergic - *see* Shock, anaphylactic
anaphylactic (from serum or
immunization) 999.4
drug or chemical - *see* Table of
adverse effects

Shock—*continued*
  anaphylactic—*continued*
    following sting(s) 989.4
  anaphylactoid - *see* Shock, anaphylactic
  anesthetic NEC 968.1
    specified agent - *see* Table of adverse
      effects
  birth, fetus or newborn NEC 768.9
  drug or chemical substance - *see* Table
    of adverse effects
  electric 994.8
  endotoxic (*see also* Bacteremia) 038.9
  following injury (immediate) (delayed)
    995.5
  hematologic 782.9
  hypovolemic 782.9
    surgical 998.0
    traumatic 995.5
  insulin 962.3
  lightning 994.0
  nervous 307
  obstetric
    with abortion - *see* Abortion, by type
    complicating delivery 661.8
      fetus or newborn - *see* categories
        768.0-768.9
  paralytic (*see also* Disease,
    cerebrovascular, acute) 436.9
  pleural (surgical) 998.0
    due to trauma 995.5
  postoperative 998.0
  psychic 307
  septic, cause unknown 039.9
  spinal - *see also* Injury, spinal, by
    region
    with spinal bone injury - *code by*
      region under Fracture,
      vertebra, with spinal cord
      lesion
  surgical 998.0
  therapeutic misadventure NEC (*see*
    also Complications) 999.9
  transfusion - *see* Complications,
    transfusion
  traumatic (immediate) (delayed) 995.5
Shoemakers' chest 738.8
Short, shortening, shortness
  arm 738.2
    congenital 755.2
  breath 783.2
  common bile duct, congenital 751.6
  cord (umbilical) - *see* Complications,
    umbilical cord
  cystic duct, congenital 751.6
  esophagus (congenital) 750.8
  femur (acquired) 738.5
    congenital 755.3

Short, etc. — *continued*
  frenulum linguae 750.0
  frenum linguae 750.0
  hamstrings 733.9
  hip (acquired) 738.4
    congenital 755.7
  leg (acquired) 738.5
    congenital 755.3
  metatarsus (congenital) 754.9
    acquired 738.6
  organ or site, congenital NEC - *see*
    Distortion
  palate (congenital) 750.8
  radius (acquired) 738.2
    congenital 755.2
  round ligament 615.9
  stature, constitutional (hereditary)
    793.8
  tendon 733.9
    Achilles (acquired) 733.4
      congenital 754.9
    congenital 756.8
  thigh (acquired) 738.5
    congenital 755.3
  tibialis anticus 733.9
  umbilical cord - *see* Complications,
    umbilical cord
  urethra 599.9
  uvula (congenital) 750.8
  vagina 629.9
Shortsightedness 370.0
Shoulder - *see* condition
Shovel shaped incisors 520.2
Shower, thrombo-embolic - *see* Embolism
Shrinking vitreous, nutritional 378.9
Shunt
  arteriovenous, pulmonary (acquired)
    NEC 458.9
    congenital 747.6
    traumatic (complication) 995.3
  surgical, prosthetic with complication -
    see categories 997.5, 997.6
Shutdown, renal (*see also* Lesion, kidney)
  593.2
Sialadenitis (any gland) (chronic)
  (suppurative) 527.2
  epidemic 136
Sialadenosis
  periodic 527.2
Sialitis 527.2
Sialo-adenitis (*see also* Sialadenitis)
  527.2
Sialo-angitis 527.2
Sialodochitis 527.2
  fibrinosa 527.2
Sialodocholithiasis 527.5
Sialolithiasis 527.5

Sialorrhea (*see also* Ptyalism)   527.7
Sialosis   527.8
Siamese twin   759.1
Sick   796.0
Sickle cell anemia or trait (*see also*
    Disease, sickle cell)   282.5
Sicklemia (trait) (*see also* Disease, sickle
    cell)   282.5
Sickness
  air (travel)   994.6
  airplane   994.6
  alpine   993.2
  altitude   993.2
  aviators'   993.2
  balloon   993.2
  car   994.6
  compressed air   993.3
  decompression   993.3
  milk   988.9
  morning - *see* Hyperemesis, gravidarum
  motion   994.6
  mountain   993.2
  protein (*see also* Complications,
    vaccination)   999.5
  radiation - *see* Effect, adverse,
    radioactivity
  roundabout (motion)   994.6
  sea   994.6
  serum NEC (*see also* Complications,
    vaccination)   999.5
  sleeping   065
    African   087.8
      by Trypanosoma   087.8
        gambiense   087.0
        rhodesiense   087.1
    late effects   066
  sweating   136
  swing (motion)   994.6
  train (railway) (travel)   994.6
  travel (any vehicle)   994.6
Siderosis (lung)   516.0
  eye (bulbi) (corneal) (lens)   378.9
Siemens' syndrome   757.2
Sigmoid
  flexure - *see* condition
  kidney   753.3
Sigmoiditis - *see* Enteritis
Silicosis, silicotic   515.0
  with tuberculosis   010
  non-nodular   516.0
  pulmonum   515.0
    with tuberculosis   010
Silicotuberculosis   010
Silo-filler's disease   516.2
Silver syndrome   759.8
Simmonds' cachexia or disease   253.1
Simon's disease   279

Simple, simplex - *see* condition
Sinding-Larsen disease   722.2
Singers' node or nodule   508.3
Single
  atrium   746.4
  umbilical artery   747.5
  ventricle   746.3
Singultus   784.6
  epidemicus   079.8
Sinus - *see also* Fistula
  arrest (*see also* Block, heart)   427.3
  arrhythmia (*see also* Action, heart,
    irregular)   427.9
  bradycardia (*see also* Action, heart,
    irregular)   427.9
  branchial cleft   745.4
  coccygeal   685
  dental   522.7
  dermal (congenital)   685
  draining - *see* Fistula
  infected, skin NEC   686.9
  marginal, ruptured or bleeding
    (complicating delivery)   651.1
    fetus or newborn   770.1
    undelivered   632.2
  pause (*see also* Block, heart)   427.3
  pericranii   743.0
  pilonidal (infected) (rectum)   685
  pre-auricular   745.4
  rectovaginal   629.8
  tachycardia (*see also* Action, heart,
    irregular)   427.9
  testis   607.9
  tract (postinfectional) - *see* Fistula
Sinuses, Rokitansky-Aschoff (*see also*
    Disease, gallbladder)   576.9
Sinusitis (accessory) (ethmoidal)
    (hyperplastic) (nasal) (nonpurulent)
    (purulent) (sphenoidal) (chronic)
    503.9
  with influenza, flu, or grippe, any sinus
    472
  acute   461.9
  allergic, any sinus   507
  antrum   503.0
    acute   461.0
  due to
    fungus, any sinus   117.9
    high altitude, any sinus   993.1
  frontal   503.1
    acute   461.1
  maxillary   503.0
    acute   461.0
  syphilitic, any sinus   095
  tuberculous, any sinus   012.9
    with pneumoconiosis (conditions in
      515)   010

Sinusitis — *continued*
  tuberculous, etc. — *continued*
    late effect or sequela 019.0
Sinusitis-bronchiectasis-situs inversus
    (syndrome) (triad) 759.0
Sirenomelia 759.2
Siriasis 992.0
Sirkari's disease 085.0
Siti 104.0
Sitophobia 300.2
Situation, psychiatric 300.9
Situational
  disturbance (transient) 307
  maladjustment, acute 307
  reaction 307
    adolescent 307
    adult 307
Situs inversus or transversus 759.0
  abdominalis 759.0
  thoracis 759.0
Sixth disease 057.1
Sjogren's syndrome 734.9
Skeletal - *see* condition
Skene's gland - *see* condition
Skenitis (*see also* Urethritis) 597
Skerljevo 104.0
Skevas-Zerfus disease 989.4
Skin - *see also* condition
  donor Y09.9
  hidebound 734.0
Slate-dressers' lung 515.0
  tuberculous 010
Slate-miners' lung 515.0
  tuberculous 010
Sleep
  disorder 780.6
    child 306.4
      nonorganic origin 306.4
  disturbance 780.6
    nonorganic origin 306.4
  rhythm inversion 780.6
  walking 306.4
    hysterical 300.1
Sleeping sickness - *see* Sickness, sleeping
Sleeplessness 306.4
Slipped, slipping
  epiphysis (postinfectional) 722.9
    traumatic (old) 722.9
      current - code as Fracture, closed
    upper femoral, nontraumatic 722.3
  intervertebral disc - *see* Displacement,
    intervertebral disc
  patella 729.8
  rib 723.9
  sacro-iliac joint 726
  tendon 733.9

Slipped, slipping — *continued*
  ulnar nerve, nontraumatic 357.3
  vertebra NEC (*see also*
    Spondylolisthesis) 756.1
Slocumb's syndrome 844
Sloughing (multiple) (skin) 686.9
  abscess - *see* Abscess
  appendix 543
  bladder 596.9
  fascia 732
  phagedena (*see also* Gangrene) 445.9
  rectum 569.2
  scrotum 607.9
  tendon 732
  ulcer (*see also* Ulcer, skin) 707.9
Sluder's neuralgia 355.0
Slurred, slurring speech 781.5
Small, smallness
  cardiac reserve - *see* Disease, heart
  introitus, vagina 629.7
  ovary 615.9
  pelvis
    complicating delivery - *see*
      Deformity, pelvis, complicating
      delivery
    noted during pregnancy (undelivered)
      634.9
  placenta - *see* Placenta, abnormal
  umbilical cord - *see* Complications,
    umbilical cord
  uterus 625.9
  white kidney (*see also* Nephritis,
    chronic) 582
Smallpox (*see also* Variola) 050.9
  malignant 050.0
  vaccination complications - *see*
    Complications, vaccination
Smith's fracture (separation) - *see*
    Fracture, radius, lower end
Smokers' throat 502.0
Smothering spells 783.2
Snapping
  finger 731.4
  hip 729.5
  jaw 524.9
  knee 724.5
Sneezing, intractable 508.9
Sniffing
  cocaine 304.4
  glue (airplane) 304.8
Snoring 783.2
Snow blindness 360
Snuffles (non-syphilitic) 460
  syphilitic (infant) 090.0
Social maladjustment without manifest
    psychiatric disorder Y13

Sodoku 026.0
Sodomy 302.0
Soft - *see also* condition
  nails 703.9
Softening
  bone 265.2
  brain (necrotic) (progressive) 438.9
    with hypertension (benign) (conditions
      in 401) 438.0
      malignant (*see also* Hypertension,
        malignant with
        cerebrovascular
        involvement) 400.2
    arteriosclerotic (*see also* Ischemia,
      cerebral) 437.9
    congenital 743.2
    due to
      embolism, precerebral artery
        (conditions in 432) (*see also*
        Occlusion, precerebral
        artery) 432.9
      occlusion, precerebral artery
        (conditions in 432) (*see also*
        Occlusion, precerebral
        artery) 432.9
      thrombosis, precerebral artery
        (conditions in 432) (*see also*
        Occlusion, precerebral
        artery) 432.9
    embolic NEC (*see also* Embolism,
      brain) 434.9
    hemorrhagic (*see also* Hemorrhage,
      brain) 431.9
    inflammatory 323
    late effects 324
    occlusive (*see also* Ischemia,
      cerebral) 437.9
    puerperal, postpartum, childbirth
      674
    thrombotic NEC (*see also*
      Thrombosis, brain) 433.9
  cartilage (joint) (*see also* Disease, joint)
    729.9
  cerebellar - *see* Softening, brain
  cerebral - *see* Softening, brain
  cerebrospinal - *see* Softening, brain
  myocardial, heart (*see also*
      Insufficiency, myocardial) 428
  spinal cord 349.9
  stomach 537.9
Soldier's heart 305.3
Solitary
  cyst
    bone 723.3
    kidney (*see also* Lesion, kidney)
      593.2
  kidney (congenital) 753.0

Solitary—*continued*
  ulcer, bladder 596.9
Somatization reaction, somatic reaction -
    see Disorder, psychosomatic
Somnambulism 306.4
  hysterical 300.1
Somnolence 306.4
  periodic 347.9
Sonne dysentery 004.3
Soor 112
Sore
  Delhi 085.1
  desert (*see also* Ulcer, skin) 707.9
  eye 369.9
  Lahore 085.1
  mouth 528.9
    canker 528.2
    denture 528.9
  muscle 717.9
  Naga (*see also* Ulcer, skin) 707.9
  oriental 085.1
  pressure 707.0
    with gangrene (*see also* Gangrene)
      445.9
  septic (*see also* Abscess) 682.9
  skin NEC 709.9
  soft 099.0
  throat 462
    with influenza, flu, or grippe 472
    acute 462
    chronic 502.0
    clergyman's 783.5
    diphtheritic 032
    epidemic 034.0
    gangrenous 462
    malignant 462
    purulent 462
    putrid 462
    septic 034.0
    streptococcal (ulcerative) 034.0
    ulcerated 462
    viral 462
  tropical (*see also* Ulcer, skin) 707.9
  veldt (*see also* Ulcer, skin) 707.9
Spacing
  tooth, teeth, anomalous 524.3
Spading nail 703.9
  congenital 757.4
Spanemia 285.9
Spanish collar 605
Sparganosis 123.5
Spasm, spastic, spasticity (*see also*
    condition) 780.3
  accommodation 370.9
  ampulla of Vater (*see also* Disease,
    gallbladder) 576.9

Spasm, spastic, etc. — *continued*
anus, ani (sphincter) (reflex) 564.9
  psychogenic 305
artery NEC 443.9
  cerebral (*see also* Ischemia, cerebral,
    transient) 435.9
Bell's 350
bladder (sphincter, external or internal)
  596.9
bowel 564.1
  psychogenic 305.5
bronchus, bronchiole 519.9
cardia 530.0
  psychogenic 305.5
cardiac - *see* Angina
carpopedal (*see also* Tetany) 788.5
cecum 564.1
cerebral (arteries) (vascular) (*see also*
  Ischemia, cerebral, transient)
  435.9
cervix, complicating delivery 657.9
  fetus or newborn - *see* categories
    767.0-767.9
ciliary body (of accommodation) 370.9
colon 564.1
  psychogenic 305.5
common duct (*see also* Disease,
  gallbladder) 576.9
conjugate 781.1
  late effect, viral encephalitis 066
coronary (artery) - *see* Angina
diaphragm (reflex) 784.6
  psychogenic 305.5
duodenum 564.9
esophagus 530.9
  psychogenic 305.5
facial 350
fallopian tube 615.9
gastrointestinal (tract) 536.1
  psychogenic 305.5
glottis 508.3
  hysterical 300.1
  psychogenic 306.0
    specified as conversion reaction
      300.1
  reflex through recurrent laryngeal
    nerve 508.3
habit 306.2
heart - *see* Angina
hourglass - *see* Hourglass contraction
hysterical 300.1
infantile 780.3
internal oblique, eye 373.9
intestinal 564.1
  psychogenic 305.5
larynx, laryngeal 508.3
  hysterical 300.1

Spasm, spastic, etc. — *continued*
larynx, etc. — *continued*
  psychogenic 306.0
    specified as conversion reaction
      300.1
levator palpebrae superioris 378.9
muscle 780.3
nervous 780.3
nodding 306.2
occupation 300.8
oculogyric 781.1
  late effect, viral encephalitis 066
ophthalmic artery 377.0
orbicularis 780.3
perineal 629.9
peroneo-extensor (*see also* Flat, foot)
  736
pharynx (reflex) 508.9
  hysterical 300.1
  psychogenic 305.2
    specified as conversion reaction
      300.1
pregnant uterus (abnormal) 634.7
psychogenic 305.1
pylorus 784.2
  congenital or infantile 750.1
  psychogenic 305.5
rectum (sphincter) 564.9
  psychogenic 305.5
retinal (artery) 377.0
sacro-iliac 726
saltatory 780.3
sigmoid 564.1
  psychogenic 305.5
sphincter of Oddi (*see also* Disease,
  gallbladder) 576.9·
stomach 536.1
  neurotic 305.5
throat 508.9
  hysterical 300.1
  psychogenic 305.2
    specified as conversion reaction
      300.1
tic 306.2
tongue 780.3
torsion 331.1
trigeminal nerve 351
ureter 593.5
urethra (sphincter) 599.9
uterus 625.9
vagina 786.7
  psychogenic 305.6
vascular NEC 443.9
vasomotor NEC 443.9
vein NEC 458.9
viscera 785.5
Spasmodic - *see* condition

Spasmophilia (*see also* Tetany) 788.5
Spasmus nutans 306.2
Spastic - *see also* Spasm
  child 343.1
Spasticity - *see also* Spasm
  cerebral, child 343.1
Speaker's throat 783.5
Specific, specified - *see* condition
Speech defect, disorder, disturbance,
    impediment NEC 306.9
  secondary to organic lesion 781.5
Spermatic cord - *see* condition
Spermatoblastoma 186
Spermatocele 607.6
  congenital 752.8
Spermatocystitis 607.5
Spermatorrhea 607.9
Sphacelus (*see also* Gangrene) 445.9
Sphenoidal - *see* condition
Sphenoiditis (chronic) (*see also* Sinusitis)
    503.9
Sphenopalatine ganglion neuralgia 355.0
Sphericity, increased, lens 370.9
Spherocytosis (familial) (hereditary)
    282.0
  hemoglobin disease 282.5
  sickle cell (disease) (trait) 282.5
Spherophakia 744.8
Sphincter - *see* condition
Sphincteritis, sphincter of Oddi (*see also*
    Cholecystitis) 575
Sphingolipidosis 272.2
Sphingomyelinosis 272.2
Spicule tooth 520.2
Spider
  finger 755.5
  nevus 448
  vascular 448
Spiegler-Fendt sarcoid 202.9
Spiegler's tumor (*see also* Adenoma,
    sweat glands) 216.2
Spielmeyer-Stock disease 333.0
Spielmeyer-Vogt disease 333.0
Spina bifida (aperta) 741.9
  with hydrocephalus 741.0
  occulta 756.2
Spindle, Krukenberg's 378.6
Spine, spinal - *see* condition
Spiradenoma (*see also* Adenoma, sweat
    glands) 216.2
Spirillosis NEC (*see also* Fever,
    relapsing) 088.9
Spirillum minus 026.0
Spirochetal - *see* condition
Spirochetosis 104.9
  bronchopulmonary 104.9
  icterohemorrhagic 100.0

Spirochetosis—*continued*
  lung 104.9
Spitting blood (*see also* Hemoptysis)
    783.1
Splanchnomegaly 569.9
Splanchnoptosis 569.9
Spleen - *see* condition
Splenic flexure syndrome 569.9
Splenitis 289.5
  interstitial 289.5
  malarial (*see also* Malaria) 084.9
  malignant 289.5
  nonspecific 289.5
  tuberculous 017.9
    late effect or sequela 019.9
Splenocele 289.5
Splenomegalia - *see* Splenomegaly
Splenomegalic - *see* condition
Splenomegaly 782.8
  congenital 758.0
  congestive - *see* Cirrhosis, liver
  Egyptian 120.1
  fibrocongestive - *see* Cirrhosis, liver
  Gaucher's 272.2
  idiopathic 782.8
  malarial (*see also* Malaria) 084.9
  neutropenic 288
  Niemann-Pick 272.2
  syphilitic 095
    congenital 090.0
Splenopathy 289.5
Splenopneumonia - *see* Pneumonia
Splenoptosis 289.5
Splinter(s) - *code by* site under Wound,
    open, complicated
Split
  heart sounds (*see also* Action, heart,
    irregular) 427.9
  lip, congenital 749.1
    with cleft palate 749.2
Splitting nails 703.9
Spoiled child reaction 308
Spondylarthrosis 713.1
Spondylitis 713.1
  ankylopoietica 712.4
  ankylosing (chronic) 712.4
  atrophic 712.4
  chronic (traumatic) 713.2
  deformans (chronic) 713.1
  gonococcal 098.3
  gouty 274
  hypertrophic 713.1
  infectious NEC (*see also* Arthritis,
    infectious) 712.4
  Kummell's 713.2
  Marie-Strumpell 712.4
  muscularis 712.4

Spondylitis — *continued*
ossificans ligamentosa   712.4
osteoarthritica   713.1
proliferative   712.4
rheumatoid   712.4
rhizomelica   712.4
sacro-iliac NEC   713.1
senescent   713.1
senile   713.1
static   713.1
traumatic (chronic)   713.2
tuberculous   015.0
late effect or sequela   019.3
typhosa   001
Spondyloarthrosis   713.1
Spondylolisthesis (congenital)
(lumbosacral)   756.1
complicating delivery - *see* Deformity,
pelvis, complicating delivery
noted during pregnancy (undelivered)
634.9
traumatic   756.1
acute (lumbar) - *see* Fracture,
vertebra, lumbar
site other than lumbosacral - *code
by* region under Fracture,
vertebra
Spondylolysis (congenital)   756.2
acquired   729.1
cervical   756.2
lumbosacral region   756.1
complicating delivery - *see*
Deformity, pelvis, complicating
delivery
noted during pregnancy (undelivered)
634.9
Spondylopathy, traumatic   713.2
Spondylose rhizomelique   712.4
Spondylosis   713.1
cervical   713.1
complicating delivery - *see* Deformity,
pelvis, complicating delivery
lumbar   713.1
noted during pregnancy (undelivered)
634.9
Sponge
inadvertently left in operation wound
998.4
kidney (medullary)   753.1
Sponge-divers' disease   989.4
Spongioblastoma (*see also* Neoplasm,
nervous system, malignant)   192.9
Spongiocytoma (*see also* Neoplasm,
nervous system, malignant)   192.9
Spontaneous - *see also* condition
fracture (cause unknown)   723.2
Spoon nail   703.9

Spoon nail — *continued*
congenital   757.4
Sporadic - *see* condition
Sporotrichosis, sporotrichotic
(disseminated) (epidermal)
(lymphatic) (mucous membranes)
(skeletal) (visceral)   117.1
Sporotrichum schenckii infection   117.1
Spots
atrophic (skin)   701.2
cafe au lait   709.9
Cayenne pepper   448
de Morgan's   448
Fuchs' black   370.0
interpalpebral   378.2
Koplik's   055
liver   709.9
Mongolian (pigmented)   757.1
Spotted fever - *see* Fever, spotted
Spotting, intermenstrual   626.6
Sprain, strain (joint) (ligament) (muscle)
(tendon)   848
with open wound - *see* Wound, open
acromioclavicular   840
ankle   845.0
arm   840
upper   840
and shoulder   840
astragalus   845.0
atlas   847.0
axis   847.0
back   847.9
specified part NEC   847.8
breast bone   848
broad ligament - *see* Injury, internal,
broad ligament
calcaneofibular   845.0
carpal   842.0
carpometacarpal   842.1
cartilage
costal   848
knee   844
semilunar (knee)   844
septal, nose   848
thyroid   848
xiphoid   848
cervical, cervicodorsal, cervicothoracic
847.0
clavicle   840
coccyx   847.8
collar bone   840
coraco-acromial   840
coracohumeral   840
coronary, knee   844
costal cartilage   848
crico-arytenoid articulation   848
cricothyroid articulation   848

Sprain, strain—*continued*
cruciate
  knee 844
deltoid
  ankle 845.0
  shoulder 840
elbow 841
  and forearm 841
femur (proximal end) 843
  distal end 844
fibula (proximal end) 844
  distal end 845.0
fibulocalcaneal 845.0
finger(s) 842.1
foot 845.1
forearm 841
  and elbow 841
glenoid 840
hand 842.1
hip 843
  and thigh 843
humerus (proximal end) 840
  distal end 841
iliofemoral 843
infraspinatus 840
innominate
  acetabulum 843
  pubic junction 848
  sacral junction 846
internal
  collateral, ankle 845.0
  semilunar cartilage 844
interphalangeal
  finger 842.1
  toe 845.1
ischiocapsular 843
jaw (cartilage) (meniscus) 848
knee 844
  and leg 844
  lateral collateral, knee 844
leg 844
  and knee 844
ligamentum teres 843
lumbar (spine) 847.8
lumbosacral 846
mandible 848
maxilla 848
medial collateral, knee 844
meniscus 844
  jaw 848
  knee (external) (internal) (lateral)
      (medial) 844
  old 724.5
  mandible 848
  specified site NEC 848
metacarpal (distal) (proximal) 842.1

Sprain, strain—*continued*
metacarpophalangeal 842.1
metatarsal 845.1
metatarsophalangeal 845.1
midtarsal 845.1
multiple sites except fingers alone or
    toes alone 848
neck 847.0
nose 848
occiput from atlas 847.0
orbicular, hip 843
patella(r) 844
pelvis 848
phalanx
  finger 842.1
  toe 845.1
radiocarpal 842.0
radiohumeral 841
radius, radial (collateral) (proximal end)
  841
  and ulna 841
  distal end 842.0
rib (cage) 848
rotator cuff 840
round ligament - *see also* Injury,
    internal, round ligament
  femur 843
sacral (spine) 847.8
sacrococcygeal 847.8
sacro-iliac (region) 846
  chronic or old 726
sacrospinous 846
sacrotuberous 846
scaphoid bone, ankle 845.0
scapula(r) 840
semilunar cartilage (knee) 844
septal cartilage (nose) 848
shoulder 840
  and arm, upper 840
  blade 840
specified site NEC 848
spine (dorsal) (lumbar) (sacral) (thoracic)
  847.8
  cervical 847.0
sternoclavicular 840
sternum 848
subglenoid 840
subscapularis 840
supraspinatus 840
symphysis
  jaw 848
  mandibular 848
  pubis 848
talofibular 845.0
tarsal 845.1
tarsometatarsal 845.1

Sprain, strain — *continued*
 temporomandibular 848
 teres
  ligamentum 843
  major or minor 840
 thigh (proximal end) 843
  and hip 843
  distal end 844
 thorax 848
 thumb 842.1
 thyroid cartilage 848
 tibia 844
  distal end 845.0
 tibiofibular
  distal 845.0
  superior 844
 toe(s) 845.1
 trachea 848
 trapezoid 840
 ulna, ulnar (collateral) (proximal end)
   841
  distal end 842.0
 ulnohumeral 841
 vertebrae (dorsal) (lumbar) (sacral)
   (thoracic) 847.8
  cervical, cervicodorsal,
    cervicothoracic 847.0
 wrist (cuneiform) (scaphoid) (semilunar)
   842.0
 xiphoid cartilage 848
Sprengel's deformity (congenital) 755.5
Sprue 269.0
 idiopathic 269.0
 meaning thrush 112
 nontropical 269.0
 tropical 269.0
Spur
 bone, except calcaneal 723.9
 calcaneal 723.7
 nose (septum) 508.9
  bone 723.9
 septal 508.9
Sputum, excessive (cause unknown)
   783.4
Squamous - *see also* condition
 cell metaplasia, bladder 596.9
 epithelium in cervical canal or uterine
   mucosa (congenital) 752.5
Squint (*see also* Strabismus) 373.9
 accomodative 373.9
Stab - *see also* Wound, open
 internal organs - *see* Injury, internal, by
   site, with open wound
Staggering gait 787.6
 hysterical 300.1
Staghorn calculus 592

Stahl's pigment line 378.9
Stain, port wine (*see also* Hemangioma)
   227.0
Staining
 tooth, teeth (hard tissues)
  due to
   accretions 523.6
   deposits (black, green, orange,
      tobacco) (soft) 523.6
   metals (copper, silver) 521.7
   pulpal bleeding 521.7
Stammering 306.0
Standstill
 auricular (*see also* Block, heart) 427.3
 cardiac (*see also* Arrest, cardiac)
   427.2
 sinoatrial (*see also* Block, heart) 427.3
 ventricular (*see also* Arrest, cardiac)
   427.2
Stanton's disease 025
Staphylitis (acute) (catarrhal) (chronic)
   (gangrenous) (membranous)
   (suppurative) (ulcerative) 528.3
Staphylococcemia 038.1
Staphylococcus, staphylococcal - *see*
   condition
Staphyloma 378.9
 anterior 378.6
 ciliary 378.6
 cornea 378.4
  due to ulcer 363.0
 equatorial 378.6
 posterior 378.6
 sclera 378.6
Starvation (inanition) (due to lack of food)
   994.2
 edema 269.9
 voluntary NEC 306.5
Stasis
 bile (*see also* Disease, gallbladder)
   576.9
 bronchus 490
 cardiac (*see also* Disease, heart) 429.9
 cecum 564.9
 colon 564.9
 dermatitis (lower extremity) 454.1
  ulcerated or with ulcer 454.0
 duodenal 536.9
 eczema - *see* Stasis, dermatitis
 foot 991.4
 gastric 536.9
 ileocecal coil 564.9
 ileum 564.9
 intestinal 564.9
 jejunum 564.9
 liver - *see* Cirrhosis, cardiac

Stasis—*continued*
  lymphatic 457
  portal (with ascites) - *see* Cirrhosis,
    cardiac
  pulmonary 514
  stomach 536.9
  ulcer 454.0
  urine 786.1
  venous 458.9

State
  agitated 306.9
  anxiety (neurotic) 300.0
  apprehension 300.0
  clouded
    epileptic 345.9
    paroxysmal (idiopathic) 345.9
  compulsive (with obsession) (mixed)
    300.3
  confusional 299
    acute 298.2
    reactive (from emotional stress,
      psychological trauma) 298.2
    subacute 298.2
  constitutional psychopathic 301.7
  convulsive (*see also* Convulsions)
    780.2
  depressive
    neurotic 300.4
    dissociative 300.1
  excitement (*see also* Excitement,
    mental) 306.9
  neurotic NEC 300.9
    with depersonalization episode
      300.6
    due to or associated with physical
      condition - *see* listing under
      Disorder, mental
  obsessional 300.3
  oneiroid 295.4
  panic 300.0
  paranoid 297.9
    climacteric 297.1
    involutional 297.1
    menopausal 297.1
    senile 297.9
  tension 300.9

Status
  absence, epileptic 345.2
  convulsivus idiopathicus 345.2
  epilepticus 345.2
    generalized (convulsive)
      (nonconvulsive) 345.2
    partial 345.2
    seizure (any type) 345.2
  grand mal 345.2
  lymphaticus 254

Status—*continued*
  marmoratus 331.9
  petit mal 345.2
  postoperative NEC 796.9
  postpartum NEC 650
  thymicolymphaticus 254
  thymicus 254
  thymolymphaticus 254
Stave fracture - *see* Fracture, metacarpus
Stealing, child problem 308
Steam burn - *see* Burn
Steatadenoma (*see also* Adenoma,
  sebaceous) 216.1
Steatocystoma multiplex 706.2
Steatoma (infected) 706.2
  eyelid (cystic) 378.2
  infected 362

Steatorrhea (chronic) 269.0
  with lacteal obstruction 269.0
  idiopathic 269.0
    adult 269.0
    infantile 269.0
  pancreatic 577.9
  primary 269.0
  secondary 269.0
  tropical 269.0

Steatosis 279
  heart (*see also* Insufficiency,
    myocardial) 428
  kidney (*see also* Lesion, kidney) 593.2
  liver - *see* Cirrhosis, portal
Stein-Leventhal syndrome 256.9
Steinbrocker's syndrome 358.9
Steinert's disease 330.4
Stenocardia (*see also* Angina) 413.9
Stenocephaly 756.0
Stenosis (cicatricial) - *see also* Stricture
  anus, anal (canal) (sphincter) 569.2
    congenital 751.3
  aorta (ascending) 747.2
    arch 747.1
    arteriosclerotic 440.0
    calcified 440.0
  aortic (valve) (*see also* Endocarditis,
    aortic) 395.9
    congenital 746.6
  aqueduct of Sylvius 742
    with spina bifida 741.0
    acquired (*see also* Hydrocephalus)
      347.9
  bile duct or biliary passage (*see also*
    Obstruction, gallbladder) 576.0
    congenital 751.5
  bladder neck 596.2
    congenital 753.6
  brain 347.9

Stenosis—*continued*
  vulva 629.7
Stercolith (*see also* Fecalith) 560.3
  appendix 543
Sterility
  female 628
  male 606
Sterilization, admission for Y09.0
Sternalgia (*see also* Angina) 413.9
Sternberg's
  disease 201
  tumor 201
Sternopagus 759.1
Sternum bifidum 756.4
Steroid effects (adverse) (iatrogenic)
      962.0
  cushingoid 962.0
  diabetes 962.0
  fever 962.0
  withdrawal 962.0
Stevens-Johnson disease 695.1
Stewart-Morel syndrome 723.4
Sticker's disease 057.0
Sticky eye 361
Stiff neck - *see* Torticollis
Stiffness, joint 727.9
  ankle 727.7
  elbow 727.2
  finger 727.4
  hip 727.5
  knee 727.6
  multiple sites 727.8
  produced by surgical fusion (*see also*
      Disease, joint) 729.9
  sacro-iliac 726
  shoulder 727.1
  specified NEC 727.8
  spine 727.0
  wrist 727.3

Stigmata congenital syphilis 090.5
Still's disease or syndrome 712.0
Stillbirth NEC 779.9
  for classification of births in hospital
      Y30.2
  early (gestation less than 20 weeks)
      Y30.0
  intermediate (gestation 20-27 weeks)
      Y30.1
  late (gestation 28 weeks or more)
      Y30.2
Stiller's disease 790.1
Stilling's syndrome 744.8
Stimulation, ovary 256.0
Sting (animal) (bee) (fish) (insect) (jellyfish)
      (Portuguese man-o-war) (wasp)
      (venomous) 989.4

Sting—*continued*
  anaphylactic shock or reaction 989.4
  plant 692.6
Stippled epiphyses 756.6
Stitch
  abscess 998.5
  burst (in operation wound) 998.3
  in back 728.9
Stocker's line 378.9
Stokes-Adams syndrome (*see also* Block,
      heart) 427.3
Stokes' disease 242.0
Stokvis(-Talma) disease 289.9
Stomach - *see* condition
Stomatitis 528.0
  angular 528.5
    due to
      dietary deficiency 263.0
      vitamin deficiency 263.0
  aphthous 528.2
  catarrhal 528.0
  diphtheritic 032
  due to
    thrush 112
  epidemic 079.4
  epizootic 079.4
  follicular 528.0
  gangrenous 528.1
  herpetic 054
  malignant 528.0
  membranous acute 528.0
  mycotic 112
  necrotic 528.1
  necrotizing ulcerative 101
  parasitic 112
  septic 528.0
  spirochetal 101
  suppurative (acute) 528.0
  ulcerative 528.0
  ulceromembranous 101
  vesicular 528.0
    with exanthem 074.9
  Vincent's 101

Stomatomycosis 112
Stomatorrhagia 528.9
Stone(s) - *see also* Calculus
  bladder (diverticulum) 594
  cystine 270.1
  kidney 592
  pulp (dental) 522.2
  ureter 592
  xanthin 270.5

Stonecutters' lung 515.0
  tuberculous 010
Stonemasons'
  asthma, disease, or lung 515.0

Stonemasons' — *continued*
  asthma, disease, etc. — *continued*
    tuberculous 010
    phthisis 010
Stoppage
  bowel or intestine (*see also*
          Obstruction, intestine) 560.9
  heart (*see also* Arrest, cardiac) 427.2
  urine 786.5
Strabismus (alternating) (any eye muscle)
          (comitant) (concomitant)
          (congenital) (latent) (noncomitant)
          (nonconcomitant) (nonparalytic)
          (paralytic) 373.9
  convergent 373.0
  divergent 373.1
  due to
    parasites 136
    Trichinella spiralis 124
  external 373.1
  internal 373.0
  vertical 373.2
Strain - *see also* Sprain
  eye NEC 370.9
  heart - *see* Disease, heart
  meaning gonorrhea - *see* Gonorrhea
  postural 733.9
Strangulation, strangulated 994.7
  appendix 543
  asphyxiation or suffocation by 994.7
  bladder neck 596.2
  bowel - *see* Strangulation, intestine
  bubonocele 552
  colon - *see* Strangulation, intestine
  cord (umbilical) - *see* Complications,
          umbilical cord
  enterocele 553.9
  epigastrocele 553.2
  epiplocele 553.9
  exomphalos 553.1
  food or foreign body (*see also*
          Asphyxia, food) 933
  hernia - *see* Hernia, by site, with
          obstruction
  intestine 560.2
    with hernia - *see* Hernia, by site, with
          obstruction
    congenital (large) (small) 751.4
  merocele 553.0
  mesentery or omentum 560.2
    with hernia - *see* Hernia, by site, with
          obstruction
  mucus (*see also* Asphyxia, mucus) 933
    newborn (*see also* Aspiration, content
          of birth canal) 776.0
  omentocele 553.9

Strangulation, etc. — *continued*
  omphalocele 553.1
  organ or site, congenital NEC - *see*
          Atresia
  ovary 615.9
  penis 607.9
    foreign body 939
  rupture 553.9
  sarco-epiplocele 553.9
  sarco-epiplomphalocele 553.1
  stomach due to hernia (*see also* Hernia,
          by site, with obstruction) 553.9
  umbilical cord - *see* Complications,
          umbilical cord
  vesico-urethral orifice 596.2
Strangury 786.0
Strawberry
  gallbladder (*see also* Disease,
          gallbladder) 576.9
  mark (*see also* Hemangioma) 227.0
Strephosymbolia 306.1
  secondary to organic lesion 781.5
Streptobacillus moniliformis 026.1
Streptococcemia 038.0
Streptococciosis 039.9
Streptococcus, streptococcal - *see*
          condition
Streptomycosis 113
Streptothricosis (general) 113
Streptothrix 113
Streptotrichosis 113
Stress reaction (gross) 307
Stretching, nerve - *see* Injury, nerve, by
          site
Striae
  albicantes 701.2
  atrophicae 701.2
  distensae (cutis) 701.2
Stricture 796.0
  anus (sphincter) 569.2
    congenital 751.3
    infantile 751.3
  aorta (ascending) (*see also* Stenosis,
          aorta) 747.2
  aortic (valve) (*see also* Endocarditis,
          aortic) 395.9
    congenital 746.6
  aqueduct of Sylvius 742
    with spina bifida 741.0
    acquired (*see also* Hydrocephalus)
          347.9
  artery 447
    congenital (peripheral) 747.6
      cerebral 747.8
      coronary 746.8
      retinal 744.8

Stricture—*continued*
  artery—*continued*
    congenital—*continued*
      umbilical 747.5
    coronary (*see also* Ischemia, heart)
      412.9
    pulmonary 747.3
  auditory canal (external) (congenital)
    745.0
    acquired 387.9
  bile duct or passage (*see also*
    Obstruction, gallbladder) 576.0
    congenital 751.5
  bladder 596.2
  bowel (*see also* Obstruction, intestine)
    560.9
  bronchus 519.9
    syphilitic 095
    tuberculous (*see also* Tuberculosis,
      pulmonary) 011.9
  cardia (stomach) 537.9
    congenital 750.8
  cardiac - *see also* Disease, heart
    orifice (stomach) 537.9
  cecum (*see also* Obstruction, intestine)
    560.9
  cervix, cervical (canal) 621.5
    complicating delivery 657.2
      fetus or newborn - *see* categories
        764.0-764.9
    congenital 752.5
  colon (*see also* Obstruction, intestine)
    560.9
    congenital 751.4
  common duct (*see also* Obstruction,
    gallbladder) 576.0
    congenital 751.5
  coronary (artery) (*see also* Ischemia,
    heart) 412.9
    congenital 746.8
  cystic duct (*see also* Obstruction,
    gallbladder) 576.0
    congenital 751.5
  duodenum 537.9
    congenital 751.4
  ear canal (external) (congenital) 745.0
    acquired 387.9
  ejaculatory duct 607.9
  esophagus 530.3
    congenital 750.3
    syphilitic 095
      congenital 090.5
  eustachian tube 387.9
    congenital 745.2
  fallopian tube 615.9
    gonococcal 098.1
    tuberculous 016.2

Stricture—*continued*
  fallopian tube—*continued*
    tuberculous—*continued*
      late effect or sequela 019.2
  gallbladder (*see also* Obstruction,
    gallbladder) 576.0
    congenital 751.6
  glottis (*see also* Stricture, larynx)
    508.3
  heart - *see also* Disease, heart
    valve - *see also* Endocarditis
    congenital (any) 746.6
  hepatic duct (*see also* Obstruction,
    gallbladder) 576.0
    congenital 751.5
  hymen 629.7
  hypopharynx 508.9
  intestine (*see also* Obstruction,
    intestine) 560.9
    congenital (large) (small) 751.4
    malignant - *see* Neoplasm, intestine,
      malignant
  lachrymal, lacrimal apparatus or gland
    368
    congenital 744.8
  larynx 508.3
    congenital 748.3
    syphilitic 095
      congenital 090.5
  lung 519.2
  malignant, internal NEC 199.1
  meatus
    ear (congenital) 745.0
      acquired 387.9
    osseous (ear) (congenital) 745.0
      acquired 387.9
    urinarius (*see also* Stricture, urethra)
      598
      congenital 753.6
  mitral (valve) (*see also* Endocarditis,
    mitral) 394.9
    congenital 746.6
  nares (anterior) (posterior) 508.9
    congenital 748.0
  nasal duct 368
    congenital 744.8
  nasolachrymal, nasolacrimal duct 368
    congenital 744.8
  nasopharynx 508.9
    syphilitic 095
  nose 508.9
  nostril (anterior) (posterior) 508.9
    congenital 748.0
  organ or site, congenital NEC - *see*
    Atresia
  os uteri (*see also* Stricture, cervix)
    621.5

Stricture—*continued*
  osseous meatus (ear) (congenital)
      745.0
    acquired   387.9
  oviduct - *see* Stricture, fallopian tube
  pharynx (dilatation)   508.9
  prostate   602
  pulmonary
    artery   747.3
    valve (*see also* Endocarditis,
        pulmonary)   424.9
      congenital   746.6
  punctum lacrimale   368
    congenital   744.8
  pylorus (hypertrophic)   537.0
    congenital   750.1
    infantile   750.1
  rectosigmoid   569.2
  rectum (sphincter)   569.2
    congenital   751.3
    due to
      chemical burn - *see* Table of
          adverse effects
      irradiation (*see also* Effect,
          adverse, radiotherapy)
          990.6
      lymphogranuloma venereum
          099.1
    gonococcal   098.8
    inflammatory   099.1
    syphilitic   095
    tuberculous   014
      late effect or sequela   019.9
  renal artery   440.1
  salivary duct or gland (any)   527.9
  sigmoid (flexure) (*see also* Obstruction,
      intestine)   560.9
  spermatic cord   607.9
  stoma
    following
      colostomy   998.7
      enterostomy   998.7
      gastrostomy   998.9
  stomach   537.9
    congenital   750.8
  subglottic (*see also* Stricture, larynx)
      508.3
  syphilitic NEC   095
  tendon (sheath)   733.9
  trachea   519.9
    congenital   748.3
    syphilitic   095
    tuberculous   012.9
      with pneumoconiosis (conditions in
          515)   010
      late effect or sequela   019.0

Stricture—*continued*
  tricuspid (valve) (*see also* Endocarditis,
      tricuspid)   397.0
    congenital   746.6
  tunica vaginalis   607.9
  ureter   593.3
    congenital   753.2
    tuberculous   016.1
      late effect or sequela   019.2
  ureteropelvic junction   593.3
    congenital   753.2
  ureterovesical orifice   593.3
    congenital   753.2
  urethra (anterior) (meatal) (organic)
      (posterior) (spasmodic)   598
    complicating delivery   657.9
      fetus or newborn - *see* categories
          764.0-764.9
    congenital (valvular)   753.6
    gonorrheal   098.1
    late effect of gonorrhea   098.1
    syphilitic   095
    valvular, congenital   753.6
  uterus, uterine   625.9
    complicating delivery   657.9
      fetus or newborn - *see* categories
          764.0-764.9
    os (external) (internal) - *see* Stricture,
        cervix
  vagina (outlet)   629.7
    congenital   752.6
  valve (cardiac) (heart) (*see also*
      Endocarditis)   424.9
    congenital   746.6
  valvular (*see also* Endocarditis)   424.9
    congenital (cardiac) (heart)   746.6
    urethra   753.6
  vas deferens   607.9
    congenital   752.8
  vein   458.9
  vena cava (inferior) (superior) NEC
      458.1
    congenital   747.4
  vesico-urethral orifice   596.2
    congenital   753.6
  vulva (acquired)   629.7
Stridor   783.6
  larynx (congenital)   748.3
Stridulous - *see* condition
Stroke (*see also* Disease, cerebrovascular,
    acute)   436.9
  apoplectic (*see also* Disease,
      cerebrovascular, acute)   436.9
  brain (*see also* Disease,
      cerebrovascular, acute)   436.9
  epileptic - *see* Epilepsy

Stroke—*continued*
  heart - *see* Disease, heart
  heat 992.0
  lightning 994.0
  paralytic (*see also* Disease,
    cerebrovascular, acute) 436.9
Strongyloides stercoralis infestation
  127.1
Strongyloidiasis 127.1
Strongyloidosis 127.1
Strongylus (gibsoni) infestation 128.8
Strophulus 778.9
  pruriginosus 698.2
Struck by lightning 994.0
Struma (*see also* Goiter) 240.9
  Hashimoto 245.1
  lymphomatosa 245.1
  nodosa (simplex) 241.9
    endemic 241.0
    sporadic 241.1
    toxicosa 242.1
  ovary 220.0
    functionally active 256.0
    malignant 183.0
  Riedel's 245.1
  scrofulous 017.1
  tuberculous 017.1
    abscess 017.1
    adenitis 017.1
    late effect or sequela 019.9
    lymphangitis 017.1
    ulcer 017.1
Strumipriva cachexia (*see also*
    Hypothyroidism) 244
Strumitis - *see* Thyroiditis
Strumpell-Marie spine 712.4
Strumpell Westphal pseudosclerosis
  273.3
Stuart-Prower factor deficiency (*see also*
    Defect, coagulation) 286.9
Student's elbow 731.2
Stupor 780.0
  catatonic 295.2
  circular 296.3
  episodic 573.9
  manic 296.8
  manic-depressive (*see also* Psychosis,
    manic-depressive) 296.9
  mental (anergic) (delusional) 299
  traumatic NEC - *see also* Injury,
    intracranial
    with spinal (cord)
      lesion - *see* Injury, spinal, by
        region
      shock - *see* Injury, spinal, by
        region

Sturge-Kalischer-Weber syndrome 759.8
Sturge(-Weber)(-Dimitri) disease or
    syndrome 759.8
Stuttering 306.0
Sty, stye 362
  external 362
  internal 362
  meibomian 362
Subacidity, gastric 536.0
  psychogenic 305.5
Subacute - *see* condition
Subarachnoid - *see* condition
Subcortical - *see* condition
Subcutaneous, subcuticular - *see*
    condition
Subdelirium (*see also* Delirium) 780.1
Subdural - *see* condition
Subendocardium - *see* condition
Subglossitis - *see* Glossitis
Subinvolution (uterus) 625.1
  chronic 625.1
  puerperal 677.9
Sublingual - *see* condition
Sublinguitis 527.2
Subluxation - *see also* Dislocation
  congenital NEC - *see also* Malposition,
    congenital
    hip 755.6
    joint
      lower limb 755.7
      shoulder 755.5
      upper limb 755.5
  lens 378.8
  rotary, cervical region of spine - *see*
    Fracture, vertebra, cervical
Submaxillary - *see* condition
Submersion (fatal) (nonfatal) 994.1
Submucous - *see* condition
Subnormal accommodation 370.9
Subphrenic - *see* condition
Subscapular nerve - *see* condition
Subseptus uterus 752.5
Substernal thyroid (*see also* Goiter)
  240.9
  congenital 758.2
Substitution disorder 300.1
Subtentorial - *see* condition
Subthyroidism (acquired) 244
  congenital 243
Succenturiata placenta - *see* Placenta,
    abnormal
Sucking thumb, child 308
Sudamen 705.1
Sudamina 705.1
Sudanese kala-azar 085.0

Sudden
  death, cause unknown   795
    puerperal, postpartum, childbirth
      677.0
  heart failure (*see also* Failure, heart)
      782.4
Sudeck's atrophy, disease, or syndrome
    723.0
Suffocation - *see also* Asphyxia
  by
    bed clothes   994.7
    bunny bag   994.7
    cave-in   994.7
    constriction   994.7
    drowning   994.1
    inhalation
      food or foreign body (*see also*
        Asphyxia, food or foreign
        body)   933
      gases, fumes, or vapors NEC (*see
        also* Table of adverse
        effects)   987.9
      oil or gasoline (*see also* Asphyxia,
        food or foreign body)   933
    overlying   994.7
    plastic bag   994.7
    pressure   994.7
    strangulation   994.7
  during birth (*see also* Asphyxia,
      newborn)   776.9
  mechanical   994.7
Sugar
  blood
    high - *see* category 250
    low   251
  in urine   789.5
Suicide, suicidal (attempted)
  by poisoning - *see* Table of adverse
      effects
  risk   300.9
  tendencies   300.9
  trauma NEC (*see also* nature and site
      of injury)   996.9
Sulfatidosis   333.1
Sulfhemoglobinemia, sulphemoglobinemia
    (acquired) (congenital)   289.9
Summer - *see* condition
Sunburn   692.8
Sunken acetabulum   738.8
Sunstroke   992.0
Superfecundation   634.9
Superfetation   634.9
Superinvolution uterus   625.9
Supernumerary (congenital)
  aortic cusps   746.6
  auditory ossicles   745.0

Supernumerary—*continued*
  bone   756.9
  breast   757.2
  carpal bones   755.5
  cusps, heart valve (any)   746.6
  digit(s)   755.0
  ear   745.1
  fallopian tube   752.5
  finger   755.0
  hymen   752.6
  kidney   753.3
  lachrymonasal, lacrimonasal duct
      744.8
  lobule (ear)   745.1
  muscle   756.8
  nipple(s)   757.2
  organ or site not listed - *see* Accessory
  ovary   752.5
  oviduct   752.5
  pulmonic cusps   746.6
  rib   756.4
    cervical or first   756.3
      syndrome   756.3
  roots (of teeth)   520.2
  tarsal bones   755.7
  teeth   520.1
    causing crowding   524.3
  testicle   752.8
  thumb   755.0
  toe   755.0
  uterus   752.5
  vagina   752.6
  vertebra   756.2
Supplemental teeth   520.1
  causing crowding   524.3
Suppression
  menstruation   626.9
  ovarian secretion   256.1
  renal (*see also* Lesion, kidney)   593.2
  urinary secretion   786.5
  urine   786.5
Suppuration, suppurative - *see also*
      condition
  accessory sinus (chronic) (*see also*
      Sinusitis)   503.9
  adrenal (gland)   255.9
  antrum (chronic) (*see also* Sinusitis,
      antrum)   503.0
  bladder (*see also* Cystitis)   595
  bowel   569.9
  brain   322
    late effects   324
  breast   611.0
    puerperal, postpartum   678
  dental periosteum   526.5
  ear (middle) - *see also* Otitis media

Suppuration, etc. — *continued*
  ear — *continued*
    external   380
    internal   384.0
  ethmoidal (chronic) (sinus) (*see also*
      Sinusitis)   503.9
  fallopian tube (*see also* Salpingo-
      oophoritis)   614
  frontal (chronic) (sinus) (*see also*
      Sinusitis, frontal)   503.1
  gallbladder (*see also* Cholecystitis)
    575
  gum   523.3
  hernial sac - *see* Hernia, by site
  intestine   569.9
  joint (*see also* Disease, joint)   729.9
  labyrinthine   384.0
  lung   513
  mammary gland   611.0
    puerperal, postpartum   678
  maxilla, maxillary   526.4
    sinus (chronic) (*see also* Sinusitis,
      maxillary)   503.0
  muscle   732
  nasal sinus (chronic) (*see also* Sinusitis)
    503.9
  pancreas   577.0
  parotid gland   527.2
  pelvis, pelvic
    female (*see also* Disease, pelvis,
      inflammatory)   616.0
    male (*see also* Peritonitis)   567.9
  pericranial (*see also* Osteomyelitis)
    720.2
  salivary duct or gland (any)   527.2
  sinus - *see* Sinusitis
  sphenoidal (chronic) (sinus) (*see also*
      Sinusitis)   503.9
  thymus (gland)   254
  thyroid (gland)   246
  tonsil   500
  uterus (*see also* Endometritis)   622.0
  wound - code as Wound, open,
      complicated
    dislocation - code as Dislocation,
      compound
    fracture - code as Fracture, open
    scratch or other superficial injury -
      code as Injury. superficial,
      infected

Suprarenal (gland) - *see* condition
Suprascapular nerve - *see* condition
Suprasellar - *see* condition
Surfer knots   918.0
Surgical
  abortion - *see* Abortion, therapeutic

Surgical — *continued*
  emphysema   998.9
  kidney (*see also* Pyelitis)   590.1
  operation NEC   796.9
  procedures, complication or
      misadventure - *see*
      Complications, surgical
      procedures
  shock   998.0
  treatment, plastic (*see also* Plastic
      surgery)   Y11.9
Suspected
  respiratory tuberculosis on radiological
      evidence alone   011.5
    with pneumoconiosis (conditions in
      515)   010
    late effect or sequela   019.0
Suspended
  uterus
    complicating delivery   657.9
      fetus or newborn - *see* categories
        764.0-764.9
    noted during pregnancy (undelivered)
      634.9
Sutton and Gull's disease - *see*
    Hypertension, kidney
Sutton's disease   709.9
Suture
  burst (in operation wound)   998.3
  inadvertently left in operation wound
    998.4
Swab inadvertently left in operation
    wound   998.4
Swallowed foreign body   938
Swallowing
  difficulty (*see also* Dysphagia)   784.4
Swan neck hand (intrinsic)   738.2
Sweat
  fetid   705.9
  gland disease NEC   705.9
Sweating
  disease or sickness   136
  excessive   788.1
  miliary   136
Sweats, night   788.1
Swelling
  abdominal (not referable to any
      particular organ)   785.0
  adrenal gland, cloudy   255.9
  ankle   787.4
  arm   787.2
  Calabar   125.2
  cervical gland   782.7
  extremity (lower) (upper)   787.2
  finger   787.2
  foot   787.2

Swelling—*continued*
  glands 782.7
  hand 787.2
  inflammatory - *see* Inflammation
  joint 787.4
    tuberculous - *see* Tuberculosis, joint
  kidney, cloudy (*see also* Lesion, kidney)
      593.2
  leg 787.2
  limb 787.2
  liver, cloudy 573.9
  scrotum 607.9
  testicle 607.9
  toe 787.2
  tubular (*see also* Lesion, kidney) 593.2
  wandering, due to Gnathostoma
      spinigerum 128.8
  white - *see* Tuberculosis, arthritis
Swift-Feer disease 985.0
Swift's disease 985.0
Swimmers' itch 120.3
Swollen - *see* Swelling
Sycosis 704
  barbae (not parasitic) 704
  contagiosa 110.0
  lupoides 704
  parasitic 110.0
  vulgaris 704
Sydenham's chorea - *see* Chorea
Symblepharon 378.3
  congenital 744.8
Sympathetic - *see* condition
Sympatheticotonia 358.9
Sympathicoblastoma (*see also*
      Neuroblastoma) 192.5
Sympathicogonioma (*see also*
      Neuroblastoma) 192.5
Sympathoblastoma (*see also*
      Neuroblastoma) 192.5
Sympathogonioma (*see also*
      Neuroblastoma) 192.5
Symphalangy 755.1
Symptoms specified NEC 788.9

  neurotic 300.9
    due to or associated with physical
        condition - *see* listing under
        Disorder, mental
  nonorganic origin 306.9
  psychogenic 306.9
Sympus 759.2
Synarthrosis (*see also* Disease, joint)
      729.9
Syncephalus 759.1
Synchondrosis, abnormal 756.9
Synchysis (vitreous humor) 378.6
  nutritional 378.6

Synchysis—*continued*
  scintillans 378.6
  senile 378.6
Syncope 782.5
  bradycardia (*see also* Action, heart,
      irregular) 427.9
  cardiac 782.5
  carotid sinus 358.1
  complicating delivery 661.8
  due to lumbar puncture 997.0
  fatal 782.5
  heart 782.5
  heat 992.1
  tussive 783.3
  vasoconstriction 782.5

Syncytioma (malignum) 181
Syndactylism, syndactyly (finger or toe)
      755.1

Syndrome - *see also* Disease
  abdominal
    acute 785.5
    migraine 346
    muscle deficiency 756.8
  abducens nerve palsy 382.0
  Achard-Thiers 255.0
  acute abdominal 785.5
  Adair-Dighton 756.6
  Adams-Stokes (*see also* Block, heart)
      427.3
  Adie(-Holmes) 378.6
  adiposogenital 253.1
  adrenal
    hemorrhage 036.1
      with meningitis 036.0
    meningococcic 036.1
      with meningitis 036.0
  adrenocortical 255.0
  adrenogenital (acquired) 255.0
    congenital 273.6
    iatrogenic 761.7
  afferent loop NEC 537.9
  air blast concussion - *see* Injury,
      internal
  Albright-Bantam 273.4
  Albright-Martin 273.4
  Albright-McCune)(-Sternberg) 756.7
  Aldrich(-Wiskott) 275.1
  Alport's 759.8
  Alvarez (*see also* Ischemia, cerebral,
      transient) 435.9
  alveolar capillary block (*see also*
      Fibrosis, lung) 517
  amnestic (confabulatory) 291.1
  amyostatic 273.3
  amyotrophic lateral sclerosis, residual
      of viral encephalitis 066

Syndrome—*continued*
  angina (*see also* Angina) 413.9
  anterior
    chest wall 783.7
    spinal artery (*see also* Ischemia,
      cerebral, transient) 435.9
    tibial 844
  antibody deficiency 275.0
    agammaglobulinemic 275.0
    congenital 275.0
    hypogammaglobulinemic 275.1
  aortic
    arch 446.6
    bifurcation 444.0
  Apert's 756.0
  argentaffin 258.9
  Argyll Robertson's (syphilitic) 094.0
    nonsyphilitic 378.6
  arm shoulder 358.9
  Arnold-Chiari 741.0
  Arrillaga-Ayerza 426
  arteriomesenteric duodenum occlusion
    537.9
  aspiration, massive, newborn (*see also*
    Aspiration, content of birth
    canal) 776.0
  ataxia-telangiectasia 275.0
  auriculotemporal 356
  Avellis' 344.9
  Ayerza's 426
  Babinski-Nageotte 344.1
  Babinski's 093.9
  Bagratuni's 446.4
  Banti's (with cirrhosis) (with portal
    hypertension) - *see* Cirrhosis,
    liver
  Bard-Pic's 157.0
  Baron Munchausen 306.9
  Barre-Guillian 354
  Barre-Lieou 728.1
  basilar artery (*see also* Ischemia,
    cerebral, transient) 435.9
  Bassen-Kornzweig 272.1
  battered baby or child NEC 996.8
  Baumgarten-Cruveilhier 571.8
  Behcet's 136
  Benedikt's 344.9
  Bernard-Horner 358.0
  Bernhardt-Roth 355.1
  Bernheim's (*see also* Failure, heart,
    congestive) 427.0
  Bertolotti's 756.1
  Bianchi's 781.5
  Biedl-Bardet 759.8
  big heart 425
  bilateral polycystic ovarian 256.9

Syndrome—*continued*
  black widow spider bite 989.4
  blast (concussion) - *see* Blast, injury
  blind loop 269.0
  Bloch-Sulzberger 757.2
  blue diaper 778.9
  Bonnevie-Ullrich 759.5
  Bonnier's 387.9
  Bouillaud's 391.9
  Bouveret's (*see also* Tachycardia,
    paroxysmal) 427.5
  brachial plexus 357.0
  brain (acute) (chronic) (organic) (non-
      psychotic) (with neurotic
      reaction) (with behavioral
      reaction) 309.9
    with psychosis, psychotic reaction
      (*see also* Psychosis, organic)
      294.9
    congenital - *see* Retardation, mental
    due to or associated with specified
      physical condition - *see* listing
      under Disorder, mental
  Brenneman's 289.2
  Briquet's 300.1
  Brock's 519.0
  Brown-Sequard 349.5
  Brugsch's 757.2
  bubbly lung (*see also* Syndrome,
    respiratory distress) 776.2
  Budd-Chiari 453
  bulbar 349.9
  Burnett's 999.9
  burning feet 261
  Bywater's 995.6
  Caffey's 756.7
  Caplan 515.9
    with tuberculosis 010
  carcinoid 258.9
  cardiopulmonary-obesity 277
  cardiorenal (*see also* Hypertension,
    cardiorenal) 404
  cardiovascular renal (*see also*
    Hypertension, cardiorenal) 404
  carotid
    artery (internal) (*see also* Ischemia,
      cerebral, transient) 435.9
    sinus 358.1
  carpal tunnel 357.2
  cat-cry 759.4
  cauda equina 728.9
  causalgia 355.9
  cerebellar, acute 780.4
  cerebellomedullary malformation
    741.0
  cervical (root) (spine) NEC 728.4
    disc 725.0

Syndrome — *continued*
  cervical — *continued*
    posterior, sympathicus 728.1
    rib 756.3
    sympathetic paralysis 358.0
    traumatic (acute) NEC 847.0
  cervicobrachial (diffuse) 728.2
  cervicocranial 728.1
  cervicodorsal outlet 357.9
  Cestan's 344.1
  Charcot-Marie-Tooth 330.0
  Charcot's 443.9
  Chediak-Higashi 270.8
  Chiari-Frommel 678
  Chiari's 453
  Clarke-Hadfield 577.9
  Claude Bernard-Horner 358.0
  Claude's 347.9
  cloudy cornea 378.6
  Cogan's 363.9
  cold injury 778.3
  Collet-Sicard 347.9
  Collet's 347.9
  compression 995.6
    cauda equina 728.9
  concussion 850.9
  congenital
    affecting more than one system
        759.8
    facial diplegia 350
    muscular hypertrophy-cerebral
        759.8
  congestion-fibrosis (pelvic) 616.2
  Conn's 255.0
  conus medullaris 349.9
  coronary, insufficiency or intermediate
        (*see also* Insufficiency, coronary)
        411.9
  Costen's 524.9
  costochondral junction 729.9
  costoclavicular 357.9
  cranio-vertebral 728.1
  Creutzfeldt-Jakob 333.9
    with dementia 290.1
  cri-du-chat 759.4
  Crigler-Najjar 273.5
  crush 995.6
  Cruveilhier-Baumgarten 571.8
  Cushing's (pituitary) 258.0
  Da Costa's 305.3
  Dana-Putnam 281.0
  Dandy-Walker 742
    with spina bifidia 741.0
  Danlos' 757.2
  de Lange's 759.8
  de Toni-Fanconi(-Debre) 270.2

Syndrome — *continued*
  Dejerine-Roussy 347.9
  demyelinating 341
  diabetes-dwarfism-obesity - *see*
        category 250
  discogenetic - *see* Displacement,
        intervertebral disc
  disseminated platelet thrombosis 448
  Donohue's 258.1
  dorsolateral medullary (*see also*
        Disease, cerebrovascular, acute)
        436.9
  Down's 759.3
  Dressler's (*see also* Ischemia, heart)
        412.9
  Duane's 744.8
  Dubin-Johnson 273.5
  Duchenne's 348.1
  due to abnormality
    autosomal, except 21 759.4
        21 759.3
    chromosomal 759.4
        sex 759.5
  dumping (postgastrectomy) 997.9
  dystonic, residual of encephalitis 066
  dystrophia dystocia 657.9
  ectopic ACTH 258.0
  Eddowes' 756.6
  efferent loop 537.9
  effort (psychogenic) 305.3
  Ehlers-Danlos 757.2
  Eisenmenger's 746.3
  Ekbom 781.6
  Ellis-van Creveld 756.7
  Ellison-Zollinger 251
  entrapment 357.9
  Epstein's - *see* Nephrosis
  Erb-Goldflam 733.0
  erythrocyte fragmentation 283.9
  exhaustion 300.5
  extrapyramidal 347.9
  eye retraction 744.8
  eyelid-malar-mandible 756.0
  Faber's 280
  facet 729.1
  falx (*see also* Hemorrhage, brain)
        431.9
  familial eczema-thrombocytopenia
        275.1
  Fanconi(-de Toni)(-Debre) 270.2
  fatigue 300.5
  Feil-Klippel 756.2
  Felty's 712.1
  Fitzhugh-Curtis 098.8
  Forbes-Albright 253.9
  Foville's (peduncular) 344.9

Syndrome — *continued*
 Franceschetti 756.0
 Francois' 378.4
 Frey's 356
 Friderichsen-Waterhouse 036.1
  with meningitis 036.0
 Frohlich's 253.1
 Froin's 349.9
 Frommel-Chiari 678
 functional
  bowel 564.9
  prepuberal castrate 752.8
 ganglion (basal ganglion brain) 347.9
 Ganser's - *see* Ganser's syndrome
 Gardner-Diamond 283.9
 gastrojejunal loop obstruction 537.9
 Gelineau's 347:0
 genito-anorectal 099.1
 Gerhardt's 508.0
 Gerstmann's 781.5
 Gilbert's 273.5
 glucuronyl transferase 273.5
 Goldberg-Maxwell 257.9
 Goldflam-Erb 733.0
 Goodpasture's 446.1
 Goodwin-Harrison 426
 Gopalan's 261
 Gower's 782.5
 Gradenigo's 382.0
 gray 960.2
 Guerin-Stern 755.8
 Guillain-Barre 354
 Gunn's 743.8
 gustatory sweating 356
 Hallerman-Streiff 756.0
 Hallervorden-Spatz 331.9
 Hamman-Rich (*see also* Fibrosis, lung)
  517
 Hand-Schuller-Christian 279
 Hanot-Chauffard(-Troisier) 273.2
 Harada's 366
 harlequin color-change 757.2
 Hayem-Widal 283.9
 head, traumatic NEC 854.9
 Hegglin's (*see also* Thrombocytopenia)
  287.1
 Heller's 295.8
 hemolytic 283.9
  uremia - *see* Uremia
 Henoch-Schonlein 287.0
 hepatic flexure 569.9
 hepatorenal 573.9
 Herter-Gee 269.0
 Heyd's 573.9
 Holmes' 781.0
 Horner's 358.0

Syndrome — *continued*
 Horner's — *continued*
  traumatic - *see* Injury, nerve, cervical
   sympathetic
 Horton's 346
 Hunt's 053.1
  dyssynergia cerebellaris myoclonica
   347.9
  herpetic geniculate ganglionitis
   053.1
 Hunter-Hurler 273.8
 Hurler's (in bones) 273.8
 Hutchinson-Boeck 135
 Hutchinson-Gilford 258.9
 Hutchinson's 194.0
 hydralazine 973.5
 hydraulic concussion (abdominal) (*see
   also* Injury, internal, abdomen)
  868.0
 hyperabduction 447
 hyperkalemic 788.0
 hyperkinetic heart (*see also* Disease,
   heart) 429.9
 hypersomnia-bulimia 347.9
 hypersympathetic 358.9
 hypokalemic 788.0
 hypopituitarism 253.1
 hypoplastic left-heart 746.6
 hypopotassemia 788.0
 infantilism 253.1
 inferior vena cava 458.1
 influenza-like 470
 intermediate coronary (*see also*
   Insufficiency, coronary) 411.9
 interspinous ligament 729.1
 intestinal polyposis-cutaneous
  pigmentation 211.9
 irritable
  heart 305.3
  weakness 300.5
 Jackson's 344.9
 Jaffe-Lichtenstein 723.9
 Jakob-Creutzfeldt 333.9
  with dementia 290.1
 jugular foramen 344.9
 Kartagener's 759.0
 Kast's 756.5
 Kennedy's 238.1
 Kimmelstiel(-Wilson) - *see* category 250
 Klein-Wardenburg 270.8
 Kleine-Levin 347.9
 Klinefelter's 759.5
 Klippel-Feil 756.2
 Klippel-Trenaunay 759.8
 Klumpke(-Dejerine) (birth injury)
   (newborn) (*see also* Birth injury,
   bone or nerve) 772.2

Syndrome—*continued*
  Korsakoff's (alcoholic) 291.1
    nonalcoholic 299
  Kunkel's 573.0
  labyrinthine 385
  Langdon Down 759.3
  lateral medullary (*see also* Disease,
      cerebrovascular, acute) 436.9
  Launois' 253.0
  Laurence-Moon(-Biedl) 759.8
  Legg-Calve-Perthes 722.1
  lenticular 273.3
  Leriche's 444.0
  Lermoyez's 389.9
  Lichtheim's 281.0
  Lignac(-de Toni)(-Fanconi)(-Debre)
      270.3
  Lloyd's 258.1
  Loeffler's 519.2
  Looser-Milkman 265.2
  Lorain(-Levi) 253.1
  Louis-Bar 275.0
  low
    atmospheric pressure 993.2
    back 728.7
      psychogenic 305.1
  Lowe's 270.8
  lower radicular, newborn (*see also* Birth
      injury, bone or nerve) 772.2
  Lutembacher's 746.4
  Lyell's 695.1
    due to drug (*see also* Table of
        adverse effects) 977.9
  Maffucci's 756.5
  magnesium-deficiency 788.5
  malabsorption 269.1
    postgastrectomy 998.9
  Mallory-Weiss 530.9
  mandibulofacial dysostosis 756.0
  maple syrup (urine) 270.4
  Marchiafava-Bignami 341
  Marchiafava-Micheli 283.9
  Marcus Gunn 743.8
  Marfan's 759.8
    meaning congenital syphilis 090.4
  Marie's 253.0
  Maroteaux-Lamy 273.8
  Martin-Albright 273.4
  Masters-Allen 616.9
  mastocytosis 757.2
  Mauriac - *see* category 250
  McQuarrie 251
  meconium plug (newborn) NEC 778.9
  Meigs' 220.9
  Melkersson's 350
  Menetriere's 269.9
  Meniere's 385

Syndrome—*continued*
  menopause 627
  menstruation 626.9
  mesenteric
    artery, superior 537.9
    vascular insufficiency (with gangrene)
        444.2
  micrognathia-glossoptosis 756.0
  midbrain 347.9
  middle lobe (lung) 519.0
  migraine 346
    epilepsy (*see also* Epilepsy) 345.9
  Mikulicz's 527.8
  milk-alkali 999.9
  milk-drinker's 999.9
  Milkman's 265.2
  Millard-Gubler 344.1
  Minkowski-Chauffard (*see also*
        Spherocytosis) 282.0
  Moebius 350
  Moore's 345.9
  morbid hunger 347.9
  Morel-Moore 723.4
  Morel-Morgagni 723.4
  Morgagni-Stokes-Adams (*see also*
        Block, heart) 427.3
  Morgagni's 723.4
  Morquio 273.8
  Morton's (metatarsalgia) 357.9
  multiple
    deficiency 267
    operations 306.9
  Munchausen's 306.9
  ʌurdock's 273.8
  myasthenic, residual of viral
        encephalitis 066
  myelitic, residual of viral encephalitis
        066
  myeloproliferative 209
  Naffziger's 357.0
  nephrotic - *see* Nephrosis
  Niemann-Pick 272.2
  Nothnagel's 373.9.
  oculomotor 781.1
    residual of viral encephalitis 066
  opthalmoplegia-cerebellar ataxia 373.9
  osteoporosis-osteomalacia 265.2
  Ostrum-Furst 756.7
  otolith 387.9
  ovarian-ascites-pleural effusion 220.9
  pain - *see* Pain
  Pancoast's 162.1
    benign 212.3
  papillary muscle (*see also* Infarct,
        myocardium) 410.9
  paralysis agitans 342
    postencephalitic 066

Syndrome—*continued*
  Parinaud's 781.1
    oculoglandular 360
  Parkinson's (*see also* Parkinsonism)
    342
  parkinsonian (*see also* Parkinsonism)
    342
  Parry-Romberg 356
  Paterson(-Brown)(-Kelly) 280
  Pelger-Huet 289.9
  pellagroid 262
  Pellegrini-Stieda 729.8
  Pellizzi's 258.9
  pelvic congestion-fibrosis 616.2
  Pendred's 243
  Pepper's 194.0
  peptic ulcer - *see* Ulcer, peptic
  periodic 276
  Petges-Clejat or Petges-Clegat 716.0
  Peutz-Jeghers 211.9
  phantom limb 781.6
  Pick's
    heart 423
    liver 423
  Pickwickian 277
  Pierre Robin 756.0
  pineal 258.9
  placental
    dysfunction 770.9
    insufficiency 770.9
  Plummer-Vinson 280
  pluricarential of infancy 267
  plurideficiency 267
  pluriglandular (compensatory) 258.1
  polycarential of infancy 267
  polyglandular 258.1
  pontine 347.9
  postcardiotomy 997.1
  postcholecystectomy 998.9
  postcommissurotomy 997.1
  postencephalitic 066
    Parkinson's 066
  posterior cervical sympathicus 728.1
  postgastrectomy (dumping) 997.9
  postinfarction (*see also* Ischemia, heart)
    412.9
  postmastectomy lymphedema 997.3
  postmature 778.1
  postmyocardial infarct (*see also*
    Ischemia, heart) 412.9
  postoperative NEC 796.9
  postpartum panhypopituitary 253.1
  postphlebitic 458.9
  postvalvulotomy 997.1
  postviral NEC 790.1
  potassium intoxication 788.0
  Potter's 753.0

Syndrome—*continued*
  pre-infarction (*see also* Insufficiency,
    coronary) 411.9
  premature senility 258.9
  pre-ulcer 536.9
  Profichet's 729.9
  progressive pallidal degeneration
    331.9
  prolonged gestation 778.1
  pseudo-Paget's 723.0
  pulmonary
    arteriosclerosis 426
    distress (*see also* Syndrome,
      respiratory distress) 776.2
    renal (hemorrhagic) 446.1
    sulcus, superior 162.1
  pulseless 446.6
  pyloroduodenal 537.9
  pyramidopallidonigral 342
    residual of viral encephalitis 066
  radicular NEC 728.9
    lower
      limbs 728.8
    upper limbs 728.3
    newborn, due to or with birth
      injury (*see also* Birth injury,
      bone or nerve) 772.2
  Ramsay Hunt's - *see* Syndrome Hunt's
  Raymond-Cestan (*see also* Occlusion,
    precerebral artery) 432.9
  Refsum's 332.9
  Reiter's 136
  Rendu-Osler-Weber 448
  Renon-Delille 253.9
  respiratory distress 776.2
    with
      abnormality of bones, organs or
        tissues of pelvis - *see*
        categories 764.0-764.4
      abnormality of forces of labor - *see*
        categories 767.0-767.4
      difficult labor NEC - *see* categories
        768.0-768.4
      disproportion, fetopelvic - *see*
        categories 765.0-765.4
      with abnormality of bones,
        organs or tissues of pelvis
        - *see* categories 764.0-
        764.4
      malposition of fetus - *see* categories
        766.0-766.4
  restless leg 781.6
  retraction 744.8
  Reye's 347.9
  Riddoch's 781.0
  right ventricular obstruction - *see*
    Failure, heart, congestive

Syndrome—*continued*
  Turck's 744.8
  Turner-Varny 759.5
  Turner's 759.5
  Ullrich-Feichtiger 759.8
  Ullrich(-Bonnevie)(-Turner) 759.5
  underwater blast injury (abdominal) (*see also* Injury, internal, abdomen) 868.0
  Unverricht-Wagner 716.0
  Unverricht(-Lundborg) 331.2
  upward gaze 781.1
    postencephalitic 066
  uremia, chronic - *see* Uremia
  urethro-oculo-articular 136
  urohepatic 573.9
  vago-hypoglossal 344.9
  van der Hoeve's 756.6
  vasomotor 443.9
  vasovagal 782.5
  vena cava (inferior) (superior) (obstruction) 458.1
  Vernet's 344.9
  vertebral
    artery (*see also* Ischemia, cerebral, transient) 435.9
      compression 728.4
      lumbar 728.8
    steal (*see also* Ischemia, cerebral, transient) 435.9
  vertebrogenic (pain) - *see* category 728
  Villaret's 356
  Vinson-Plummer 280
  virus 079.9
  visceral larva migrans 128.0
  visual disorientation 781.0
  Vogt-Koyanagi 366
  Vogt's 331.9
  von Bechterew-Strumpell 712.4
  von Hippel-Lindau 759.8
  Wagner(-Unverricht) 716.0
  Waldenstrom 275.5
  Wallenberg's (*see also* Disease, cerebrovascular, acute) 436.9
  Wardenburg-Klein 270.8
  Waterhouse(-Friderichsen) 036.1
    with meningitis 036.0
  Weber-Christian 686.9
  Weber-Cockayne 757.2
  Weber-Gubler 344.1
  Weber-Osler 448
  Weber's 344.1
  Wegener's 446.3
  Weiss-Baker 358.1
  Werdnig-Hoffman 330.1
  Werner 258.9

Syndrome—*continued*
  Wernicke's 263.9
  Westphal-Strumpell 273.3
  whiplash 847.0
  Wilson-Mikity (*see also* Syndrome, respiratory distress) 776.2
  Wilson's 273.3
  Wolff-Parkinson-White (*see also* Tachycardia, paroxysmal) 427.5
  Wright 447
  xiphoidalgia 355.1
  yellow vernix 770.9
  Zieve's 571.0
  Zollinger-Ellison 251
Synechia (anterior) (posterior) (pupil) 378.6
Synesthesia (*see also* Disturbance, sensation) 781.6
Synophthalmus 759.2
Synorchidism 752.1
Synorchism 752.1
Synostosis (congenital) 756.7
  astragalo-scaphoid 755.7
  radio-ulnar 755.5
Synovial - *see* condition
Synovioma (*see also* Neoplasm, connective tissue, malignant) 171.9
  benign 215
Synoviosarcoma (*see also* Neoplasm, connective tissue, malignant) 171.9
Synovitis (crepitating) (infective) (pigmented villonodular) (pneumococcal) (purulent) (septic) (staphylococcal) (streptococcal) (suppurative) (traumatic (old)) (villous) 731.9
  ankle 731.7
  buttock 731.5
  elbow 731.2
  finger 731.4
  foot 731.8
  gonococcal 098.3
  gouty 274
  hand 731.4
  hip 731.5
  knee 731.6
  shoulder 731.1
  spine 731.0
  syphilitic 095
    congenital 090.0
  toe 731.8
  traumatic, current - *see* Sprain
  tuberculous - *see* Tuberculosis, synovitis
  wrist 731.3

Syphilide   091.2
  congenital   090.0
  newborn   090.0
  tubercular   095
    congenital   090.0
Syphilis, syphilitic (acquired)   097.9
  abdomen (late)   095
  acoustic nerve   094.9
  adrenal (gland)   095
    with cortical hypofunction   095
  age under 1 year NEC   090.9
    acquired   097.9
  alopecia (secondary)   091.8
  anemia   095
  aneurysm (artery) (ruptured)   093.9
    aorta   093.0
    central nervous system   094.9
    congenital   090.5
  anus   095
  aorta (arch) (abdominal) (pulmonary)
      (thoracic)   093.9
    aneurysm   093.0
  aortic (insufficiency) (regurgitation)
      (stenosis)   093.9
  arachnoid (adhesive)   094.9
  arrested, follow-up examination   Y03.9
  artery   093.9
    cerebral   094.9
    spinal   094.9
  asymptomatic - see Syphilis, latent
  ataxia (locomotor)   094.0
  atrophoderma maculatum   091.2
  auricular fibrillation   093.9
  Bell's palsy   094.9
  bladder   095
  bone   095
  brain   094.9
  breast   095
  bronchus   095
  bubo   091.0
  bulbar palsy   094.9
  bursa (late)   095
  cardiac decompensation   093.9
  cardiovascular (early) (late) (primary)
      (secondary) (tertiary)   093.9
  causing death under 1 year of age (see
      also Syphilis, congenital)   090.9
    stated to be acquired NEC   097.9
  central nervous system (any site)
      (asymptomatic) (early) (late)
      (latent) (primary) (recurrent)
      (relapse) (secondary) (tertiary)
      094.9
    with
      ataxia   094.0

Syphilis, etc. — continued
  central nervous system, etc. — continued
    with — continued
      paralysis general   094.1
        juvenile   090.4
      paresis (general)   094.1
        juvenile   090.4
      tabes (dorsalis)   094.0
        juvenile   090.4
      taboparesis   094.1
        juvenile   090.4
    aneurysm   094.9
    congenital   090.4
    remission in (sustained)   094.9
    serology doubtful, negative, or
        positive   094.9
    vascular   094.9
  cerebral   094.9
    meningovascular   094.9
    nerves   094.9
    sclerosis   094.9
    thrombosis   094.9
  cerebrospinal   094.9
    tabetic type   094.0
  cerebrovascular   094.9
  cervix   095
  chancre (multiple)   091.0
    extragenital   091.1
    Rollet's   091.0
  Charcot's joint   094.0
  choked disc   094.9
  choroid (late)   095
    vessels   093.9
  choroiditis (late)   095
    congenital   090.0
    prenatal   090.0
  choroidoretinitis   095
  ciliary body   095
    secondary   091.8
  colon (late)   095
  combined sclerosis   094.9
  condyloma (latum)   091.2
  congenital   090.9
    with
      paresis (general)   090.4
      tabes (dorsalis)   090.4
      taboparesis   090.4
    early, or less than 5 years after birth
        NEC   090.2
      with manifestations   090.0
      latent (without manifestations)
          090.1
        negative spinal fluid test   090.1
        serology, positive   090.1
      symptomatic   090.0
    interstitial keratitis   090.3

Syphilis, etc. — *continued*
  congenital — *continued*
    juvenile neurosyphilis   090.4
    late, or 5 years or more after birth
      NEC   090.7
      latent (without manifestations)
        090.6
        negative spinal fluid test   090.6
        scrology, positive   090.6
      symptomatic or with manifestations
        NEC   090.5
        interstitial keratitis   090.3
        juvenile neurosyphilis   090.4
  conjugal   097.9
    tabes   094.0
  conjunctiva   095
  cord bladder   094.0
  cornea, late   095
  coronary (artery)   093.9
    sclerosis   093.9
  cranial nerve   094.9
  cutaneous - *see* Syphilis, skin
  d'emblee   095
  dacryocystitis   095
  degeneration, spinal cord   094.9
  dementia
    paralytica   094.1
      juvenilis   090.4
  destruction of bone   095
  dilatation, aorta   093.0
  due to blood transfusion   097.9
  dura mater   094.9
  ear   095
    inner   095
      nerve (eighth)   094.9
      neurorecurrence   094.9
  early   091.9
    cardiovascular   093.9
    central nervous system   094.9
      paresis   094.1
      tabes   094.0
    latent (without manifestations) (less
      than 2 years after infection)
      092.9
      negative spinal fluid test   092.9
      serological relapse after treatment
        092.0
      serology positive   092.9
    paresis   094.1
    relapse (treated, untreated)   091.3
    skin   091.2
    symptomatic NEC   091.8
      extragenital chancre   091.1
      primary, except extragenital
        chancre   091.0
      secondary skin, mucous membrane
        091.2

Syphilis, etc. — *continued*
  early — *continued*
    symptomatic NEC — *continued*
      secondary skin, etc. — *continued*
        relapse (treated, untreated)
          091.3
      tabes   094.0
      ulcer   091.2
  eighth nerve   094.9
  epididymis (late)   095
  epiglottis   095
  epiphysitis (congenital)   090.0
  esophagus   095
  eustachian tube   095
  eye   095
    neuromuscular mechanism   094.9
  eyelid   095
    with gumma   095
    ptosis   094.9
  fallopian tube   095
  fracture   095
  gallbladder (late)   095
  gastric   095
    crisis   094.0
    polyposis   095
  general   097.9
    paralysis   094.1
      juvenile   090.4
  gumma   095
    cardiovascular system   093.9
    central nervous system   094.9
    congenital   090.5
  heart   093.9
    block   093.9
    decompensation   093.9
    disease   093.9
    failure   093.9
  hemianesthesia   094.9
  hemianopsia   095
  hemiparesis   094.9
  hemiplegia   094.9
  hepatic artery   093.9
  hepatis   095
  hereditaria tarda (*see also* Syphilis,
    congenital, late)   090.7
  hereditary (*see also* Syphilis, congenital)
    090.9
    interstitial keratitis   090.3
  hyalitis   095
  inactive - *see* Syphilis, latent
  infantum NEC   090.9
  inherited - *see* Syphilis, congenital
  internal ear   095
  intestine (late)   095
  iris, iritis   095
    secondary   091.8

Syphilis, etc. — *continued*
  optic nerve (atrophy) (neuritis) (papilla) 094.9
  orbit (late) 095
  organic 097.9
  osseous (late) 095
  osteochondritis (congenital) 090.0
  osteoporosis 095
  ovary 095
  oviduct 095
  palate 095
  pancreas (late) 095
  pancreatitis 095
  paralysis 094.9
    general 094.1
    juvenile 090.4
  paresis (general) 094.1
    juvenile 090.4
  paresthesia 094.9
  Parkinson's disease or syndrome 094.9
  paroxysmal tachycardia 093.9
  pemphigus (congenital) 090.0
  penis 091.0
    chancre 091.0
    late 095
  pericardium 093.9
  perichondritis, larynx 095
  periosteum 095
    congenital 090.0
    early 091.8
  peripheral nerve 095
  petrous bone (late) 095
  pharynx 095
  pituitary (gland) 095
  placenta 095
  pleura (late) 095
  pontine lesion 094.9
  portal vein 093.9
  primary 091.0
    and secondary 091.2
    cardiovascular 093.9
    central nervous system 094.9
    extragenital chancre 091.1
  prostate 095
  ptosis (eyelid) 094.9
  pulmonary (late) 095
    artery 093.9
  pulmonum 095
  pyelonephritis 095
  recently acquired, symptomatic NEC 091.8
  rectum 095
  respiratory tract 095
  retina (late) 095
    neurorecidive 094.9

Syphilis, etc. — *continued*
  retrobulbar neuritis 094.9
  salpingitis 095
  sclera (late) 095
  sclerosis
    cerebral 094.9
    coronary 093.9
    multiple 094.9
    subacute 094.9
  scotoma (central) 095
  scrotum 095
  secondary (and primary) 091.2
    cardiovascular 093.9
    central nervous system 094.9
    mucous membranes 091.2
    relapse (treated, untreated) 091.3
    skin 091.2
    ulcer 091.2
  seminal vesicle (late) 095
  seronegative
    with signs or symptoms - *code by* site and stage under Syphilis
    follow-up of latent syphilis (not needing further care) Y03.9
  seropositive
    with signs or symptoms - *code by* site and stage under Syphilis
    follow-up of latent syphilis - *see* Syphilis, latent
    only finding - *see* Syphilis, latent
  seventh nerve (paralysis) 094.9
  sinus 095
  sinusitis 095
  skeletal system 095
  skin (with ulceration) (early) (secondary) 091.2
    late or tertiary 095
  small intestine 095
  spastic spinal paralysis 094.0
  spermatic cord (late) 095
  spinal (cord) 094.9
    with
      paresis 094.1
      tabes 094.0
  spleen 095
  splenomegaly 095
  spondylitis 095
  staphyloma 095
  stigmata (congenital) 090.5
  stomach 095
  tabes dorsalis (early) (late) 094.0
    juvenile 090.4
  tabetic type 094.0
    juvenile 090.4
  taboparesis 094.1
    juvenile 090.4

T

Tab - *see* Tag
Tabacism 989.9
Tabacosis 989.9

Tabardillo 080
  flea-borne 081.0
  louse-borne 080

Tabes, tabetic
  with
    central nervous system syphilis
      094.0
    Charcot's joint 094.0
    cord bladder 094.0
    crisis, viscera (any) 094.0
    paralysis, general 094.1
    paresis (general) 094.1
    perforating ulcer 094.0
  arthropathy 094.0
  bladder 094.0
  bone 094.0
  cerebrospinal 094.0
  congenital 090.4
  conjugal 094.0
  dorsalis 094.0
    neurosyphilis 094.0
  early 094.0
  juvenile 090.4
  latent 094.0
  mesenterica 014
    late effect or sequela 019.9
  paralysis insane, general 094.1
  spasmodic 094.0
    not dorsal or dorsalis - *see* Palsy,
      cerebral
  syphilis (cerebrospinal) 094.0

Taboparalysis 094.1

Taboparesis (remission) 094.1
  with
    Charcot's joint 094.1
    cord bladder 094.1
    perforating ulcer 094.1
  juvenile 090.4

Tachycardia 782.2
  atrial (*see also* Action, heart, irregular)
    427.9
  auricular (*see also* Action, heart,
    irregular) 427.9
  nodal (*see also* Action, heart, irregular)
    427.9
  paroxysmal (atrium) (auricle) (junctional)
    (nodal) (supraventricular) 427.5

Tachycardia — *continued*
  paroxysmal — *continued*
    with
      hypertension (benign) (conditions in
        401) (*see also* Hypertension,
        heart) 402
      malignant (*see also*
        Hypertension, malignant
        with heart involvement)
        400.1
    psychogenic 305.3
  psychogenic 305.3
  sino-auricular (*see also* Action, heart,
    irregular) 427.9
  sinus (*see also* Action, heart, irregular)
    427.9
  supraventricular (*see also* Action, heart,
    irregular) 427.9
  ventricular (paroxysmal) (*see also*
    Action, heart, irregular) 427.9

Tachypnea 783.2
  hysterical 300.1
  psychogenic 305.2

Taenia (infection) (infestation) (*see also*
  Infestation, taenia) 123.3
  diminuta 123.6
  nana 123.6
  saginata 123.2
  solium (intestinal form) 123.0
    larval form 123.1

Taeniasis (intestine) (*see also* Infestation,
  taenia) 123.3

Taenzer's disease 757.2

Tag (hypertrophied skin) (infected) 701.9
  adenoid 500
  anus (bleeding) (external) (internal)
    (prolapsed) (strangulated)
    (thrombosed) (ulcerated) 455
  hemorrhoidal 455
  hymen 629.9
  perineal 629.9
  rectum (bleeding) (external) (internal)
    (prolapsed) (strangulated)
    (thrombosed) (ulcerated) 455
  skin 701.9
    accessory 757.2
    congenital 757.2
  tonsil 500
  urethra, urethral 599.9
  vulva 629.9

Takayasu's disease or syndrome 446.6

Talipes (congenital) 754.9
  acquired (any type except planus)
      738.6
  calcaneovalgus 754.2
  calcaneovarus 754.8
  calcaneus 754.8
  cavus 754.0
  equinovalgus 754.8
  equinovarus 754.1
  equinus 754.8
  percavus 754.0
  planovalgus 754.8
  planus (acquired) (any degree) 736
    congenital 755.7
    due to rickets 265.1
  postpoliomyelitic 044
  valgus 754.8
  varus 754.8
Talma's disease 733.9
Tamponade heart (Rose's) (see also
      Pericarditis) 423
Tangier disease 272.1
Tantrum (childhood) 308
Tapeworm (infection) (infestation) (see
      also Infestation, tapeworm) 123.9
Tapia's syndrome 344.9
Tar cancer - see Neoplasm, skin,
      malignant
Tarsalgia 355.1
Tarsitis 361
  eyelid 361
    syphilitic 095
    tuberculous 017.0
  syphilis, syphilitic 095
  tuberculous 015.8
    late effect or sequela 019.6
Tartar (teeth) 523.6
Tattoo (mark) 709.1
Taurodontism 520.2
Taussig-Bing heart or syndrome 746.1
Tay-Sachs
  amaurotic familial idiocy 333.0
  disease 333.0
Tay's choroiditis 365
Taylor's disease 701.9
Tear-stone 378.3
Tear, torn (traumatic) - see also Wound,
      open
  anus, anal (sphincter) - see also Injury,
      internal, anus
    complicating delivery - see
        Laceration, perineum,
        complicating delivery
    nontraumatic, nonpuerperal 565.0
  articular cartilage, old - see
      Derangement, joint

Tear, torn, etc. - continued
  bladder, complicating delivery - see
      Obstetrical trauma
  capsule, joint - see Sprain
  cartilage - see also Sprain
    articular, old - see Derangement, joint
    knee - see Dislocation, knee
  cervix, complicating delivery - see
      Laceration, cervix, complicating
      delivery
  internal organ (abdomen, chest, or
      pelvis) - see Injury, internal, by
      site
  ligament - see Sprain
  meniscus (knee) (current injury) 836.0
    with open wound - see Wound, open
    late effect 836.9
    old 724.5
      elbow 724.3
      shoulder 724.1
    site other than knee - code as Sprain
  muscle - see Sprain
  pelvic
    floor, complicating delivery - see
        Laceration, perineum,
        complicating delivery
    organ, complicating delivery - see
        Obstetrical trauma
  perineum, complicating delivery - see
      Laceration, perineum,
      complicating delivery
  rectovaginal septum, complicating
      delivery - see Laceration,
      perineum, complicating delivery
  retina, retinal (nontraumatic) 376
  semilunar cartilage, knee - see also
      Dislocation, knee
    old 724.5
  tendon - see Sprain
  tentorial, at birth (see also Birth injury,
      brain) 772.0
  umbilical cord - see Complications,
      umbilical cord
  urethra, complicating delivery - see
      Laceration, urethra, complicating
      delivery
  uterus, complicating delivery - see
      Obstetrical trauma
  vagina, complicating delivery - see
      Laceration, perineum,
      complicating delivery
  vulva, complicating delivery - see
      Laceration, perineum,
      complicating delivery
Teeth - see condition
Teething 520.7

Teething—*continued*
syndrome 520.7
Telangiectasia, telangiectasis (congenital)
(hemorrhagic) (hereditary) (senile)
(simple) (spider) 448
ataxic (cerebellar) 275.0
Telescoped
bowel or intestine (*see also*
Intussusception) 560.0
Teletherapy, adverse effect 990.4
Temperature
body, high (of unknown origin) (*see also*
Pyrexia) 788.6
cold, trauma from NEC 991.9
newborn 778.3
Temple - *see* condition
Temporal - *see* condition
Temporosphenoidal - *see* condition
Tendency
bleeding (*see also* Defect, coagulation)
286.9
homosexual 302.0
paranoid 301.0
suicide 300.9
Tendinitis, tendonitis - *see also*
Tenosynovitis
adhesive (scapulohumeral) (shoulder)
717.1
Tendon - *see* condition
Tendosynovitis - *see* Tenosynovitis
Tendovaginitis - *see* Tenosynovitis
Tenesmus 785.5
rectal 785.5
vesical 786.0
Tennis elbow 731.2
Tenonitis - *see also* Tenosynovitis
eye (capsule) 369.9
Tenontosynovitis - *see* Tenosynovitis
Tenontothecitis - *see* Tenosynovitis
Tenophyte 733.9
Tenosynovitis (calcareous) (calcific)
(crepitans) (fibrinous) (purulent)
(serous) (stenosans) (suppurative)
(villous) 731.9
adhesive (shoulder) 717.1
ankle 731.7
bicipital (calcifying) 731.1
buttock 731.5
elbow 731.2
finger 731.4
foot 731.8
gonococcal 098.3
hand 731.4
hip 731.5
knee 731.6

Tenosynovitis—*continued*
shoulder 731.1
adhesive 717.1
spine 731.0
supraspinatous 731.1
toe 731.8
tuberculous - *see* Tuberculosis,
tenosynovitis
wrist 731.3
Tenovaginitis - *see* Tenosynovitis
Tension
arterial, high (*see also* Hypertension)
401
headache 306.8
nervous 790.0
premenstrual 626.9
state 300.9
Tentorium - *see* condition
Teratencephalus 759.2
Teratism 759.2
Teratocarcinoma (*see also* Neoplasm,
malignant) 199.1
liver 155.0
Teratoma (cystic) (benign) - *see also*
Neoplasm, benign
bladder 223.3
broad ligament 221.0
coccygeal body 226.8
craniobuccal pouch 226.2
embryonal - *see also* Neoplasm,
malignant
liver 155.0
fallopian tube 221.0
kidney 223.0
pelvis 223.1
malignant - *see also* Neoplasm,
malignant
liver 155.0
mediastinum 212.5
orbit 224
ovary (solid) 220.0
oviduct 221.0
palate 210.4
pharynx 210.9
pineal gland 226.3
prostate 222.8
sacrococcygeal 228
scrotum 222.8
seminal vesicle 222.8
suprasellar 225.0
testis 186
benign 222.0
thymus (gland) 226.1
thyroid (gland) 226.8
uterus 219.9

Termination
  anomalous - *see also* Malposition,
        congenital
    portal vein   747.4
    right pulmonary vein   747.4
  pregnancy - *see* Abortion by type
    fetus NEC   773
Ternidens diminutus infestation   127.4
Terrors, night (child)   308
Tertiary - *see* condition
Tessellated fundus, retina (tigroid)   377.4
Test(s)
  allergy (skin sensitization)   Y01
  basal metabolic rate   Y00.0
  dextrose tolerance   Y00.3
  laboratory   Y00.3
  only (type unspecified)   Y00.3
  sensitization   Y01
  skin immunity   Y01
  tuberculin   Y01
  Wasserman
    positive   097.1
Testicle, testicular, testis - *see* condition
Tetanus, tetanic (cephalic) (convulsions)
        (neonatorum)   037
  with
    abortion - *see* Abortion, by type, with
        sepsis
    ectopic gestation - *see* categories
        631.0-631.3
  inoculation
    reaction (due to serum) - *see*
        Complications, vaccination
  puerperal, postpartum, childbirth   670
Tetany   788.5
  alkalosis   788.0
  associated with rickets   265.0
  convulsions   788.5
    hysterical   300.1
  functional (hysterical)   300.1
  hyperkinetic   788.5
    hysterical   300.1
  hyperpnea   783.2
    hysterical   300.1
    psychogenic   305.2
  hyperventilation   783.2
    hysterical   300.1
    psychogenic   305.2
  hysterical   300.1
  parathyroid (gland)   252.1
  parathyroprival   252.1
  postoperative   998.9
  post-thyroidectomy   998.9
  pseudo   788.5
    hysterical   300.1
  psychogenic   305.2

Tetany — *continued*
  psychogenic — *continued*
    specified as conversion reaction
        300.1
Tetralogy of Fallot   746.2
Tetraplegia - *see* Quadriplegia
Thalassanemia (*see also* Thalassemia)
        282.4
Thalassemia (disease) (Hb C) (Hb D) (Hb
        E) (Hb H) (Hb I) (Hb S) (high fetal
        gene) (high fetal hemoglobin)
        (major) (minor) (mixed) (sickle cell)
        282.4
  with other abnormal hemoglobin NEC
        282.4
Thalassemic variants (*see also*
        Thalassemia)   282.4
Thecoma (ovary)   256.0
  malignant   183.0
Thelitis   611.0
  puerperal, postpartum   678
Therapeutic - *see* condition
Thermic - *see* condition
Thermoplegia   992.0
Thesaurismosis, glycogen (*see also*
        Disease, glycogen storage)   271.1
Thiaminic deficiency   261
Thibierge-Weissenbach syndrome   734.0
Thickening
  bone   723.9
  breast   611.1
  hymen   629.9
  larynx   508.3
  nail   703.9
    congenital   757.4
  periosteal   723.9
  pleura (*see also* Pleurisy)   511.0
  subepiglottic   508.3
  tongue   529.9
  valve, heart - *see* Endocarditis
Thiele syndrome   728.9
Thigh - *see* condition
Thinning vertebra   723.9
Thirst   994.3
Thomsen's disease   330.9
Thomson's disease   757.2
Thoracic - *see also* condition
  kidney   753.3
  stomach - *see* Hernia, diaphragm
Thoracogastroschisis (congenital)   758.8
Thoracopagus   759.1
Thorax - *see* condition
Thorn syndrome (*see also* Lesion, kidney)
        593.2
Thornwaldt's
  cyst   508.9
  disease   508.9

Thorson-Biorck syndrome   258.9
Threadworm (infection) (infestation)
    127.1
Threatened
    abortion (undelivered)   632.3
        with subsequent abortion - see
            Abortion, by type
        complicating subsequent delivery
            651.9
        fetus or newborn   769.9
    miscarriage (undelivered)   632.3
        with subsequent abortion - see
            Abortion, spontaneous
        complicating subsequent delivery
            651.9
        fetus or newborn   769.9
    premature delivery (undelivered)   632.3
        complicating subsequent delivery
            651.9
        fetus or newborn   769.9
Thrix annulata (congenital)   757.3
Throat - see condition
Thrombasthenia (Glanzmann)   287.3
Thrombo-angiitis   443.1
    obliterans (general)   443.1
        cerebral (see also Ischemia, cerebral)
            437.9
        vessels
            brain (see also Ischemia, cerebral)
                437.9
            spinal cord (see also Ischemia,
                cerebral)   437.9
Thrombo-arteritis - see Arteritis
Thrombocytasthenia (Glanzmann)   287.3
Thrombocythemia   289.9
    hemorrhagic   287.2
Thrombocytopathy   287.3
    dystrophic   287.3
    granulopenic   287.3
Thrombocytopenia, thrombocytopenic
        (acute) (allergic) (amegakaryocytic,
        primary) (anemia) (chronic)
        (congenital) (essential) (Frank's)
        (hereditary) (hypoplastic)
        (idiopathic) (infectional) (secondary)
        (splenic) (with hemangioma) (with
        skeletal abnormalities)   287.1
    puerperal, postpartum   675
Thrombocytosis, essential   289.9
Thrombo-embolism - see Embolism
Thrombopathy (Bernard-Soulier)   287.3
    constitutional   286.3
    Willebrand-Jurgens'   286.3
Thrombopenia (essential) (primary)
        (purpura) (see also
        Thrombocytopenia)   287.1

Thrombophlebitis   451.9
    with
        abortion - see Abortion, by type, with
            sepsis
        ectopic gestation - see categories
            631.0-631.3
    cavernous (venous) sinus - see
        Thrombophlebitis, intracranial
        venous sinus
    cerebral (sinus) (vein)   321
        late effects   324
        nonpyogenic (see also Disease,
            cerebrovascular NEC)   438.9
    complicating pregnancy   634.9
        fetus or newborn   763.9
    femoral   451.0
    hepatic (vein)   451.9
    idiopathic, recurrent   453
    ilio-femoral   451.0
    intracranial venous sinus (any)   321
        late effects   324
        nonpyogenic (see also Disease,
            cerebrovascular NEC)   438.9
    lateral (venous) sinus - see
        Thrombophlebitis, intracranial
        venous sinus
    leg   451.0
    longitudinal (venous) sinus - see
        Thrombophlebitis, intracranial
        venous sinus
    lower extremity   451.0
    migrans, migrating   453
    portal (vein)   572
    puerperal, postpartum, childbirth
        671.9
        intracranial venous sinus   674
        lower extremities   671.0
        pelvic (vein)   671.9
        specified site NEC   677.9
    sinus (intracranial) - see
        Thrombophlebitis, intracranial
        venous sinus
    specified site NEC   451.9
Thrombosis, thrombotic (marantic)
        (multiple) (progressive) (septic)
        (vein) (vessel)   453
    with
        abortion - see Abortion, by type, with
            sepsis
        childbirth or during the puerperium
            - see Thrombosis, puerperal,
            postpartum, childbirth
        ectopic gestation - see categories
            631.0-631.3
    aorta, aortic   444.1
        abdominal   444.0

Thrombosis, etc. — *continued*
  aorta, aortic — *continued*
    bifurcation 444.0
    saddle 444.0
    thoracic 444.1
    valve - *see* Endocarditis, aortic
  apoplexy (*see also* Thrombosis, brain)
      433.9
  appendix, septic 540.9
    with peritonitis, perforation, or
        rupture 540.0
  arteries of extremities 444.4
  artery (postinfectional) 444.9
    auditory, internal (*see also* Occlusion,
        precerebral artery) 432.9
    basilar (*see also* Occlusion,
        precerebral artery) 432.9
    carotid (common) (internal) (*see also*
        Occlusion, precerebral artery)
        432.9
    cerebellar (anterior inferior) (posterior
        inferior) (superior) (*see also*
        Occlusion, precerebral artery)
        432.9
    cerebral (*see also* Thrombosis, brain)
        433.9
    choroidal (anterior) (*see also*
        Occlusion, precerebral artery)
        432.9
    communicating posterior (*see also*
        Occlusion, precerebral artery)
        432.9
    coronary (*see also* Infarct,
        myocardium) 410.9
      due to syphilis 093.9
    hepatic 444.9
    hypophyseal (*see also* Occlusion,
        precerebral artery) 432.9
    lower extremity 444.4
    meningeal, anterior or posterior (*see
        also* Occlusion, precerebral
        artery) 432.9
    mesenteric (with gangrene) 444.2
    ophthalmic 377.0
    pontine (*see also* Occlusion,
        precerebral artery) 432.9
    pulmonary 450
    retinal 377.0
    spinal, anterior or posterior (*see also*
        Occlusion, precerebral artery)
        432.9
    traumatic (complication) (early)
        995.3
    vertebral (left) (right) (*see also*
        Occlusion, precerebral artery)
        432.9

Thrombosis, etc. — *continued*
  auricular (*see also* Infarct, myocardium)
      410.9
  basilar (artery) (*see also* Occlusion,
      precerebral artery) 432.9
  bland NEC 453
  brain (artery) (stem) 433.9
    with
      hypertension (benign) (conditions in
          401) 433.0
        malignant (*see also*
            Hypertension, malignant
            with cerebrovascular
            involvement) 400.2
    due to
      syphilis 094.9
    puerperal, postpartum, childbirth
        674
    sinus (*see also* Thrombosis,
        intracranial venous sinus) 321
  capillary 448
  cardiac (*see also* Infarct, myocardium)
      410.9
    due to syphilis 093.9
    valve - *see* Endocarditis
  carotid (artery) (common) (internal) (*see
      also* Occlusion, precerebral
      artery) 432.9
  cavernous (venous) sinus - *see*
      Thrombosis, intracranial venous
      sinus
  cerebral (*see also* Thrombosis, brain)
      433.9
  complicating pregnancy 634.9
  coronary (artery) (*see also* Infarct,
      myocardium) 410.9
    due to syphilis 093.9
  corpus cavernosum 607.9
  cortical (*see also* Thrombosis, brain)
      433.9
  endocardial - *see* Infarct, myocardium
  eye 377.0
  femoral 453
    artery 444.4
  heart (chamber) (*see also* Infarct,
      myocardium) 410.9
  hepatic 453
    artery 444.9
  iliac 453
    artery 444.9
  intestine (with gangrene) 444.2
  intracranial (*see also* Thrombosis, brain)
      433.9
    venous sinus (any) 321
      late effects 324

Thrombosis, etc. — *continued*
  intracranial — *continued*
    venous sinus — *continued*
      nonpyogenic origin (*see also*
        Disease, cerebrovascular
        NEC) 438.9
  intramural - *see* Infarct, myocardium
  jugular (bulb) 453
  kidney (*see also* Lesion, kidney) 593.2
    artery 444.3
  lateral (venous) sinus - *see* Thrombosis,
    intracranial venous sinus
  liver 453
    artery 444.9
  longitudinal (venous) sinus - *see*
    Thrombosis, intracranial venous
    sinus
  lung 450
  meninges (brain) (*see also* Thrombosis,
    brain) 433.9
  mesenteric (artery) (with gangrene)
    444.2
  mitral - *see* Endocarditis, mitral
  mural (*see also* Infarct, myocardium)
    410.9
    due to syphilis 093.9
  omentum (with gangrene) 444.2
  ophthalmic (artery) 377.0
  parietal (*see also* Infarct, myocardium)
    410.9
  penis, penile 607.9
  peripheral arteries 444.4
  portal 452
    due to
      syphilis 093.9
  precerebral artery (*see also* Occlusion,
    precerebral artery) 432.9
  puerperal, postpartum, childbirth
    671.9
    brain or cerebral (artery) 674
    cardiac 677.9
    intracranial venous sinus 674
    lower extremity 671.0
    pelvic 671.9
    pulmonary (artery) 673.9
    septic (any site) 670
    specified site NEC 677.9
  pulmonary (artery) 450
  renal (*see also* Lesion, kidney) 593.2
    artery 444.3
  resulting from insertion of shunt or
    other internal prosthetic device
    997.6
  retina, retinal (artery) 377.0
  scrotum 607.9
  seminal vesicle 607.9

Thrombosis, etc. — *continued*
  sigmoid (venous) sinus - *see*
    Thrombosis, intracranial venous
    sinus
  silent NEC 453
  sinus, intracranial (any) (*see also*
    Thrombosis, intracranial venous
    sinus) 321
  spermatic cord 607.9
  spinal cord (*see also* Disease,
    cerebrovascular NEC) 438.9
    due to syphilis 094.9
    pyogenic origin 322
      late effects 324
  spleen, splenic 289.5
    artery 444.9
  testis 607.9
  traumatic (complication) (early) 995.3
  tricuspid - *see* Endocarditis, tricuspid
  tunica vaginalis 607.9
  umbilical cord - *see* Complications,
    umbilical cord
  vas deferens 607.9
  vena cava (inferior) (superior) 453
Thrombus - *see* Thrombosis
Thrush (any site) 112
Thumb - *see also* condition
  sucking (child problem) 308
Thymergasia (*see also* Psychosis, manic-
  depressive) 296.9
Thymitis 254
Thymoma 226.1
  malignant 194.2
Thymus, thymic (gland) - *see* condition
Thyrocele 240.9
Thyroglossal - *see also* condition
  cyst 758.2
  duct, persistent 758.2
Thyroid (gland) (body) - *see* condition
Thyroiditis (auto-immune) (suppurative)
  245.9
  acute 245.0
    nonsuppurative 245.0
  chronic (lymphomatous) 245.1
    lymphadenoid 245.1
    lymphocytic 245.1
  de Quervain 245.0
  giant
    cell 245.0
    follicular 245.0
  granulomatous (subacute) (de Quervain)
    245.0
  invasive 245.1
  ligneous 245.1
  lymphoid 245.1
  pseudotuberculous 245.0

Thyroiditis—*continued*
  Riedel's 245.1
  subacute 245.0
  tuberculous 017.9
    late effect or sequela 019.9
  woody 245.1
Thyrolingual duct, persistent 758.2
Thyrosarcoma 193
Thyrotoxic
  heart failure (*see also* Thyrotoxicosis)
    242.2
  storm (*see also* Thyrotoxicosis) 242.2
Thyrotoxicosis (recurrent) 242.2
  with
    adenoma, thyroid (gland) 242.1
    goiter (diffuse) 242.0
      adenomatous 242.1
        nodular 242.1
Tibia vara 738.5
Tic 306.2
  breathing 306.2
  child problem 306.2
  compulsive 300.3
  convulsive 306.2
  degenerative (generalized) 347.9
    localized 347.9
      facial 350
  douloureux 351
  habit 306.2
  lid 306.2
  occupational 300.8
  orbicularis 306.2

  postchoreic - *see* Chorea
  residual of viral encephalitis 066
  spasm 306.2
Tick-borne - *see* condition
Tics and spasms, compulsive 300.3
Tietze's disease or syndrome 729.9
Tight fascia (lata) 733.9
Tightness
  anus 564.9
  foreskin (congenital) 605
  hymen 629.9
  rectal sphincter 564.9
  tendon 733.9
    Achilles (heel) 733.4
  urethral sphincter 599.9
Tilting vertebra 735.9
Tin miners' lung 516.0
Tinea (circinata (corporis)) (corporis)
    (cruris) (favosa) (glabrosa)
    (imbricata) (intersecta) (tarsi)
    (trichophytina) (ungium) 110.9
  amiantacea 110.0
  asbestina 110.0
  barbae 110.0

Tinea—*continued*
  beard 110.0
  blanca 111.2
  capitis 110.0
  decalvans (*see also* Alopecia) 704
  flava 111.0
  foot 110.1
  furfuracea 110.0
  lepothrix 111.8
  nigra 111.1
  nodosa 111.2
  pedis 110.1
  scalp 110.0
  sycosis 110.0
  tonsurans 110.0
  versicolor 111.0
Tinnitus (audible) (aurium) (subjective)
    781.3
Tipping pelvis 738.8
  complicating delivery - *see* Deformity,
    pelvis, complicating delivery
  noted during pregnancy (undelivered)
    634.9
Tissue - *see* condition
Tobacco heart 989.9
Tocopherol deficiency 266.8
Todd's
  cirrhosis - *see* Cirrhosis, biliary
  paralysis 345.5
Toe - *see* condition
Tokelau ringworm - *see* Dermatophytosis
Tollwut 071
Tommaselli's disease 961.3
Tongue - *see also* condition
  works 134.2
Tonguetie 750.0
Toni-Fanconi syndrome 270.2
Tonic
  pupil 378.6
Tonsil - *see* condition
Tonsillitis (acute) (catarrhal) (croupous)
    (follicular) (gangrenous) (infective)
    (lacunar) (lingual) (malignant)
    (membranous) (phlegmonous)
    (pneumococcal)
    (pseudomembranous) (purulent)
    (septic) (staphylococcal) (subacute)
    (suppurative) (toxic) (ulcerative)
    (vesicular) (viral) 463
  with
    influenza, flu, or grippe 472
  chronic 500
  diphtheritic 032
  hypertrophic 500
  influenzal 472
  parenchymatous 501

Tonsillitis — *continued*
  streptococcal 034.0
  tuberculous 012.9
    with pneumoconiosis (conditions in
      515) 010
    late effect or sequela 019.0
  Vincent's 101
Tonsillopharyngitis 465
Tooth, teeth - *see* condition
Toothache 525.9
Topagnosis 781.6
Tophi 274
  gouty 274
Torn - *see* Tear, torn
Torpid liver 573.9
Torsion
  adnexa (female) 615.9
  aorta (congenital) 747.2
  bile duct (*see also* Disease, gallbladder)
    576.9
    congenital 751.5
  bowel, colon or intestine 560.2
    with hernia - *see* Hernia, by site, with
      obstruction
  cervix (*see also* Malposition, uterus)
    624.9
  dystonia 331.1
  epididymis 607.7
    appendix 607.7
  fallopian tube 615.9
  gallbladder (*see also* Disease,
    gallbladder) 576.9
    congenital 751.6
  hydatid of Morgagni 752.8
  kidney (pedicle) (*see also* Lesion,
    kidney) 593.2
  Meckel's diverticulum (congenital)
    751.0
  mesentery or omentum 560.2
    with hernia - *see* Hernia, by site, with
      obstruction
  organ or site, congenital NEC - *see*
    Anomaly, specified type NEC
  ovary (pedicle) 615.0
    congenital 752.5
  oviduct 615.9
  penis 607.9
    congenital 752.8
  spasm 331.1
  spermatic cord 607.7
  spleen 289.5
  testicle, testis 607.7
  tibia 738.5
  umbilical cord - *see* Complications,
    umbilical cord
  uterus (*see also* Malposition, uterus)
    624.9

Torticollis (intermittent) (spasmodic)
  (spastic) 717.2
  congenital 756.8
  due to birth injury (*see also* Birth injury
    NEC) 772.9
  hysterical 300.1
  psychogenic 305.1
    specified as conversion reaction
      300.1
  rheumatic 717.2
  rheumatoid 717.2
  traumatic, current NEC 847.0
Tortuous
  artery 447
  organ or site, congenital NEC - *see*
    Distortion
  retina vessel (congenital) 744.8
  ureter 593.5
  urethra 599.9
  vein - *see* Varicose vein
Torula, torular (infection) 116.0
  histolytica 116.0
  lung 116.0
Torulosis 116.0
Torus
  mandibularis 526.9
  palatinus 526.9
Tower skull 756.0
  with exophthalmos 756.0
Toxemia 796.0
  with abortion - *see* Abortion, by type,
    with toxemia
  antenatal (fetus or newborn) - *see*
    Toxemia, maternal
  antepartum - *see* Toxemia, arising
    during pregnancy
  arising during pregnancy 637.9
    eclamptic (nephritic) (uremic) 637.1
      fetus or newborn 762.2
    fetus or newborn NEC 762.3
    nephritic 636
      fetus or newborn 762.0
    pre-eclamptic (nephritic) (uremic)
      637.0
      fetus or newborn 762.1
    uremic 636
      fetus or newborn 762.0
  bacterial - *see* Septicemia
  biliary (*see also* Disease, gallbladder)
    576.9
  burn - *see* Burn
  congenital NEC 778.9
  eclampsia, eclamptic
    with abortion - *see* Abortion, by type,
      with toxemia

Toxemia — *continued*
  eclampsia, etc. — *continued*
    arising during pregnancy or
        puerperium   637.1
  erysipelatous (*see also* Erysipelas)   035
  fatigue   796.0
  fetus or newborn NEC   778.9
  food (*see also* Poisoning, food)   005.9
  gastric   537.9
  gastro-intestinal   569.9
  intestinal   569.9
  kidney (*see also* Lesion, kidney)   593.2
  lung   519.2
  malarial NEC (*see also* Malaria)   084.9
  maternal (of pregnancy), affecting fetus
        or newborn   762.3
    eclamptic   762.2
    nephritic   762.0
    not of pregnancy   761.9
    pre-eclamptic   762.1
    uremic   762.0
  myocardial - *see* Myocarditis, toxic
  pre-eclamptic
    with abortion - *see* Abortion, by type,
        with toxemia
    arising during pregnancy or
        puerperium   637.0
  puerperal, postpartum   637.9
    eclamptic (nephritic) (uremic)   637.1
    nephritic   636
    pre-eclamptic (nephritic) (uremic)
        637.0
    uremic   636
  pulmonary   519.2
  septic (*see also* Septicemia)   038.9
  small intestine   569.9
  staphylococcal, due to food   005.0
  stasis   796.0
  stomach   537.9
  uremic (*see also* Uremia)   792
    with abortion - *see* Abortion, by type,
        with toxemia
    arising during pregnancy or
        puerperium   636
  urinary   596.9
Toxic (poisoning) - *see also* condition
  from drug or poison - *see* Table of
        adverse effects
  thyroid (gland) (*see also* Thyrotoxicosis)
        242.2
Toxicemia - *see* Toxemia
Toxicity
  fava bean   282.2
  from drug or poison - *see* Table of
        adverse effects
Toxicosis (*see also* Toxemia)   796.0

Toxicosis — *continued*
  capillary
    hemorrhagic   287.0
Toxinfection   796.0
  gastro-intestinal   569.9
Toxoplasmosis   130.9
  acquired   130.0
  congenital, active   130.1
    late effects of intra-uterine infection
        130.2
  late effects of intra-uterine infection
        130.2
  maternal, affecting fetus or newborn
        761.4
  manifest toxoplasmosis in infant or
        fetus   130.1
Trabeculation, bladder   596.2
Trachea - *see* condition
Tracheitis (acute) (catarrhal) (infantile)
        (membranous) (plastic)
        (pneumococcal) (viral)   464
  with
    bronchitis   490
      acute or subacute   466
      chronic   491
      tuberculous - *see* Tuberculosis,
          pulmonary
    laryngitis (acute)   464
      chronic   506
      tuberculous   012.3
        with pneumoconiosis (conditions
            in 515)   010
        late effect or sequela   019.0
  chronic   491
    with
      bronchitis (chronic)   491
      laryngitis (chronic)   506
    diphtheritic   032
    streptococcal   034.0
    syphilitic   095
    tuberculous   012.9
      with pneumoconiosis (conditions in
          515)   010
      late effect or sequela   019.0
Trachelitis (nonvenereal) (*see also*
        Cervicitis)   620.9
  trichomonal   131
Tracheobronchial - *see* condition
Tracheobronchitis (*see also* Bronchitis)
        490
  acute or subacute   466
  chronic   491
  senile   491
Tracheobronchopneumonitis - *see*
        Pneumonia, broncho
Tracheocele (external) (internal)   519.9

Tracheocele — *continued*
  congenital 748.3
Tracheomalacia 519.9
  congenital 748.3
Tracheopharyngitis (acute) 465
  chronic 508.9
Tracheostenosis 519.9
Trachoma, trachomatous (active) 076
  contraction of conjunctiva 076
    late effect 077
  healed 077
    late effect 077
  Turck's 506
Train sickness 994.6
Trait
  hemoglobin
    abnormal NEC 282.5
      with thalassemia 282.4
    C (*see also* Disease, hemoglobin C)
      282.5
      with elliptocytosis 282.5
    Lepore 282.4
      with other abnormal hemoglobin
        NEC 282.4
    sickle cell - *see also* Disease, sickle cell
      with
        elliptocytosis 282.5
        spherocytosis 282.5
Traits
  paranoid 301.0
Trance 796.0
  hysterical 300.1
Transfusion reaction (adverse) - *see*
    Complications, transfusion
Transient - *see* condition
Transitional, lumbosacral joint or vertebra
    756.1
Translocation
  autosomes, except 21 759.4
    involving additional 21 759.3
  chromosomes NEC 759.4
Transmission of chemical substances
    through the placenta, affecting fetus
    or newborn 761.7
Transplanted organ, complication or
    rejection 997.7
Transplants, ovarian, endometrial 625.3
Transposed - *see* Transposition
Transposition (congenital) - *see also*
    Malposition, congenital
  abdominal viscera 759.0
  aorta 746.1
  appendix 751.4
  arterial trunk 746.1
  colon 751.4
  great vessels (complete) (partial) 746.1

Transposition — *continued*
  heart 746.8
    with complete transposition of viscera
      759.0
  intestine (large) (small) 751.4
  stomach 750.8
    with general transposition of viscera
      759.0
  tooth, teeth 524.3
  vessels (complete) (partial) 746.1
  viscera (abdominal) (thoracic) 759.0
Transverse - *see* condition
Transvestism, transvestitism 302.3
Trauma, traumatism (*see also* Injury)
    996.9
  during delivery NEC - *see* Obstetrical
    trauma
  maternal, during pregnancy, affecting
    fetus or newborn 761.5
Traumatic - *see* condition
Treacher-Collins syndrome 756.0
Treitz's hernia - *see* Hernia, Treitz's
Trematode infestation NEC 121.9
Trematodiasis NEC 121.9
Trembles 988.9
Tremor 780.3
  encephalitic 066
  familial 333.9
  flapping (liver) 573.9
  hereditary 333.9
  hysterical 300.1
  intention 780.4
  mercurial 985.0
  muscle 780.3
  Parkinson's 342
    late effect, viral encephalitis 066
  psychogenic 305.1
    specified as conversion reaction
      300.1
  senilis 794
Trench
  foot 991.4
  mouth 101
  nephritis - *see* Nephritis, acute
Treponema pallidum infection (*see also*
    Syphilis) 097.9
Treponematosis 102.9
  due to
    T. pallidum - *see* Syphilis
    T. pertenue (yaws) (*see also* Yaws)
      102.9
Triad
  Kartagener 759.0
  Saint's (*see also* Hernia, diaphragm)
    551.3

Trichiasis 704
· cicatricial 704
eyelid 704
late effect of trachoma (healed) 077
Trichinella spiralis (infection) (infestation)
124
Trichinelliasis 124
Trichiniasis 124
Trichinosis 124
Trichobezoar 938
intestine 936
stomach 935
Trichocephaliasis 127.2
Trichocephalosis 127.2
Trichocephalus infestation 127.2
Trichoclasis 704
Trichoepithelioma (benign) (skin) 216.1
breast 217
external area or site NEC 216.1
genital organ NEC - code as Neoplasm,
benign, by site
malignant - see Neoplasm, skin,
malignant
scrotum 216.1
Trichomoniasis 131
bladder 131
intestinal 007.9
prostate 131
seminal vessels 131
specified site NEC 136
urethra 131
urogenitalis 131
vagina 131
Trichomycosis 111.9
axillaris 111.8
nodosa 111.2
nodularis 111.2
rubra 111.8
Trichonocardiosis (axillaris) (palmellina)
111.8
Trichonodosis 704
Trichophytid, Trichophyton infection -
see Dermatophytosis
Trichophytide infection - see
Dermatophytosis
Trichophytobezoar 938
intestine 936
stomach 935
Trichophytosis - see Dermatophytosis
Trichoptilosis 704
Trichorrhexis (nodosa) 704
Trichosporosis nodosa 111.8
Trichostasis spinulosa (congenital) 757.3
Trichostrongyliasis (small intestine)
127.1
Trichostrongylosis 127.1

Trichostrongylus instabilis infection
127.1
Trichotillomania 300.3
Trichromat, anomalous (congenital)
377.3
Trichromatopsia, anomalous (congenital)
377.3
Trichuriasis 127.2
Trichuris trichiura (infection) (infestation)
(any site) 127.2
Tricuspid (valve) - see condition
Trifid - see also Accessory
kidney (pelvis) 753.3
tongue 750.0
Trigger finger (acquired) 731.4
congenital 756.8
Trigonitis (bladder) (pseudomembranous)
(see also Cystitis) 595
Trigonocephaly 756.0
Trilocular heart 746.8
Tripartita placenta - see Placenta,
abnormal
Triple - see also Accessory
kidneys 753.3
uteri 752.5
X female 759.5
Triplegia - see Paralysis
Triplet (low birthweight) 769.4
for classification of births in hospital -
see Newborn
pregnancy
complicating delivery 657.0
undelivered 634.9
Triplication - see Accessory
Trismus 781.4
neonatorum 037
newborn 037
Trisomy (syndrome) (see also Syndrome,
trisomy) 759.4
autosomes, except 21 759.4
D (group) 759.4
E (group) 759.4
21 (partial) 759.3
Trombidiosis 133.9
Trophedema (hereditary) 757.0
Trophic changes 357.9
Trophoblastic disease (see also
Hydatidiform mole) 634.0
Trophoneurosis 357.9
disseminated 734.0
Tropical - see also condition
eosinophilia 519.2
maceration feet (syndrome) 991.4
wet foot (syndrome) 991.4
Trouble - see also Disease
bowel 569.9

Trouble — *continued*
  heart - *see* Disease, heart
  intestine 569.9
  kidney (*see also* Lesion, kidney) 593.2
  nervous 790.0
  sinus (*see also* Sinusitis) 503.9
Truancy, childhood 308
Truncus
  arteriosus (persistent) 746.0
  communis 746.0
Trunk - *see* condition
Trypanosoma infestation - *see*
    Trypanosomiasis
Trypanosomiasis 087.9
  African 087.8
    by Trypanosoma 087.8
      gambiense 087.0
      rhodesiense 087.1
  American 086.9
    with
      heart involvement 086.0
      other organ involvement 086.8
    without mention of organ
        involvement 086.9
  Brazilian - *see* Trypanosomiasis,
      American
  by Trypanosoma
    cruzi - *see* Trypanosomiasis,
        American
    gambiense 087.0
    rhodesiense 087.1
  gambiensis, Gambian 087.0
  nervous system NEC 087.9
  rhodesiensis, Rhodesian 087.1
  South American - *see* Trypanosomiasis,
      American
T-shaped incisors 520.2
Tube, tubal, tubular - *see* condition
Tubercle - *see also* Tuberculosis
  brain, solitary 013.9
  Darwin's 745.2
  Ghon, primary infection (with
      symptoms) (*see also*
      Tuberculosis, primary, complex)
      012.0
Tuberculid, tuberculide (indurating,
    subcutaneous) (lichenoid) (miliary)
    (papulonecrotic) (primary) (skin)
    017.0
  late effect or sequela 019.9
Tuberculoma - *see also* Tuberculosis
  brain (any part) (calcified) 013.9
    late effect or sequela 019.1
  meninges (cerebral) (spinal) 013.0
    late effect or sequela 019.1

Tuberculosis, tubercular, tuberculous
    (calcification) (calcified) (caseous)
    (chromogenic acid fast bacilli)
    (congenital) (degeneration) (disease)
    (fibrocaseous) (fibroid) (fibrosis)
    (fistula) (gangrene) (interstitial)
    (isolated circumscribed lesions)
    (necrosis) (parenchymatous)
    (ulcerative) 011.9

Note — The following fourth-digit subdivisions of category 019 are used for classifying any condition specified as a late effect or sequela of (tuberculosis of):
  .0 *Respiratory tuberculosis* (i.e., any condition classifiable to 011 or 012)
  .1 *Central nervous system* (i.e., any condition classifiable to 013)
  .2 *Genito-urinary system* (i.e., any condition classifiable to 016)
  .3 *Vertebral column* (i.e., any condition classifiable to 015.0)
  .4 *Hip* (i.e., any condition classifiable to 015.1)
  .5 *Knee* (i.e., any condition classifiable to 015.2)
  .6 *Other bones and joints* (i.e., any condition classifiable to 015.8 or 015.9)
  .9 *Other specified organs* (i.e., any condition classifiable to 014, 017, or 018)
The appropriate fourth-digit subdivision of category Y03 given below is used for the classification of follow-up examination or prophylactic treatment of inactive tuberculosis in persons not needing further medical care:
  .0 *Of inactive pulmonary tuberculosis, after treatment*
  .1 *Of inactive pulmonary tuberculosis, not known to have been active*
  .2 *Of other cases of inactive tuberculosis*

Tuberculosis, etc. — *continued*
  with pneumoconiosis (conditions in 515)
      010
  abdomen 014
    lymph gland 014
  abscess 011.9
    arm 017.9
    bone 015.9
      hip 015.1

Tuberculosis, etc — *continued*
bowel — *continued*
  miliary 014
brain (miliary) (diffuse) 013.9
  calcified 013.9
breast 017.9
broad ligament 016.2
bronchi (*see also* Tuberculosis,
    pulmonary) 011.9
bronchial (*see also* Tuberculosis,
    pulmonary) 011.9
  gland (with symptoms) 012.9
    with pneumoconiosis (conditions in
      515) 010
    lymph gland or node (with symptoms)
      012.9
    with pneumoconiosis (conditions in
      515) 010
bronchiectasis (*see also* Tuberculosis,
    pulmonary) 011.9
bronchitis (*see also* Tuberculosis,
    pulmonary) 011.9
bronchopleural 012.1
  with pneumoconiosis (conditions in
    515) 010
bronchopneumonia, bronchopneumonic
    (*see also* Tuberculosis,
    pulmonary) 011.9
bronchorrhagia (*see also* Tuberculosis,
    pulmonary) 011.9
bronchotracheal (*see also* Tuberculosis,
    pulmonary) 011.9
bronchus (*see also* Tuberculosis,
    pulmonary) 011.9
bronze disease 017.9
buccal cavity 017.9
bulbo-urethral gland 016.1
bursa (*see also* Tuberculosis, joint)
    015.9
cachexia NEC (*see also* Tuberculosis,
    pulmonary) 011.9
caries (*see also* Tuberculosis, bone)
    015.9
cartilage (*see also* Tuberculosis, bone)
    015.9
  intervertebral 015.0
catarrhal (*see also* Tuberculosis,
    pulmonary) 011.9
cecum 014
cellular tissue (primary) 017.0
cellulitis (primary) 017.0
central nervous system 013.9
cerebellum 013.9
cerebral 013.9
  meninges 013.0
cerebrospinal 013.9

Tuberculosis, etc. — *continued*
cerebrospinal — *continued*
  meninges 013.0
cerebrum 013.9
cervical 017.1
  gland 017.1
  lymph nodes 017.1
cervicis uteri 016.2
cervicitis (uteri) 016.2
cervix 016.2
chest (*see also* Tuberculosis,
    pulmonary) 011.9
childhood type or first infection - *see*
    Tuberculosis, primary complex
choroid 017.2
choroiditis (circumscribed) (plastic)
    017.2
ciliary body 017.2
colitis 014
colliers' 010
colliquativa (primary) 017.0
colon 014
  ulceration 014
complex, primary (with symptoms)
    012.0
conjunctiva 017.2
connective tissue 017.9
  bone - *see* Tuberculosis, bone
cornea (ulcer) 017.2
Cowper's gland 016.1
coxae 015.1
coxalgia 015.1
cul-de-sac of Douglas 014
curvature, spine 015.0
cutis (colliquativa) (primary) 017.0
cyst, ovary 016.2
cystitis 016.1
dacrocystitis 017.2
dactylitis 015.8
diarrhea 014
diffuse (*see also* Tuberculosis, miliary)
    018.9
digestive tract 014
disseminated (*see also* Tuberculosis,
    miliary) 018.9
duodenum 014
dura (mater) 013.0
dysentery 014
ear (inner) (middle) 017.3
  bone 015.8
  external (primary) 017.0
  skin (primary) 017.0
elbow 015.8
emphysema (*see also* Tuberculosis,
    pulmonary) 011.9

Tuberculosis, etc. — *continued*
   empyema 012.1
      with pneumoconiosis (conditions in
         515) 010
   encephalitis 013.9
   endarteritis 017.9
   endocarditis 017.9
   endocardium 017.9
   endocrine glands 017.9
   endometrium 016.2
   enteric, enterica 014
   enteritis 014
   enterocolitis 014
   epididymis 016.2
   epididymitis 016.2
   epidural abscess 013.0
   epiglottis 012.3
      with pneumoconiosis (conditions in
         515) 010
   episcleritis 017.2
   erythema (induratum) (nodosum)
      (primary) 017.0
   esophagus 017.9
   eustachian tube 017.3
   exudative 012.1
      with pneumoconiosis (conditions in
         515) 010
   eye 017.2
   eyelid (primary) 017.0
   fallopian tube 016.2
   fascia 017.9
   fauces 012.9
      with pneumoconiosis (conditions in
         515) 010
   finger 017.9
   first infection 012.0
      with pneumoconiosis (conditions in
         515) 010
   florida (*see also* Tuberculosis,
      pulmonary) 011.9
   foot 017.9
   gallbladder 017.9
   galloping (*see also* Tuberculosis,
      pulmonary) 011.9
   ganglionic 015.9
   gastritis 017.9
   gastrocolic fistula 014
   gastro-enteritis 014
   gastro-intestinal tract 014
   general, generalized 018.9
      acute 018.1
         lung 011.4
            with pneumoconiosis (conditions
               in 515) 010
         nonpulmonary 018.0
      lung 011.4

Tuberculosis, etc. — *continued*
   general, etc. — *continued*
      lung — *continued*
         with pneumoconiosis (conditions in
            515) 010
   genital organs 016.2
   genito-urinary NEC 016.9
   genu 015.2
   glandulae suprarenalis 017.9
   glandular, general 017.1
   glottis 012.3
      with pneumoconiosis (conditions in
         515) 010
   grinders' 010
   groin 017.1
   gum 017.9
   hand 017.9
   heart 017.9
   hematogenous - *see* Tuberculosis,
      miliary
   hemoptysis (*see also* Tuberculosis,
      pulmonary) 011.9
   hemorrhage NEC (*see also*
      Tuberculosis, pulmonary) 011.9
   hemothorax 012.1
      with pneumoconiosis (conditions in
         515) 010
   hepatitis 017.9
   hilar lymph nodes 012.9
      with pneumoconiosis (conditions in
         515) 010
   hip (joint) (disease) 015.1
   hydrocephalus 013.0
   hydropneumothorax 012.1
      with pneumoconiosis (conditions in
         515) 010
   hypo-adrenalism 017.9
   hypopharynx 012.9
      with pneumoconiosis (conditions in
         515) 010
   ileocecal (hyperplastic) 014
      coil 014
   ileocolitis 014
   ileum 014
   iliac spine (superior) 015.0
   incipient NEC (*see also* Tuberculosis,
      pulmonary) 011.9
   indurativa (primary) 017.0
   infantile - *see* Tuberculosis, primary
      complex
   infraclavicular gland 017.1
   inguinal gland 017.1
   inguinalis 017.1
   intestine (any part) 014
      abscess 014
      hyperplastic 014

Tuberculosis, etc. — *continued*
 intestine — *continued*
  miliary 014
 iris 017.2
 iritis 017.2
 ischiorectal 014
 jaw 015.8
 jejunum 014
 joint 015.9
  hip 015.1
  knee 015.2
  specified NEC 015.8
  vertebral 015.0
 keratitis (interstitial) 017.2
 kidney 016.0
 knee (joint) 015.2
 kyphoscoliosis 015.0
 kyphosis 015.0
 lachrymal, lacrimal apparatus, gland
   017.2
 laryngitis 012.3
  with pneumoconiosis (conditions in
    515) 010
 larynx 012.3
  with pneumoconiosis (conditions in
    515) 010
 leptomeninges, leptomeningitis
   (cerebral) (spinal) 013.0
 lichenoides (primary) 017.0
 linguae 017.9
 lip 017.9
 liver 017.9
 lordosis 015.0
 lung - *see* Tuberculosis, pulmonary
 luposa 017.0
 lymph gland or node (peripheral) 017.1
  abdomen 014
  bronchial (with symptoms) 012.9
   with pneumoconiosis (conditions in
     515) 010
  cervical 017.1
  hilar 012.9
   with pneumoconiosis (conditions in
     515) 010
  mediastinal (with symptoms) 012.9
   with pneumoconiosis (conditions in
     515) 010
  mesenteric 014
  retroperitoneal 014
  tracheobronchial (with symptoms)
    012.9
   with pneumoconiosis (conditions in
     515) 010
 lymphadenitis - *see* Tuberculosis, lymph
   gland

Tuberculosis, etc. — *continued*
 lymphangitis - *see* Tuberculosis, lymph
   gland
 lymphatic (gland) (vessel) - *see*
   Tuberculosis, lymph gland
 malignant NEC (*see also* Tuberculosis,
   pulmonary) 011.9
 mammary gland 017.9
 marasmus NEC (*see also* Tuberculosis,
   pulmonary) 011.9
 mastoiditis 015.8
 mediastinal (lymph) gland or node (with
   symptoms) 012.9
  with pneumoconiosis (conditions in
    515) 010
 mediastinitis 012.9
  with pneumoconiosis (conditions in
    515) 010
 mediastino-pericarditis 017.9
 mediastinum 012.9
  with pneumoconiosis (conditions in
    515) 010
 medulla 013.9
 melanosis, addisonian 017.9
 membrane, brain 013.0
 meninges (cerebral) (spinal) (miliary)
   013.0
 meningitis (basilar) (brain) (cerebral)
   (cerebrospinal) (spinal) 013.0
 meningo-encephalitis 013.0
 mesentery, mesenteric 014
  lymph gland or node 014
 miliary 018.9
  acute 018.1
   lung 011.4
    with pneumoconiosis (conditions
      in 515) 010
   meninges (cerebral) (spinal) 013.0
   multiple sites 018.0
    lung included 011.4
     with pneumoconiosis
       (conditions in 515) 010
   nonpulmonary 018.0
   pulmonary 011.4
    with pneumoconiosis (conditions
      in 515) 010
   single site - *code by* site under
     Tuberculosis
  bilateral 011.4
   with pneumoconiosis (conditions in
     515) 010
  brain 013.9
  chronic 018.9
   brain 013.9
   intestine 014
   lung 011.4

Tuberculosis, etc. — *continued*
  miliary — *continued*
    chronic — *continued*
      lung — *continued*
        with pneumoconiosis (conditions
            in 515)   010
      meninges (cerebral) (spinal)   013.0
      multiple sites   018.9
        lung included   011.4
          with pneumoconiosis
              (conditions in 515)   010
        pulmonary   011.4
          with pneumoconiosis (conditions
              in 515)   010
        single site - *code by* site under
            Tuberculosis
    intestine (chronic)   014
    lung   011.4
      with pneumoconiosis (conditions in
          515)   010
      meninges (cerebral) (spinal)   013.0
      single site - *code by* site under
          Tuberculosis
  millstone makers'   010
  miner's   010
  moulders'   010
  mouth   017.9
  multiple   018.9
    lung included   011.4
      with pneumoconiosis (conditions in
          515)   010
    round foci NEC   011.4
      with pneumoconiosis (conditions in
          515)   010
  muscle   017.9
  myelitis   013.9
  myocarditis, chronic   017.9
  myocardium   017.9
  nasal (passage) (sinus)   012.9
    with pneumoconiosis (conditions in
        515)   010
  nasopharynx   012.9
    with pneumoconiosis (conditions in
        515)   010
  neck gland   017.1
  nephritis   016.0
  nerve   017.9
  nose (septum)   012.9
    with pneumoconiosis (conditions in
        515)   010
  ocular   017.2
  old NEC   019.0
  omentum   014
  oophoritis   016.2
  optic   017.2
    nerve trunk   017.2
    papilla, papillae   017.2

Tuberculosis, etc. — *continued*
  orbit   017.2
  orchitis   016.2
  organ, specified NEC   017.9
  orificialis (primary)   017.0
  osseous (*see also* Tuberculosis, bone)
      015.9
  osteitis (*see also* Tuberculosis, bone)
      015.9
  osteomyelitis (*see also* Tuberculosis,
      bone)   015.9
  otitis (media)   017.3
  ovaritis   016.2
  ovary   016.2
  oviduct   016.2
  pachymeningitis   013.0
  palate (soft)   017.9
  pancreas   017.9
  papulonecrotic(a) (primary)   017.0
  parathyroid glands   017.9
  paronychia (primary)   017.0
  parotid gland or region   017.9
  pelvic organ NEC
    female   016.2
    male   016.9
  pelvis (bony)   015.8
  penis   016.2
  peribronchitis (*see also* Tuberculosis,
      pulmonary)   011.9
  pericarditis   017.9
  pericardium   017.9
  perichondritis, larynx   012.3
    with pneumoconiosis (conditions in
        515)   010
  perineum   017.9
  periostitis (*see also* Tuberculosis, bone)
      015.9
  periphlebitis   017.9
    eye vessel   017.2
    retina   017.2
  perirectal fistula   014
  peritoneal gland   014
  peritoneum   014
  peritonitis   014
  pernicious NEC (*see also* Tuberculosis,
      pulmonary)   011.9
  pharyngitis   012.9
    with pneumoconiosis (conditions in
        515)   010
  pharynx   012.9
    with pneumoconiosis (conditions in
        515)   010
  phlyctenulosis (conjunctiva)   017.2
  phthisis NEC (*see also* Tuberculosis,
      pulmonary)   011.9
  pituitary gland   017.9

Tuberculosis, etc.—*continued*

placenta 016.2

pleura, pleural, pleurisy, pleuritis
(fibrinous) (obliterative) (purulent)
(simple plastic) (with effusion)
012.1
with pneumoconiosis (conditions in
515) 010
radiological evidence suggestive of
012.1

pneumonia, pneumonic (*see also*
Tuberculosis, pulmonary) 011.9

pneumothorax (spontaneous) (tense
valvular) (*see also* Tuberculosis,
pulmonary) 011.9

polyserositis 018.9
with
lung (*see also* Tuberculosis,
pulmonary) 011.9

potters' 010

prepuce 016.2

primary 012.0
with pneumoconiosis (conditions in
515) 010
complex (with symptoms) 012.0
with pneumoconiosis (conditions in
515) 010
skin 017.0

proctitis 014

prostate 016.2

prostatitis 016.2

pulmonaris (*see also* Tuberculosis,
pulmonary) 011.9

pulmonary (artery) (florida) (incipient)
(malignant)
(pernicious) (reinfection stage)
011.9
with pneumoconiosis (conditions in
515) 010
active
far advanced 011.2
minimal 011.0
moderately advanced 011.1
stage unspecified 011.3
childhood type or first infection - *see*
Tuberculosis, primary complex
miliary 011.4
old 019.0
primary - *see* Tuberculosis, primary
complex
radiological evidence alone,
suggestive of 011.5
status following surgical collapse of
lung NEC 011.9

pyelitis 016.0

pyelonephritis 016.0

Tuberculosis, etc.—*continued*

pyemia - *see* Tuberculosis, miliary

pyonephrosis 016.0

pyopneumothorax 012.1
with pneumoconiosis (conditions in
515) 010

pyothorax 012.1
with pneumoconiosis (conditions in
515) 010

rectum (with abscess) 014
fistula 014

reinfection stage (*see also* Tuberculosis,
pulmonary) 011.9

renal 016.0

renis 016.0

reproductive organ 016.2

respiratory NEC (*see also*
Tuberculosis, pulmonary) 011.9
specified site NEC 012.9
with pneumoconiosis (conditions in
515) 010

retina 017.2

retroperitoneal 014
gland 014
lymph gland or node 014

rheumatism NEC 015.9

rhinitis 012.9
with pneumoconiosis (conditions in
515) 010

sacro-iliac (joint) 015.8

sacrum 015.0

salivary gland 017.9

salpingitis 016.2

sandblasters' 010

sclera 017.2

scoliosis 015.0

scrofulous 017.1

scrotum 016.2

seminal tract or vesicle 016.2

senile NEC (*see also* Tuberculosis,
pulmonary) 011.9

septic NEC (*see also* Tuberculosis,
miliary) 018.9

shoulder 015.8

sigmoid 014

sinus (any nasal) 012.9
with pneumoconiosis (conditions in
515) 010
bone (*see also* Tuberculosis, bone)
015.9
epididymis 016.2

skeletal NEC 015.9

skin (any site) (primary) 017.0

spermatic cord 016.2

spinal
column 015.0

Tuberculosis, etc. — *continued*
  spinal — *continued*
    cord (miliary) 013.9
    disease 015.0
    medulla 013.9
    membrane 013.0
    meninges 013.0
  spine 015.0
  spleen 017.9
    acute miliary 017.9
  splenitis 017.9
  spondylitis 015.0
  sternoclavicular joint 015.8
  stomach 017.9
  stonemasons' 010
  struma 017.1
  subcutaneous tissue (cellular) (primary)
    017.0
  subcutis (primary) 017.0
  subdeltoid bursa 017.9
  submaxillary 017.9
    region 017.9
  supraclavicular gland 017.1
  suprarenal (capsule) (gland) 017.9
  suspected
    respiratory, on radiological evidence
      alone 011.5
  swelling, joint (*see also* Tuberculosis,
    joint) 015.9
  symphysis pubis 015.8
  synovitis 015.9
    hip 015.1
    knee 015.2
    specified site NEC 015.8
    spine or vertebra 015.0
  systemic - *see* Tuberculosis, miliary
  tarsitis (ankle) (bone) 015.8
    eyelid 017.0
  tendon (sheath) - *see* Tuberculosis,
    tenosynovitis
  tenosynovitis 015.9
    hip 015.1
    knee 015.2
    specified site NEC 015.8
    spine or vertebra 015.0
  testicle 016.2
  testis 016.2
  throat 012.9
    with pneumoconiosis (conditions in
      515) 010
  thymus gland 017.9
  thyroid gland 017.9
  toe 017.9
  tongue 017.9
  tonsil (lingual) 012.9

Tuberculosis, etc. — *continued*
  tonsil — *continued*
    with pneumoconiosis (conditions in
      515) 010
  tonsillitis 012.9
    with pneumoconiosis (conditions in
      515) 010
  trachea, tracheal 012.9
    with pneumoconiosis (conditions in
      515) 010
    gland (with symptoms) 012.9
  tracheobronchial (*see also* Tuberculosis,
    pulmonary) 011.9
    glandular (with symptoms) 012.9
      with pneumoconiosis (conditions in
        515) 010
    lymph gland or node (with symptoms)
      012.9
      with pneumoconiosis (conditions in
        515) 010
  tubal 016.2
  tunica vaginalis 016.2
  typhlitis 014
  ulcer (skin) (primary) 017.0
    bowel or intestine 014
    other specified sites - code according
      to site under Tuberculosis
  unspecified site - *see* Tuberculosis,
    pulmonary
  ureter 016.1
  urethra, urethral 016.1
    gland 016.1
  urinary organ or tract 016.1
  uterus 016.2
  uveal tract 017.2
  uvula 017.9
  vagina 016.2
  vas deferens 016.2
  vein 017.9
  verruca (primary) 017.0
  verrucosa (cutis) (primary) 017.0
  vertebra (column) 015.0
  vesiculitis 016.2
  viscera NEC 014
  vulva 016.2
  wrist 015.8
Tuberculum
  anomale carabelli 520.2
  occlusal 520.2
  paramolare 520.2
Tuberous sclerosis (brain) 759.6
Tubo-ovarian - *see* condition
Tubotympanitis 384.0
Tularemia 021
  opthalmic 021
  pneumonia (any) 021

Turner's
  hypoplasia, hypoplasis (tooth)   520.4
  syndrome   759.5
  tooth   520.4
Turricephaly   756.0
Tussis convulsiva (*see also* Whooping
        cough)   033.9
Twin (low birthweight)   769.4
  conjoined   759.1
  for classification of births in hospital -
        see Newborn
  pregnancy
    complicating delivery   657.0
    undelivered   634.9
Twist, twisted
  bowel, colon or intestine   560.2
    with hernia - *see* Hernia, by site, with
        obstruction
  hair (congenital)   757.3
  mesentery or omentum   560.2
    with hernia - *see* Hernia, by site, with
        obstruction
  organ or site, congenital NEC - *see*
        Anomaly, specified type NEC
  ovarian pedicle   615.0
    congenital   752.5
  umbilical cord - *see* Complications,
        umbilical cord
Tylosis   700
  linguae   529.7
  palmaris et plantaris   757.2
Tympanites (abdominal) (intestine)   785.4
Tympanitis - *see* Otitis media
Tympanosclerosis   387.9
Tympanum - *see* condition
Typhlitis (*see also* Appendicitis)   541
Typho-enteritis   001
Typhoid (abortive) (ambulant) (any site)
        (fever) (hemorrhagic) (infection)
        (intermittent) (malignant)
        (rheumatic)   001
  abdominal   001
  carrier (state) (suspected)   Y05.1
  clinical (Widal and blood test negative)
        001
  inoculation reaction - *see*
        Complications, vaccination
  mesenteric lymph nodes   001

Typhoid—*continued*
  spine   001
  Widal negative   001
Typhomalaria (fever) (*see also* Malaria)
        084.9
Typhomania   001
Typhoperitonitis   001
Typhus (fever)   081.9
  abdominal, abdominalis   001
  African tick   082.1
  brain   081.9
  cerebral   081.9
  classical   080
  endemic (flea-borne)   081.0
  epidemic (louse-borne)   080
  exanthematic NEC   080
  exanthematicus SAI   080
    brillii SAI   081.1
    mexicanus SAI   081.9
    pediculo vestimenti causa   080
    typus murinus   081.0
  flea-borne   081.0
  India tick   082.1
  Kenya tick   082.1
  louse-borne   080
  Mexican   081.9
    flea-borne   081.0
    louse-borne   080
    tabardillo   080
  mite-borne   081.2
  murine   081.0
  North Asian tick-borne   082.2
  petechial   081.9
  Queensland tick   082.9
  rat   081.0
  recrudescent   081.1
  recurrent (*see also* Fever, relapsing)
        088.9
  Sao Paulo   082.0
  scrub (China) (India) (Malay) (New
        Guinea)   081.2
  shop (of Malaya)   081.0
  Siberian tick   082.2
  tick-borne NEC   082.9
  tropical   081.2
Tyroma - *see* Neoplasm
Tyrosinosis   270.8
Tyrosinuria   270.8

U

Ulcer, ulcerated, ulcerating, ulceration,
  ulcerative 707.9
  with gangrene (see also Gangrene)
    445.9
  abdomen (wall) - see Ulcer, skin
  ala, nose 508.9
  alveolar process 526.5
  amebic (intestine) (skin) 006.9
    with liver abscess 006.0
  anastomotic - see Ulcer, gastrojejunal
  anorectal 569.2
  antral - see Ulcer, stomach
  anus (sphincter) 569.2
    varicose 455
  aphthous (oral) (recurrent) 528.2
    genital organ(s)
      female 629.9
      male 607.9
  arm - see Ulcer, skin
  artery 447
  atrophic NEC - see Ulcer, skin
  bile duct (see also Disease, gallbladder)
    576.9
  bladder (solitary) (sphincter) 596.9
    submucosal (see also Cystitis) 595
    tuberculous 016.1
      late effect or sequela 019.2
  bleeding (see also Ulcer, peptic) 533.9
    specified site - code by site under
      Ulcer
  bone 723.9
  bowel (see also Ulcer, intestine) 569.4
  breast 611.0
  bronchus 519.9
  buccal (cavity) (traumatic) 528.9
  burn (acute) - see Ulcer, duodenum
  buttock - see Ulcer, skin
  cancerous - see Neoplasm, malignant
  cardia (with melena) - see Ulcer,
    stomach
  cardio-esophageal (peptic) 530.1
  cecum (see also Ulcer, intestine) 569.4
  cervix (uteri) (decubital) (trophic)
    621.3
  chancroidal 099.0
  chest (wall) - see Ulcer, skin
  chin - see Ulcer, skin
  chronic (cause unknown) - see Ulcer,
    skin
  Cochin-China 085.1
  colon (see also Ulcer, intestine) 569.4
  conjunctiva (postinfectional) 360

Ulcer, etc. — continued
  cornea 363.0
    with perforation 363.0
    annular 363.0
    catarrhal 363.0
    dentritic 054
    infectional 363.0
    marginal 363.0
    phlyctenular, tuberculous 017.2
      late effect or sequela 019.9
    ring 363.0
    rodent 363.0
    serpent, serpiginous 363.0
    superficial marginal 363.0
    tuberculous 017.2
      late effect or sequela 019.9
  corpus cavernosum (chronic) 607.2
  crural - see Ulcer, lower extremity
  Curling's (with melena) - see Ulcer,
    duodenum
  Cushing's - see also Ulcer, stomach
  duodenal - see Ulcer, duodenum
  decubitus (any site) 707.0
    with gangrene (see also Gangrene)
      445.9
  dentritic 054
  diabetes, diabetic (mellitus) - see
    category 250
  Dieulafoy's (with melena) - see Ulcer,
    stomach
  due to
    infection NEC - see Ulcer, skin
    radiation - see Effect, adverse,
      radiation
    trophic disturbance (any region) - see
      Ulcer, skin
    x-ray - see Effect, adverse, x-rays
  duodenum, duodenal (eroded) (peptic)
    (with melena) 532.9
    with
      hemorrhage 532.0
        and perforation 532.2
      perforation 532.1
        and hemorrhage 532.2
    asymptomatic or inactive, follow-up
      examination Y03.9
    bleeding (recurrent) - see Ulcer,
      duodenum, with hemorrhage
    healed or old, follow-up examination
      Y03.9
    penetrating - see Ulcer, duodenum,
      with perforation

Ulcer, etc. — *continued*
  duodenum, etc. — *continued*
    perforating - *see* Ulcer, duodenum,
      with perforation
  dysenteric NEC 009.0
  elusive (*see also* Cystitis) 595
  epiglottis 508.3
  eroding - *code by* site under Ulcer
  esophagus (peptic) 530.1
    infectional 530.1
    varicose 456.0
  eye NEC 369.9
    dentritic 054
  eyelid (region) 361
  face - *see* Ulcer, skin
  fauces 508.9
  fistulous NEC - *see* Ulcer, skin
  foot (indolent) (*see also* Ulcer, lower
    extremity) 707.1
    perforating 707.1
      hereditary 349.0
      leprous 030.1
      syphilitic 094.0
      varicose 454.0
  gallbladder or duct (*see also* Disease,
    gallbladder) 576.9
  gangrenous (*see also* Gangrene) 445.9
  gastric (with melena) - *see* Ulcer,
    stomach
  gastrocolic - *see* Ulcer, gastrojejunal
  gastroduodenal (with melena) - *see*
    Ulcer, peptic
  gastro-esophageal (with melena) - *see*
    Ulcer, stomach
  gastrohepatic (with melena) - *see* Ulcer,
    stomach
  gastro-intestinal - *see* Ulcer,
    gastrojejunal
  gastrojejunal (peptic) (with melena)
    534.9
    with
      hemorrhage 534.0
        and perforation 534.2
      perforation 534.1
        and hemorrhage 534.2
    bleeding (recurrent) - *see* Ulcer,
      gastrojejunal, with hemorrhage
    penetrating - *see* Ulcer, gastrojejunal,
      with perforation
    perforating - *see* Ulcer, gastrojejunal,
      with perforation
  gastrojejunocolic - *see* Ulcer,
    gastrojejunal
  gingiva 523.9
  gingivitis 523.1
  glottis 508.3
  groin - *see* Ulcer, skin

Ulcer, etc. — *continued*
  gum 523.9
  hand - *see* Ulcer, skin
  hemorrhage (*see also* Ulcer, peptic)
    533.9
    specified site - *code by* site under
      Ulcer
  hip - *see* Ulcer, skin
  Hunner's (*see also* Cystitis) 595
  hypopharynx 508.9
  hypopyon (chronic) (subacute) 363.0
  hypostaticum - *see* Ulcer, varicose
  ileum (*see also* Ulcer, intestine) 569.4
  intestine, intestinal 569.4
    amebic 006.9
      with liver abscess 006.0
    duodenal - *see* Ulcer, duodenum
    granulocytopenic (with hemorrhage)
      288
    malignant - *see* Neoplasm, intestine,
      malignant
    marginal 569.4
    perforating 569.4
    stercoraceous 569.4
    stercoral 569.4
    tuberculous 014
      late effect or sequela 019.9
    typhoid (fever) 001
    varicose 456.9
  Jacob's - *see* Neoplasm, skin, malignant
  jejunum, jejunal - *see* Ulcer,
    gastrojejunal
  keratitis 363.0
  knee - *see* Ulcer, lower extremity
  labium (majus) (minus) 629.9
  larynx (aphthous) (contact) 508.3
    diphtheritic 032
  leg - *see* Ulcer, lower extremity
  lip 528.5
  Lipschutz 629.9
  lower extremity (atrophic) (chronic)
    (neurogenic) (perforating)
    (pyogenic) (trophic) (tropical)
    707.1
    with gangrene (*see also* Gangrene)
      445.9
    decubitus 707.0
      with gangrene (*see also* Gangrene)
        445.9
    varicose 454.0
  luetic - *see* Ulcer, syphilitic
  lung 519.2
    tuberculous (*see also* Tuberculosis,
      pulmonary) 011.9
  malignant - *see* Neoplasm, malignant
  marginal NEC - *see* Ulcer, gastrojejunal

Ulcer, etc. — *continued*
  meatus (urinarius) 599.9
  Meckel's diverticulum 751.0
  Meleney's (chronic undermining)
    686.0
  Mooren's (cornea) 363.0
  mouth (traumatic) 528.9
  nasopharynx 508.9
  navel cord (newborn) 686.9
  neck - *see* Ulcer, skin
  neurogenic NEC - *see* Ulcer, skin
  nose, nasal (passage) (infectional)
    508.9
    septum 508.9
     varicose 456.9
    skin - *see* Ulcer, skin
    spirochetal NEC 104.9
  oral mucosa (traumatic) 528.9
  palate 528.9
    soft 528.9
  penis (chronic) 607.2
  peptic (with hemorrhage) (with melena)
    (site unspecified) 533.9
    penetrating 533.0
    perforating or with perforation
     533.0
    specified site - *code by* site under
     Ulcer
  perforating
    specified site or type - *code by* site or
     type under Ulcer
    unspecified site - *see* Ulcer, skin
  perineum - *see* Ulcer, skin
  peritonsillar 500
  phagedenic (tropical) NEC - *see* Ulcer,
    skin
  pharynx 508.9
  phlebitis - *see* Phlebitis
  plaster (*see also* Ulcer, decubitus)
    707.0
  popliteal space - *see* Ulcer, lower
    extremity
  postpyloric - *see* Ulcer, duodenum
  prepuce 607.2
  prepyloric (with melena) - *see* Ulcer,
    stomach
  pressure (*see also* Ulcer, decubitus)
    707.0
  pseudopeptic (*see also* Ulcer, peptic)
    533.9
  pyloric (with melena) - *see* Ulcer,
    stomach
  rectosigmoid 569.2
  rectum (sphincter) 569.2
    stercoraceous, stercoral 569.2
    varicose 455

Ulcer, etc. — *continued*
  retina 367
  rodent - *see also* Neoplasm, skin,
    malignant
    cornea 363.0
  round - *see* Ulcer, stomach
  sacrum (region) - *see* Ulcer, skin
  scalp - *see* Ulcer, skin
  sclera 369.9
  scrofulous 017.1
    late effect or sequela 019.9
  scrotum 607.9
    tuberculous 016.2
     late effect or sequela 019.9
    varicose 456.1
  seminal vesicle 607.9
  sigmoid 569.4
  skin (atrophic) (chronic) (neurogenic)
    (perforating) (pyogenic) (trophic)
    707.9
    with gangrene (*see also* Gangrene)
     445.9
    decubitus 707.0
     with gangrene (*see also* Gangrene)
      445.9
    in granulocytopenia 288
    lower extremity 707.1
     with gangrene (*see also* Gangrene)
      445.9
     decubitus - *see* Ulcer, skin,
      decubitus
    tuberculous (primary) 017.0
     late effect or sequela 019.9
    varicose - *see* Ulcer, varicose
  sloughing NEC - *see* Ulcer, skin
  sore throat 462
    streptococcal 034.0
  spermatic cord 607.9
  spine (tuberculous) 015.0
    late effect or sequela 019.3
  stasis (venous) 454.0
  stercoral, stercoraceous 569.4
    rectum 569.2
  stoma, stomal - *see* Ulcer, gastrojejunal
  stomach (eroded) (peptic) (round) (with
    melena) 531.9
    with
     hemorrhage 531.0
      and perforation 531.2
     perforation 531.1
      and hemorrhage 531.2
    asymptomatic or inactive, follow-up
     examination Y03.9
    bleeding (recurrent) - *see* Ulcer,
     stomach, with hemorrhage

Ulcer, etc. — *continued*
  stomach — *continued*
    healed or old, follow-up examination
      Y03.9
    penetrating - *see* Ulcer, stomach,
      with perforation
    perforating - *see* Ulcer, stomach, with
      perforation
  stomatitis 528.0
  stress - *see also* Ulcer, stomach
    duodenal - *see* Ulcer, duodenum
  strumous (tuberculous) 017.1
    late effect or sequela 019.9
  submental - *see* Ulcer, skin
  syphilitic (any site) (early) (secondary)
      091.2
    late 095
    perforating 095
      foot 094.0
  testis 607.9
  thigh - *see* Ulcer, lower extremity
  throat 508.9
    diphtheritic 032
  toe - *see* Ulcer, lower extremity
  tongue (traumatic) 529.0
  tonsil 500
    diphtheritic 032
  trachea 519.9
  trophic - *see* Ulcer, skin
  tropical NEC (*see also* Ulcer, skin)
      707.9
  tuberculous - *see* Tuberculosis, ulcer
  tunica vaginalis 607.9
  turbinate 723.9
  typhoid (fever) 001
    perforating 001
  unspecified site NEC - *see* Ulcer, skin
  urethra (meatus) (*see also* Urethritis)
      597
  uterus 625.9
    cervix 621.3
    neck 621.3
  vagina 629.9
  valve, heart 421.0
  varicose (lower extremity, any part)
      454.0
    anus 455
    esophagus 456.0
    nasal septum 456.9
    rectum 455
    scrotum 456.1
    specified site NEC 456.9
  vas deferens 607.9
  vulva (acute) (infectional) 629.9
  vulvobuccal, recurring 629.9
  x-ray - *see* Effect, adverse, x-rays
  yaws 102.4

Ulcus - *see also* Ulcer
  cutis tuberculosum 017.0
    late effect or sequela 019.9
  duodeni (with melena) - *see* Ulcer,
    duodenum
  durum 091.0
    extragenital 091.1
  gastrojejunale - *see* Ulcer, gastrojejunal
  hypostaticum - *see* Ulcer, varicose
  molle (cutis) (skin) 099.0
  serpens corneae (pneumococcal) 363.0
  ventriculi (with melena) - *see* Ulcer,
    stomach
Ulegyria 743.2
Ulerythema
  acneiforme 695.9
  ophryogenes 757.2
Ullrich-Feichtiger syndrome 759.8
Ullrich(-Bonnevie)(-Turner) syndrome
    759.5
Ulnar - *see* condition
Ulorrhagia 523.9
Umbilicus, umbilical - *see also* condition
  cord complications (during delivery) -
      see Complications, umbilical
      cord
Uncinariasis (*see also* Ancylostomiasis)
    126.9
Unconscious 780.0
Under observation - *see* Observation
Underdevelopment - *see also*
      Undeveloped
    sexual 258.9

Undernourishment 269.9
Undernutrition 269.9
Underweight 269.9
Underwood's disease 778.9
Undescended - *see also* Malposition,
      congenital
    cecum 751.1
    colon 751.1
    testicle 752.1
Undetermined cause 796.9

Undeveloped, undevelopment - *see also*
      Hypoplasia
    brain (congenital) 743.1
    cerebral (congenital) 743.1
    fetus or newborn 778.9
    heart 746.8
    lung 748.6
    testicle 257.1
    uterus 258.9

Undiagnosed (disease) 796.9
Unequal leg (length) (acquired) 738.5
  congenital 755.3
Unerupted tooth, teeth 520.6

Unextracted dental root 525.9
Unguis incarnatus 703.0
Unicollis uterus 752.5
Unicornis uterus 752.5
Unicorporeus uterus 752.5
Uniformis uterus 752.5
Unilateral - *see also* condition
  development, breast 611.9
  organ or site, congenital NEC - *see*
    Agenesis
  vagina 752.6
Unilateralis uterus 752.5
Unilocular heart 746.8
Uninhibited
  neurogenic
    bladder NEC 596.9
Union, abnormal - *see also* Fusion
  larynx and trachea 748.3
Universal mesentery 751.1
Unknown 796.9
  cause 796.9
  diagnosis 796.9
Unna's
  disease 690
  nevus (*see also* Hemangioma) 227.0
Unsoundness of mind (*see also* Psychosis)
  299
Unspecified cause 796.9
Unstable
  back NEC 729.1
  colon 569.9
  joint (*see also* Disease, joint) 729.9
  lumbosacral joint (congenital) 756.1
    acquired 729.1
  sacro-iliac 726
  spine NEC 729.1
Untruthfulness, child problem 308
Unverricht-Wagner syndrome 716.0
Unverricht(-Lundborg) disease or epilepsy
  331.2
Upper respiratory - *see* condition
Upset
  gastro-intestinal 536.9
    psychogenic 305.5
    virus (*see also* Enteritis, viral) 008.9
  intestinal (large) (small) 564.9
    psychogenic 305.5
  menstruation 626.9
  mental 300.9
  stomach 536.9
    psychogenic 305.5
Urachus - *see also* condition
  patent 753.8
  persistent 753.8
Uratic arthritis 274
Urbach-Oppenheim disease - *see* category
  250

Urbach-Wiethe disease 279
Urbach's lipoid proteinosis 279
Urea, blood, high - *see* Uremia
Uremia, uremic (absorption) (amaurosis)
  (amblyopia) (aphasia) (apoplexy)
  (coma) (delirium) (dementia)
  (dropsy) (dyspnea) (fever)
  (intoxication) (mania) (paralysis)
  (poisoning) (toxemia) (vomiting)
  792
  with
    abortion - *see* Abortion, by type, with
      toxemia
    hypertension, malignant (*see also*
      Hypertension, malignant, with
      renal involvement) 400.3
  arising during pregnancy 636
    fetus or newborn 762.0
  congenital 778.9
  convulsions 792
    arising during pregnancy 637.1
      fetus or newborn 762.2
    puerperal, postpartum 637.1
  eclampsia 792
    arising during pregnancy 637.1
      fetus or newborn 762.2
    puerperal, postpartum 637.1
  extrarenal 788.9
  hypertensive (*see also* Hypertension,
    kidney) 403
  maternal NEC, affecting fetus or
    newborn 762.0
  pericarditis - *see* Nephritis, chronic
  puerperal, postpartum 636
  pyelitic (*see also* Pyelitis) 590.1
Ureter, ureteral - *see* condition
Ureteralgia 786.0
Ureterectasis 593.5
Ureteritis 593.5
  cystica 593.5
  due to
    calculus 592
  gonococcal (acute) 098.0
    chronic or duration of 2 months or
      over 098.1
  nonspecific 593.5
Ureterocele 593.5
  congenital 753.2
Ureterolith 592
Ureterolithiasis 592
Urethra, urethral - *see* condition
Urethralgia 786.0
Urethritis (abacterial) (acute) (allergic)
  (anterior) (chronic) (nongonorrheal)
  (nonvenereal) (posterior) (recurrent)
  (simple) (subacute) (ulcerative)
  (undifferentiated) 597

Urethritis — *continued*
  diplococcal 098.0
    chronic or duration of 2 months or
      over 098.1
  gonococcal 098.0
    chronic or duration of 2 months or
      over 098.1
  Reiter's 136
  trichomonal or due to Trichomonas
    (vaginalis) 131
  venereal NEC 099.9
Urethrocele
  female 623.2
  male 599.9
Urethrorectal - *see* condition
Urethrorrhagia 599.9
Urethrotrigonitis (*see also* Cystitis) 595
Urethrovaginal - *see* condition
Urhidrosis, uridrosis 705.9
Uric acid
  diathesis 274
  in blood 274
  poisoning 274
Uricacidemia 274
Uricemia 274
Uricosuria 789.9
Urinary - *see* condition
Urine
  blood in 789.3
  discharge excessive 786.4
  extravasation 596.9
  incontinence 786.2
    nonorganic origin 306.6
  pus in 789.1
  retention or stasis 786.1
    psychogenic 305.6
  secretion
    deficient 786.5
    excessive 786.4
Urinemia - *see* Uremia
Uroarthritis
  infectious 136
Urodialysis 786.5
Urolithiasis 594
  right or left 592

Uronephrosis (*see also* Lesion, kidney)
  593.2
Uropathy 599.9
  obstructive 599.9
Urosepsis 596.9
  Pseudomonas 596.9
Urticaria 708.9
  with angioneurotic edema 708.0
  allergic 708.9
  cholinergic 708.9
  factitia 709.9
  giant 708.0
  gigantea 708.0
  larynx 708.0
  nonallergic 708.9
  papulosa (Hebra) 698.2
  perstans hemorrhagica 757.2
  pigmentosa 757.2
  solare 692.7
Usher-Senear disease 694
Uta 085.2
Uteromegaly 625.9
Uterovaginal - *see* condition
Uterovesical - *see* condition
Utriculitis (utriculus prostaticus) 599.9
Uveal - *see* condition
Uveitis (allergic) (anterior) (endogenous)
    (exogenous) (granulomatous)
    (healed) (heterochromic)
    (nongranulomatous) (posterior)
    (recurrent) (sympathetic) 366
  due to toxoplasmosis (acquired) 130.0
    congenital (active) 130.1
      late effects 130.2
  syphilitic 095
    congenital 090.0
    secondary 091.8
  tuberculous 017.2
    late effect or sequela 019.9
Uveokeratitis (*see also* Uveitis) 366
Uveoparotitis 135
Uvula - *see* condition
Uvulitis (acute) (catarrhal) (chronic)
    (gangrenous) (membranous)
    (suppurative) (ulcerative) 528.3

V

Vaccination Y02
  complication or reaction - *see*
      Complications, vaccination
Vaccinia (generalized) 999.0
  conjunctiva 999.3
  eyelids 999.3
  localized 999.3
  nose 999.3
  not from vaccination 051
  sine vaccinatione 051
  without vaccination 051
Vacuum
  in sinus - *see* Sinusitis
Vagabondage 301.7
Vagabonds' disease 132
Vagina, vaginal - *see* condition
Vaginalitis (tunica) 607.5
Vaginismus (reflex) 786.7
  hysterical 300.1
  psychogenic 305.6
Vaginitis (acute) (atrophic) (chronic)
      (circumscribed) (diffuse)
      (emphysematous) (Hemophilus
      vaginalis) (nonspecific)
      (nonvenereal) (senile) (ulcerative)
      622.1
  with
    abortion - *see* Abortion, by type, with
        sepsis
    ectopic gestation - *see* categories
        631.0-631.3
  adhesive, congenital 752.6
  arising during pregnancy 630
    fetus or newborn 763.1
  blennorrhagic 098.0
    chronic or duration of 2 months or
        over 098.1
  due to Trichomonas (vaginalis) 131
  gonococcal 098.0
    chronic or duration of 2 months or
        over 098.1
  granuloma 099.2
  monilia 112
  mycotic 112
  puerperal, postpartum, childbirth 670
  syphilitic (early) 091.0
    late 095
  trichomonal 131
  tuberculous 016.2
    late effect or sequela 019.2
  venereal NEC 099.9

Vagotonia 356
Vagrancy 301.7
Vallecula - *see* condition
Valley fever 114
Valsuani's disease
  of pregnancy 633.0
    fetus or newborn 769.9
  puerperal, postpartum, childbirth 676
Valve, valvular (formation) - *see also*
      condition
  cervix, internal os 752.5
  colon 751.4
  formation, congenital NEC - *see*
      Atresia
  heart defect 746.6
  ureter (pelvic junction) (vesical orifice)
      753.2
  urethra 753.6
Valvulitis (*see also* Endocarditis) 424.9
  rheumatic (chronic) (inactive) (with
      chorea) 397.9
    active or acute (aortic) (mitral)
        (pulmonary) (tricuspid) 391.1
Valvulopathy - *see* Endocarditis
Van Bogaert's leuko-encephalitis
      (sclerosing) (subacute) 065
  late effects 066
Van Creveld-von Gierke disease 271.0
Van der Hoeve's syndrome 756.6
Van Neck's disease 722.2
Vanillism 692.9
Vapor asphyxia or suffocation NEC
      987.9
  specified agent - *see* Table of adverse
      effects
Vaquez-Osler disease 208
Vaquez's disease 208
Variants
  thalassemic (*see also* Thalassemia)
      282.4
Varicella 052
Varices - *see* Varix
Varicocele (thrombosed) (scrotum) 456.1
  ovary 456.9
  spermatic cord (ulcerated) 456.1
Varicose
  aneurysm (ruptured) (*see also*
      Aneurysm) 442
  dermatitis (lower extremity) 454.1
    ulcerated or with ulcer 454.0
  eczema - *see* Varicose, dermatitis

Varicose—*continued*
  phlebitis - *see* Varicose vein
  placental vessel - *see* Placenta,
      abnormal
  tumor - *see* Varicose vein
  ulcer (lower extremity, any part) 454.0
    anus 455
    esophagus 456.0
    nasal septum 456.9
    rectum 455
    scrotum 456.1
    specified site NEC 456.9
  vein (infected) (lower extremity)
      (ruptured) (*see also* Varix)
      454.9
    with
      stasis dermatitis 454.1
        with ulcer 454.0
        ulcerated 454.0
      ulcer 454.0
    anus (ulcerated) 455
    complicating pregnancy (undelivered)
        634.9
    congenital (any site) 747.6
    esophagus (ulcerated) 456.0
    puerperal, postpartum (current)
        677.9
      infected 671.0
    rectum (ulcerated) 455
    scrotum (ulcerated) 456.1
    ulcerated 454.0
    umbilical cord - *see* Complications,
        umbilical cord
  vessel - *see also* Varix
    amnion - *see* Placenta, abnormal
    chorion - *see* Placenta, abnormal
    placenta - *see* Placenta, abnormal
    syncytium - *see* Placenta, abnormal
Varicosis, varicosities, varicosity (*see also*
    Varix) 454.9
Variola 050.9
  major 050.0
  minor 050.1
Varioloid 050.1
Varix (infected) (lower extremity)
      (ruptured) 454.9
  with
    stasis dermatitis 454.1
      ulcerated or with ulcer 454.0
    ulcer 454.0
  aneurysmal (*see also* Aneurysm) 442
  anus (ulcerated) 455
  arteriovenous 747.6
  bladder 456.9
  broad ligament 456.9
  complicating pregnancy 634.9

Varix—*continued*
  congenital (any site) 747.6
  esophagus (ulcerated) 456.0
    congenital 747.6
  labia (majora) 456.9
  orbit 456.9
    congenital 747.6
  ovary 456.9
  papillary 448
  pelvis 456.9
  pharynx 456.9
  placenta - *see* Placenta, abnormal
  puerperal, postpartum (current) 677.9
    infected 671.0
  rectum (ulcerated) 455
  renal papilla 456.9
  scrotum (ulcerated) 456.1
  sigmoid colon 456.9
  specified site NEC 456.9
  spinal (cord) (vessels) 456.9
  spleen, splenic (vein) (with phlebolith)
      456.9
  ulcerated 454.0
  umbilical cord - *see* Complications,
      umbilical cord
  uterine ligament 456.9
  vocal cord 456.9
  vulva 456.9
    complicating
      delivery 657.9
      pregnancy (undelivered) 634.9
Vas deferens - *see* condition
Vas deferentitis 607.5
Vasa praevia - *see* Placenta, previa
Vascular - *see also* condition
  loop on papilla (optic) 744.8
  spider 448
Vascularity, pulmonary, congenital
    747.6
Vasculitis 447
  allergic 446.2
  disseminated 447
  kidney 446.9
  nodular 695.2
  rheumatic - *see* Fever, rheumatic
Vasitis 607.5
  nodosa 607.5
  tuberculous 016.2
    late effect or sequela 019.2
Vasodilation 443.9
Vasomotor - *see* condition
Vasospasm 443.9
  cerebral (artery) (*see also* Ischemia,
      cerebral, transient) 435.9
  nerve
    autonomic 358.9

Vasospasm—*continued*
  nerve—*continued*
    peripheral - *see* Angiospasm, nerve
    spinal - *see* Angiospasm, nerve
    sympathetic 358.9
  peripheral NEC 443.9
  retina (artery) 377.0
Vasospastic - *see* condition
Vasovagal attack (paroxysmal) 782.5
  psychogenic 305.3
Vater's ampulla - *see* condition
Vegetation, vegetative
  adenoid (nasal fossa) 500
  endocarditis (acute) (any valve) (chronic)
      (subacute) 421.0
  heart (mycotic) (valve) 421.0
Veil
  Jackson's 751.1
  over face (causing asphyxia) (*see also*
      Asphyxia, newborn) 776.9
Vein, venous - *see* condition
Veldt sore (*see also* Ulcer, skin) 707.9
Velpeau's hernia - *see* Hernia, Velpeau's
Venofibrosis 458.9
Venom poisoning 989.4
Venomous bite or sting (animal or insect)
      989.4
Venous - *see* condition
Ventral - *see* condition
Ventricle, ventricular - *see also* condition
  escape - *see* Action, heart, irregular
Ventriculitis, cerebral (*see also*
      Meningitis) 320.9
Vernet's syndrome 344.9
Verneuil's disease 095
Verruca (filiformis) (plana) (plana juvenilis)
      (plantaris) (vulgaris) 079.1
  acuminata (any site) 099.9
  necrogenica (primary) 017.0
    late effect or sequela 019.9
  peruana 089.0
  peruviana 089.0
  seborrheica (*see also* Keratosis,
      seborrheic) 216.0
  senile (*see also* Keratosis, seborrheic)
      216.0
  tuberculosa (primary) 017.0
    late effect or sequela 019.9
  venereal 099.9
  viral 079.1
Verrucosities (*see also* Verruca) 079.1
  hyaline, papilla 377.6
Verse's disease 279
Version
  cervix (*see also* Malposition, uterus)
      624.9

Version—*continued*
  during labor
    fetus or newborn (*see also* Birth
        injury NEC) 772.9
    uterus (postinfectional) (postpartal, old)
        (*see also* Malposition, uterus)
        624.9
  during delivery - *see* Obstetrical
      trauma
    forward - *see* Anteversion, uterus
    lateral - *see* Lateroversion, uterus
Vertebra, vertebral - *see* condition
Vertigo 780.5
  auditory 385
  aural 385
  epidemic 079.8
  epileptic - *see* Epilepsy
  hysterical 300.1
  labyrinthine 385
  laryngeal 783.3
  Meniere's 385
  menopausal 627
Verumontanitis (chronic) (*see also*
      Urethritis) 597
Vesania (*see also* Psychosis) 299
Vesical - *see* condition
Vesicle
  cutaneous 709.9
  seminal - *see* condition
  skin 709.9
Vesicocolic - *see* condition
Vesicoperineal - *see* condition
Vesicorectal - *see* condition
Vesico-urethrorectal - *see* condition
Vesicovaginal - *see* condition
Vesicular - *see* condition
Vesiculitis (seminal) 607.4
  amebic 006.9
    with liver abscess 006.0
  gonorrheal (acute) 098.0
    chronic or duration of 2 months or
        over 098.1
  trichomonal 131
  tuberculous 016.2
    late effect or sequela 019.2
Vestibulitis 384.0
  ear 384.0
  nose (external) 508.9
Vestige, vestigial - *see also* Persistence
  branchial 745.4
  structures in vitreous 744.8
Vibriosis NEC 027.9
Vidal's disease 698.3
Villaret's syndrome 356
Villous - *see* condition
Vincent's
  angina 101

Vincent's—*continued*
 bronchitis 101
 disease 101
 gingivitis 101
 infection (any site) 101
 laryngitis 101
 stomatitis 101
 tonsillitis 101
Vinson-Plummer syndrome 280
Viosterol deficiency (*see also* Deficiency,
  calciferol) 265.9
Virchow's
 degeneration (any site) 276
 disease 723.4
Viremia 079.9
Virilism (adrenal) NEC 255.0
 with
  adrenal hyperplasia or tumor 255.0
  adrenal insufficiency (congenital)
   273.6
  cortical hyperfunction 255.0
  11 hydroxylase defect 273.6
  21 hydroxylase defect 273.6
  3B hydroxysteroid dehydrogenase
   defect 273.6
Virilization (female) (*see also* Virilism)
  255.0
Virus, viral (*see also* condition) 079.9
 infection (*see also* Infection, virus)
  079.9
  Coxsackie (*see also* Coxsackie)
   079.9
 lung - *see* Pneumonia, virus
 septicemia 079.9
Viscera, visceral - *see* condition
Visceroptosis 569.9
Visible peristalsis 785.8
Vision, visual
 blurred, blurring 781.0
  hysterical 300.1
 defect, defective NEC 370.9
 disorientation (syndrome) 781.0
 disturbance NEC 781.0
  hysterical 300.1
 field, limitation 781.0
Vitality, lack or want of 790.1
 newborn 778.9
Vitamin deficiency NEC (*see also*
  Deficiency, vitamin) 266.9
Vitelline duct, persistent 751.0
Vitiligo 709.9
 eyelid 709.9
 vulva 629.9
Vitreous - *see* condition
Vocal cord - *see* condition
Vogt-Koyanagi syndrome 366

Vogt-Spielmeyer
 amaurotic familial idiocy 333.0
 disease 333.0
Vogt's (Cecile) disease or syndrome
  331.9
Voice
 change (*see also* Dysphonia) 783.5
 loss (*see also* Aphonia) 783.5
Volhard-Fahr disease (*see also*
  Hypertension, malignant with renal
  involvement) 400.3
Volkmann's ischemic contracture or
  paralysis (complicating trauma)
  995.7
Voluntary starvation 306.5
Volvulus (bowel) (colon) (intestine) 560.2
 with
  hernia - *see* Hernia, by site, with
   obstruction
 congenital 751.4
 duodenum 537.9
 fallopian tube 615.9
 oviduct 615.9
 stomach (due to absence of gastrocolic
  ligament) 537.9
Vomiting 784.1
 allergic 535
 arising during pregnancy - *see*
   Hyperemesis, gravidarum
 bilious (cause unknown) 784.1
 blood (*see also* Hematemesis) 784.5
 causing asphyxia, choking, or
   suffocation (*see also* Asphyxia,
   food) 933
 cyclical 305.5
 epidemic 079.8
 fecal matter 569.9
 functional 536.9
  psychogenic 305.5
 hysterical 300.1
 nervous 305.5
 neurotic 305.5
 pernicious or persistent 536.9
  with abortion - *see* Abortion, by type,
   with toxemia
  arising during pregnancy - *see*
    Hyperemesis, gravidarum
  psychogenic 305.5
  puerperal, postpartum - *see*
    Hyperemesis, gravidarum
 physiological 784.1
 psychic 305.5
 stercoral 569.9
 uncontrollable 536.9
  pregnancy - *see* Hyperemesis,
   gravidarum

Vomiting — *continued*
 uncontrollable — *continued*
  psychogenic 305.5
 uremic - *see* Uremia
 winter 079.8
Vomito negro (*see also* Fever, yellow)
  060.9
Von Bechterew's disease 712.4
Von Bergmann's hypopituitarism 253.1
Von Bezold's abscess - *see* Mastoiditis
Von Economo's disease 065
 late effects 066
Von Gierke's disease 271.0
Von Gies' joint 095
Von Graefe's disease 373.9
Von Hippel-Lindau disease 759.8
Von Hippel's disease 224
Von Jaksch's
 anemia 285.8
 disease 285.8
Von Recklinghausen-Applebaum disease
  273.2
Von Recklinghausen's
 disease (nerves) (skin) 743.4
  bones 252.0
 tumor 743.4
Von Willebrand(-Jurgens') disease 286.3
Vossius' ring 921
Voyeurism 302.5

Vrolik's disease 756.6
Vulva - *see* condition
Vulvitis (acute) (allergic) (aphthous)
   (atrophic) (chronic) (gangrenous)
   (hypertrophic) (intertriginous)
   (senile) 622.1
 with
  abortion - *see* Abortion, by type, with
    sepsis
  ectopic gestation - *see* categories
    631.0-631.3
 adhesive, congenital 752.6
 arising during pregnancy 630
  fetus or newborn 763.1
 blennorrhagic 098.0
  chronic or duration of 2 months or
    over 098.1
 diabetic - *see* category 250
 due to Ducrey's bacillus 099.0
 gonococcal 098.0
  chronic or duration of 2 months or
    over 098.1
 leukoplakic 629.2
 monilial 112
 puerperal, postpartum, childbirth 670
 syphilitic (early) 091.0
  late 095
 trichomonal 131
Vulvorectal - *see* condition
Vulvovaginitis (*see also* Vulvitis) 622.1

W

Wagner-Unverricht syndrome 716.0
Wagner's disease 709.9
Waldenstrom's
  disease 722.1
  macroglobulinemia 275.5
  syndrome 275.5
Walking
  difficulty 787.5
    psychogenic 306.3
  sleep 306.4
    hysterical 300.1
Wall, abdominal - see condition
Wallenberg's syndrome (see also Disease,
    cerebrovascular, acute) 436.9
Wallgren's meningitis (see also Meningitis,
    aseptic) 045.9
Wandering
  acetabulum 723.9
  gallbladder 751.6
  kidney, congenital 753.3
  organ or site, congenital NEC - see
    Malposition, congenital
  pacemaker (heart) (see also Action,
    heart, irregular) 427.9
  spleen 289.5
War neurosis 300.1
Wardenburg-Klein syndrome 270.8
Wardrop's disease (with lymphangitis)
  681
Wart (common) (digitate) (filiform)
    (infectious) (juvenile) (plantar) (viral)
    079.1
  external genital organs (venereal)
    099.9
  Henle's (of cornea) 378.4
  Peruvian 089.0
  prosector 017.0
    late effect or sequela 019.9
  seborrheic (see also Keratosis,
    seborrheic) 216.0
  senile (see also Keratosis, seborrheic)
    216.0
  tuberculous 017.0
    late effect or sequela 019.9
  venereal 099.9
Warthin's tumor (salivary gland) 210.2
Washerwoman's itch 692.4
Wasting
  disease 796.0
  extreme (due to malnutrition) 268
Water
  deprivation of 994.3

Water—continued
  in joint (see also Disease, joint) 729.9
  intoxication 788.0
  itch 120.3
  lack of 994.3
  loading 788.0
  on brain - see Hydrocephalus
  on chest 511.2
  poisoning 788.0
Waterbrash 784.7
Water-hammer pulse (see also
    Endocarditis, aortic) 395.9
Waterhouse(-Friderichsen) syndrome or
    disease 036.1
  with meningitis 036.0
Wax in ear 387.1
Waxy
  degeneration, any site 276
  kidney 276
  liver (large) 276
  spleen 276
Weak, weakness 790.1
  arches (acquired) 736
    congenital 755.7
  bladder sphincter 786.2
  congenital 778.9
  foot (double) - see Weak, arches
  heart, cardiac (congenital) (see also
    Failure, heart) 782.4
  mind - see Retardation, mental, mild
  muscle 733.9
  myocardium (see also Failure, heart)
    782.4
  newborn 778.9
  senile 794
  valvular - see Endocarditis
Wear, worn
  tooth, teeth (hard tissues)
    (interproximal) (occlusal) 521.1
Weather
  effects of
    cold NEC 991.9
    hot NEC (see also Heat) 992.9
  skin 709.9
Web, webbed (congenital) - see also
    Anomaly, specified type NEC
  canthus 744.8
  esophagus 750.3
  fingers 755.1
  larynx 748.2
  neck 745.5
  toes 755.1
Weber-Christian disease 686.9

Weber-Cockayne syndrome 757.2
Weber-Gubler syndrome 344.1
Weber-Osler syndrome 448
Weber's paralysis or syndrome 344.1
Wedge-shaped or wedging vertebrae
 729.1
Wegener's granulomatosis or syndrome
 446.3
Weight
 gain (excessive) 277
  during pregnancy 634.9
 loss (cause unknown) 788.4
 5 1/2 pounds (2,500 grams) or less 777
  .in multiple birth 769.4
Weil's disease 100.0
Weingarten's syndrome 519.2
Weiss-Baker syndrome 358.1
Wen (see also Cyst, sebaceous) 706.2
Wenckebach's phenomenon (see also
  Block, heart) 427.3
Werdnig-Hoffman
 atrophy, muscle 330.1
 syndrome 330.1
Werlhof's disease (see also
  Thrombocytopenia) 287.1
Werner's disease or syndrome 258.9
Wernicke's
 encephalopathy 263.9
 polioencephalitis, superior 263.9
West African fever 084.4
Westphal-Strumpell syndrome 273.3
Wet
 brain (alcoholic) 303.9
 feet, tropical (syndrome) (maceration)
  991.4
Wharton's duct - see condition
Wheal 709.9
Wheezing 783.2
Whiplash injury or syndrome 847.0
Whipple's disease 039.9
Whipworm 127.2
White - see also condition
 kidney
  large - see Nephrosis
  small (see also Nephritis, chronic)
   582
 leg, puerperal, postpartum, childbirth
  671.0
 mouth 112
 spot lesions, teeth 521.0
Whitehead 706.2
Whites 629.3
Whitlow (with lymphangitis) 681
 melanotic 172.9
  fingernail 172.7
  toenail 172.8

Whitmore's disease or fever 025
Whooping cough 033.9
 Bordetella
  bronchoseptica 033.9
  parapertussis 033.1
  pertussis 033.0
Wickman's influenzal encephalitis 474
Widening aorta (see also Aneurysm,
  aorta) 441.9
Willan's lepra 696.1
Willebrand-Jurgens thrombopathy 286.3
Wilms'
 neoplasm 189.0
 tumor 189.0
Wilson-Mikity syndrome (see also
  Syndrome, respiratory distress)
  776.2
Wilson's
 disease or syndrome 273.3
 hepatolenticular degeneration 273.3
 lichen ruber 697.0
Winckel's disease (see also Septicemia)
  038.9
Window - see also Imperfect closure
 aorticopulmonary 746.0
Winged scapula 723.9
Winter - see condition
Withdrawal symptoms, syndrome (drug)
  (narcotic) NEC 304.9
 specified drug - see listing under
   Dependence, if not listed see
   Table of adverse effects
 steroid NEC 962.0
Witts' anemia 280
Witzelsucht 301.9
Wolff-Parkinson-White syndrome (see
  also Tachycardia, paroxysmal)
  427.5
Wolhynian fever 083.2
Woolly, wooly hair (congenital) (nevus)
  757.3
Word
 blindness (congenital) (developmental)
  306.1
  secondary to organic lesion 781.5
 deafness (congenital) (developmental)
  306.1
  secondary to organic lesion 781.5
Worm-eaten soles 102.3
Worm(s) (colic) (fever) (infection)
  (infestation) (see also Infestation)
  128.9
 guinea 125.8
 in intestine NEC 127.9
Worn out (see also Exhaustion) 790.1

Wound, open (by cutting or piercing instrument) (by firearms) (dissection) (incised) (penetrating) (perforating) (puncture) (with initial hemorrhage, not internal) (with involvement of ligament, muscle or tendon) 907

Note—For open wounds of any of the following sites with open wounds of any of the other sites—*see* Wound, open, multiple.

For open wounds penetrating to internal organs of abdomen, chest, or pelvis—*see* Injury, internal, by site, with open wound.

The following fourth-digit subdivisions are for use with categories 870, 872, 874–878, 880–887, 890–897, 900–907:

.0 *Without mention of complication*
.1 *Complicated*
.2 *With tendon involvement* (for use with categories 880–884, 890–894 and 900–906 only)
.9 *Late effect*

"Complicated" includes open wounds with mention of delayed healing, delayed treatment, foreign body, or major infection.

Wound, open—*continued*
abdomen, abdominal (external) (muscle) (wall) 879.0
  complicated 879.1
  late effect 879.9
alveolar (process) - *see* Wound, open, face
ankle 891
anterior chamber, eye 870
anus - *see* Injury, internal, anus
arm 884
  forearm 881
  upper 880
auditory canal (external) (meatus) 872
auricle, ear 872
axilla 880
back 876
breast 879.0
  complicated 879.1
  late effect 879.9
brow - *see* Wound, open, face
buttock 877
calf 891
canaliculus lacrimalis 870
canthus, eye 870
cauda equina 958.5
  late effect 958.9
cheek(s) - *see* Wound, open, face
chest (wall) (external) 875

Wound, open—*continued*
chin - *see* Wound, open, face
choroid 870
ciliary body (eye) 870
clitoris 878
conjunctiva 870
cornea (non-penetrating) 870
costal region 875
Descemet's membrane 870
digit(s)
  foot 893
  hand 883
ear (auricle) (canal) (drum) (external) 872
elbow 881
epididymis 878
epigastric region 879.0
  complicated 879.1
  late effect 879.9
epiglottis 874
eustachian tube 872
extremity
  lower (multiple) NEC 894
  upper (multiple) NEC 884
eye(s) (lid) (muscle) (globe) 870
eyeball 870
eyebrow - *see* Wound, open, face
eyelid 870
face (except ear, eye and nose) (multiple sites) 873.7
  complicated 873.8
  late effect 873.9
feet 901
finger(s) (nail) (subungual) 883
flank 879.0
  complicated 879.1
  late effect 879.9
foot (any part except toe(s) alone) 892
forearm 881
forehead - *see* Wound, open, face
genital organs (external) NEC 878
globe (eye) 870
groin 879.0
  complicated 879.1
  late effect 879.9
gum(s) - *see* Wound, open, face
hand 882
head NEC 854.1
  laceration or cut (superficial) - *see* Wound, open, scalp
  scalp - *see* Wound, open, scalp
heel 892
hip 890
hymen 878
iliac region 879.0
  complicated 879.1
  late effect 879.9

Wound, open—*continued*
  incidental to
    dislocation - code as Dislocation,
      compound
    fracture - code as Fracture, open
    intracranial injury - code as Injury,
      intracranial, with open wound
    nerve injury - code as Injury, nerve,
      with open wound
  inguinal region 879.0
    complicated 879.1
    late effect 879.9
  instep 892
  intra-ocular 870
  iris 870
  jaw (fracture not involved) - *see* Wound,
    open, face
  knee 891
  labium (majus) (minus) 878
  lacrimal apparatus, gland, or sac 870
  larynx 874
  leg (except thigh) (multiple) 891
  lens (eye) 870
  limb
    lower (multiple) NEC 894
    upper (multiple) NEC 884
  lip - *see* Wound, open, face
  loin 876
  lumbar region 876
  malar region - *see* Wound, open, face
  mastoid region - *see* Wound, open, face
  midthoracic region 875
  mouth - *see* Wound, open, face
  multiple 907

Note—Multiple open wounds of sites classifiable to the same three- or four-digit category should be classified to that category unless they are in different limbs.

Multiple open wounds of sites classifiable to different three- or four-digit categories, or in different limbs, should be coded according to the following list.

Wound, open—*continued*
  multiple—*continued*
    arm(s) (site(s) classifiable to 880, 881,
      884)
      both 900
      one 884
      one or both with
        face (site(s) classifiable to 870-
          872, 873.2, 873.7) 906
        hand(s) (site(s) classifiable to 882,
          883) (same limb only)
          884
        other or both limb(s) 900

Wound, open—*continued*
  multiple—*continued*
    arm(s)—*continued*
      one or both with—*continued*
        lower limb(s) (site(s) classifiable
          to 890-894) 902
        neck (site(s) classifiable to 874)
          905
        scalp (site(s) classifiable to 873.0)
          904
        trunk (site(s) classifiable to 875-
          878, 879.0, 879.7) 905
      face (site(s) classifiable to 870-872,
        873.2, 873.7)
      with
        limb(s) (site(s) classifiable to 880-
          884, 890-894) 906
        scalp, neck or trunk (site(s)
          classifiable to 873.0, 874-
          878, 879.0, 879.7) 879.7
        complicated 879.8
        late effect 879.9
    finger(s) (site(s) classifiable to 883)
      both hands (with other part(s) of
        hand(s) (site(s) classifiable to
        882) 903
      one hand, with
        part(s) of hand other than
          finger(s) (site(s) classifiable
          to 882) (of same hand
          only) 884
        other or both hand(s) 903
      one or both hand(s), with
        arm(s) (site(s) classifiable to 880,
          881, 884) (same limb only)
          884
        other or both limb(s) 900
        other site(s) - *see* listing under
          Wound, open, multiple,
          arm, one or both with
    hand(s) (site(s) classifiable to 882)
      both (with finger(s)) (site(s)
        classifiable to 884) 903
      one or both, with
        arm(s) (site(s) classifiable to 880,
          881, 884) (same limb only)
          884
        other or both limb(s) 900
        other site(s) - *see* listing under
          Wound, open, multiple,
          arm, one or both with
      one, with
        finger(s) (site(s) classifiable to
          883) (of same hand only)
          884
        other or both hand(s) 903

Wound, open—*continued*
  multiple—*continued*
    lower limb(s) (site(s) classifiable to
        890-894)
      both   901
      one   894
      one or both with
        face (site(s) classifiable to 870-
            872, 873.2, 873.7)   906
        neck (site(s) classifiable to 874)
            905
        scalp (site(s) classifiable to 873.0)
            904
        trunk (site(s) classifiable to 875-
            878, 879.0, 879.7)   905
        upper limb (site(s) classifiable to
            880-884)   902
    neck (site(s) classifiable to 874)
      with
        face, scalp or trunk (site(s)
            classifiable to 870-873,
            875-878, 879.0, 879.7) 879.7
          complicated   879.8
          late effect   879.9
        limb(s) (site(s) classifiable to 880-
            884, 890-894)   905
    scalp (site(s) classifiable to 873.0)
      with
        face, neck or trunk (site(s)
            classifiable to 870-872,
            873.2, 873.7, 874-878,
            879.0, 879.7)   879.7
          complicated   879.8
          late effect   879.9
        limb(s) (site(s) classifiable to 880-
            884, 890-894)   904
    sites of one upper limb   884
    trunk (site(s) classifiable to 875-878,
        879.0, 879.7)   879.7
      with
        face, scalp or neck (site(s)
            classifiable to 870-874)879.7
          complicated   879.8
          late effect   879.9
        limb(s) (site(s) classifiable to 880-
            884, 890-894)   905
      complicated   879.8
      late effect   879.9
  nail
    finger(s)   883
    thumb   883
    toe(s)   893
  nasal (septum) (sinus) - *see* Wound,
      open, nose
  nasopharynx - *see* Wound, open, nose
  neck   874

Wound, open—*continued*
  nerve - *see* Injury, nerve, by site, with
      open wound
  nose (septum) (sinus)   873.2
    complicated   873.3
    late effect   873.9
  ocular muscle   870
  orbit   870
  orbital region   870
  palate - *see* Wound, open, face
  palm   882
  parathyroid (gland)   874
  pelvic floor or region   879.0
    complicated   879.1
    late effect   879.9
  penis   878
  perineum   879.0
    complicated   879.1
    late effect   879.9
  pharynx   874
  pinna   872
  popliteal space   891
  prepuce   878
  pubic region   879.0
    complicated   879.1
    late effect   879.9
  pudenda   878
  rectovaginal septum   878
  retina   870
  sacral region   877
  sacroiliac region   877
  salivary (ducts) (glands) - *see* Wound,
      open, face
  scalp   873.0
    complicated   873.1
    late effect   873.9
  scapular region   880
  sclera   870
  scrotum   878
  shin   891
  shoulder   880
  skin NEC   907
  skull (without skull fracture)   854.1
  spermatic cord   878
  spinal cord (*see also* Injury, spinal, by
      region, with open wound)   958.7
    late effect   958.9
  sternal region   875
  subconjunctival   870
  subcutaneous NEC   907
  submaxillary region - *see* Wound, open,
      face
  submental region - *see* Wound, open face
  supraclavicular region   874
  supraorbital - *see* Wound, open, face

Wound, open—*continued*
  temple - *see* Wound, open, face
  temporal region - *see* Wound, open,
    face
  testicle   878
  testis   878
  thigh   890
  thorax, thoracic (external)   875
  throat   874
  thumb (nail) (subungual)   883
  thyroid (gland)   874
  toe(s) (nail) (subungual)   893
  tongue - *see* Wound, open, face
  trachea   874
  trunk (multiple) NEC   879.7
    complicated   879.8
    late effect   879.9
    specified part NEC   879.0
      complicated   879.1
      late effect   879.9
  tunica vaginalis   878
  tympanic membrane   872

Wound, open—*continued*
  tympanum   872
  unspecified site(s)   907
  uvula - *see* Wound, open, face
  vagina   878
  vitreous (humor)   870
  vulva   878
  wrist   881
Wright's syndrome   447
Wrist - *see also* condition
  drop   738.2
Wrong drug (given in error) NEC   977.9
  specified drug or substance - *see* Table
    of adverse effects
Wry neck - *see* Torticollis
Wuchereria infestation   125.0
  bancrofti   125.0
  Brugia malayi   125.1
  malayi   125.1
Wuchereriasis   125.0
Wuchereriosis   125.0

X

X-ray
  cancer - *see* Neoplasm, skin, malignant
  effects, adverse - *see* Effect, adverse, x-
    rays
Xanthelasma   272.0
  eyelid   272.0
  palpebrarum   272.0
Xanthelasmoidea   757.2
Xanthinuria   270.5
Xanthoma(s), xanthomatosis (bone)
    (cutaneotendinous) (disseminatum)
    (familial) (hereditary)
    (hypercholesterinemic)
    (hypercholesterolemic)
    (hyperlipemic) (infantile, of skin)
    (joint) (juvenile) (multiple) (pituitary
    gland) (splenomegalic) (tendon
    sheath) (tuberosum multiplex)
    272.0

Xanthoma(s), etc.—*continued*
  diabeticorum - *see* category 250
Xanthosarcoma - *see* Neoplasm,
    connective tissue, malignant
Xanthosis   709.9
Xenophobia   300.2
Xeroderma (congenital) (*see also*
    Ichthyosis)   757.2
  acquired   701.1
  pigmentosum   757.2
Xerophthalmia, vitamin A deficiency
    260.1
Xerosis
  conjunctiva   378.3
    vitamin A deficiency   260.1
  skin   706.3
Xerostomia   527.7
Xiphopagus   759.1
Xylulosuria   271.8

Y

Yawning
  psychogenic   305.2
Yaws   102.9
  bone or joint lesions   102.6
  butter   102.1
  chancre   102.0
  cutaneous, less than five years after
        infection   102.2
  early (cutaneous) (macular)
        (maculopapular) (micropapular)
        (papular)   102.2
    frambeside   102.2
  ganglion   102.6
  gangosis, gangosa   102.5
  gumma, gummata   102.4
    bone   102.6
  gummatous
    frambeside   102.4
    osteitis   102.6
    periostitis   102.6
  hydrarthrosis   102.6
  hyperkeratosis (early) (late)   102.3
  initial lesions   102.0
  juxta-articular nodules   102.7
  late nodular (ulcerated)   102.4
  latent (without clinical manifestations)
        (with positive serology)   102.8

Yaws − *continued*
  mother   102.0
  mucosal   102.7
  multiple papillomata   102.1
  nodular, late (ulcerated)   102.4
  osteitis   102.6
  papilloma, plantar or palmar   102.1
  periostitis (hypertrophic)   102.6
  ulcers   102.4
  wet crab   102.1
Yellow
  atrophy (acute) (congenital) (liver)
        (subacute) (*see also* Necrosis,
        liver)   570
    chronic   573.9
    healed - *see* Cirrhosis, postnecrotic
  resulting from
    administration of blood, plasma,
        serum or other biological
        substance (within 8 months
        of administration)   999.2
  fever - *see* Fever, yellow
  jack (*see also* Fever, yellow)   060.9
  jaundice (*see also* Jaundice)   785.2
Yersinia septica   027.9

Z

Zenker's diverticulum (esophagus)   530.2
Ziehen-Oppenheimer disease   331.1
Zieve's syndrome   571.0
Zollinger-Ellison syndrome   251
Zona - *see* Herpes, zoster

Zoophobia   300.2
Zoster (herpes) - *see* Herpes, zoster
Zuelzer(-Ogden) anemia (megaloblastic)
      281.2
Zymotic - *see* Condition

SECTION II

ALPHABETICAL INDEX TO EXTERNAL CAUSES OF INJURY (E CODE)

SECTION II

ALPHABETICAL INDEX TO EXTERNAL CAUSES OF INJURY (E CODE)

Note — See Volume 1, pp. 451–455, for definitions and examples related to transport accidents.

See end of Section II, Volume 2, pp. 546–550, for fourth-digit subdivisions which are for use with categories E800–E845 to identify the injured person.

For complications resulting from an overdose of a drug (except anesthesia) or a wrong drug given in error and for intoxication or poisoning by a drug or other chemical substance — *see* Table of adverse effects (Section III).

For allergy, dermatitis and unspecified reaction due to external medicaments or to contact with drugs or other chemical substances — *see* Category 692, Volume 1.

See "Introduction" for other important explanations about the use of the index.

A

Abandonment
  child, with intent to injure or kill E968
  newborn E904
    with intent to injure or kill E968
Abortion, criminal, injury to child E968
Abuse, child E968
Accident (to) E929
  aircraft (in transit) (powered) E841
    at landing, take-off E840
    late effect of E941
    unpowered E842
    while alighting, boarding E843
  amphibious vehicle
    on
      land - *see* Accident, motor vehicle
      water - *see* Accident, watercraft
  animal, ridden NEC E827
    in sport E906
  balloon E842
  caused by, due to
    animal (in sport) E906
      ridden, in transport NEC E827
    avalanche NEC E909
    cataclysm E908
    cold (excessive) (*see also* Cold)
      E901
    conflagration - *see* Conflagration
    corrosive liquid, substance NEC
      E924

Accident (to) — *continued*
  caused by, due to — *continued*
    corrosive liquid, etc. — *continued*
      in therapeutic procedure - *see*
        categories E930, E931
    cutting or piercing instrument (*see also* Cut) E920.9
    electric current (*see also* Electric shock) E925.9
    environmental factor NEC E909
    explosive material (*see also* Explosion) E923.9
    fire, flames - *see also* Fire
      conflagration - *see* Conflagration
    firearm missile (by other person)
      E922.9
      self-inflicted E922.0
    heat (excessive) (*see also* Heat)
      E900
    hot object, liquid, substance (not producing fire or flames)
      E924
      in therapeutic procedure - *see*
        categories E930, E931
    in transport accident - *see*
      categories E800-E845
    ignition - *see* Ignition
    landslide NEC E909
    lightning NEC E907
    natural factor NEC E909
    radiation - *see* Radiation
    thunderbolt NEC E907

Accident (to)—*continued*
  railway—*continued*
    involving—*continued*
      derailment (*see also* Derailment,
          railway)   E802
      explosion (*see also* Explosion,
          railway engine)   E803
      fall (*see also* Fall from railway
          rolling stock)   E804
      fire (*see also* Explosion, railway
          engine)   E803
      hitting by, being struck by
        object falling in, on, from, rolling
            stock, train, vehicle
            E806
        rolling stock, train, vehicle
            E805
      overturning, railway rolling stock,
          train, vehicle (*see also*
          Derailment, railway)   E802
      running off rails, railway (*see also*
          Derailment, railway)   E802
      specified circumstances NEC
          E806
      train or vehicle hit by
        avalanche   E806
        falling
          earth   E806
          object   E806
          rock   E806
          tree   E806
        landslide   E806
  ski(ing)   E885
    jump   E884
  spacecraft   E845
  street car   E825
  traffic NEC   E819
  vehicle, nonroad NEC   E927
  watercraft
    with
      drowning or submersion resulting
          from
        accident other than to watercraft
            E832
        accident to watercraft   E830
      injury, except drowning or
          submersion, resulting from
        accident other than to watercraft
            - *see* categories E833-
            E838
        accident to watercraft   E831
    machinery   E836
Acid throwing   E961
Aero-otitis media   E902
Aerosinusitis   E902
After-effect, late - *see* Late effect

Air
  blast in war operations   E993
  embolism (traumatic) NEC   E902
    in medical, surgical procedure - *see*
        Complication, procedure
        involved
  sickness   E903
Alpine sickness   E902
Anaphylactic shock, anaphylaxis   E931.9
  due to bite or sting (venomous)   E905
  following, in, specified medical or
      surgical procedure - *see*
      Complication, procedure
      involved
Andes disease   E902
Anoxia
  due to high altitude   E902
  in anesthesia (*see also* Complication,
      anesthesia)   E930.1
Apoplexy
  heat   E900
Arachnidism   E905
Arthritis, serum   E931.9
  following, in, specified medical or surgical
      procedure - *see* Complication,
      procedure involved
Asphyxia, asphyxiation
  by
    chemical in war operations   E997
    explosion - *see* Explosion
    gas - *see also* Table of adverse
        effects
      in war operations   E997
      legal
        execution   E978
        intervention (tear)   E972
    mechanical means (*see also*
        Suffocation)   E913.9
  from
    conflagration - *see* Conflagration
    fire - *see also* Fire
      in war operations   E990
    ignition - *see* Ignition
  in
    anesthesia - *see* Complication,
        anesthesia
Aspiration
  during medical, surgical procedure
      (mucus) (phlegm) (vomitus) - *see*
      Complication, procedure
      involved
  foreign body - *see* Foreign body,
      aspiration
  mucus, not of newborn (with asphyxia,
      obstruction respiratory passage,
      suffocation)   E912

Aspiration—*continued*
  phlegm (with asphyxia, obstruction
     respiratory passage, suffocation)
     E912
  vomitus (with asphyxia, obstruction
     respiratory passage, suffocation)
     E911
Assassination (attempt) (*see also* Assault)
    E968
Assault (homicidal) (by) (in) E968
  acid E961
    swallowed E962
  bite (of human being) E968
  brawl (hand) (fists) (foot) E960
  burning, burns (by hot liquid, substance,
     fire) E968
    acid E961
     swallowed E962
    caustic, corrosive substance E961
     swallowed E962
    chemical from swallowing caustic,
     corrosive substance E962
    vitriol E961
     swallowed E962
  caustic, corrosive substance E961
    swallowed E962
  cut, any part of body E966
  dagger E966
  drowning E964
  explosive(s) E965
  fight (hand) (fists) (foot) E960
    with weapon (blunt) E968
     cutting or piercing E966
     firearm E965
  fire E968
  firearm(s) E965
  garrotting E963
  gunshot (wound) E965
  hanging E963
  hitting (by blunt instrument) on head
     E968
  injury NEC E968
    to child due to criminal abortion
     E968
  knife E966
  late effect of E969
  ligature E963
  poisoning (gas) (liquid) (solid) E962
  puncture, any part of body E966
  pushing
    before moving object, train, vehicle
     E968
    from high place E967
  rape E960
  scalding - *see* Assault, burning
  shooting E965

Assault (homicidal)—*continued*
  stab, any part of body E966
  strangulation E963
  submersion E964
  suffocation E963
  violence NEC E968
  vitriol E961
    swallowed E962
  weapon (blunt) E968
    cutting or piercing E966
    firearm E965
  wound E968
    cutting E966
    gunshot E965
    knife E966
    piercing E966
    puncture E966
    stab E966
Atrophy, liver, subacute, yellow,
    following, in, specified medical or
    surgical procedure - *see*
    Complication, procedure involved
Attack by animal E906
Avalanche E909
  falling on or hitting
    motor vehicle (in motion) (on public
     highway) E818
     not on public highway E823
    railway train E806
Aviators' disease E902

B

Barotrauma (otitic) (sinus) E902
Battered baby or child (syndrome) E968
Bayonet wound (*see also* Cut) E920.8
  in
    legal intervention E974
    war operations E995
Bean in nose E912
Beheading (by guillotine)
  homicide E966
  legal execution E978
Bending, injury in E919
Bends E902
Bite
  animal (nonvenomous) E906
    venomous (sea) E905
  cat E906
  centipede E905
  dog E906
  human being E968
  insect (nonvenomous) E906
    venomous E905

Bite — *continued*
late effect of - *see* Late effect
rat E906
serpent E905
snake (venomous) E905
spider E905
venomous E905
Blast (air) in war operations E993
from nuclear explosion E996
underwater E992
Blow E929
by law-enforcing agent, police (on duty) E975
with blunt object E973
from being hit or struck by specified object or vehicle - *see* Hit by
Blowing up (*see also* Explosion) E923.9
Brawl (hand) (fists) (foot) E960
Breakage (accidental)
ladder (causing fall) E881
part (any) of
ladder (causing fall) E881
motor vehicle
in motion (on public highway) E818
not on public highway E823
nonmotor road vehicle E827
pedal cycle E826
scaffolding (causing fall) E881
Broken glass, injury by E920.8
Bumping against, into (accidentally)
object (moving) (projected) (stationary) E917
person E917
with fall E886
Burning, burns (accidental) (by) (from) (on) E899
acid (any kind) E924
swallowed - *see* Table of adverse effects
bedclothes (*see also* Fire, specified NEC) E898
blowlamp (*see also* Fire, specified NEC) E898
boat, ship, watercraft - *see* categories E830, E831, E837
bonfire (controlled) E897
uncontrolled E892
brazier fire (controlled) E897
caustic liquid, substance E924
swallowed - *see* Table of adverse effects
chemical E924
from swallowing caustic, corrosive substance - *see* Table of adverse effects
in war operations E997

Burning, burns, etc. — *continued*
cigar(s) or cigarette(s) (*see also* Fire, specified NEC) E898
clothes, clothing, nightdress E893
with conflagration - *see* Conflagration
conflagration - *see* Conflagration
corrosive liquid, substance E924
swallowed - *see* Table of adverse effects
electric current (*see also* Electric shock) E925.9
fire, flames (*see also* Fire) E899
flare, Verey pistol E922.9
accidentally self-inflicted E922.0
heat
from appliance (electrical) E924
in medical, surgical procedure - *see* Complication, procedure involved
homicide (attempt) (*see also* Assault, burning) E968
hot liquid, object E924
ignition - *see also* Ignition
clothes, clothing, nightdress E893
with conflagration - *see* Conflagration
highly inflammable material (benzine) (gasoline) (kerosene) (matches, box or packet) (petrol) E894
in war operations (from fire-producing device or conventional weapon) E990
from nuclear explosion E996
inflicted by other person
in accidental circumstances - code as accidental
stated as
homicidal, intentional E968
undetermined whether accidental or intentional E988
internal, from swallowed caustic, corrosive liquid, substance - *see* Table of adverse effects
late effect of NEC E944
lighter (cigar) (cigarette) (*see also* Fire, specified NEC) E898
lightning E907
liquid (boiling) (hot) (molten) E924
caustic, corrosive (external) E924
swallowed - *see* Table of adverse effects
local application of externally applied medicaments E931.3
matches (*see also* Fire, specified NEC) E898
ignition of box or packet E894

Burning, burns, etc. - *continued*
  medical, surgical procedure - *see*
    Complication, procedure
    involved
  medicament, externally applied
    E931.3
  metal, molten E924
  object (hot) E924
    producing fire or flames - *see* Fire
  pipe (smoking) (*see also* Fire, specified
    NEC) E898
  radiation, radioactive substance (*see*
    also Radiation) E926.1
    in medical, surgical procedure - *see*
      Complication, irradiation
  railway engine, locomotive, train (*see*
    also Explosion, railway engine)
    E803
  self-inflicted injury from
    accidental circumstances - code as
      accidental
    stated as intentional, purposeful
      E958
    unspecified whether accidental or
      intentional E988
  stated as undetermined whether
    accidental or intentional E988
  steam E924
  substance (boiling) (hot) (molten) E924
    caustic, corrosive (external) E924
    swallowed - *see* Table of adverse
      effects
  suicidal (attempt) NEC E958
    late effect of E959
  therapeutic misadventure - *see*
    categories E930, E931
  torch, welding (*see also* Fire, specified
    NEC) E898
  trash fire (*see also* Burning, bonfire)
    E897
  vapor E924
  vitriol E924
  x-rays E926.1
    in medical, surgical procedure - *see*
      Complication, irradiation

C

Cachexia, lead or saturnine E866
  from pesticide E865
Caisson disease E902
Capital punishment (any means) E978

Car sickness E903
Casualty (not due to war) NEC E929
  war (*see also* War operations) E995
Cat scratch or bite E906
Cataclysm (any injury) E908
Catching fire - *see* Ignition
Caught
  between
    objects (moving) (stationary and
      moving) E918
  in
    door - *see* Trapped by door
    object E918
Cave-in (causing asphyxia, suffocation (by
    pressure)) E913.9
  with injury other than asphyxia or
    suffocation E916
  struck or crushed by E916
    with asphyxiation or suffocation
      E913.9
Choking (on) (any object except food or
    vomitus) E912
  apple E911
  food, any type (regurgitated) E911
  mucus or phlegm E912
  seed E911
Civil insurrection - *see* War operations
Cloudburst (any injury) E908
Cold, exposure to (accidental) (excessive)
    (extreme) (place) E901
  in surgery, complication of use of
    E930.9
  late effect of NEC E945
  suicide E958
Colic, lead, painter's or saturnine - *see*
    category E866
Collapse
  building E916
    burning E891
      private E890
  due to heat E900
  during medical, surgical procedure - *see*
    Complication, procedure
    involved
  machinery E928
  structure, burning NEC E891
Collision (accidental)

Note - In the case of collisions between
different types of vehicles, persons, and
objects, priority in classification is in the
following order and in the listing below
the combinations are listed only under the
vehicle, etc., having priority. For definitions see Vol. 1, pages 451-455.
  Aircraft

Watercraft
Motor vehicle
Railway vehicle
Street car
Pedal cycle
Other nonmotor road vehicle
Pedestrian or person (using pedestrian
    conveyance)
Other vehicle
Object (except where falling from or set
    in motion by vehicle, etc., listed
    above)

Collision—continued
aircraft (with object or vehicle) (fixed)
        (movable) (moving) E841
    with
        person (while landing, taking off)
                (without accident to aircraft)
                E844
        powered (in transit) E841
            while landing, taking off E840
        unpowered E842
        while landing, taking off E840
    motor vehicle (on public highway)
            (traffic accident) E812
        after leaving, running off, public
                highway (without antecedent
                collision) E816
            with antecedent collision on public
                highway - see categories
                E810-E815
        and
            abutment (bridge) E815
            animal (herded) (unattended) E815
                carrying person, property E813
            animal-drawn vehicle E813
            another motor vehicle E812
            any object, person or vehicle off
                    the public highway resulting
                    from a noncollision motor
                    vehicle traffic accident E816
            avalanche E815
            culvert E815
            fallen
                stone E815
                tree E815
            guard post or guard rail E815
            landslide E815
            machinery (road) E815
            nonmotor road vehicle NEC
                    E813
            object (fallen) (fixed) (movable)
                    (moving) (normally on public
                    highway) not falling from, set
                    in motion by, aircraft NEC
                    E815

Collision—continued
    motor vehicle, etc.—continued
        and—continued
            object —continued
                off, normally not on, public
                    highway resulting from a
                    noncollision motor vehicle
                    traffic accident E816
            pedal cycle E813
            pedestrian (conveyance) E814
            person (using pedestrian
                    conveyance) E814
            post (lamp) (light) (signal)
                    (telephone) E815
            railway rolling stock, train, vehicle
                    E810
            street car E811
            traffic signal or sign E815
            tree E815
            tricycle E813
        not on public highway, nontraffic
                accident E820
            and
                animal (carrying person,
                        property) (herded)
                        (unattended) E820
                animal-drawn vehicle E820
                another motor vehicle (moving)
                        E820
                    stationary E821
                avalanche E821
                landslide E821
                nonmotor vehicle (moving)
                        E820
                    stationary E821
                object (fallen) ((normally) fixed)
                        (movable but not in
                        motion) (stationary) E821
                    moving, except when falling
                        from, set in motion by,
                        aircraft E820
                pedal cycle (moving) E820
                    stationary E821
                pedestrian (conveyance) E820
                person (using pedestrian
                        conveyance) E820
                railway rolling stock, train,
                        vehicle (moving) E820
                    stationary E821
                road vehicle (any) (moving)
                        E820
                    stationary E821
                tricycle (moving) E820
                    stationary E821
        pedal cycle E826

Combustion, spontaneous - *see* Ignition
Complication (from administration of)
(during) (in) (of) (use of)

Note— For complications resulting from
an overdose of a drug (except anesthesia)
or a wrong drug given in error and for intoxication or poisoning by a drug—*see*
Table of adverse effects.

For allergy, dermatitis, and unspecified
reaction due to external medicaments or
to contact with drugs—*see* Category 692.3.

Complication, etc.—*continued*
  anesthesia, anesthetic (drug) (in
        operative or surgical (therapeutic)
        procedure or management)
        E930.1
    cosmetic   E936.1
    diagnostic   E932.1
    esthetic   E936.1
    nontherapeutic NEC   E936.1
    prophylactic   E935.1
  biological(s) -*see* Complication, drug
  blood sampling   E932.8
  catheterization (bladder) (urethral)
        E931.8
    diagnostic   E932.8
  circumcision (prophylactic)   E935.0
    anesthesia, anesthetic (drug)   E935.1
    ritual   E936.0
  cosmetic procedure (*see also*
        Complication, esthetic procedure)
        E936.9
    surgical   E936.0
      anesthesia, anesthetic (drug)
        E936.1
  diagnostic procedure   E932.9
    biological(s)   E932.3
    blood sampling   E932.8
    catheterization   E932.8
    drug(s)   E932.3
    radioactive substance   E932.2
    specified procedure NEC   E932.8
    surgical   E932.0
      anesthesia, anesthetic (drug)
        E932.1
    x-rays   E932.2
  drug(s) or biological(s)   E931.1
    anesthetic - *see* Complication,
        anesthesia
    contraceptive (nontherapeutic)
        E936.9
    diagnostic (procedure)   E932.3
    during operative or surgical
        therapeutic procedure   E930.9

Complication, etc.—*continued*
  drug(s) or biological(s)—*continued*
    nontherapeutic NEC   E936.9
    prophylactic (procedure)   E935.3
  esthetic procedure   E936.9
    biological(s)   E936.9
    drug(s)   E936.9
    radioactive substances   E936.9
    surgical   E936.0
      anesthesia, anesthetic (drug)
        E936.1
    x-rays   E936.9
  immunization (*see also* Complication,
        prophylactic, vaccination)
        E934.9
  infusion, transfusion (therapeutic) (with
        onset of serum hepatitis within
        eight months after)   E931.2
    during
      nontherapeutic procedure NEC
        E936.9
      operative or surgical (therapeutic)
        procedure   E930.2
      prophylactic procedure   E935.9
  injection (with onset of serum hepatitis
        within eight months after)
    drug or biological (therapeutic)
        E931.1
      diagnostic procedure   E932.3
      during surgical procedure   E930.9
        anesthesia   E930.1
      nontherapeutic procedure NEC
        E936.9
      prophylactic procedure - *see*
        categories E933-E935
  needle in blood test   E932.8
  skin test   E932.8
  vaccine (prophylactic) (*see also*
        Complication, prophylactic
        vaccination)   E934.9
    therapeutic   E931.1
  irradiation, radiation (ionizing) (from
        isotope, radioactive substance,
        radium or x-rays)
    diagnostic   E932.2
    heat (lamp), therapeutic   E931.8
    in unspecified medical procedure
        E931.0
    non-ionizing (infra-red lamp) (ultra-
        violet lamp), therapeutic
        E931.8
    nontherapeutic procedure NEC
        E936.9
    prophylactic   E935.2
    therapeutic   E931.0
      during operative or surgical
        procedure   E930.9

Complication, etc. — *continued*
  isotope - *see* Complication, irradiation
  late effect of
    irradiation, classifiable to E931.0,
        E932.2, E935.2, E936.9
        E948
    procedures classifiable to E930-E936,
        except as in E947, E948
        E949
    surgery, classifiable to E930.0,
        E932.0, E935.0, E936.0
        E947
  local application (therapeutic)   E931.3
  nontherapeutic procedure NEC
        E936.9
    biological(s)   E936.9
    drug(s)   E936.9
    operative, surgical   E936.0
      anesthesia   E936.1
    other specified   E936.9
    radioactive substance(s)   E936.9
    x-rays   E936.9
  prophylactic (procedure), prophylaxis
        (with)   E935.9
    appendectomy, appendicectomy
        E935.0
      anesthesia, anesthetic (drug)
        E935.1
    biologicals   E935.3
    circumcision   E935.0
      anesthesia, anesthetic (drug)
        E935.1
    drug(s)   E935.3
    infusion or transfusion, during
        E935.9
    operative, surgical   E935.0
      anesthesia, anesthetic (drug)
        E935.1
    radioactive substance(s)   E935.2
    specified NEC   E935.9
    sterilization   E935.0
      anesthesia, anesthetic (drug)
        E935.1
    vaccination, vaccine   E934.9
      bacterial NEC   E933.8
        mixed (without pertussis
            component)   E933.9
        with pertussis component
            E933.6
      BCG   E933.0
      cholera   E933.2
      diphtheria   E933.5
      measles   E934.4
      mixed
        bacterial, no pertussis component
            E933.9

Complication, etc. — *continued*
  prophylactic, etc. — *continued*
    vaccination, vaccine — *continued*
      mixed — *continued*
        pertussis and other   E933.6
        viral-rickettsial and bacterial, no
            pertussis component
            E934.7
      nonbacterial NEC   E934.9
      pertussis   E933.6
      plague   E933.3
      poliomyelitis   E934.5
      rabies   E934.1
      rickettsial NEC   E934.6
      smallpox   E934.0
      specified NEC   E934.9
      TAB   E933.1
      tetanus   E933.4
      typhoid, (and) paratyphoid   E933.1
      typhus   E934.2
      viral NEC   E934.6
      yellow fever   E934.3
    x-rays   E935.2
  radioactive substance(s) - *see*
        Complication, irradiation
  surgery (therapeutic), surgical treatment
        (not in anesthetic management)
        E930.0
    anesthesia (*see also* Complication,
        anesthesia)   E930.1
    cosmetic   E936.0
    diagnostic   E932.0
    drug(s), biological(s) during   E930.9
    esthetic   E936.0
    in disease carrier   E936.0
    infusion, transfusion during   E930.2
    nontherapeutic NEC   E936.0
    prophylactic   E935.0
    x-rays, radioactive substance(s)
        during   E930.9
  therapeutic procedure (nonoperative)
        E931.9
    biological(s)   E931.1
    drug(s)   E931.1
    infusion, transfusion during   E931.2
    local application (fomentations)
        (medicaments) (plasters)
        E931.3
    operative, surgical   E930.0
      anesthesia, anesthetic (drug)
        E930.1
      biological(s) during   E930.9
      drug(s) during   E930.9
      infusion, transfusion during
        E930.2
      procedure NEC during   E930.9

Complication, etc. — *continued*
  therapeutic procedure — *continued*
    operative, surgical — *continued*
      radioactive substance during
          E930.9
      x-rays during   E930.9
    radioactive isotope(s), substance
        E931.0
      specified NEC   E931.8
      x-rays   E931.0
    vaccination (prophylactic) - *see also*
        Complication, prophylactic
        vaccination
      therapeutic   E931.1
    x-rays - *see* Complication, irradiation
Compression, divers' squeeze   E902
Conflagration
  building or structure, except private
      dwelling (church) (convalescent
      or residential home) (factory)
      (hospital) (hotel) (institution
      (educational) (dormitory)
      (residental)) (school) (shop) (store)
      (theatre)   E891
  not in building or structure   E892
  private dwelling (apartment) (boarding
      house) (camping place) (caravan)
      (home (private)) (house) (lodging
      house) (rooming house)
      (tenement)   E890
Cramp(s)
  heat   E900
  swimmers'   E910.0
    not in recreation   E910.9
Cranking (car) (truck) (bus) (engine) injury
      by   E917
Crash
  aircraft (in transit) (powered)   E841
    at landing, take-off   E840
    in war operations   E994
    on runway NEC   E840
    unpowered   E842
  glider   E842
Crushed (accidentally)   E929
  between
    boat(s), ship(s), watercraft (and dock
        or pier) (without accident to
        watercraft)   E838
      after accident to, or collision,
          watercraft   E831
    objects (moving) (stationary and
        moving)   E918
  by
    avalanche NEC   E909
    boat, ship, watercraft after accident
        to, collision, watercraft   E831

Crushed (accidentally) — *continued*
  by — *continued*
    cave-in   E916
      with asphyxiation or suffocation
          E913.9
    falling
      aircraft (*see also* Accident, aircraft)
          E841
        in war operations   E994
      earth, material   E916
        with asphyxiation or suffocation
            E913.9
      object   E916
        on ship, watercraft   E838
        while loading, unloading
            watercraft   E838
    landslide NEC   E909
    lifeboat after abandoning ship   E831
    machinery as listed in E928   E928
    railway rolling stock, train, vehicle
        (part of)   E805
    street car   E825
    vehicle as listed in E927   E927
  in
    machinery   E918
    object   E918
    transport accident - *see* categories
        E800-E845
  late effect of NEC   E946
Cut, cutting (any part of body) (accidental)
      E920.9
  by
    axe   E920.1
    bayonet (*see also* Bayonet wound)
        E920.8
    broken glass   E920.8
    circular saw   E920.2
    cutting or piercing instrument - *see*
        also category E920
      late effect of   E946
    garden fork   E920.1
    hand saw or tool (not powered)
        E920.1
      powered   E920.0
    hedge clipper   E920.1
      powered   E920.0
    hoe   E920.1
    knife   E920.1
    lawn mower   E920.1
      powered   E920.0
      riding   E920.2
    machine (cutting) (metal cutting)
        E920.2
    meat
      grinder   E920.2
      slicer   E920.2
    nails   E920.8

Drowning - *see* Submersion
Dust in eye   E914

E

Earth falling (on) (with asphyxia or
        suffocation (by pressure))   E913.9
    with injury other than asphyxia,
        suffocation   E916
    motor vehicle (in motion) (on public
        highway)   E818
        not on public highway   E823
    nonmotor road vehicle NEC   E827
    pedal cycle   E826
    railway rolling stock, train, vehicle
        E806
    street car   E825
    struck or crushed by   E916
        with asphyxiation or suffocation
            E913.9
Earthquake (any injury)   E908
Effect(s) (adverse) of
    air pressure
        high   E902
        low   E902
    altitude (in aircraft)   E902
    chemical substance NEC - *see* Table of
        adverse effects
    cold, excessive (exposure to) (*see also*
        Cold, exposure)   E901
    drug - *see* Complication, drug
    heat (excessive) (*see also* Heat)   E900
    high pressure   E902
    hot
        place   E900
        weather   E900
    insolation   E900
    insulation   E900
    late - *see* Late effect of
    low pressure (in aircraft)   E902
    medical procedure - *see* Complication,
        procedure involved
    motion   E903
    nuclear explosion or weapon in war
        operations (blast) (fireball) (heat)
        (radiation) (direct) (secondary)
        E996
    poisonous substance NEC - *see* Table
        of adverse effects

Effect(s) (adverse) of - *continued*
    radiation - *see* Radiation
    surgical procedure - *see* Complication,
        surgery
    travel   E903
Electric shock, electrocution (accidental)
        (from exposed wire, faulty
        appliance, high voltage cable, live
        rail, open socket) (by) (in)   E925.9
    appliance or wiring
        factory   E925.1
        farm (building)   E925.8
            house   E925.0
        home   E925.0
        industrial   E925.1
        outdoors   E925.8
        public building   E925.8
        resident institution   E925.8
        school   E925.8
        specified place NEC   E925.8
    caused by other person
        in accidental circumstances - code as
            accidental
        stated as
            intentional, homicidal   E968
            undetermined whether accidental
                or intentional   E988
    homicidal (attempt)   E968
    legal execution   E978
    lightning   E907
    machinery   E925.9
        factory   E925.1
        farm   E925.8
        home   E925.0
    misadventure in therapeutic procedure
        - *see* Electric shock, therapeutic
    self-inflicted injury from
        in accidental circumstances - code as
            accidental
        stated as intentional   E958
        unspecified whether accidental or
            intentional   E988
        stated as undetermined whether
            accidental or intentional   E988
    suicidal (attempt)   E958
    therapeutic (adverse effect)   E931.8
        during operative, surgical procedure
            E930.9
Electrocution - *see* Electric shock
Embolism
    air (traumatic) NEC   E902
        in medical, surgical procedure - *see*
            Complication, procedure
            involved
Encephalitis
    lead or saturnine   E866

Encephalitis—*continued*
  lead or saturnine—*continued*
    from pesticide E865
  postvaccinal - *see* Complication,
    prophylactic vaccination
Entanglement
  in
    bedclothes, causing suffocation
      E913.0
    wheel of pedal cycle E826
Entry of foreign body, material, any - *see*
  Foreign body
Error in administration of drug (overdose)
  (wrong drug) - code as accidental
  - *see* Table of adverse effects
Execution, legal (any method) E978
Exhaustion
  cold E901
  due to excessive exertion E919
  heat E900
Explosion (accidental) (in) (of) (on)
  E923.9
  acetylene E923.2
  air tank (compressed) (in machinery)
    E921.1
  aircraft (in transit) (powered) E841
    at landing, take-off E840
    in war operations E994
    unpowered E842
  anesthetic gas in operating theatre
    E923.2
  blasting (cap) (materials) E923.1
  boiler (machinery), not on transport
    vehicle E921.0
    steamship - *see* Explosion, watercraft
  bomb E923.8
    in war operations E993
      after cessation of hostilities E998
      atom, hydrogen or nuclear E996
      injury by fragments from E991
  butane E923.2
  caused by other person
    in accidental circumstances - code as
      accidental
    stated as
      intentional, homicidal E965
      undetermined whether accidental
        or homicidal E985
  coal gas E923.2
  detonator E923.1
  dynamite E923.1
  explosive (material) NEC E923.9
    gas(es) E923.2
    missile E923.8
      in war operations E993
        injury by fragments from E991

Explosion—*continued*
  explosive (material) NEC—*continued*
    used in blasting operations E923.1
  fire-damp E923.2
  fireworks E923.0
  gas E923.2
    cylinder (in machinery) E921.1
    pressure tank (in machinery) E921.1
  gasoline (fumes) (tank) not in motor
    vehicle E923.2
  grain store E923.8
  grenade E923.8
    in war operations E993
      injury by fragments from E991
  homicide (attempt) E965
  hot water heater, tank (in machinery)
    E921.0
  in mine (of explosive gases) NEC
    E923.2
  late effect of NEC E946
  methane E923.2
  missile E923.8
    in war operations E993
      injury by fragments from E991
  motor vehicle (part of)
    in motion (on public highway) E818
    not on public highway E823
  munitions (dump) (factory) E923.8
    in war operations E993
  of mine E923.8
    in war operations
      after cessation of hostilities E998
      at sea or in harbor E992
      land E993
        after cessation of hostilities
          E998
        injury by fragments from E991
      marine E992
  own weapons in war operations E993
    injury by fragments from E991
  pressure
    cooker E921.8
    gas tank (in machinery) E921.1
    vessel (in machinery), specified type
      NEC E921.8
    on transport vehicle - *see*
      categories E800-E845
  propane E923.2
  railway engine, locomotive, train (boiler)
    (with subsequent collision,
      derailment, fall) E803
    with
      collision (antecedent) (*see also*
        Collision, railway) E800
      derailment (antecedent) E802
      fire (without collision or derailment
        (antecedent)) E803

Explosion—*continued*
  secondary fire resulting from - *see* Fire
  self-inflicted injury from
    in accidental circumstances - code as
        accidental
    stated as intentional, purposeful
        E955
    unspecified whether accidental or
        intentional   E985
  shell (artillery)   E923.8
    in war operations   E993
      injury by fragments from   E991
    stated as undetermined whether caused
        accidentally or purposely
        inflicted   E985
  steam or water lines (in machinery)
      E921.0
  suicide (attempted)   E955
  torpedo   E923.8
    in war operations   E992
  transport accident - *see* categories
      E800-E845
  war operations - *see* War operations,
      explosion
  watercraft (boiler)   E837
    causing drowning, submersion (after
        jumping from watercraft)
        E830
Exposure (weather) (conditions) (rain)
      (wind)   E904
  excessive
    cold   E901
      homicidal intent   E968
    heat   E900
  radiation - *see* Radiation
  resulting from transport accident - *see*
      categories E800-E845

F

Fall, falling (accidental)   E887
  building   E916
    burning   E891
      private   E890
  down
    escalator   E880
    ladder   E881
      in boat, ship, watercraft   E833
    staircase   E880
    stairs, steps - *see* Fall from stairs
  earth (with asphyxia or suffocation (by
      pressure)) (*see also* Earth, falling)
      E913.9

Fall, falling, etc.—*continued*
  from, off
    aircraft (at landing, take-off) (in
        transit) (while alighting,
        boarding)   E843
      resulting from accident to aircraft
        - *see* categories E840-E842
    balcony   E882
    bed   E884
    bicycle   E826
    boat, ship, watercraft (into water)
        E832
      after accident to, collision, fire on
          E830
        and subsequently struck by (part
            of) boat   E831
      and subsequently struck by (part
          of) boat   E838
      burning, crushed, sinking   E830
        and subsequently struck by (part
            of) boat   E831
      gangplank   E832
    bridge   E882
    building   E882
      burning   E891
        private   E890
    bunk in boat, ship, watercraft   E834
      due to accident to watercraft
          E831
    car - *see* Fall from motor vehicle
    chair   E884
    cliff   E884
    elevation aboard ship   E834
      due to accident to ship   E831
    embankment   E884
    escalator   E880
    flagpole   E882
    furniture   E884
    gangplank (into water) (*see also* Fall
        from boat)   E832
      to deck, dock   E834
    hammock on ship   E834
      due to accident to watercraft
          E831
    haystack   E884
    high place NEC   E884
      stated as undetermined whether
          accidental or intentional
          E987
    horse (while riding)   E827
      in sport   E906
    ladder   E881
      in boat, ship, watercraft   E833
      due to accident to watercraft
          E831
    machinery as listed in E928   E884

Fall, falling, etc. — continued
  in, on — continued
    street car E825
    water transport (see also Fall in boat)
        E835
  into
    cavity E883
    dock E883
    from boat, ship, watercraft (see
        also Fall from boat) E832
    hold (of ship) E834
      due to accident to watercraft
          E831
    hole E883
    moving part of machinery E918
    opening in surface E883
    pit E883
    quarry E883
    shaft E883
    tank E883
    water - see Submersion
    well E883
  late effect of NEC E943
  object (see also Hit by object, falling)
      E916
  out of - see Fall from
  over
    animal E885
    cliff E884
    embankment E884
    small object E885
  overboard (see also Fall from boat)
      E832
  rock E916
  same level NEC E887
    aircraft (any kind) E843
      resulting from accident to aircraft
          - see categories E840-E842
    boat, ship, watercraft E835
      due to accident to, collision,
          watercraft E831
    from
      collision, pushing, shoving, by or
          with other person E886
      slipping, stumbling, tripping E885
    snow E916
    stone E916
    through
      hatch (on ship) E834
        due to accident to watercraft
            E831
      window E882
    timber E916
  while alighting from, boarding, entering, ·
      leaving
      aircraft (any kind) E843

Fall, falling, etc. — continued
  while alighting from, etc. — continued
    motor bus, motor vehicle (on public
        highway) E817
      not on public highway E822
    nonmotor road vehicle NEC E827
    railway train E804
    street car E825
Fallen on by
  animal (in sport) E906
    ridden in transport E827
  horse (in sport) E906
    ridden in transport E827
Fell or jumped from high place, so stated
    E987
Felo-de-se (see also Suicide) E958
Fever
  heat E900
  thermic E900
Fight (hand) (fists) (foot) (see also Assault,
    fight) E960
Fire (accidental) (caused by heat from
    appliance (electrical), hot object or
    hot substance) (secondary, resulting
    from explosion) E899
  conflagration - see Conflagration
  controlled, normal (in fireplace, furnace
      or stove) (charcoal) (coal) (coke)
      (electric) (gas) (wood)
    bonfire E897
    brazier E897
    in building or structure, except
        private dwelling (church)
        (convalescent or residential
        home) (factory) (hospital)
        (hotel) (institution (educational)
        (dormitory) (residential))
        (school) (shop) (store) (theatre)
        E896
    in private dwelling (apartment)
        (boarding house) (camping
        place) (caravan) (home
        (private)) (house) (lodging
        house) (rooming house)
        (tenement) E895
    not in building or structure E897
    trash E897
  forest (uncontrolled) E892
  grass (uncontrolled) E892
  hay (uncontrolled) E892
  homicide (attempt) E968
    late effect of E969
  in, of, on, starting in
    aircraft (in transit) (powered) E841
      at landing, take-off E840
      stationary E892
    unpowered (balloon) (glider) E842

Fire, etc. — *continued*
in, of, on, etc. — *continued*
balloon E842
boat, ship, watercraft - *see* categories
E830, E831, E837
building or structure, except private
dwelling (church) (convalescent
or residential home) (factory)
(hospital) (hotel) (institution
(educational) (dormitory)
(residential)) (school) (shop)
(store) (theatre) (uncontrolled)
E891
forest (uncontrolled) E892
glider E842
grass (uncontrolled) E892
hay (uncontrolled) E892
lumber (uncontrolled) E892
mine (uncontrolled) E892
motor vehicle (in motion) (on public
highway) E818
not on public highway E823
stationary E892
prairie (uncontrolled) E892
private dwelling (apartment) (boarding
house) (camping place)
(caravan) (home (private))
(house) (lodging house)
(rooming house) (tenement)
(uncontrolled) E890
railway rolling stock, train, vehicle
(*see also* Explosion, railway
engine) E803
stationary E892
street car (in motion) E825
stationary E892
transport vehicle, stationary NEC
E892
tunnel (uncontrolled) E892
war operations (by fire-producing
device or conventional
weapon) E990
from nuclear explosion E996
late effect of NEC E944
lumber (uncontrolled) E892
mine (uncontrolled) E892
prairie (uncontrolled) E892
self-inflicted injury from
in accidental circumstances - code as
accidental
stated as intentional, purposeful
E958
unspecified whether accidental or
intentional E988
specified NEC E898

Fire, etc. — *continued*
specified NEC — *continued*
with
conflagration - *see* Conflagration
ignition (of)
clothing E893
highly inflammable material
(benzine) (gasoline)
(kerosene) (matches, box
or packet) (petrol) E894
started by other person
in accidental circumstances - code as
accidental
stated as
with intent to injure or kill E968
undetermined whether or not with
intent to injure or kill E988
suicide (attempted) E958
late effect of E959
tunnel (uncontrolled) E892
Fireball effects from nuclear explosion in
war operations E996
Fireworks (explosion) E923.0
Flash burns from explosion (*see also*
Explosion) E923.9
Flood (any injury) E908
Forced landing (aircraft) E840
Foreign body, object or material (entrance
into (accidental))
air passage (causing injury) E915
with asphyxia, obstruction,
suffocation E912
food or vomitus E911
nose (with asphyxia, obstruction,
suffocation) E912
causing injury without asphyxia,
obstruction, suffocation
E915
alimentary canal (causing injury) (with
obstruction) E915
with asphyxia, obstruction respiratory
passage, suffocation E912
food E911
mouth E915
with asphyxia, obstruction,
suffocation E912
food E911
pharynx E915
with asphyxia, obstruction,
suffocation E912
food E911
aspiration (with asphyxia, obstruction
respiratory passage, suffocation)
E912
causing injury without asphyxia,
obstruction respiratory
passage, suffocation E915

Foreign body, etc. — *continued*
  aspiration, etc. — *continued*
    food (regurgitated) (vomited) E911
      causing injury without asphyxia,
        obstruction respiratory
        passage, suffocation E915
    mucus (not of newborn) E912
    phlegm E912
  bladder (causing injury or obstruction)
    E915
  bronchus, bronchi - *see* Foreign body,
    air passage
  conjunctival sac E914
  digestive system - *see* Foreign body,
    alimentary canal
  ear (causing injury or obstruction)
    E915
  esophagus (causing injury or
    obstruction) E915
  eye (any part) E914
  eyelid E914
  hairball (stomach) (with obstruction)
    E915
  ingestion - *see* Foreign body, alimentary
    canal
  inhalation - *see* Foreign body,
    aspiration
  intestine (causing injury or obstruction)
    E915
  iris E914
  lacrimal apparatus E914
  larynx - *see* Foreign body, air passage
  late effect of NEC E946
  lung - *see* Foreign body, air passage
  mouth - *see* Foreign body, alimentary
    canal, mouth
  nasal passage - *see* Foreign body, air
    passage, nose
  nose - *see* Foreign body, air passage,
    nose
  ocular muscle E914
  oesophagus (causing injury or
    obstruction) E915
  operation wound (left in) (*see also*
    Complication, surgery) E930.0
  orbit E914
  pharynx - *see* Foreign body, alimentary
    canal, pharynx
  rectum (causing injury or obstruction)
    E915
  stomach (hairball) (causing injury or
    obstruction) E915
  tear ducts or glands E914
  trachea - *see* Foreign body, air passage
  urethra (causing injury or obstruction)
    E915

Foreign body, etc. — *continued*
  vagina (causing injury or obstruction)
    E915
Found dead, injured
  from exposure (to) E904
  on
    public highway E819
    railway right-of-way E807
Fracture (circumstances unknown or
    unspecified) E887
  due to specified external means - *see*
    manner of accident
  late effect of NEC E943
  occurring in water transport NEC
    E835
Freezing E901
Frostbite E901
Frozen E901

G

Garrotting, homicidal (attempted) E963
Gored E906
Gunshot wound (*see also* Shooting)
    E922.9

H

Hailstones, injured by E909
Hairball (stomach) (with obstruction)
    E915
Hanged himself (*see also* Hanging, self-
    inflicted) E983
Hanging (accidental) (*see also*
    Strangulation) E913.9
  caused by other person
    in accidental circumstances E913.9
    stated as
      intentional, homicidal E963
      undetermined whether accidental
        or intentional E983
  homicide (attempt) E963
  legal execution E978
  self-inflicted injury from
    in accidental circumstances E913.9
    stated as intentional, purposeful
      E953
    unspecified whether accidental or
      intentional E983

Hanging (accidental) — *continued*
  stated as undetermined whether
      accidental or intentional E983
  suicidal (attempt) E953
Heat (apoplexy) (collapse) (cramps)
  (effects of) (excessive) (exhaustion)
  (fever) (generated in transport
  vehicle, except in boiler, engine,
  evaporator, fire room of boat, ship,
  watercraft) (prostration) (stroke)
  E900
  from
    electric heating apparatus causing
      burning E924
    nuclear explosion in war operations
      E996
  generated in, in, boiler, engine,
    evaporator, fire room of boat,
    ship, watercraft E838
  in medical, surgical procedure - *see*
    Complication, procedure
    involved
  late effect of NEC E945
Hemolysis
  due to infusion, transfusion (*see also*
    Complication, infusion) E931.2
Hemorrhage, delayed, in surgical
    treatment (*see also* Complication,
    surgery) E930.0
Hepatitis, serum (onset within eight
    months after)
  infusion, transfusion - *see* Complication,
    infusion
  injection - *see* Complication, injection
  unspecified procedure (therapeutic)
    E931.9
High
  altitude, effects E902
  level of radioactivity, effects - *see*
    Radiation
  pressure, effects E902
  temperature, effects E900
Hit, hitting (accidental) by
  aircraft (propeller) (without accident to
    aircraft) E844
  avalanche E909
  being thrown against object in or part
    of
    motor vehicle (in motion) (on public
      highway) E818
      not on public highway E823
    nonmotor road vehicle NEC E827
    street car E825
  boat, ship, watercraft
    after fall from watercraft E838
    damaged, involved in accident
      E831

Hit, hitting (accidental) by — *continued*
  boat, ship, etc. — *continued*
    while swimming, water ski-ing E838
  bullet (automatic weapon) (pistol) (rifle)
    (*see also* Shooting) E922.9
    from air gun E917
    in war operations E991
  flare, Verey pistol (*see also* Shooting)
    E922.9
  hailstones E909
  landslide E909
  law-enforcing agent (on duty) E975
    with blunt object (baton) (stave)
      (truncheon) E973
  missile
    firearm (*see also* Shooting) E922.9
    in war operations - *see* War
      operations, missile
  motor vehicle (on public highway)
    (traffic accident) E814
    not on public highway, nontraffic
      accident E820
  nonmotor road vehicle NEC E827
  object
    falling E916
      from, in, on
        aircraft E844
          due to accident to aircraft - *see*
            categories E840-E842
        boat, ship, watercraft E838
          due to accident to watercraft
            E831
        building E916
          burning E891
            private E890
        cataclysm E908
        cave-in E916
          with asphyxiation or
            suffocation E913.9
        earthquake E908
        motor vehicle (in motion) (on
          public highway) E818
          not on public highway E823
        nonmotor road vehicle NEC
          E827
        pedal cycle E826
        railway rolling stock, train,
          vehicle E806
        street car E825
        structure, burning NEC E891
    moving NEC E917
    projected NEC E917
    set in motion by
      compressed air or gas E917
      explosion - *see* Explosion
      spring E917

Hit, hitting (accidental) by—*continued*
  object—*continued*
    set in motion by—*continued*
      striking E917
      throwing E917
    thrown into or towards
      motor vehicle (in motion) (on public
        highway) E818
        not on public highway E823
      nonmotor road vehicle NEC
        E827
      pedal cycle E826
      street car E825
    other person E917
      with blunt object E917
        intentionally, homicidal E968
        on head, homicidal E968
    pedal cycle E826
    police (on duty) E975
      with blunt object (baton) (stave)
        (truncheon) E973
    railway rolling stock, train, vehicle (part
      of) E805
    shot (shotgun) - *see* Shooting
    street car E825
Homicide (homicidal) (attempt) (justifiable)
  (*see also* Assault) E968
Hot
  liquid, object, substance, accident
    caused by E924
    late effect of E946
  place, effects E900
  weather, effects E900
Hunger E904
  resulting from transport accident - *see*
    categories E800-E845
Hurricane (any injury) E908
Hypobaropathy E902
Hypothermia E901
  in surgery, complication of E930.9

I

Ictus
  caloris E900
  solaris E900
Ignition (accidental)
  anesthetic gas in operating theatre
    E923.2
  bedclothes E898
    with
      conflagration - *see* Conflagration

Ignition (accidental)—*continued*
  bedclothes—*continued*
    with—*continued*
      ignition (of)
        clothing E893
        highly inflammable material
          (benzine) (gasoline)
          (kerosene) (matches, box
          or packet) (petrol) E894
    benzine E894
    clothes, clothing E893
      with conflagration - *see* Conflagration
    explosive material - *see* Explosion
    gasoline E894
    kerosene E894
    matches, box or packet E894
    material
      explosive - *see* Explosion
      highly inflammable E894
    nightdress E893
      with conflagration - *see* Conflagration
    petrol E894
Immersion - *see* Submersion
Inanition from hunger, thirst E904
  resulting from homicidal intent E968
Inattention after, at birth E904
  homicidal, infanticidal intent E968
Infanticide (*see also* Assault) E968
Infection (following) (from) medical,
  surgical procedure - *see*
    Complication, procedure involved
Ingestion
  drug, adverse effect - *see* Complication,
    drug
  foreign body (causing injury) (with
    obstruction) - *see* Foreign body,
    alimentary canal
  isotope, adverse effect - *see*
    Complication, irradiation
  poisonous substance NEC - *see* Table
    of adverse effects
Inhalation
  foreign body - *see* Foreign body,
    aspiration
  in medical, surgical procedure (mucus)
    (phlegm) - *see* Complication,
    procedure involved
  mucus, not of newborn (with asphyxia,
    obstruction respiratory passage,
    suffocation) E912
  phlegm (with asphyxia, obstruction
    respiratory passage, suffocation)
    E912
  poisonous gas - *see* Table of adverse
    effects

Injury, injured, etc. — *continued*
homicidal E968
in, on
  civil insurrection - *see* War
      operations
  collision - *see* Collision
  parachute descent (voluntary)
      (without accident to aircraft)
      E844
    with accident to aircraft - *see*
      categories E840-E842
  public highway E819
  railway right-of-way E807
  war operations - *see* War operations
inflicted (by)
  in course of arrest (attempted),
    suppression of disturbance,
    maintenance of order, by law-
    enforcing agents - *see* Legal
    intervention
  law-enforcing agent (on duty) - *see*
    Legal intervention
  other person
    stated as
      accidental E929
      homicidal, intentional E968
      undetermined whether
        accidentally or purposely
        E988
  police (on duty) - *see* Legal
    intervention
late effect of E946
purposely (inflicted) by other person(s)
  E968
self-inflicted
  stated as
    accidental E929
    intentionally, purposely E958
    undetermined whether accidentally
      or purposely E988
stated as
  undetermined whether accidentally or
    purposely inflicted (by) E988
  cut (any part of body) E986
  cutting or piercing instrument
    (classifiable to E920) E986
  drowning E984
  explosive(s) (missile) E985
  falling from high place E987
  firearm, explosive (classifiable to
    E922-E923) E985
  hanging E983
  knife E986
  late effect of E989

Injury, injured, etc. — *continued*
  stated as — *continued*
    undetermined whether accidentally
      or purposely inflicted
      (by) — *continued*
    poisoning (by)
      gas
        in domestic use (classifiable to
          E870-E872) E981
        not in domestic use
          (classifiable to E873-
          E877) E982
      solid or liquid substance - *see*
        Table of adverse effects,
        undetermined
    puncture (any part of body) E986
    shooting E985
    specified means NEC E988
    stab (any part of body) E986
    strangulation E983
    submersion E984
    suffocation (in plastic bag) E983
  to child due to criminal abortion E968
Inoculation - *see* Complication,
  prophylactic, vaccination
Insufficient nourishment E904
  homicidal intent E968
Insulation, effects E900
Intervention, legal - *see* Legal
  intervention
Intoxication, drug or poison - *see* Table
  of adverse effects
Irradiation - *see* Radiation

J

Jammed (accidentally)
  between objects (moving) (stationary
    and moving) E918
  in object E918
Jaundice, serum E931.9
  following, in, specified medical or
    surgical procedure - *see*
    Complication, procedure
    involved
Jumped or fell from high place, so stated
  E987
Jumping
  before train, vehicle or other moving
    object
    stated as
      intentional, purposeful E958
      suicidal (attempt) E958
      undetermined whether accidental
        or intentional E988

Late effect of—*continued*
  fall, accidental (accident classifiable to
    E880-E887) E943
  fire, accident caused by (accident
    classifiable to E890-E899)
    E944
  homicide, attempt (any means) E969
  injury undetermined whether
    accidentally or purposely
    inflicted (injury classifiable to
    E980-E988) E989
  legal intervention (injury classifiable to
    E970-E976) E977
  motor vehicle accident (accident
    classifiable to E810-E823)
    E940
  natural or environmental factor,
    accident due to (accident
    classifiable to E900-E909)
    E945
  poisoning, accidental (accident
    classifiable to E850-E877)
    E942
  suicide, attempt (any means) E959
  transport accident NEC (accident
    classifiable to E800-E807, E825-
    E845) E941
  war operations, injury due to (injury
    classifiable to E990-E998)
    E999
Launching pad accident E845
Legal
  execution, any method E978
  intervention (by) (injury from) E976
    baton E973
    bayonet E974
    blow E975
    blunt object E973
    cutting or piercing instrument E974
    dynamite E971
    execution, any method E978
    explosive(s) (shell) E971
    firearm(s) E970
    gas (asphyxiation) (poisoning) (tear)
      E972
    grenade E971
    late effect of E977
    machine gun E970
    man-handling E975
    mortar bomb E971
    revolver E970
    rifle E970
    specified means NEC E975
    stabbing E974
    stave E973
    truncheon E973

Lifting, injury in E919
Lightning (shock) (stroke) (struck by)
  E907
Liquid (noncorrosive) in eye E914
  corrosive E924
Loss of control
  motor vehicle (on public highway)
    (without antecedent collision)
    E816
  with
    antecedent collision on public
      highway - *see* Collision,
      motor vehicle
    subsequent collision
      involving any object, person or
        vehicle not on public
        highway E816
      on public highway - *see*
        Collision, motor vehicle
    not on public highway, nontraffic
      accident E823
      with antecedent collision - *see*
        Collision, motor vehicle, not
        on public highway
Lost at sea E832
  with accident to watercraft E830
  in war operations E995
Low
  pressure, effects E902
  temperature, effects E901
Lynching (*see also* Assault) E968

M

Malfunction, atomic power plant in water
  transport E838
Man-handling (in brawl, fight) E960
  legal intervention E975
Mangled (accidentally) NEC E929
Manslaughter (nonaccidental) - *see also*
  Assault
  stated as, or in circumstances indicating
    accidental - code as accident by
      means of injury
    due to negligence - code as accident
      by means of injury
    undetermined whether accidental or
      homicidal - code as injury
      undetermined whether
      accidental or purposeful
    without intent to injure or kill - code
      as accident by means of injury

Overheated (*see also* Heat) E900
Overlaid E913.0
Overturning (accidental)
  boat, ship, watercraft
    causing
      drowning, submersion E830
      injury except drowning, submersion
        E831
    machinery as listed in E928 E928
    motor vehicle (*see also* Loss of control,
      motor vehicle) E816
      with antecedent collision on public
        highway - *see* Collision, motor
        vehicle
      not on public highway, nontraffic
        accident E823
        with antecedent collision - *see*
          Collision, motor vehicle, not
          on public highway
    nonmotor road vehicle NEC E827
    pedal cycle E826
    railway rolling stock, train, vehicle (*see
      also* Derailment, railway) E802
    street car E825
    vehicle as listed in E927 E927

P

Palsy, diver's E902
Parachuting (voluntary) (without accident
    to aircraft) E844
  due to accident to aircraft - *see*
    categories E840-E842
Paralysis
  divers' E902
  lead or saturnine E866
    from pesticide E865
Phlegm aspiration or inhalation (with
    asphyxia, obstruction respiratory
    passage, suffocation) E912
Piercing (*see also* Cut) E920.9
Pinched
  between objects (moving) (stationary
    and moving) E918
  in object E918
Plumbism E866
  from insecticide E865
Poisoning (accidental) (by) - *see also*
    Table of adverse effects
  carbon monoxide
    generated by
      aircraft in transit E844

Poisoning (accidental) (by) — *continued*
  carbon monoxide — *continued*
    generated by — *continued*
      motor vehicle
        in motion (on public highway)
          E818
        not on public highway E823
      watercraft (in transit) (not in transit)
        E838
  fumes or smoke due to
    conflagration - *see* Conflagration
    explosion or fire - *see* Fire
    ignition - *see* Ignition
  gas
    in legal intervention E972
    legal execution, by E978
    on watercraft E838
    used as anesthetic - *see*
      Complication, anesthesia
  in war operations E997
  late effect of - *see* Late effect
  legal
    execution E978
    intervention
      by gas E972
Pressure, external, causing asphyxia,
    suffocation (*see also* Suffocation)
    E913.9
Privation E904
  late effect of NEC E945
  resulting from transport accident - *see*
    categories E800-E845
Projected objects, striking against or
    struck by E917
Prostration
  heat E900
Pulling, injury in E919
Puncture, puncturing (*see also* Cut)
    E920.9
Pushing (injury in) (overexertion) E919
  by other person (accidental) E917
    with fall E886
    before moving vehicle or object
      in accidental circumstances - code
        as collision
      stated as
        intentional, homicidal E968
        undetermined whether accidental
          or intentional E988
    from
      high place
        in accidental circumstances - *see*
          categories E880-E884
        stated as
          intentional, homicidal E967
          undetermined whether
            accidental or intentional
            E987

Pushing, etc. — *continued*
by other person, etc. — *continued*
from — *continued*
motor vehicle (*see also* Fall, from, motor vehicle) E818
stated as
intentional, homicidal E968
undetermined whether accidental or intentional E988

R

Radiation (effects of) (overexposure to) (ionizing) (from isotope, radioactive substance, radium or x-rays) E926.1
from atomic power plant (malfunction) E926.1
in water transport E838
in
medical or surgical procedure (complications of) - *see* Complication, irradiation
war operations (from or following nuclear explosion) (direct) (secondary) E996
water transport E838
late effect of NEC E946
natural E926.0
non-ionizing (from infra-red lamp, natural radiation, ultra-violet lamp or welding torch) E926.0
in therapy E931.8
Rape E960
Reaction
drug (idiosyncratic) (*see also* Complication, drug) E931.1
infusion, transfusion (*see also* Complication, infusion) E931.2
Residual (effect) - *see* Late effect
Rock falling on or hitting (accidentally)
motor vehicle (in motion) (on public highway) E818
not on public highway E823
nonmotor road vehicle NEC E827
pedal cycle E826
person E916
railway rolling stock, train, vehicle E806
Run over (accidentally) (by)
animal E906

Run over (accidentally) (by) — *continued*
animal — *continued*
in transport accident E827
horse E906
in transport accident E827
machinery as listed in E928 E917
motor vehicle (on public highway) E814
not on public highway E820
nonmotor road vehicle NEC E827
object (moving) E917
railway train E805
street car E825
vehicle as listed in E927 E917
Running off, away
animal
being ridden E827
in sport E906
rails, railway (*see also* Derailment) E802
roadway
motor vehicle (without antecedent collision) E816
with
antecedent collision - *see* Collision, motor vehicle
subsequent collision
involving any object, person or vehicle not on public highway E816
on public highway - *see* Collision, motor vehicle
nontraffic accident E823
with antecedent collision - *see* Collision, motor vehicle, not on public highway
nonmotor road vehicle NEC E827
pedal cycle E826

S

Saturnism E866
from insecticide E865
Scald, scalding (accidental) (by) (from) (in) E924
acid - *see* Scald, caustic
caustic or corrosive liquid, substance E924
swallowed - *see* Table of adverse effects
homicide (attempt) - *see* Assault, burning

Scald, scalding (accidental) — *continued*
  inflicted by other person
    in accidental circumstances - code as
        accidental
    stated as
      intentional or homicidal   E968
      undetermined whether accidental
          or intentional   E988
  late effect of NEC   E946
  liquid (boiling) (hot)   E924
  local application of externally applied
      medicament   E931.3
  medical, surgical procedure - *see*
      Complication, procedure
      involved
  molten metal   E924
  self-inflicted injury
    in accidental circumstances - code as
        accidental
    stated as intentional, purposeful
        E958
    unspecified whether accidental or
        intentional   E988
  stated as undetermined whether
      accidental or intentional   E988
  steam   E924
  transport accident - *see* categories
      E800-E845
  vapor   E924
Scratch, cat   E906
Sea
  sickness   E903
Self-mutilation - *see* Suicide
Sepsis
  postvaccinal - *see* Complication,
      prophylactic vaccination
  resulting from medical or surgical
      procedure - *see* Complication,
      procedure involved
Serum
  arthritis   E931.9
    following, in, specified medical or
        surgical procedure - *see*
        Complication, procedure
        involved
  hepatitis (onset within eight months
      after)
    infusion, transfusion - *see*
        Complication, infusion
    injection - *see* Complication, injection
    unspecified procedure (therapeutic)
        E931.9
  jaundice   E931.9
    following, in, specified medical or
        surgical procedure - *see*
        Complication, procedure
        involved

Serum — *continued*
  sickness   E931.9
    following, in, specified medical or
        surgical procedure - *see*
        Complication, procedure
        involved
Shock
  anaphylactic   E931.9
    due to bite or sting (venomous)
        E905
    following, in, specified medical or
        surgical procedure - *see*
        Complication, procedure
        involved
  electric (*see also* Electric shock)
      E925.9
  from electric appliance or current (*see*
      also Electric shock)   E925.9
Shooting, shot (accidental(ly))   E922.9
  down, aircraft, in war operations   E994
  himself (*see also* Shooting, self-inflicted)
      E985
  homicide (attempt)   E965
  in war operations   E991
  inflicted by other person
    in accidental circumstances   E922.9
    stated as
      intentional, homicidal   E965
      undetermined whether accidental
          or intentional   E985
  legal
    execution   E978
    intervention   E970
  self-inflicted
    accidental   E922.0
    stated as
      intentional, purposeful   E955
    unspecified whether accidental or
        intentional   E985
  stated as undetermined whether
      accidental or intentional   E985
  suicidal (attempt)   E955
Shoving (accidentally) by other person
    (*see also* Pushing by other person)
    E917
Sickness
  air   E903
  alpine   E902
  car   E903
  motion   E903
  mountain   E902
  sea   E903
  travel   E903
Sinking (accidental)
  boat, ship, watercraft (causing
      drowning, submersion)   E830

Sinking (accidental) — *continued*
  boat, ship, watercraft — *continued*
    causing injury except drowning,
        submersion   E831
Siriasis   E900
Skin eruption, postvaccinal - *see*
        Complication, prophylactic
        vaccination
Skydiving   E844
Slashed wrists (*see also* Cut, self-inflicted)
        E986
Slipping (accidental)
  on
    deck (of boat, ship, watercraft) (icy)
        (oily) (wet)   E835
    ice   E885
    ladder of ship   E833
      due to accident to watercraft
          E831
    mud   E885
    oil   E885
    snow   E885
    stairs of ship   E833
      due to accident to watercraft
          E831
    surface
      slippery   E885
      wet   E885
Sliver, wood, injury by   E920.8
Smothering, smothered (*see also*
        Suffocation)   E913.9
Solid substance in eye (any part) or
        adnexa   E914
Splinter, injury by   E920.8
Stab, stabbing   E966
  accidental - *see* Cut
Starvation   E904
  homicidal intent   E968
  late effect of NEC   E945
  resulting from accident connected with
        transport - *see* categories E800-
        E845
Stepped on by
  animal   E906
Stepping on
  object (moving) (projected) (stationary)
        E917
  person   E917
Sting
  bee   E905
  insect   E905
  scorpion   E905
  venomous   E905
  wasp   E905
Storm   E908
Straining, injury in   E919

Strangling - *see* Strangulation
Strangulation (accidental) (due to hanging)
        (*see also* Suffocation)   E913.9
  caused by other person
    in accidental circumstances - *see*
        category E913
    stated as
      intentional, homicidal   E963
      undetermined whether accidental
          or intentional   E983
  due to, by
    baby harness in baby carriage or
        perambulator   E913.0
    bars of cot or crib   E913.0
    bedclothes   E913.0
    bib   E913.0
    ligature, homicidal (attempt)   E963
    pressure NEC   E913.9
    sheet (plastic)   E913.0
    specified means NEC   E913.9
  homicide (attempt)   E963
  in
    baby carriage   E913.0
    bed   E913.0
    cot, cradle   E913.0
    perambulator   E913.0
    place other than bed, cradle   E913.9
  self-inflicted
    in accidental circumstances - *see*
        category E913
    stated as intentional, purposeful
        E953
    unspecified whether accidental or
        intentional   E983
  stated as undetermined whether
        accidental or intentional   E983
  suicidal (attempted)   E953
Strenuous movement(s)   E919
Striking
  against
    object (moving) (stationary)   E917
    person   E917
      with fall   E886
Stroke
  heat   E900
  lightning   E907
Struck by - *see also* Hit by
  lightning   E907
  thunderbolt   E907
Stumbling over animal, carpet, curb, kerb,
        rug or (small) object (with fall)
        E885
  without fall   E917
Submersion (accidental)   E910.9
  boat, ship, watercraft (causing
        drowning, submersion)   E830

Submersion (accidental) — *continued*
  boat, ship, watercraft — *continued*
    causing injury except drowning,
      submersion E831
  by other person
    in accidental circumstances - *see*
      category E910 ·
    intentional, homicidal E964
    stated as undetermined whether
      accidental or intentional
      E984
  due to
    accident
      to boat, ship, watercraft E830
      transport - *see* categories E800-
        E845
    avalanche (*see also* Avalanche)
      E909
    cataclysm E908
    cloudburst E908
    cyclone E908
    fall
      from
        boat, ship, watercraft (not
          involved in accident)
          E832
          burning, crushed E830
          involved in accident, collision
            E830
          gangplank (into water) E832
          overboard NEC E832
    flood E908
    hurricane E908
    jumping into water E910.9
      from boat, ship, watercraft
        burning, crushed, sinking E830
        involved in accident, collision
          E830
      in recreational activity E910.0
    landslide (*see also* Landslide) E909
    overturning boat, ship, watercraft
      E830
    sinking boat, ship, watercraft E830
    submersion boat, ship, watercraft
      E830
    tidal wave E908
    torrential rain E908
  homicide (attempt) E964
  in
    recreational activity E910.0
    specified activity, not in transport or
      recreational E910.9
    war operations E995
    water transport E832
      due to accident to boat, ship,
        watercraft E830

Submersion (accidental) — *continued*
  late effect of NEC E946
  self-inflicted injury from
    in accidental circumstances - *see*
      category E910
    stated as intentional, purposeful
      E954
    unspecified whether accidental or
      intentional E984
  stated as undetermined whether
    accidental or intentional E984
  suicidal (attempted) E954
  while
    fishing, not from boat E910.0
    hunting, not from boat E910.0
    ice skating E910.0
    playing in water E910.0
    skin diving E910.0
    snorkel diving E910.0
    surfboarding E910.0
    swimming E910.0
    wading (in water) E910.0
    water ski-ing E910.0
Sucked
  into
    jet (aircraft) E844
Suffocation (accidental) (by external
  means) (by pressure) (mechanical)
  E913.9
  caused by other person
    in accidental circumstances - *see*
      category E913
    stated as
      intentional, homicidal E963
      undetermined whether accidental
        or intentional E983
  due to, by
    avalanche (*see also* Avalanche)
      E909
    bedclothes E913.0
    bib E913.0
    blanket E913.0
    cave-in E913.9
    conflagration - *see* Conflagration
    explosion - *see* Explosion
    falling earth, other substance
      E913.9
    fire - *see* Fire
    food, any type (ingestion) (inhalation)
      (regurgitated) (vomited) E911
    foreign body, except food (ingestion)
      (inhalation) E912
    ignition - *see* Ignition
    landslide (*see also* Landslide) E909
    material, object except food entering
      by nose or mouth, ingested,
      inhaled E912

Suffocation — *continued*
  due to, by — *continued*
    mucus (aspiration) (inhalation), not of
        newborn E912
    phlegm (aspiration) (inhalation) E912
    pillow E913.0
    plastic bag E913.9
      in bed, cradle or perambulator
          E913.0
    sheet (plastic) E913.0
    vomitus (aspiration) (inhalation)
        E911
  homicidal (attempt) E963
  in
    baby carriage E913.0
    bed E913.0
    closed place E913.9
    cot, cradle E913.0
    perambulator E913.0
    plastic bag
      homicidal, purposely inflicted by
          other person E963
      in accidental circumstances - *see*
          category E913
      stated as undetermined whether
          accidentally or purposely
          inflicted E983
      suicidal, purposely self-inflicted
          E953
    refrigerator E913.9
  self-inflicted injury from (in plastic bag)
    in accidental circumstances - *see*
        category E913
    stated as intentional, purposeful
        E953
    unspecified whether accidental or
        intentional E983
  stated as undetermined whether
      accidental or intentional E983
  suicidal (attempted) E953
Suicide, suicidal (attempted) (by) E958
  burning, burns E958
  caustic substance E958
    poisoning (*see also* Table of adverse
        effects) E950.9
    swallowed (*see also* Table of adverse
        effects) E950.9
  cold, extreme E958
  cut (any part of body) E956
  cutting or piercing instrument
      (classifiable to E920) E956
  drowning E954
  electrocution E958
  explosive(s) (classifiable to E923)
      E955
  fire E958

Suicide, suicidal, etc. — *continued*
  firearm (classifiable to E922) E955
  hanging E953
  jumping
    before moving object, train, vehicle
        E958
    from high place E957
  knife E956
  late effect of E959
  motor vehicle E958
  poison(ing) (by) - *see also* Table of
      adverse effects
    gas (any)
      in domestic use (classifiable to
          E870-E872) E951
  puncture (any part of body) E956
  scald E958
  shooting E955
  specified means NEC E958
  stab (any part of body) E956
  strangulation E953
  submersion E954
  suffocation (in plastic bag) E953
  wound NEC E958
Sunstroke E900
Surgical procedure, complication of - *see*
    Complication, surgery
Swallowed, swallowing
  foreign body - *see* Foreign body,
      alimentary canal
  poison - *see* Table of adverse effects
  substance
    caustic - *see* Table of adverse effects
    corrosive - *see* Table of adverse
        effects
    poisonous - *see* Table of adverse
        effects
Swimmers' cramp E910.0
  not in recreation E910.9
Syndrome, battered baby or child E968

T

Tackle in sport E886
Thermic fever E900
Thermoplegia E900
Thirst E904
  resulting from accident connected with
      transport - *see* categories E800-
      E845
Thrown (accidentally)
  against object in, part of vehicle
    by motion of vehicle
      aircraft E844

Thrown (accidental) — *continued*
  against object in, etc. — *continued*
    by motion of vehicle — *continued*
      boat, ship, watercraft   E838
      motor vehicle (on public highway)
        E818
        not on public highway   E823
      due to accident to vehicle - *see*
        manner of accident
      nonmotor road vehicle NEC   E827
      railway rolling stock, train, vehicle
        E806
      street car   E825
  from
    high place, homicide (attempt)   E967
    machinery as listed in E928   E928
    vehicle as listed in E927   E927
    off animal, horse (in transport)   E827
      in sport   E906
    overboard (by motion of boat, ship,
      watercraft)   E832
      by accident to boat, ship, watercraft
        E830
Thunderbolt NEC   E907
Tidal wave (any injury)   E908
Took
  overdose of drug
    in accidental circumstances - code as
      accidental - *see* Table of
      adverse effects
    stated as intentional, suicidal (*see
      also* Table of adverse effects,
      suicide)   E950.3
    unspecified whether accidental or
      suicidal (*see also* Table of
      adverse effects, undetermined)
      E980.3
  poison
    in accidental circumstances - code as
      accidental - *see* Table of
      adverse effects
    stated as intentional, suicidal (*see.
      also* Table of adverse effects,
      suicide)   E950.9
    unspecified whether accidental or
      suicidal (*see also* Table of
      adverse effects, undetermined)
      E980.9
Tornado (any injury)   E908
Torrential rain (any injury)   E908
Traffic accident NEC   E819
Trapped (accidentally)
  between
    objects (moving) (stationary and
      moving)   E918

Trapped (accidental) — *continued*
  by
    door of
      elevator   E918
      motor vehicle (on public highway)
        (while alighting, boarding,
        entering, leaving)   E817
        not on public highway   E822
      railway train (underground)   E806
      street car   E825
      subway train   E806
  in object   E918
Travel (effects)   E903
  sickness   E903
Tree
  falling on or hitting   E916
    motor vehicle (in motion) (on public
      highway)   E818
      not on public highway   E823
    nonmotor road vehicle NEC   E827
    pedal cycle   E826
    person   E916
    railway rolling stock, train, vehicle
      E806
    street car   E825
Trench foot   E901
Tripping over animal, carpet, curb, kerb,
  rug or (small) object (with fall)
  E885
  without fall   E917
Twisting, injury in   E919

V

Vaccinia, generalized   E934.0
Violence, nonaccidental (*see also* Assault)
  E968
Volcanic eruption (any injury)   E908
Vomitus in air passages (with asphyxia,
  obstruction or suffocation)   E911

W

War operations (during hostilities) (injury)
  (by) (in)   E995
  after cessation of hostilities, injury due
    to   E998
  air blast   E993

War operations, etc. — *continued*
mustard gas E997
nerve gas E997
phosgene E997
poisoning (chemical) (gas) E997
radiation, ionizing from nuclear
explosion E996
rocket (explosion) E993
fragments, injury by E991
saber, sabre E995
screening smoke E997
shell (aircraft) (artillery) (cannon) (land-
based) (explosion) E993
fragments, injury by E991
sea-based E992
shrapnel E991
submersion E995
torpedo E992
unconventional warfare, except by
nuclear weapon E997
underwater blast E992
vesicant (chemical) (gas) E997
weapon burst E993
Washed
away by flood, tidal wave E908
overboard E832
Weather exposure, except as result of
accident connected with transport
E904
cold E901
hot E900
Wound (accidental) NEC (*see also* Injury)
E929

Wound (accidental) NEC — *continued*
battle (*see also* War operations) E995
bayonet E920.8
in
legal intervention E974
war operations E995
gunshot E922.9
homicidal (attempt) E965
inflicted by other person
in accidental circumstances
E922.9
stated as
intentional, homicidal E965
undetermined whether accidental
or intentional E985
self-inflicted
in accidental circumstances
E922.0
stated as intentional, purposeful
E955
unspecified whether accidental or
intentional E985
stated as undetermined whether
accidentally or intentionally
caused E985
suicidal (attempt) E955
incised - *see* Cut
saber, sabre E920.8
in war operations E995
Wrong drug given in error - code as
accidental - *see* Table of adverse
effects

FOURTH DIGIT SUBDIVISIONS FOR
THE EXTERNAL CAUSE (E) CODE

Injured person involved in railway accident
(fourth digits for code numbers E800–E807)

.0 Railway employee

Any person who by virtue of his employment in connection with a railway, whether by the railway company or not, is at increased risk of involvement in a railway accident

Includes: catering staff on train
            driver
            fireman
            guard

porter
postal staff on train
shunter
sleeping car attendant

.1 Passenger on railway

Any authorized person travelling on a train, except a railway employee

Excludes: intending passenger waiting at station (.8)
            unauthorized rider on railway vehicle (.8)

.2 Pedestrian

See definition (q), Vol. 1, page 455

.3 Pedal cyclist

See definition (o), Vol. 1, page 454

.8 Other specified person

Includes: intending passenger waiting at station
            occupant of road vehicle other than railway vehicle, motor vehicle,
                pedal cycle
            person accompanying passenger to train
            unauthorized rider on railway vehicle

.9 Unspecified person

**Injured person involved in motor vehicle traffic
and non-traffic accidents**
(fourth digits for code numbers E810–E819 and E820–E823)

.0 Driver of motor vehicle other than motorcycle

See definition (k), Vol. 1, page 454

.1 Passenger in motor vehicle other than motorcycle

See definition (k), Vol. 1, page 454

.2 Motorcyclist

See definition (k), Vol. 1, page 454

.3 Passenger on motorcycle

See definition (k), Vol. 1, page 454

.4 Occupant of street car

.5 Rider of animal; occupant of animal-drawn vehicle

.6 Pedal cyclist

See definition (o), Vol. 1, page 454

.7 Pedestrian

See definition (q), Vol. 1, page 455

.8 Other specified person

Includes: occupant of vehicle other than above
person on railway train involved in accident
unauthorized rider of motor vehicle

.9 Unspecified person

Injured person involved in other road vehicle accident
(street car, pedal cycle and other non-motor road vehicle accident)

(fourth digits for code numbers E825, E826, E827)

.0 Pedestrian

   See definition (q), Vol. 1, page 455

.1 Pedal cyclist (does not apply to code E827)

   See definition (o), Vol. 1, page 454

.2 Occupant of street car (does not apply to codes E826, E827)

.8 Other specified person

   Includes: occupant of non-motor road vehicle, except street car or pedal
                cycle
                rider of animal

.9 Unspecified person

Injured person in water transport accident

(fourth digits for code numbers E830–E838)

.0 Occupant of small boat

See definition(s), Vol. 1, page 455

.1 Occupant of other water craft-crew

Includes: persons:
>>> engaged in the operation of water craft
>>> providing passenger services (cabin attendants,
>>>> ship physician, catering personnel)
>>> working on ship during voyage in other capacity
>>>> (musician in band, operators of shops and
>>>> beauty parlors)

.2 Occupant of other water craft-other than crew

Includes: passenger
>>> occupant of lifeboat other than crew after abandoning ship

.3 Dockers, stevedores

Includes: longshoreman employed in the dock in loading and unloading ships

.8 Other specified person

Includes: person:
>>> accompanying passenger or member of crew
>>> visiting boat
>> immigration and customs officials on board ship
>> pilot (guiding ship into port)
>> swimmer }
>> water skier } struck by boat or part thereof

.9 Unspecified person

Injured person involved in air and space transport accidents
(fourth digits for code numbers E840–E845)

.0 Occupant of spacecraft

.1 Occupant of military aircraft

Includes: crew   } in military aircraft
        passenger (civilian) (military) }   (army) (navy)
        troops   }   (air force)

.2 Occupant of commercial aircraft, crew

Includes: air hostess   navigator
        captain   pilot
        co-pilot   steward

.3 Other occupant of commercial aircraft

Includes: flight personnel:
           on familiarization flight
           not part of crew
        passenger on plane

.4 Occupant of other and unspecified aircraft

Includes: crew   } of aircraft not military or commercial
        passenger }   police
                  }   private

.5 Ground crew, airline employee

Includes: persons employed at airfields (civilian or military) or launching
        pads, not occupants of aircraft

.8 Other specified person

Includes: parachutist making voluntary descent
        person not at airfield
        visitor to airfield

.9 Unspecified person

SECTION III

ALPHABETICAL INDEX TO ADVERSE EFFECTS OF DRUGS AND OTHER CHEMICAL SUBSTANCES

(Table of Adverse Effects)

SECTION III

ALPHABETICAL INDEX TO
ADVERSE EFFECTS OF DRUGS AND OTHER CHEMICAL SUBSTANCES

(Table of Adverse Effects)

This table is for the classification of adverse effects of drugs and other chemical substances and contains an extensive but not exhaustive list of drugs, alcohols, petroleum products, industrial solvents, corrosives, metals, gases, noxious plants, household cleansing agents, pesticides and other chemicals. For a general definition of what constitutes adverse effects, *see* notes in Volume 1 preceding categories 960, E850 and E860.

Each of the listed substances is given a code assignment according to the nature of injury classification (960–977 and 980–989). Also shown are the codes for suicide or self-inflicted injury by means of drugs or chemicals (E950–E952), for accidents involving drugs or chemicals (E850–E877 and E905), and for cases in which it could not be determined whether the adverse effect or poisoning was accidental, suicidal, or homicidal, as in E980–E982. The external causes (or circumstances) not classifiable to the categories cited, are indexed in Section II.

Not included in this table are adverse effects of two or more medicinal agents in specified combinations, and of alcohol in combination with specified medicinal agents. For the classification of these agents according to the nature of injury, *see* categories 978 and 979 in the Tabular List, Volume 1.

Also excluded are immunological agents, and radium and other radioactive substances. The classification of adverse effects and complications due to these substances will l found in Sections I and II of the Index.

Anesthetic gases are indexed in the table to categories 968.1, E856.2, E952.9 and E982. Category E856.2 is applicable only when the gas was given in error or resulted in adverse effects in circumstances other than medical treatment. In the E-Classification, "overdose" of an anesthetic gas is to be regarded as a complication of medical or surgical procedures in contrast to "overdose" of drugs which is classifiable to the categories shown in the table.

Specific symptoms and diseases constituting an adverse effect of the listed substances are not shown in this table. These can be found in Section I. Also to be found in Section I under "Effects, adverse" are the American Hospital Formulary numbers which can be used to classify new drugs listed by the American Hospital Formulary Service.

Although certain substances are indexed with one or more subentries, the great majority are listed in the table according to some one usage or state. However, it is recognized that many substances can be used in various ways – both in medicine and in industry – and may cause adverse effects as liquids and also in terms of their fumes or dusts. In cases in which the reported data indicates clearly a usage or state not shown in the table, or which is plainly different from the one shown, an attempt should be made to classify the substance in the form which more nearly expresses the reported facts.

Substance	Nature of Injury	External Cause (E-Code)		
		Accident	Suicide (attempt)	Undetermined
ABOB	961.9	E850.9	E950.3	E980.3
Abrus (seed)	988.2	E868	E950.9	E980.9
Absinthe	980.0	E860	E950.9	E980.9
Acemorphan	965.0	E853.0	E950.3	E980.3
Acenocoumarin, acenocoumarol	964.2	E852.6	E950.3	E980.3
Acepromazine	970.1	E855.1	E950.2	E980.2
Acetal	982.9	E864	E950.9	E980.9
Acetaldehyde (vapor)	987.9	E876	E952.9	E982
liquid	989.9	E869	E950.9	E980.9
Acetaminophen	965.4	E853.4	E950.3	E980.3
Acetaminosalol	965.1	E853.1	E950.1	E980.1
Acetanilid(e)	965.4	E853.4	E950.3	E980.3
Acetarsol, acetarsone	961.1	E850.6	E950.3	E980.3
Acetazolamide	975.2	E859.3	E950.3	E980.3
Acetic				
acid	983.1	E867	E950.9	E980.9
lotion	977.0	E859.7	E950.3	E980.3
anhydride	983.1	E867	E950.9	E980.9
ester	982.9	E864	E950.9	E980.9
vapor	987.9	E876	E952.9	E982
ether	982.9	E864	E950.9	E980.9
vapor	987.9	E876	E952.9	E982
Acetohexamide	962.3	E851.3	E950.3	E980.3
Acetomenaphthone	964.3	E852.7	E950.3	E980.3
Acetone (oils)	982.9	E864	E950.9	E980.9
vapor	987.9	E876	E952.9	E982
Acetophenazine (maleate)	970.1	E855.1	E950.2	E980.2
Acetophenetidin	965.4	E853.4	E950.3	E980.3
Acetophenone	982.9	E864	E950.9	E980.9
Acetorphine	965.0	E853.0	E950.3	E980.3
Acetrizoate (sodium)	977.2	E859.8	E950.3	E980.3
Acetylcarbromal	967.3	E854.3	E950.3	E980.3
Acetylcholine (chloride)	972.0	E855.3	E950.3	E980.3
Acetylcysteine	977.8	E859.8	E950.3	E980.3
Acetyldihydrocodeine	965.0	E853.0	E950.3	E980.3
Acetyldihydrocodeinone	965.0	E853.0	E950.3	E980.3
Acetylene (gas)	987.1	E872	E951	E981
industrial	987.1	E876	E952.9	E982
tetrachloride	982.9	E864	E950.9	E980.9
vapor	987.9	E876	E952.9	E982
Acetyliodosalicylic acid	965.1	E853.1	E950.1	E980.1
Acetylphenylhydrazine	963.1	E852.1	E950.3	E980.3
Acetylsalicylic acid	965.1	E853.1	E950.1	E980.1
Achromycin	960.5	E850.3	E950.3	E980.3

Substance	Nature of Injury	External Cause (E-Code)		
		Accident	Suicide (attempt)	Undetermined
Acid (corrosive) NEC	983.1	E867	E950.9	E980.9
Acidifying agents	963.2	E852.2	E950.3	E980.3
Acinitrazole	961.9	E850.9	E950.3	E980.3
Aconite (wild)	988.2	E868	E950.9	E980.9
Aconitine (liniment)	977.0	E859.5	E950.3	E980.3
Aconitum ferox	988.2	E868	E950.9	E980.9
Acridine	983.0	E867	E950.4	E980.4
vapor	987.9	E876	E952.9	E982
Acriflavine	961.9	E850.9	E950.3	E980.3
Acrolein (gas)	987.9	E876	E952.9	E982
liquid	989.9	E869	E950.9	E980.9
Actaea spicata	988.2	E868	E950.9	E980.9
Acterol	963.6	E852.3	E950.3	E980.3
ACTH	962.4	E851.4	E950.3	E980.3
Actinomycin	963.1	E852.1	E950.3	E980.3
Adalin	967.3	E854.3	E950.3	E980.3
Adicillin	960.0	E850.0	E950.3	E980.3
Adiphenine	976.1	E859.4	E950.3	E980.3
Adrenal (extract, cortex or medulla) (glucocorticoids) (hormones) (mineralocorticoids)	962.0	E851.0	E950.3	E980.3
Adrenalin(e)	972.2	E855.5	E950.3	E980.3
Adrenergics	972.2	E855.5	E950.3	E980.3
Adrenochrome	964.4	E852.8	E950.3	E980.3
Adrenocorticotropic hormone	962.4	E851.4	E950.3	E980.3
Adronol	980.9	E860	E950.9	E980.9
Aerosol spray — see Sprays				
Aethusa cynapium	988.2	E868	E950.9	E980.9
Aflatoxin	988.2	E868	E950.9	E980.9
African boxwood	988.2	E868	E950.9	E980.9
Agar (-agar)	974.5	E858.5	E950.3	E980.3
Agrypnal	967.0	E854.0	E950.0	E980.0
Air contaminant(s), source or type not specified	987.9	E877	E952.9	E982
specified type — see substance specified				
Akee	988.2	E868	E950.9	E980.9
Albamycin	960.9	E850.4	E950.3	E980.3
Alcohol	980.9	E860	E950.9	E980.9
absolute	980.0	E860	E950.9	E980.9
amyl	980.9	E860	E950.9	E980.9
antifreeze	980.1	E860	E950.9	E980.9
butyl	980.9	E860	E950.9	E980.9
dehydrated	980.0	E860	E950.9	E980.9
denatured	980.9	E860	E950.9	E980.9

Substance	Nature of Injury	External Cause (E-Code)		
		Accident	Suicide (attempt)	Undeter- mined
Alcohol — *continued*				
ethyl	980.0	E860	E950.9	E980.9
grain	980.0	E860	E950.9	E980.9
industrial	980.9	E860	E950.9	E980.9
isopropyl	980.2	E860	E950.9	E980.9
methyl	980.1	E860	E950.9	E980.9
propyl	980.2	E860	E950.9	E980.9
radiator	980.1	E860	E950.9	E980.9
rubbing	980.2	E860	E950.9	E980.9
surgical	980.9	E860	E950.9	E980.9
vapor (from any type of alcohol)	987.9	E876	E952.9	E982
wood	980.1	E860	E950.9	E980.9
Aldomet	973.5	E857.5	E950.3	E980.3
Aldosterone	962.0	E851.0	E950.3	E980.3
Aldrin (dust)	989.2	E865	E950.9	E980.9
Algeldrate	974.0	E858.0	E950.3	E980.3
Alkali (caustic)	983.2	E867	E950.6	E980.6
Alkalinizing agents (medicinal)	963.3	E852.2	E950.3	E980.3
Alka-seltzer	963.3	E852.2	E950.3	E980.3
Alkavervir	973.5	E857.5	E950.3	E980.3
Allegron	970.0	E855.0	E950.2	E980.2
Allobarbital, allobarbitone	967.0	E854.0	E950.0	E980.0
Allomethadione	966.0	E856.0	E950.3	E980.3
Allonal	967.0	E854.0	E950.0	E980.0
Allopurinol	977.8	⁻859.8	E950.3	E980.3
Allylestrenol	962.6	E851.6	E950.3	E980.3
Allylisopropylacetylurea	967.9	E854.9	E950.3	E980.3
Allyltribromide	967.3	E854.3	E950.3	E980.3
Aloe, aloes, aloin	974.1	E858.1	E950.3	E980.3
Aloxidone	966.0	E856.0	E950.3	E980.3
Aloxiprin	965.1	E853.1	E950.1	E980.1
Alpha amylase	963.5	E852.4	E950.3	E980.3
Alpha tocopherol	963.6	E852.3	E950.3	E980.3
Alphaprodine (hydrochloride)	965.0	E853.0	E950.3	E980.3
Alseroxylon	970.1	E855.1	E950.2	E980.2
Alum (ammonium) (potassium)	983.9	E867	E950.9	E980.9
medicinal (external) NEC	977.0	E859.7	E950.3	E980.3
Aluminium, aluminum (hydroxide) (gel)	974.0	E858.0	E950.3	E980.3
medicinal NEC	977.0	E859.7	E950.3	E980.3
Alurate	967.0	E854.0	E950.0	E980.0
Alvodine	965.0	E853.0	E950.3	E980.3
Amantadine (hydrochloride)	961.9	E850.9	E950.3	E980.3
Ambazone	961.9	E850.9	E950.3	E980.3
Ambenonium	972.0	E855.3	E950.3	E980.3

Substance	Nature of Injury	External Cause (E-Code)		
		Accident	Suicide (attempt)	Undeter- mined
Ambutonium bromide................................	972.1	E855.4	E950.3	E980.3
Amesec...	975.1	E859.2	E950.3	E980.3
Ametazole..	977.2	E859.8	E950.3	E980.3
Amethocaine..	969	E859.0	E950.3	E980.3
Amethopterin...	963.1	E852.1	E950.3	E980.3
Amidone...	965.0	E853.0	E950.3	E980.3
Amidopyrine..	965.5	E853.5	E950.3	E980.3
Amimethyline...	970.0	E855.0	E950.2	E980.2
Aminacrine..	961.9	E850.9	E950.3	E980.3
Amino acids...	963.4	E852.2	E950.3	E980.3
Aminocaproic acid....................................	964.4	E852.8	E950.3	E980.3
Aminoethylisothiourium............................	963.9	E852.4	E950.3	E980.3
Aminoglutethimide...................................	966.9	E856.0	E950.3	E980.3
Aminometradine.......................................	975.3	E859.3	E950.3	E980.3
Aminopentamide.......................................	972.1	E855.4	E950.3	E980.3
Aminophenol..	983.0	E867	E950.4	E980.4
Aminophenylpyridone...............................	970.1	E855.1	E950.2	E980.2
Aminophylline..	975.1	E859.2	E950.3	E980.3
Aminopterin...	963.1	E852.1	E950.3	E980.3
Aminopyrine...	965.5	E853.5	E950.3	E980.3
Aminosalicylic acid..................................	961.9	E850.9	E950.3	E980.3
Amiphenazole..	971	E856.8	E950.3	E980.3
Amiquinsin..	973.5	E857.5	E950.3	E980.3
Amisometradine.......................................	975.3	E859.3	E950.3	E980.3
Amitriptyline...	970.0	E855.0	E950.2	E980.2
Ammonia (fumes) (gas) (vapor)..................	987.9	E876	E952.9	E982
liquid (household) NEC.........................	983.2	E862	E950.6	E980.6
Ammonium				
chloride (diuretic).................................	975.3	E859.3	E950.3	E980.3
compounds (household) NEC..................	983.2	E862	E950.6	E980.6
fumes (any usage).............................	987.9	E876	E952.9	E982
industrial...	983.2	E867	E950.6	E980.6
Amobarbital...	967.0	E854.0	E950.0	E980.0
Amodiaquin(e)..	961.3	E850.8	E950.3	E980.3
Amopyroquin(e).......................................	961.3	E850.8	E950.3	E980.3
Amphenidone...	970.1	E855.1	E950.2	E980.2
Amphetamine...	971	E856.4	E950.3	E980.3
Amphomycin..	960.9	E850.4	E950.3	E980.3
Amphotericin (B)......................................	960.1	E850.1	E950.3	E980.3
Ampicillin..	960.0	E850.0	E950.3	E980.3
Amprotropine...	972.1	E855.4	E950.3	E980.3
Amygdalin..	977.8	E859.8	E950.3	E980.3
Amyl				
acetate..	982.9	E864	E950.9	E980.9

Substance	Nature of Injury	External Cause (E-Code)		
		Accident	Suicide (attempt)	Undetermined
Amyl—*continued*				
acetate—*continued*				
vapor	987.9	E876	E952.9	E982
alcohol	980.9	E860	E950.9	E980.9
chloride	982.9	E864	E950.9	E980.9
formate	982.9	E864	E950.9	E980.9
nitrite (medicinal)	973.4	E857.4	E950.3	E980.3
propionate	982.9	E864	E950.9	E980.9
Amylase	963.5	E852.4	E950.3	E980.3
Amylene				
dichloride	982.9	E864	E950.9	E980.9
hydrate	980.9	E860	E950.9	E980.9
Amylobarbitone	967.0	E854.0	E950.0	E980.0
Amylobenzamide	961.9	E850.9	E950.3	E980.3
Amylocaine	968.9	E856.3	E950.3	E980.3
Amytal (sodium)	967.0	E854.0	E950.0	E980.0
Anadin	965.9	E853.9	E950.3	E980.3
Analgesic drug NEC	965.9	E853.9	E950.3	E980.3
Anamirta cocculus	988.2	E868	E950.9	E980.9
Ancillin	960.0	E850.0	E950.3	E980.3
Androgens	962.1	E851.1	E950.3	E980.3
Androstalone	962.1	E851.1	E950.3	E980.3
Androsterone	962.1	E851.1	E950.3	E980.3
Anemone pulsatilla	988.2	E868	E950.9	E980.9
Anesthesia, anesthetic (gas) (general) NEC	968.1	E856.2	E952.9	E982
intravenous	968.9	E856.3	E950.3	E980.3
local	969	E859.0	E950.3	E980.3
rectal	968.9	E856.3	E950.3	E980.3
spinal	968.9	E856.3	E950.3	E980.3
Aneurine	963.6	E852.3	E950.3	E980.3
Angiotensin	972.2	E855.5	E950.3	E980.3
Anileridine	965.0	E853.0	E950.3	E980.3
Aniline (dye) (liquid)	983.0	E867	E950.4	E980.4
analgesic	965.4	E853.4	E950.3	E980.3
vapor	987.9	E876	E952.9	E982
Anisindione	964.2	E852.6	E950.3	E980.3
Anisotropine	972.1	E855.4	E950.3	E980.3
Anorexia producing drugs NEC	971	E856.4	E950.3	E980.3
Ant poisons—*see* Pesticides				
Antabuse	977.8	E859.8	E950.3	E980.3
Antacids	974.0	E858.0	E950.3	E980.3
Antazoline	963.0	E852.0	E950.3	E980.3
Anthramycin	960.9	E850.4	E950.3	E980.3
Antiaris toxicaria	988.2	E868	E950.9	E980.9

Substance	Nature of Injury	External Cause (E-Code)		
		Accident	Suicide (attempt)	Undetermined
Antibiotics NEC..	960.9	E850.4	E950.3	E980.3
Anticancer agents.....................................	963.1	E852.1	E950.3	E980.3
Anticholinergics.......................................	972.1	E855.4	E950.3	E980.3
Anticoagulants...	964.2	E852.6	E950.3	E980.3
Anticonvulsants NEC................................	966.9	E856.0	E950.3	E980.3
Antidepressants.......................................	970.0	E855.0	E950.2	E980.2
Antidiabetic agents...................................	962.3	E851.3	E950.3	E980.3
Antidiarrhea agents..................................	974.0	E858.0	E950.3	E980.3
Antiemetic agents.....................................	963.0	E852.0	E950.3	E980.3
Antifertility pills.....................................	962.6	E851.6	E950.3	E980.3
Antiflatulents..	974.9	E858.9	E950.3	E980.3
Antifreeze...	989.9	E869	E950.9	E980.9
alcohol..	980.1	E860	E950.9	E980.9
ethylene glycol....................................	982.9	E864	E950.9	E980.9
Antifungals (nonmedicinal) (sprays)..............	989.9	E865	E950.9	E980.9
medicinal NEC....................................	961.9	E850.9	E950.3	E980.3
antibiotic...	960.1	E850.1	E950.3	E980.3
Antihistamines...	963.0	E852.0	E950.3	E980.3
Anti-infectives NEC..................................	961.9	E850.9	E950.3	E980.3
Antiknock (tetraethyl lead).........................	984	E866	E950.9	E980.9
Antimony (compounds) (vapor) NEC............	985.9	E866	E950.9	E980.9
anti-infectives....................................	961.9	E850.9	E950.3	E980.3
pesticides (vapor)................................	989.3	E865	E950.9	E980.9
potassium tartrate (emetic).....................	974.6	E858.6	E950.3	E980.3
tartrated...	974.6	E858.6	E950.3	E980.3
Antineoplastic agents................................	963.1	E852.1	E950.3	E980.3
Antipruritics (local).................................	969	E859.0	E950.3	E980.3
Antipyretics NEC.....................................	965.9	E853.9	E950.3	E980.3
Antipyrine..	965.5	E853.5	E950.3	E980.3
Antiseptics (medicinal) (external) NEC	977.0	E859.7	E950.3	E980.3
Antistine...	963.0	E852.0	E950.3	E980.3
Antithyroid agents...................................	962.8	E851.8	E950.3	E980.3
Antituberculars..	961.9	E850.9	E950.3	E980.3
Antitussives—see Cough mixtures				
Antrol—see Pesticides				
Apomorphine (emetic)...............................	974.6	E858.6	E950.3	E980.3
Aprobarbital, aprobarbitone.......................	967.0	E854.0	E950.0	E980.0
Apronal	967.9	E854.9	E950.3	E980.3
Aqua fortis...	983.1	E867	E950.9	E980.9
Arachis oil (medicinal) NEC.......................	974.2	E858.2	E950.3	E980.3
Aralen...	961.3	E850.8	E950.3	E980.3
Arginine (salts)..	963.4	E852.2	E950.3	E980.3
Argyrol..	961.2	E850.7	E950.3	E980.3
Aromatics, corrosive.................................	983.0	E867	E950.4	E980.4

Substance	Nature of Injury	External Cause (E-Code)		
		Accident	Suicide (attempt)	Undetermined
Arsenate of lead	985.1	E865	E950.7	E980.7
Arsenic, arsenicals, (compounds) (dust)				
(vapor) NEC	985.1	E866	E950.7	E980.7
medicinal NEC	985.1	E859.8	E950.3	E980.3
anti-infective	961.1	E850.6	E950.3	E980.3
pesticide (dust) (fumes)	985.1	E865	E950.7	E980.7
Arsine (gas)	985.1	E866	E950.7	E980.7
Arsphenamine (silver)	961.1	E850.6	E950.3	E980.3
Arsthinol	961.1	E850.6	E950.3	E980.3
Artane	972.1	E855.4	E950.3	E980.3
Ascaridole	961.9	E850.9	E950.3	E980.3
Ascorbic acid	963.6	E852.3	E950.3	E980.3
Asiaticoside	961.9	E850.9	E950.3	E980.3
Aspidium (oleoresin)	961.9	E850.9	E950.3	E980.3
Aspirin	965.1	E853.1	E950.1	E980.1
Astringents NEC	977.0	E859.7	E950.3	E980.3
Atabrine	961.3	E850.8	E950.3	E980.3
Ataractics	970.1	E855.1	E950.2	E980.2
Atophan	965.2	E853.2	E950.3	E980.3
Atropine	972.1	E855.4	E950.3	E980.3
Attapulgite	974.0	E858.0	E950.3	E980.3
Aureomycin	960.5	E850.3	E950.3	E980.3
Aurothioglucose	976.2	E859.4	E950.3	E980.3
Aurothioglycanide	976.2	E859.4	E950.3	E980.3
Aurothiomalate	976.2	E859.4	E950.3	E980.3
Avertin (bromide)	968.9	E856.3	E950.3	E980.3
Avlosulfon	961.9	E850.9	E950.3	E980.3
Avomine	967.9	E854.9	E950.3	E980.3
Azacyclonol	970.1	E855.1	E950.2	E980.2
Azadirachta	989.9	E869	E950.9	E980.9
Azapetine	973.5	E857.5	E950.3	E980.3
Azaserine	963.1	E852.1	E950.3	E980.3
Azathioprine	963.1	E852.1	E950.3	E980.3
Azosulfamide	961.0	E850.5	E950.3	E980.3
Azulfidine	961.0	E850.5	E950.3	E980.3
Azuresin	977.2	E859.8	E950.3	E980.3
Bacitracin	960.9	E850.4	E950.3	E980.3
Baking soda	963.3	E852.2	E950.3	E980.3
BAL	963.9	E852.4	E950.3	E980.3
Bamethan (sulfate)	973.4	E857.4	E950.3	E980.3
Bamipine	963.0	E852.0	E950.3	E980.3
Baneberry	988.2	E868	E950.9	E980.9
Banewort	988.2	E868	E950.9	E980.9
Barbenyl	967.0	E854.0	E950.0	E980.0

Substance	Nature of Injury	External Cause (E-Code)		
		Accident	Suicide (attempt)	Undetermined
Barbital, barbitone...................................	967.0	E854.0	E950.0	E980.0
Barbiturates, barbituric acid.......................	967.0	E854.0	E950.0	E980.0
anesthetic (intravenous)..........................	968.9	E856.3	E950.3	E980.3
Barium (carbonate) (chloride) (sulfate)..........	985.9	E869	E950.9	E980.9
diagnostic agent...................................	977.2	E859.8	E950.3	E980.3
pesticide..	989.3	E865	E950.9	E980.9
Barrier cream...	977.0	E859.6	E950.3	E980.3
Battery acid or fluid................................	983.1	E867	E950.9	E980.9
Bay rum...	980.9	E860	E950.9	E980.9
Bearsfoot...	988.2	E868	E950.9	E980.9
Beclamide..	966.9	E856.0	E950.3	E980.3
Belladonna (alkaloids)..............................	972.1	E855.4	E950.3	E980.3
Bemegride...	971	E856.8	E950.3	E980.3
Benactyzine..	970.9	E855.2	E950.2	E980.2
Benadryl..	963.0	E852.0	E950.3	E980.3
Bendrofluazide......................................	975.3	E859.3	E950.3	E980.3
Bendroflumethiazide................................	975.3	E859.3	E950.3	E980.3
Benethamine penicillin..............................	960.0	E850.0	E950.3	E980.3
Benoxinate...	969	E859.0	E950.3	E980.3
Bentonite...	974.0	E858.0	E950.3	E980.3
Benzalkonium (chloride)............................	961.9	E850.9	E950.3	E980.3
Benzamidosalicylate (calcium)....................	961.9	E850.9	E950.3	E980.3
Benzathine penicillin................................	960.0	E850.0	E950.3	E980.3
Benzcarbimine.......................................	963.1	E852.1	E950.3	E980.3
Benzdiazepin...	970.1	E855.1	E950.2	E980.2
Benzedrex..	972.2	E855.5	E950.3	E980.3
Benzedrine (amphetamine).........................	971	E856.4	E950.3	E980.3
Benzene (acetyl) (dimethyl) (methyl) (solvent)..	982.0	E864	E950.9	E980.9
hexachloride (gamma) (insecticide) (vapor)..	989.2	E865	E950.9	E980.9
vapor NEC...	987.9	E876	E952.9	E982
Benzethonium.......................................	961.9	E850.9	E950.3	E980.3
Benzhexol..	972.1	E855.4	E950.3	E980.3
Benzilonium..	972.1	E855.4	E950.3	E980.3
Benzin(e) — see Ligroin				
Benziodarone..	973.4	E857.4	E950.3	E980.3
Benzocaine...	969	E859.0	E950.3	E980.3
Benzoic acid (anti-infective)......................	961.9	E850.9	E950.3	E980.3
Benzol...	982.0	E864	E950.9	E980.9
vapor...	987.9	E876	E952.9	E982
Benzomorphan.......................................	965.0	E853.0	E950.3	E980.3
Benzonatate..	977.8	E859.8	E950.3	E980.3
Benzperidol..	970.1	E855.1	E950.2	E980.2

Substance	Nature of Injury	External Cause (E-Code)		
		Accident	Suicide (attempt)	Undetermined
Benzphetamine..	971	E856.4	E950.3	E980.3
Benzpyrinium...	972.0	E855.3	E950.3	E980.3
Benzthiazide..	975.3	E859.3	E950.3	E980.3
Benztropine...	972.1	E855.4	E950.3	E980.3
Benzyl				
acetate...	982.9	E864	E950.9	E980.9
benzoate (anti-infective).........................	961.9	E850.9	E950.3	E980.3
morphine..	965.0	E853.0	E950.3	E980.3
penicillin..	960.0	E850.0	E950.3	E980.3
Bephenium hydroxynaphthoate...................	961.9	E850.9	E950.3	E980.3
Bergamot oil...	989.9	E869	E950.9	E980.9
Berries, poisonous...................................	988.2	E868	E950.9	E980.9
Beryllium (compounds).............................	985.3	E869	E950.9	E980.9
Beta-chlor...	967.1	E854.1	E950.3	E980.3
Betamethasone.......................................	962.0	E851.0	E950.3	E980.3
Betazole...	977.2	E859.8	E950.3	E980.3
Bethanechol...	972.0	E855.3	E950.3	E980.3
Bethanidine...	973.5	E857.5	E950.3	E980.3
Bhang..	967.9	E854.9	E950.3	E980.3
Bialamicol (hydrochloride)........................	961.9	E850.9	E950.3	E980.3
Bichloride of mercury — see Mercuric chloride				
Bichromates (calcium) (potassium) (sodium)				
(crystals)...	983.9	E867	E950.9	E980.9
fumes..	987.9	E876	E952.9	E982
Bidormal..	967.0	E854.0	E950.0	E980.0
Biligrafin...	977.2	E859.8	E950.3	E980.3
Biliposol..	961.9	E850.9	E950.3	E980.3
Binitrobenzol...	983.0	E867	E950.4	E980.4
Biperiden...	972.1	E855.4	E950.3	E980.3
Bisacodyl...	974.5	E858.5	E950.3	E980.3
Bishydroxycoumarin................................	964.2	E852.6	E950.3	E980.3
Bismarsen...	961.1	E850.6	E950.3	E980.3
Bismuth (compounds) NEC........................	985.9	E866	E950.9	E980.9
medicinal (anti-infective) NEC.................	961.9	E850.9	E950.3	E980.3
sulfarsphenamine.................................	961.1	E850.6	E950.3	E980.3
Bithionol..	961.9	E850.9	E950.3	E980.3
Bitter almond oil.....................................	989.0	E869	E950.9	E980.9
Bittersweet...	988.2	E868	E950.9	E980.9
Black				
flag...	989.3	E865	E950.9	E980.9
henbane..	988.2	E868	E950.9	E980.9
leaf (40)...	989.3	E865	E950.9	E980.9
Blast furnace gas (carbon monoxide from).....	986	E875	E952.1	E982
Bleach...	983.9	E869	E950.9	E980.9

Substance	Nature of Injury	External Cause (E-Code)		
		Accident	Suicide (attempt)	Undeter-mined
Blood, dried	989.9	E865	E950.9	E980.9
Blue velvet	965.0	E853.0	E950.3	E980.3
Bone meal	989.9	E865	E950.9	E980.9
Bonine	963.0	E852.0	E950.3	E980.3
Boracic acid	977.0	E859.7	E950.3	E980.3
Borate (sodium) (cleanser)	989.9	E861	E950.9	E980.9
Borax (cleanser)	989.9	E861	E950.9	E980.9
Boric acid	977.0	E859.7	E950.3	E980.3
Boron hydride NEC	989.9	E869	E950.9	E980.9
fumes or gas	987.9	E876	E952.9	E982
Brass (fumes)	985.9	E866	E950.9	E980.9
Brasso	989.9	E861	E950.9	E980.9
Bretylium (tosylate)	973.5	E857.5	E950.3	E980.3
Brevital	968.9	E856.3	E950.3	E980.3
Bromal (hydrate)	967.3	E854.3	E950.3	E980.3
Bromelains, bromelins	963.5	E852.4	E950.3	E980.3
Bromides NEC	967.3	E854.3	E950.3	E980.3
Bromine (vapor)	987.9	E876	E952.9	E982
compounds (medicinal)	967.3	E854.3	E950.3	E980.3
Bromisovalum	967.3	E854.3	E950.3	E980.3
Bromobenzylcyanide	987.9	E876	E952.9	E982
Bromodiphenhydramine	963.0	E852.0	E950.3	E980.3
Bromoform	967.3	E854.3	E950.3	E980.3
Bromosalicylhydroxamic acid	961.9	E850.9	E950.3	E980.3
Bromo-seltzer	967.3	E854.3	E950.3	E980.3
Brompheniramine	963.0	E852.0	E950.3	E980.3
Bromural	967.3	E854.3	E950.3	E980.3
Bromvaletone	967.3	E854.3	E950.3	E980.3
Brucea	988.2	E868	E950.9	E980.9
Brucine	989.1	E869	E950.5	E980.5
Brunswick green — see Copper				
Bryonia (alba) (dioica)	988.2	E868	E950.9	E980.9
Buclizine	970.1	E855.1	E950.2	E980.2
Bufferin	965.1	E853.1	E950.1	E980.1
Bufotenine	970.9	E855.2	E950.2	E980.2
Buphenine	972.2	E855.5	E950.3	E980.3
Busulphan	963.1	E852.1	E950.3	E980.3
Butabarbital (sodium)	967.0	E854.0	E950.0	E980.0
Butabarpal	967.0	E854.0	E950.0	E980.0
Butacaine	969	E859.0	E950.3	E980.3
Butallylonal	967.0	E854.0	E950.0	E980.0
Butane (distributed in mobile container)	987.0	E871	E951	E981
distributed through pipes	987.0	E870	E951	E981

Substance	Nature of Injury	External Cause (E-Code)		
		Accident	Suicide (attempt)	Undetermined
Butane (distributed in mobile container) — *continued*				
incomplete combustion — *see* Carbon monoxide, butane				
Butanol	980.9	E860	E950.9	E980.9
Butanone	982.9	E864	E950.9	E980.9
Butazolidin	965.5	E853.5	E950.3	E980.3
Butethal	967.0	E854.0	E950.0	E980.0
Butethamate	972.1	E855.4	E950.3	E980.3
Buthalitone (sodium)	967.0	E854.0	E950.0	E980.0
Butisol	967.0	E854.0	E950.0	E980.0
Butobarbital, butobarbitone	967.0	E854.0	E950.0	E980.0
Butol	982.9	E864	E950.9	E980.9
Butriptyline	970.0	E855.0	E950.2	E980.2
Butter of antimony — *see* Antimony				
Buttercups	988.2	E868	E950.9	E980.9
Butyl				
acetate (secondary)	982.9	E864	E950.9	E980.9
alcohol	980.9	E860	E950.9	E980.9
butyrate	982.9	E864	E950.9	E980.9
carbinol	980.9	E860	E950.9	E980.9
carbitol	982.9	E864	E950.9	E980.9
cellosolve	982.9	E864	E950.9	E980.9
chloral (hydrate)	967.1	E854.1	E950.3	E980.3
formate	982.9	E864	E950.9	E980.9
lactate	982.9	E864	E950.9	E980.9
propionate	982.9	E864	E950.9	E980.9
scopolammonium bromide	972.1	E855.4	E950.3	E980.3
Butyrophenone	970.1	E855.1	E950.2	E980.2
Cacodyl, cacodylic acid — *see* Arsenic				
Cadmium (chloride) (fumes) (oxide)	985.9	E866	E950.9	E980.9
sulfide (medicinal) NEC	977.0	E859.7	E950.3	E980.3
Caffeine	971	E856.8	E950.3	E980.3
Calabar bean	988.2	E868	E950.9	E980.9
Caladium seguinium	988.2	E868	E950.9	E980.9
Calamine (lotion)	977.0	E859.7	E950.3	E980.3
Calciferol	963.6	E852.3	E950.3	E980.3
Calcium				
benzamide salicylate	961.9	E850.9	E950.3	E980.3
carbimide (citrated)	977.8	E859.8	E950.3	E980.3
carbonate (antacid)	974.0	E858.0	E950.3	E980.3
dioctyl sulfosuccinate	974.4	E858.4	E950.3	E980.3
disodium edetate	963.9	E852.4	E950.3	E980.3
hydrate, hydroxide	983.2	E867	E950.6	E980.6
oxide	983.2	E867	E950.6	E980.6

Substance	Nature of Injury	External Cause (E-Code)		
		Accident	Suicide (attempt)	Undetermined
Calcium—*continued*				
salts NEC..	963.4	E852.2	E950.3	E980.3
Calomel—*see* Mercurous chloride				
Caloric agents NEC................................	963.4	E852.2	E950.3	E980.3
Camoquin(e)..	961.3	E850.8	E950.3	E980.3
Camphor (oil).......................................	969	E859.0	E950.3	E980.3
Candicidin...	960.1	E850.1	E950.3	E980.3
Cannabinols...	967.9	E854.9	E950.3	E980.3
Cannabis (indica) (sativa).........................	967.9	E854.9	E950.3	E980.3
Canned heat...	980.1	E860	E950.9	E980.9
Cantharides, cantharidin, cantharis.............	977.0	E859.7	E950.3	E980.3
Capreomycin..	960.9	E850.4	E950.3	E980.3
Captodiame, captodiamine........................	970.1	E855.1	E950.2	E980.2
Caramiphen..	972.1	E855.4	E950.3	E980.3
Carbachol..	972.0	E855.3	E950.3	E980.3
Carbacrylamine resins.............................	963.4	E852.2	E950.3	E980.3
Carbamazepine......................................	966.9	E856.0	E950.3	E980.3
Carbarsone..	961.1	E850.6	E950.3	E980.3
Carbaspirin..	965.1	E853.1	E950.1	E980.1
Carbazochrome.....................................	964.4	E852.8	E950.3	E980.3
Carbenoxolone......................................	974.9	E858.9	E950.3	E980.3
Carbimazole...	962.8	E851.8	E950.3	E980.3
Carbinol..	980.1	E860	E950.9	E980.9
Carbinoxamine......................................	963.0	E852.0	E950.3	E980.3
Carbitol..	982.9	E864	E950.9	E980.9
Carbocaine..	969	E859.0	E950.3	E980.3
Carbofluorine.......................................	972.1	E855.4	E950.3	E980.3
Carbolic acid (*see also* Phenol)...................	983.0	E867	E950.4	E980.4
Carbomycin..	960.9	E850.4	E950.3	E980.3
Carbon				
bisulfide (liquid)...............................	982.2	E864	E950.9	E980.9
vapor..	987.9	E876	E952.9	E982
dioxide (gas)...................................	987.9	E876	E952.9	E982
disulfide (liquid)..............................	982.2	E864	E950.9	E980.9
vapor..	987.9	E876	E952.9	E982
monoxide (from incomplete combustion of)				
(in) NEC....................................	986	E875	E952.1	E982
blast furnace gas............................	986	E875	E952.1	E982
butane (distributed in mobile container)...	986	E871	E951	E981
distributed through pipes...................	986	E870	E951	E981
charcoal fumes..............................	986	E874	E952.1	E982
coal				
gas (piped).................................	986	E870	E951	E981
solid (in domestic stoves, fireplaces)...	986	E874	E952.1	E982

Substance	Nature of Injury	External Cause (E-Code)		
		Accident	Suicide (attempt)	Undeter-mined
Carbon—*continued*				
monoxide, etc.—*continued*				
coke (in domestic stoves, fireplaces)......	986	E874	E952.1	E982
exhaust gas (motor) not in transit..........	986	E873	E952.0	E982
combustion engine, any, not in water-				
craft......................................	986	E873	E952.0	E982
farm tractor, not in transit.................	986	E873	E952.0	E982
gas engine...................................	986	E873	E952.0	E982
motor pump.................................	986	E873	E952.0	E982
motor vehicle, not in transit..............	986	E873	E952.0	E982
fuel (in domestic use)..........................	986	E874	E952.1	E982
gas (piped)....................................	986	E870	E951	E981
in mobile container.....................	986	E871	E951	E981
illuminating gas...............................	986	E870	E951	E981
industrial fuels or gases, any.................	986	E875	E952.1	E982
kerosene (in domestic stoves, fireplaces)..	986	E874	E952.1	E982
kiln vapor..........................	986	E875	E952.1	E982
motor exhaust gas, not in transit...........	986	E873	E952.0	E982
piped gas...................................	986	E870	E951	E981
producer gas....................................	986	E875	E952.1	E982
propane (distributed in mobile container)..	986	E871	E951	E981
distributed through pipes...................	986	E870	E951	E981
stove gas (piped).............................	986	E870	E951	E981
utility gas (piped).............................	986	E870	E951	E981
water gas......................................	986	E872	E951	E981
wood (in domestic stoves, fireplaces).....	986	E874	E952.1	E982
tetrachloride (vapor) NEC......................	987.9	E876	E952.9	E982
liquid (cleansing agent) NEC................	982.1	E861	E950.9	E980.9
solvent..	982.1	E864	E950.9	E980.9
Carbonic acid (gas).................................	987.9	E876	E952.9	E982
anhydrase inhibitors..............................	975.2	E859.3	E950.3	E980.3
Carbrital...	967.0	E854.0	E950.0	E980.0
Carbromal...	967.3	E854.3	E950.3	E980.3
Cardiac				
depressants..	973.0	E857.0	E950.3	E980.3
tonics..	973.1	E857.1	E950.3	E980.3
Cardrase...	975.2	E859.3	E950.3	E980.3
Carfenazine (maleate).............................	970.1	E855.1	E950.2	E980.2
Carisoprodol.......................................	968.0	E856.1	E950.3	E980.3
Carotene...	963.6	E852.3	E950.3	E980.3
Carphenazine (maleate)............................	970.1	E855.1	E950.2	E980.2
Cascara (sagrada)...................................	974.1	E858.1	E950.3	E980.3
Cassava..	988.2	E868	E950.9	E980.9
Castor bean..	988.2	E868	E950.9	E980.9
Castor oil..	974.1	E858.1	E950.3	E980.3

Substance	Nature of Injury	External Cause (E-Code)		
		Accident	Suicide (attempt)	Undeter- mined
Catha (edulis)	971	E856.8	E950.3	E980.3
Cathartics NEC	974.5	E858.5	E950.3	E980.3
emollient	974.2	E858.2	E950.3	E980.3
intestinal irritants	974.1	E858.1	E950.3	E980.3
saline	974.3	E858.3	E950.3	E980.3
Cathomycin	960.9	E850.4	E950.3	E980.3
Caustic(s) NEC	983.9	E867	E950.9	E980.9
alkali	983.2	E867	E950.6	E980.6
hydroxide	983.2	E867	E950.6	E980.6
potash	983.2	E867	E950.6	E980.6
soda	983.2	E867	E950.6	E980.6
Celestone	962.0	E851.0	E950.3	E980.3
Cellosolve	982.9	E864	E950.9	E980.9
Cellulose derivatives, cathartic	974.5	E858.5	E950.3	E980.3
Cephaloridine	960.9	E850.4	E950.3	E980.3
Cephalosporins NEC	960.9	E850.4	E950.3	E980.3
N, or adicillin	960.0	E850.0	E950.3	E980.3
Cephalothin (sodium)	960.9	E850.4	E950.3	E980.3
Cerbera (odallam)	988.2	E868	E950.9	E980.9
Cerberine	973.1	E857.1	E950.3	E980.3
Cetalkonium (chloride)	961.9	E850.9	E950.3	E980.3
Cetoxime	963.0	E852.0	E950.3	E980.3
Cetrimide	961.9	E850.9	E950.3	E980.3
Cetylpyridinium	961.9	E850.9	E950.3	E980.3
Cevadilla — *see* Sabadilla				
Charcoal				
fumes (carbon monoxide)	986	E874	E952.1	E982
industrial	986	E875	E952.1	E982
medicinal (activated)	974.0	E858.0	E950.3	E980.3
Chelidonium majus	988.2	E868	E950.9	E980.9
Chemical substance NEC	989.9	E869	E950.9	E980.9
Chenopodium (oil)	961.9	F850.9	E950.3	E980.3
Cherry laurel	988.2	E868	E950.9	E980.9
Chiniofon	961.3	E850.8	E950.3	E980.3
Chlophedianol	977.8	E859.8	E950.3	E980.3
Chloral (betaine) (hydrate)	967.1	E854.1	E950.3	E980.3
Chloralamide	967.9	E854.9	E950.3	E980.3
Chloralformamide	967.9	E854.9	E950.3	E980.3
Chloralose	967.1	E854.1	E950.3	E980.3
Chlorambucil	963.1	E852.1	E950.3	E980.3
Chloramphenicol	960.2	E850.2	E950.3	E980.3
Chlorate(s) (potassium) (sodium) NEC	983.9	E867	E950.9	E980.9
Chlorbenzene, chlorbenzol	982.0	E864	E950.9	E980.9
Chlorcylizine	963.0	E852.0	E950.3	E980.3

Substance	Nature of Injury	External Cause (E-Code)		
		Accident	Suicide (attempt)	Undetermined
Chlordan(e) (dust)	989.2	E865	E950.9	E980.9
Chlordiazepoxide	970.1	E855.1	E950.2	E980.2
Chlorethyl—see Ethyl chloride				
Chloretone	967.1	E854.1	E950.3	E980.3
Chlorex	982.9	E864	E950.9	E980.9
Chlorguanide	961.9	E850.9	E950.3	E980.3
Chlorhexadol	967.9	E854.9	E950.3	E980.3
Chlorhexidine (hydrochloride)	961.9	E850.9	E950.3	E980.3
Chloride of lime (bleach)	983.2	E869	E950.6	E980.6
Chlorinated				
camphene	989.2	E865	E950.9	E980.9
diphenyl	989.9	E869	E950.9	E980.9
hydrocarbons NEC	982.9	E864	E950.9	E980.9
lime (bleach)	983.2	E869	E950.6	E980.6
naphthalene—see Naphthalene				
pesticides NEC	989.2	E865	E950.9	E980.9
soda—see Sodium hypochlorite				
Chlorine (fumes) (gas)	987.9	E876	E952.9	E982
bleach	983.9	E869	E950.9	E980.9
compound NEC	983.9	E867	E950.9	E980.9
disinfectant	983.9	E862	E950.9	E980.9
releasing agents NEC	983.9	E862	E950.9	E980.9
Chlorisondamine	973.3	E857.3	E950.3	E980.3
Chlormadinone	962.6	E851.6	E950.3	E980.3
Chlormerodrin(e)	975.0	E859.1	E950.3	E980.3
Chlormethiazole	967.9	E854.9	E950.3	E980.3
Chlormethylenecycline	960.5	E850.3	E950.3	E980.3
Chlormezanone	968.0	E856.1	E950.3	E980.3
Chloroaniline	983.0	E867	E950.4	E980.4
Chlorobenzene, chlorobenzol	982.0	E864	E950.9	E980.9
Chlorobutanol	967.1	E854.1	E950.3	E980.3
Chlorodinitrobenzene	983.0	E867	E950.4	E980.4
dust or vapor	987.9	E876	E952.9	E982
Chlorodyne	965.9	E853.9	E950.3	E980.3
Chloroethane—see Ethyl chloride				
Chloroform (fumes) (vapor)	987.9	E876	E952.9	E982
anesthetic (gas)	968.1	E856.2	E952.9	E982
liquid NEC	968.9	E856.3	E950.3	E980.3
solvent	982.9	E864	E950.9	E980.9
Chloromycetin	960.2	E850.2	E950.3	E980.3
Chloronitrobenzene	983.0	E867	E950.4	E980.4
dust or vapor	987.9	E876	E952.9	E982
Chlorophenol	983.0	E867	E950.4	E980.4
Chlorophenothane	989.2	E865	E950.9	E980.9

Substance	Nature of Injury	External Cause (E-Code)		
		Accident	Suicide (attempt)	Undeter-mined
Chlorophyll	977.0	E859.7	E950.3	E980.3
Chloropicrin (fumes)	987.9	E876	E952.9	E982
pesticide (fumes)	989.3	E865	E950.9	E980.9
Chloroprocaine	969	E859.0	E950.3	E980.3
Chloropurine	963.1	E852.1	E950.3	E980.3
Chloroquine (phosphate)	961.3	E850.8	E950.3	E980.3
Chlorothen	963.0	E852.0	E950.3	E980.3
Chlorothiazide	975.3	E859.3	E950.3	E980.3
Chlorotrianisene	962.2	E851.2	E950.3	E980.3
Chlorovinyldichloroarsine — see Lewisite				
Chloroxylenol	961.9	E850.9	E950.3	E980.3
Chlorphenesin	961.9	E850.9	E950.3	E980.3
carbamate	968.0	E856.1	E950.3	E980.3
Chlorpheniramine	963.0	E852.0	E950.3	E980.3
Chlorphenoxamine	972.1	E855.4	E950.3	E980.3
Chlorphentermine	971	E856.4	E950.3	E980.3
Chlorproguanil	961.9	E850.9	E950.3	E980.3
Chlorpromazine	970.1	E855.1	E950.2	E980.2
Chlorpropamide	962.3	E851.3	E950.3	E980.3
Chlorprothixene	970.1	E855.1	E950.2	E980.2
Chlorquinaldol	961.9	E850.9	E950.3	E980.3
Chlortetracycline	960.5	E850.3	E950.3	E980.3
Chlorthalidone	975.9	E859.3	E950.3	E980.3
Chlortrimeton	963.0	E852.0	E950.3	E980.3
Chlorzoxazone	968.0	E856.1	E950.3	E980.3
Choke damp	987.9	E876	E952.9	E982
Cholic acid	974.9	E858.9	E950.3	E980.3
Choline				
salicylate	965.1	E853.1	E950.1	E980.1
theophyllinate	975.1	E859.2	E950.3	E980.3
Cholinergics	972.0	E855.3	E950.3	E980.3
Chorionic gonadotropin	962.9	E851.9	E950.3	E980.3
Chromates	983.9	E867	E950.9	E980.9
dust or mist	987.9	E876	E952.9	E982
lead (see also Lead)	984	E866	E950.9	E980.9
Chromic acid	983.9	E867	E950.9	E980.9
dust or mist	987.9	E876	E952.9	E982
Chromium	985.9	E866	E950.9	E980.9
compounds — see Chromates				
Chromonar	973.4	E857.4	E950.3	E980.3
Chromyl chloride	983.9	E867	E950.9	E980.9
Chrysarobin (ointment)	977.0	E859.6	E950.3	E980.3
Chymar	963.5	E852.4	E950.3	E980.3
Chymotrypsin	963.5	E852.4	E950.3	E980.3

Substance	Nature of Injury	External Cause (E-Code)		
		Accident	Suicide (attempt)	Undeter-mined
Cicuta maculata or virosa	988.2	E868	E950.9	E980.9
Cigarette lighter fluid	981.2	E864	E950.9	E980.9
Cinchocaine	969	E859.0	E950.3	E980.3
Cinchona	961.3	E850.8	E950.3	E980.3
Cinchonine alkaloids	961.3	E850.8	E950.3	E980.3
Cinchophen	965.2	E853.2	E950.3	E980.3
Cinnarizine	963.0	E852.0	E950.3	E980.3
Citric acid	989.9	E869	E950.9	E980.9
Citrovorum factor	963.6	E852.3	E950.3	E980.3
Claviceps purpurea	988.2	E868	E950.9	E980.9
Cleaner, cleansing agent NEC	989.9	E861	E950.9	E980.9
of paint or varnish	982.9	E864	E950.9	E980.9
Clematis vitalba	988.2	E868	E950.9	E980.9
Clemizole	963.0	E852.0	E950.3	E980.3
penicillin	960.0	E850.0	E950.3	E980.3
Clidinium	972.1	E855.4	E950.3	E980.3
Cliradon	965.0	E853.0	E950.3	E980.3
Clocortolone	962.0	E851.0	E950.3	E980.3
Clofedanol	977.8	E859.8	E950.3	E980.3
Clofibrate	973.2	E857.2	E950.3	E980.3
Clomiphene	977.8	E859.8	E950.3	E980.3
Clopamide	975.3	E859.3	E950.3	E980.3
Clorexolone	975.9	E859.3	E950.3	E980.3
Clorox (bleach)	983.9	E869	E950.9	E980.9
Cloxacillin	960.0	E850.0	E950.3	E980.3
Coagulants NEC	964.4	E852.8	E950.3	E980.3
Coal (carbon monoxide from)—*see* Carbon monoxide, coal				
oil—*see* Kerosene				
tar NEC	983.0	E867	E950.4	E980.4
fumes	987.9	E876	E952.9	E982
medicinal (ointment)	977.0	E859.6	E950.3	E980.3
analgesics NEC	965.5	E853.5	E950.3	E980.3
naphtha (solvent)	982.0	E864	E950.9	E980.9
Cobalt (fumes) (industrial)	985.9	E866	E950.9	E980.9
Coca (leaf)	971	E856.8	E950.3	E980.3
Cocaine (hydrochloride) (salt)	969	E859.0	E950.3	E980.3
Cocculus indicus	988.2	E868	E950.9	E980.9
Cochineal	989.9	E869	E950.9	E980.9
medicinal products	977.1	E859.8	E950.3	E980.3
Codeine	965.0	E853.0	E950.3	E980.3
Codis	965.9	E853.9	E950.3	E980.3
Coffee	989.9	E869	E950.9	E980.9

Substance	Nature of Injury	External Cause (E-Code)		
		Accident	Suicide (attempt)	Undeter-mined
Coke fumes or gas (carbon monoxide)..........	986	E874	E952.1	E982
industrial use..	986	E875	E952.1	E982
Colchicine..	965.3	E853.3	E950.3	E980.3
Colchicum..	988.2	E868	E950.9	E980.9
Colistimethate..	960.9	E850.4	E950.3	E980.3
Colistin...	960.9	E850.4	E950.3	E980.3
Colocynth..	974.1	E858.1	E950.3	E980.3
Coloring matter — *see* Dye(s)				
Columbia spirit.......................................	980.1	E860	E950.9	E980.9
Combustion gas — *see* Carbon monoxide				
Compazine...	970.1	E855.1	E950.2	E980.2
Compound				
42 (warfarin)......................................	989.3	E865	E950.9	E980.9
269 (endrin).......................................	989.2	E865	E950.9	E980.9
497 (dieldrin).....................................	989.2	E865	E950.9	E980.9
1080 (sodium fluoroacetate)...................	989.3	E865	E950.8	E980.8
3422 (parathion).................................	989.3	E865	E950.9	E980.9
3911 (phorate)...................................	989.3	E865	E950.9	E980.9
3956 (toxaphene)................................	989.2	E865	E950.9	E980.9
4049 (malathion)................................	989.3	E865	E950.9	E980.9
4124 (dicapthon)................................	989.3	E865	E950.9	E980.9
Coniine, conine......................................	965.9	E853.9	E950.3	E980.3
Conium (maculatum)................................	988.2	E868	E950.9	E980.9
Contrast media (roentgenographic).............	977.2	E859.8	E950.3	E980.3
Convallaria majalis..................................	988.2	E868	E950.9	E980.9
Copaiba (oil)..	977.8	E859.8	E950.3	E980.3
Copper (dust) (fumes) (sulfate) NEC...........	985.9	E866	E950.9	E980.9
arsenate, arsenite.................................	985.1	E866	E950.7	E980.7
insecticide......................................	985.1	E865	E950.7	E980.7
emetic..	974.6	E858.6	E950.3	E980.3
insecticide	989.3	E865	E950.9	E980.9
Cordite...	989.9	E869	E950.9	E980.9
vapor...	987.9	E876	E952.9	E982
Corn cures...	977.0	E859.7	E950.3	E980.3
Corrosive NEC..	983.9	E867	E950.9	E980.9
acid NEC..	983.1	E867	E950.9	E980.9
aromatics..	983.0	E867	E950.4	E980.4
fumes NEC..	987.9	E876	E952.9	E982
sublimate — *see* Mercuric chloride				
Corticosteroids.......................................	962.0	E851.0	E950.3	E980.3
Corticotropin...	962.4	E851.4	E950.3	E980.3
Cortisone (acetate).................................	962.0	E851.0	E950.3	E980.3
Cosmetics..	989.9	E869	E950.9	E980.9
Cotarnine..	964.4	E852.8	E950.3	E980.3

Substance	Nature of Injury	External Cause (E-Code)		
		Accident	Suicide (attempt)	Undetermined
Cough mixtures (unspecified)	977.9	E859.9	E950.3	E980.3
specified type NEC	977.8	E859.8	E950.3	E980.3
containing opiates	965.0	E853.0	E950.3	E980.3
Coumadin	964.2	E852.6	E950.3	E980.3
rodenticide	989.3	E865	E950.9	E980.9
Coumarin	964.2	E852.6	E950.3	E980.3
Cowbane	988.2	E868	E950.9	E980.9
Creolin	983.0	E862	E950.4	E980.4
Creosol (compound)	983.0	E862	E950.4	E980.4
Creosote (coal tar) (beechwood)	983.0	E862	E950.4	E980.4
medicinal (expectorant)	977.8	E859.8	E950.3	E980.3
Cresol	983.0	E862	E950.4	E980.4
Cresolin	983.0	E862	E950.4	E980.4
Cresylic acid	983.0	E862	E950.4	E980.4
Cropropamide	971	E856.8	E950.3	E980.3
Crotamiton	961.9	E850.9	E950.3	E980.3
Crotethamide	971	E856.8	E950.3	E980.3
Croton				
chloral	967.1	E854.1	E950.3	E980.3
oil	974.1	E858.1	E950.3	E980.3
Crude oil	981.9	E864	E950.9	E980.9
Cryogenine	965.9	E853.9	E950.3	E980.3
Cryolite	983.9	E867	E950.8	E980.8
pesticide (vapor)	989.3	E865	E950.8	E980.8
vapor NEC	987.9	E876	E952.9	E982
Cryptenamine	973.5	E857.5	E950.3	E980.3
Cubeb(a) (oil)	977.8	E859.8	E950.3	E980.3
Cuckoopint	988.2	E868	E950.9	E980.9
Cumetarol, cumetharol	964.2	E852.6	E950.3	E980.3
Curare, curarine	976.9	E859.4	E950.3	E980.3
Cyanic acid — see Cyanide(s)				
Cyanide(s) (compounds) (hydrogen) (potassium) (sodium) NEC	989.0	E869	E950.9	E980.9
dust (inhalation) or gas NEC	987.9	E876	E952.9	E982
mercuric — see Mercury				
pesticide (dust) (fumes)	989.0	E865	E950.9	E980.9
Cyanocobalamin	963.6	E852.3	E950.3	E980.3
Cyanocol	963.6	E852.3	E950.3	E980.3
Cyanogen (chloride) (gas) NEC	987.9	E876	E952.9	E982
Cyclamen Europaeum	988.2	E868	E950.9	E980.9
Cyclandelate	973.4	E857.4	E950.3	E980.3
Cyclazocine	965.0	E853.0	E950.3	E980.3
Cyclizine	963.0	E852.0	E950.3	E980.3
Cyclobarbital, cyclobarbitone	967.0	E854.0	E950.0	E980.0

Substance	Nature of Injury	External Cause (E-Code)		
		Accident	Suicide (attempt)	Undetermined
Cyclohexane	982.9	E864	E950.9	E980.9
Cyclohexanol	980.9	E860	E950.9	E980.9
Cyclohexanone	982.9	E864	E950.9	E980.9
Cyclohexyl acetate	982.9	E864	E950.9	E980.9
Cyclomethycaine	969	E859.0	E950.3	E980.3
Cyclopentamine	972.2	E855.5	E950.3	E980.3
Cyclopenthiazide	975.3	E859.3	E950.3	E980.3
Cyclopentolate	972.1	E855.4	E950.3	E980.3
Cyclophosphamide	963.1	E852.1	E950.3	E980.3
Cyclopropane	968.1	E856.2	E952.9	E982
Cycloserine	960.9	E850.4	E950.3	E980.3
Cyclothiazide	975.3	E859.3	E950.3	E980.3
Cycrimine	972.1	E855.4	E950.3	E980.3
Cyproheptadine	963.0	E852.0	E950.3	E980.3
Cyprolidol	970.0	E855.0	E950.2	E980.2
Cytisine	971	E856.8	E950.3	E980.3
Cytisus				
laburnum	988.2	E868	E950.9	E980.9
scoparius	988.2	E868	E950.9	E980.9
Cytosine NEC	961.9	E850.9	E950.3	E980.3
antineoplastic	963.1	E852.1	E950.3	E980.3
Cytoxan	963.1	E852.1	E950.3	E980.3
Dactinomycin	963.1	E852.1	E950.3	E980.3
DADPS	961.9	E850.9	E950.3	E980.3
Dakin's solution (external)	977.0	E859.7	E950.3	E980.3
DAM	977.8	E859.8	E950.3	E980.3
Danthron, dantron	974.1	E858.1	E950.3	E980.3
Daphne (gnidium)	988.2	E868	E950.9	E980.9
Dapsone	961.9	E850.9	E950.3	E980.3
Daraprim	961.9	E850.9	E950.3	E980.3
Darnel	988.2	E868	E950.9	E980.9
Darrow's solution	963.4	E852.2	E950.3	E980.3
Darvon	965.9	E853.9	E950.3	E980.3
D-Con (rodenticide)	989.3	E865	E950.9	E980.9
D–D (vapor)	989.2	E865	E950.9	E980.9
DDS	961.9	E850.9	E950.3	E980.3
DDT (dust)	989.2	E865	E950.9	E980.9
Deadly nightshade	988.2	E868	E950.9	E980.9
Deanol	971	E856.8	E950.3	E980.3
Debrisoquine	973.5	E857.5	E950.3	E980.3
Decaborane	989.9	E869	E950.9	E980.9
fumes	987.9	E876	E952.9	E982
Decahydronaphthalene	982.0	E864	E950.9	E980.9
Decalin	982.0	E864	E950.9	E980.9

Substance	Nature of Injury	External Cause (E-Code)		
		Accident	Suicide (attempt)	Undeter- mined
Decamethonium..	976.9	E859.4	E950.3	E980.3
Declomycin...	960.5	E850.3	E950.3	E980.3
Dekalin..	982.0	E864	E950.9	E980.9
Delphinium...	988.2	E868	E950.9	E980.9
Delvinal...	967.0	E854.0	E950.0	E980.0
Demecarium (bromide)............................	972.0	E855.3	E950.3	E980.3
Demecolcine...	965.3	E853.3	E950.3	E980.3
Demerol...	965.0	E853.0	E950.3	E980.3
Demethylchlortetracycline........................	960.5	E850.3	E950.3	E980.3
Denatured alcohol...................................	980.9	E860	E950.9	E980.9
Deoxyribonuclease..................................	963.5	E852.4	E950.3	E980.3
Depressants				
cardiac..	973.0	E857.0	E950.3	E980.3
psychotherapeutic NEC........................	970.1	E855.1	E950.2	E980.2
Dequalinium...	961.9	E850.9	E950.3	E980.3
Deserpidine..	970.1	E855.1	E950.2	E980.2
Desipramine...	970.0	E855.0	E950.2	E980.2
Deslanoside..	973.1	E857.1	E950.3	E980.3
Desocodeine...	965.0	E853.0	E950.3	E980.3
Desomorphine...	965.0	E853.0	E950.3	E980.3
Desoxycorticosterone (acetate)..................	962.0	E851.0	E950.3	E980.3
Desoxyephedrine.....................................	971	E856.4	E950.3	E980.3
Detergents..	989.5	E861	E950.9	E980.9
Detrothyronine.......................................	962.7	E851.7	E950.3	E980.3
Dettol..	977.0	E859.7	E950.3	E980.3
Dexamethasone.......................................	962.0	E851.0	E950.3	E980.3
Dexamphetamine.....................................	971	E856.4	E950.3	E980.3
Dexedrine..	971	E856.4	E950.3	E980.3
Dexpanthenol...	963.6	E852.3	E950.3	E980.3
Dextran...	964.9	E852.9	E950.3	E980.3
Dextriferron...	964.0	E852.5	E950.3	E980.3
Dextromethorphan...................................	965.0	E853.0	E950.3	E980.3
Dextromoramide......................................	965.0	E853.0	E950.3	E980.3
Dextronorpseudoephedrine........................	971	E856.8	E950.3	E980.3
Dextropropoxyphene (hydrochloride)..........	965.9	E853.9	E950.3	E980.3
Dextrorphan...	965.0	E853.0	E950.3	E980.3
Dextrose NEC...	963.4	E852.2	E950.3	E980.3
DFP..	972.0	E855.3	E950.3	E980.3
DHE–45...	973.5	E857.5	E950.3	E980.3
Diacetyl monoxime..................................	977.8	E859.8	E950.3	E980.3
Diacetylmorphine....................................	965.0	E853.0	E950.3	E980.3
Diagnostic agents....................................	977.2	E859.8	E950.3	E980.3
Dial..	967.0	E854.0	E950.0	E980.0
Di-alkyl carbonate..................................	982.9	E864	E950.9	E980.9

Substance	Nature of Injury	External Cause (E-Code)		
		Accident	Suicide (attempt)	Undetermined
Diallylbarbituric acid	967.0	E854.0	E950.0	E980.0
Diaminodiphenylsulfone	961.9	E850.9	E950.3	E980.3
Diamorphine	965.0	E853.0	E950.3	E980.3
Diamox	975.2	E859.3	E950.3	E980.3
Diamthazole	961.9	E850.9	E950.3	E980.3
Diaphenylsulfone	961.9	E850.9	E950.3	E980.3
Diasone (sodium)	961.9	E850.9	E950.3	E980.3
Diatol	982.9	E864	E950.9	E980.9
Diazepam	970.1	E855.1	E950.2	E980.2
Diazomethane (gas)	987.9	E876	E952.9	E982
Dibenzheptropine	963.0	E852.0	E950.3	E980.3
Dibistin	963.0	E852.0	E950.3	E980.3
Diborane (gas)	987.9	E876	E952.9	E982
Dibromomannitol	963.1	E852.1	E950.3	E980.3
Dibucaine	969	E859.0	E950.3	E980.3
Dibutoline	972.1	E855.4	E950.3	E980.3
Dicapthon	989.3	E865	E950.9	E980.9
Dichloralphenazone	967.9	E854.9	E950.3	E980.3
Dichlorodifluoromethane	987.4	E876	E952.9	E982
local anesthetic	969	E859.0	E950.3	E980.3
Dichloroethane	982.9	E864	E950.9	E980.9
Dichloroethyl sulfide — *see* Mustard gas				
Dichloroethylene	982.9	E864	E950.9	E980.9
Dichlorohydrin	982.9	E864	E950.9	E980.9
Dichloromethane (solvent)	982.9	E864	E950.9	E980.9
vapor	987.9	E876	E952.9	E982
Dichlorophen(e)	961.9	E850.9	E950.3	E980.3
Dichlorphenamide	975.2	E859.3	E950.3	E980.3
Dichlorvos	989.3	E865	E950.9	E980.9
Diconal	965.9	E853.9	E950.3	E980.3
Dicoumarin, dicumarol	964.2	E852.6	E950.3	E980.3
Dicyanogen (gas)	987.9	E876	E952.9	E982
Dicyclomine	972.1	E855.4	E950.3	E980.3
Dieldrin (vapor)	989.2	E865	E950.9	E980.9
Dielene	982.9	E864	E950.9	E980.9
Dienestrol	962.2	E851.2	E950.3	E980.3
Diethazine	972.1	E855.4	E950.3	E980.3
Diethyl				
barbituric acid	967.0	E854.0	E950.0	E980.0
carbamazine	961.9	E850.9	E950.3	E980.3
carbinol	980.9	E860	E950.9	E980.9
carbonate	982.9	E864	E950.9	E980.9
ether (vapor) (*see also* Ether(s))	987.9	E876	E952.9	E982

Substance	Nature of Injury	External Cause (E-Code)		
		Accident	Suicide (attempt)	Undeter- mined
Diethyl – *continued*				
propion	971	E856.4	E950.3	E980.3
stilbestrol	962.2	E851.2	E950.3	E980.3
Diethylene				
dioxide	982.9	E864	E950.9	E980.9
glycol (monoacetate) (monoethyl ether)	982.9	E864	E950.9	E980.9
Diethylsulfone-diethylmethane	967.9	E854.9	E950.3	E980.3
Difencloxazine	965.0	E853.0	E950.3	E980.3
Diflos	972.0	E855.3	E950.3	E980.3
Digitalin, digitalis, digitoxin, digoxin	973.1	E857.1	E950.3	E980.3
Dihydrocodeine	965.0	E853.0	E950.3	E980.3
Dihydrocodeinone	965.0	E853.0	E950.3	E980.3
Dihydroergotamine	973.5	E857.5	E950.3	E980.3
Dihydrohydroxycodeinone	965.0	E853.0	E950.3	E980.3
Dihydrohydroxymorphinone	965.0	E853.0	E950.3	E980.3
Dihydroisocodeine	965.0	E853.0	E950.3	E980.3
Dihydromorphine	965.0	E853.0	E950.3	E980.3
Dihydromorphinone	965.0	E853.0	E950.3	E980.3
Dihydrostreptomycin	960.4	E850.3	E950.3	E980.3
Dihydrotachysterol	962.9	E851.9	E950.3	E980.3
Dihydroxyanthraquinone	974.1	E858.1	E950.3	E980.3
Dihydroxycodeinone	965.0	E853.0	E950.3	E980.3
Dihydroxyphenylisatin	974.1	E858.1	E950.3	E980.3
Diiodohydroxyquin	961.3	E850.8	E950.3	E980.3
Diiodohydroxyguinoline	961.3	E850.8	E950.3	E980.3
Dilantin	966.1	E856.0	E950.3	E980.3
Dilaudid	965.0	E853.0	E950.3	E980.3
Diloxanide	961.9	E850.9	E950.3	E980.3
Dimefline	971	E856.8	E950.3	E980.3
Dimenhydrinate	963.0	E852.0	E950.3	E980.3
Dimercaprol	963.9	E852.4	E950.3	E980.3
Dimetane	963.0	E852.0	E950.3	E980.3
Dimethindene	963.0	E852.0	E950.3	E980.3
Dimethisoquin	969	E859.0	E950.3	E980.3
Dimethisterone	962.6	E851.6	E950.3	E980.3
Dimethoxanate	977.8	E859.8	E950.3	E980.3
Dimethyl				
arsine, arsinic acid – *see* Arsenic				
carbinol	980.2	E860	E950.9	E980.9
diguanide	962.3	E851.3	E950.3	E980.3
isopropylazulene	961.9	E850.9	E950.3	E980.3
ketone	982.9	E864	E950.9	E980.9
vapor	987.9	E876	E952.9	E982
meperidine	965.0	E853.0	E950.3	E980.3

Substance	Nature of Injury	External Cause (E-Code)		
		Accident	Suicide (attempt)	Undetermined
Dimethyl—*continued*				
polysiloxane	974.9	E858.9	E950.3	E980.3
sulfate (fumes)	987.9	E876	E952.9	E982
liquid	983.9	E867	E950.9	E980.9
sulfoxide NEC	982.9	E864	E950.9	E980.9
triptamine	970.9	E855.2	E950.2	E980.2
tubocurarine	976.9	E859.4	E950.3	E980.3
Dindevan	964.2	E852.6	E950.3	E980.3
Dinitrobenzene	983.0	E867	E950.4	E980.4
vapor	987.9	E876	E952.9	E982
Dinitrobenzol	983.0	E867	E950.4	E980.4
vapor	987.9	E876	E952.9	E982
Dinitro(-ortho-)cresol (pesticide) (spray)	989.3	E865	E950.9	E980.9
Dinitrophenol (pesticide) (spray)	989.3	E865	E950.9	E980.9
Dioctyl sodium sulfosuccinate	974.4	E858.4	E950.3	E980.3
Diodoquin	961.3	E850.8	E950.3	E980.3
Dione derivatives	966.0	E856.0	E950.3	E980.3
Dionin(e)	965.0	E853.0	E950.3	E980.3
Dioxane	982.9	E864	E950.9	E980.9
Dioxyline	973.4	E857.4	E950.3	E980.3
Dipentene	982.9	E864	E950.9	E980.9
Diphemanil	972.1	E855.4	E950.3	E980.3
Diphenhydramine	963.0	E852.0	E950.3	E980.3
Diphenidol	963.0	E852.0	E950.3	E980.3
Diphenoxylate	974.0	E858.0	E950.3	E980.3
Diphenylchloroarsine (war)	985.1	....	....	.......•.
Diphenylhydantoin (sodium)	966.1	E856.0	E950.3	E980.3
Diphenylpyraline	963.0	E852.0	E950.3	E980.3
Diphenylthiourea	961.9	E850.9	E950.3	E980.3
Dipipanone	965.0	E853.0	E950.3	E980.3
Diprophylline	975.1	E859.2	E950.3	E980.3
Dipyridamole	973.4	E857.4	E950.3	E980.3
Dipyrone	965.5	E853.5	E950.3	E980.3
Disinfectant	983.9	E862	E950.9	E980.9
alkaline	983.2	E862	E950.6	E980.6
aromatic	983.0	E862	E950.4	E980.4
Disipal	972.1	E855.4	E950.3	E980.3
Disodium edetate	963.9	E852.4	E950.3	E980.3
Disulfamide	975.9	E859.3	E950.3	E980.3
Disulfanilamide	961.0	E850.5	E950.3	E980.3
Disulfiram	977.8	E859.8	E950.3	E980.3
Dithiazanine	961.9	E850.9	E950.3	E980.3
Dithranol	977.0	E859.7	E950.3	E980.3
Ditophal	961.9	E850.9	E950.3	E980.3

Substance	Nature of Injury	External Cause (E-Code)		
		Accident	Suicide (attempt)	Undeter- mined
Diuretics NEC	975.9	E859.3	E950.3	E980.3
carbonic acid anhydrase inhibitors	975.2	E859.3	E950.3	E980.3
mercurial	975.0	E859.1	E950.3	E980.3
saluretic	975.3	E859.3	E950.3	E980.3
xanthine	975.1	E859.2	E950.3	E980.3
Diuril	975.3	E859.3	E950.3	E980.3
Divinyl ether	968.1	E856.2	E952.9	E982
D-lysergic acid diethylamide	970.9	E855.2	E950.2	E980.2
DMCT	960.5	E850.3	E950.3	E980.3
DMSO	982.9	E864	E950.9	E980.9
DMT	970.9	E855.2	E950.2	E980.2
DNOC	989.3	E865	E950.9	E980.9
Dolophine	965.0	E853.0	E950.3	E980.3
Doloxene	965.9	E853.9	E950.3	E980.3
Domestic gas — see Gas, utility				
Domestos	983.2	E867	E950.6	E980.6
Domiphen (bromide)	961.9	E850.9	E950.3	E980.3
Doriden	967.9	E854.9	E950.3	E980.3
Dormiral	967.0	E854.0	E950.0	E980.0
Dormison	967.9	E854.9	E950.3	E980.3
Dornase	963.5	E852.4	E950.3	E980.3
Doxapram	971	E856.8	E950.3	E980.3
Doxylamine	963.0	E852.0	E950.3	E980.3
Dramamine	963.0	E852.0	E950.3	E980.3
Drano (drain cleaner)	983.2	E861	E950.6	E980.6
Drinamyl	971	E856.4	E950.3	E980.3
Dromoran	965.0	E853.0	E950.3	E980.3
Dromostanolone	962.1	E851.1	E950.3	E980.3
Drug				
specified type NEC	977.8	E859.8	E950.3	E980.3
unspecified	977.9	E859.9	E950.3	E980.3
Duboisine	972.1	E855.4	E950.3	E980.3
Durabolin	962.1	E851.1	E950.3	E980.3
Dyclonine	969	E859.0	E950.3	E980.3
Dydrogesterone	962.6	E851.6	E950.3	E980.3
Dye(s) NEC	989.9	E869	E950.9	E980.9
diagnostic agents	977.2	E859.8	E950.3	E980.3
pharmaceutical NEC	977.1	E859.8	E950.3	E980.3
Dyflos	972.0	E855.3	E950.3	E980.3
Dynamite	989.9	E869	E950.9	E980.9
fumes	987.9	E876	E952.9	E982
Easton's syrup	977.8	E859.8	E950.3	E980.3
Echothiopate, ecothiopate	972.0	E855.3	E950.3	E980.3

Substance	Nature of Injury	External Cause (E-Code)		
		Accident	Suicide (attempt)	Undetermined
Ectylurea	967.9	E854.9	E950.3	E980.3
Edetate, calcium disodium	963.9	E852.4	E950.3	E980.3
Edrophonium	972.0	E855.3	E950.3	E980.3
Elaterin	974.1	E858.1	E950.3	E980.3
Elaterium	974.1	E858.1	E950.3	E980.3
Elder (berry)	988.2	E868	E950.9	E980.9
Electrolytes NEC	963.4	E852.2	E950.3	E980.3
Embramine	963.0	E852.0	E950.3	E980.3
Emetics	974.6	E858.6	E950.3	E980.3
Emetine (hydrochloride)	961.9	E850.9	E950.3	E980.3
Emylcamate	970.1	E855.1	E950.2	E980.2
Encyprate	970.0	E855.0	E950.2	E980.2
Endocaine	968.9	E856.3	E950.3	E980.3
Endrin	989.2	E865	E950.9	E980.9
Enoxolone (ointment)	977.0	E859.6	E950.3	E980.3
Enzymes	963.5	E852.4	E950.3	E980.3
Epanutin	966.1	E856.0	E950.3	E980.3
Ephedra (tincture)	972.2	E855.5	E950.3	E980.3
Ephedrine	972.2	E855.5	E950.3	E980.3
Epiestriol	962.2	E851.2	E950.3	E980.3
Epinephrine	972.2	E855.5	E950.3	E980.3
Epioestriol	962.2	E851.2	E950.3	E980.3
Epsom salts	974.3	E858.3	E950.3	E980.3
Equanil	970.1	E855.1	E950.2	E980.2
Equisetum (diuretic)	975.9	E859.3	E950.3	E980.3
Ergometrine	976.0	E859.4	E950.3	E980.3
Ergonovine	976.0	E859.4	E950.3	E980.3
Ergot NEC	988.2	E868	E950.9	E980.9
medicinal NEC	976.0	E859.4	E950.3	E980.3
Ergotamine (tartrate) NEC (for migraine)	973.5	E857.5	E950.3	E980.3
Erythrityl tetranitrate	973.4	E857.4	E950.3	E980.3
Erythrol tetranitrate	973.4	E857.4	E950.3	E980.3
Erythromycins	960.3	E850.3	E950.3	E980.3
Eserine	972.0	E855.3	E950.3	E980.3
Eskabarb	967.0	E854.0	E950.0	E980.0
Estradiol (cypionate) (dipropionate) (valerate)	962.2	E851.2	E950.3	E980.3
Estriol	962.2	E851.2	E950.3	E980.3
Estrogens	962.2	E851.2	E950.3	E980.3
Estrone	962.2	E851.2	E950.3	E980.3
Etafedrine	972.2	E855.5	E950.3	E980.3
Etamivan	971	E856.8	E950.3	E980.3
Ethacrynic acid	975.9	E859.3	E950.3	E980.3
Ethambutol	961.9	E850.9	E950.3	E980.3

Substance	Nature of Injury	External Cause (E-Code)		
		Accident	Suicide (attempt)	Undetermined
Ethamivan	971	E856.8	E950.3	E980.3
Ethamsylate	964.4	E852.8	E950.3	E980.3
Ethanol	980.0	E860	E950.9	E980.9
Ethchlorvynol	967.9	E854.9	E950.3	E980.3
Ethebenecid	963.4	E852.2	E950.3	E980.3
Ether(s) (diethyl) (ethyl) (vapor)	987.9	E876	E952.9	E982
anesthetic (divinyl) (vinyl)	968.1	E856.2	E952.9	E982
liquid NEC	968.9	E856.3	E950.3	E980.3
petroleum — see Ligroin				
solvent	982.9	E864	E950.9	E980.9
Ethidine chloride (vapor)	987.9	E876	E952.9	E982
liquid (solvent)	982.9	E864	E950.9	E980.9
Ethinamate	967.9	E854.9	E950.3	E980.3
Ethinyl estradiol	962.2	E851.2	E950.3	E980.3
Ethionamide	961.9	E850.9	E950.3	E980.3
Ethisterone	962.6	E851.6	E950.3	E980.3
Ethobral	967.0	E854.0	E950.0	E980.0
Ethocaine	969	E859.0	E950.3	E980 3
Ethoglucid(e)	963.1	E852.1	E950.3	E980.3
Ethoheptazine (citrate)	965.9	E853.9	E950.3	E980.3
Ethopropazine	972.1	E855.4	E950.3	E980.3
Ethosalamide	965.1	E853.1	E950.1	E980.1
Ethosuximide	966.9	E856.0	E950.3	E980.3
Ethotoin	966.1	E856.0	E950.3	E980.3
Ethoxazene	961.9	E850.9	E950.3	E980.3
Ethoxyzolamide, ethoxzolamide	975.2	E859.3	E950.3	E980.3
Ethyl				
acetate	982.9	E864	E950.9	E980.9
vapor	987.9	E876	E952.9	E982
alcohol	980.0	E860	E950.9	E980.9
aldehyde (vapor)	987.9	E876	E952.9	E982
liquid	989.9	E869	E950.9	E980.9
aminobenzoate	969	E859.0	E950.3	E980.3 ·
benzoate	982.9	E864	E950.9	E980.9
biscoumacetate	964.2	E852.6	E950.3	E980.3
bromide NEC (local anesthetic)	969	E859.0	E950.3	E980.3
carbamate (antineoplastic)	963.1	E852.1	E950.3	E980.3
carbinol	980.2	E860	E950.9	E980.9
chaulmoograte	961.9	E850.9	E950.3	E980.3
chloride (vapor)	987.9	E876	E952.9	E982
anesthetic (local)	969	E859.0	E950.3	E980.3
inhaled	968.1	E856.2	E952.9	E982
solvent	982.9	E864	E950.9	E980.9
dichloroarsine (vapor)	985.1	E866	E950.7	E980.7

Substance	Nature of Injury	External Cause (E-Code)		
		Accident	Suicide (attempt)	Undeter-mined
Ethyl—*continued*				
estranol	962.1	E851.1	E950.3	E980.3
ether (*see also* Ether(s))	987.9	E876	E952.9	E982
formate NEC (solvent)	982.9	E864	E950.9	E980.9
hydroxyisobutyrate NEC (solvent)	982.9	E864	E950.9	E980.9
lactate NEC (solvent)	982.9	E864	E950.9	E980.9
methylcarbinol	980.9	E860	E950.9	E980.9
morphine	965.0	E853.0	E950.3	E980.3
oxybutyrate NEC (solvent)	982.9	E864	E950.9	E980.9
Ethylene (gas)	987.1	E876	E952.9	E982
anesthetic (general)	968.1	E856.2	E952.9	E982
chlorohydrin	982.9	E864	E950.9	E980.9
vapor	987.9	E876	E952.9	E982
dichloride	982.9	E864	E950.9	E980.9
vapor	987.9	E876	E952.9	E982
glycol(s) (any)	982.9	E864	E950.9	E980.9
vapor	987.9	E876	E952.9	E982
Ethylidene				
chloride NEC	982.9	E864	E950.9	E980.9
diethyl ether	982.9	E864	E950.9	E980.9
Ethynodiol	962.6	E851.6	E950.3	E980.3
Etilfen	967.0	E854.0	E950.0	E980.0
Etomide	965.9	E853.9	E950.3	E980.3
Etorphine	965.0	E853.0	E950.3	E980.3
Etoval	967.0	E854.0	E950.0	E980.0
Etryptamine	970.0	E855.0	E950.2	E980.2
Eucaine	969	E859.0	E950.3	E980.3
Eucalyptus (oil) NEC	977.8	E859.8	E950.3	E980.3
Eucatropine	972.1	E855.4	E950.3	E980.3
Eucodal	965.0	E853.0	E950.3	E980.3
Euneryl	967.0	E854.0	E950.0	E980.0
Euphorbia (extract)	977.8	E859.8	E950.3	E980.3
Euphthalmine	972.1	E855.4	E950.3	E980.3
Eusolvan	982.9	E864	E950.9	E980.9
Evipal	968.9	E856.3	E950.3	E980.3
Evipan	968.9	E856.3	E950.3	E980.3
Exalgin	965.4	E853.4	E950.3	E980.3
Exhaust gas—*see* Carbon monoxide, exhaust gas				
Expectorants—*see* Cough mixtures				
External medicaments NEC	977.0	E859.7	E950.3	E980.3
antifungal—*see* Antifungals				
liniments	977.0	E859.5	E950.3	E980.3

Substance	Nature of Injury	External Cause (E-Code)		
		Accident	Suicide (attempt)	Undeter- mined
External medicaments NEC—*continued*				
lotions	977.0	E859.7	E950.3	E980.3
ointments	977.0	E859.6	E950.3	E980.3
Famel (syrup)	977.8	E859.8	E950.3	E980.3
Fecal softeners	974.4	E858.4	E950.3	E980.3
Fenbutrazate	971	E856.4	E950.3	E980.3
Fencamfamin	971	E856.8	E950.3	E980.3
Fenfluramine	971	E856.4	E950.3	E980.3
Fentanyl	965.0	E853.0	E950.3	E980.3
Fentazin	970.1	E855.1	E950.2	E980.2
Fenticlor	961.9	E850.9	E950.3	E980.3
Ferric—*see* Iron				
Ferrocholinate	964.0	E852.5	E950.3	E980.3
Ferrous fumerate, gluconate, lactate, salt NEC, sulfate (medicinal)	964.0	E852.5	E950.3	E980.3
Ferrum—*see* Iron				
Fertilizers NEC	989.9	E865	E950.9	E980.9
Fibrinogen	964.4	E852.8	E950.3	E980.3
Fibrinolysin	963.5	E852.4	E950.3	E980.3
Filix mas	961.9	E850.9	E950.3	E980.3
Fire damp	987.1	E876	E952.9	E982
Fish, nonbacterial or noxious	988.9	E868	E950.9	E980.9
shell	988.0	E868	E950.9	E980.9
Flagyl	961.9	E850.9	E950.3	E980.3
Flaxedil	976.9	E859.4	E950.3	E980.3
Fludrocortisone	962.0	E851.0	E950.3	E980.3
Flumethiazide	975.3	E859.3	E950.3	E980.3
Flumidin	961.9	E850.9	E950.3	E980.3
Fluocinolone	962.0	E851.0	E950.3	E980.3
Fluocortolone	962.0	E851.0	E950.3	E980.3
Fluopromazine	970.1	E855.1	E950.2	E980.2
Fluorescein (sodium)	977.2	E859.8	E950.3	E980.3
Fluoride(s) (sodium) (pesticides) NEC	989.3	E865	E950.8	E980.8
hydrogen—*see* Hydrofluoric acid				
not pesticides NEC	983.9	E867	E950.8	E980.8
Fluorine (gas)	987.9	E876	E952.9	E982
salt—*see* Fluoride(s)				
Fluoroacetate	989.3	E865	E950.8	E980.8
Fluorodeoxyuridine	963.1	E852.1	E950.3	E980.3
Fluorophosphate	989.3	E865	E950.8	E980.8
Fluorouracil	963.1	E852.1	E950.3	E980.3
Fluothane	968.1	E856.2	E952.9	E982
Fluoxymesterone	962.1	E851.1	E950.3	E980.3
Fluphenazine	970.1	E855.1	E950.2	E980.2

Substance	Nature of Injury	External Cause (E-Code)		
		Accident	Suicide (attempt)	Undetermined
Fluprednisolone	962.0	E851.0	E950.3	E980.3
Flurandrenolone	962.0	E851.0	E950.3	E980.3
Flurothyl	970.9	E855.2	E950.2	E980.2
Fluthiazide	975.3	E859.3	E950.3	E980.3
Folic acid	963.6	E852.3	E950.3	E980.3
Follicle stimulating hormone	962.4	E851.4	E950.3	E980.3
Food, foodstuffs, nonbacterial or noxious NEC	988.9	E868	E950.9	E980.9
Fool's parsley	988.2	E868	E950.9	E980.9
Formaldehyde (solution)	989.9	E862	E950.9	E980.9
gas or vapor	987.9	E876	E952.9	E982
Formalin	989.9	E862	E950.9	E980.9
vapor	987.9	E876	E952.9	E982
Formic acid	983.1	E867	E950.9	E980.9
vapor	987.9	E876	E952.9	E982
Fowler's solution	985.1	E859.8	E950.3	E980.3
Foxglove	988.2	E868	E950.9	E980.9
Framycetin	960.9	E850.4	E950.3	E980.3
Frangula (extract)	974.1	E858.1	E950.3	E980.3
Freons	987.4	E876	E952.9	E982
Frusemide	975.3	E859.3	E950.3	E980.3
FSH	962.4	E851.4	E950.3	E980.3
Fuel				
automobile	981.1	E864	E950.9	E980.9
exhaust gas, not in transit	986	E873	E952.0	E982
vapor NEC	987.1	E876	E952.9	E982
gas (domestic use) — *see* Carbon monoxide, fuel				
industrial, incomplete combustion	986	E875	E952.1	E982
Fugillin	960.9	E850.4	E950.3	E980.3
Fulminate of mercury	985.0	E866	E950.9	E980.9
Fulvicin	960.1	E850.1	E950.3	E980.3
Fumadil	960.9	E850.4	E950.3	E980.3
Fumagillin	960.9	E850.4	E950.3	E980.3
Fumes (from)	987.9	E877	E952.9	E982
carbon monoxide — *see* Carbon monoxide				
charcoal (domestic use)	986	E874	E952.1	E982
chloroform — *see* Chloroform				
coke (in domestic stoves, fireplaces)	986	E874	E952.1	E982
corrosive NEC	987.9	E877	E952.9	E982
ether — *see* Ether(s)				
lead — *see* Lead				
metals — *see* Metals, or the specified metal				
pesticides — *see* Pesticides				

Substance	Nature of Injury	External Cause (E-Code)		
		Accident	Suicide (attempt)	Undeter-mined
Fumes (from) — *continued*				
specified source, other (*see also* substance specified)	987.9	E876	E952.9	E982
Fungi, noxious, used as food	988.1	E868	E950.9	E980.9
Fungicides — *see* Antifungals				
Fungizone	960.1	E850.1	E950.3	E980.3
Furadantin	961.9	E850.9	E950.3	E980.3
Furazolidone	961.9	E850.9	E950.3	E980.3
Furnace (coal burning) (domestic), gas from	986	E874	E952.1	E982
industrial	986	E875	E952.1	E982
Furniture polish	989.9	E861	E950.9	E980.9
Furosemide	975.3	E859.3	E950.3	E980.3
Furoxone	961.9	E850.9	E950.3	E980.3
Fusel oil (any) (amyl) (butyl) (propyl)	980.9	E860	E950.9	E980.9
vapor	987.9	E876	E952.9	E982
Fusidic acid	960.9	E850.4	E950.3	E980.3
Gallamine	976.9	E859.4	E950.3	E980.3
Gamboge	974.1	E858.1	E950.3	E980.3
Gamma-benzene hexachloride (vapor)	989.2	E865	E950.9	E980.9
Ganglionic blocking agents	973.3	E857.3	E950.3	E980.3
Ganja	967.9	E854.9	E950.3	E980.3
Gardenal	967.0	E854.0	E950.0	E980.0
Gardenpanyl	967.0	E854.0	E950.0	E980.0
Gas	987.9	E877	E952.9	E982
acetylene	987.1	E872	E951	E981
air contaminants, source or type not specified	987.9	E877	E952.9	E982
anesthetic (general)	968.1	E856.2	E952.9	E982
blast furnace	986	E875	E952.1	E982
butane — *see* Butane				
carbon monoxide — *see* Carbon monoxide				
chlorine	987.9	E876	E952.9	E982
coal — *see* Carbon monoxide, coal				
cyanide	987.9	E876	E952.9	E982
dicyanogen	987.9	E876	E952.9	E982
domestic — *see* Gas, utility				
exhaust — *see* Carbon monoxide, exhaust gas				
from wood- or coal-burning stove or fireplace	986	E874	E952.1	E982
fuel (domestic use) — *see* Carbon monoxide, fuel				
industrial use	986	E875	E952.1	E982
garage	986	E873	E952.0	E982

Substance	Nature of Injury	External Cause (E-Code)		
		Accident	Suicide (attempt)	Undeter- mined
Gas—*continued*				
hydrocarbon NEC	987.1	E876	E952.9	E982
hydrocyanic acid	987.9	E876	E952.9	E982
illuminating—*see* Gas, utility				
incomplete combustion, any—*see* Carbon monoxide				
kiln	986	E875	E952.1	E982
marsh	987.1	E876	E952.9	E982
motor exhaust, not in transit	986	E873	E952.0	E982
mustard—*see* Mustard gas				
natural	987.1	E870	E951	E981
nerve (war)	987.9	....	....	....
producer	986	E875	E952.1	E982
propane—*see* Propane				
refrigerant (freon)	987.4	E876	E952.9	E982
not freon	987.9	E876	E952.9	E982
sewer	987.9	E876	E952.9	E982
specified source, other (*see also* substance specified)	987.9	E876	E952.9	E982
stove—*see* Gas, utility				
utility (for cooking, heating, or lighting) (piped) NEC	986	E870	E951	E981
in mobile container	987.0	E871	E951	E981
natural	987.1	E870	E951	E981
other specified type NEC	986	E872	E951	E981
water	986	E872	E951	E981
Gaseous substance—*see* Gas				
Gasolene, gasoline	981.1	E864	E950.9	E980.9
vapor	987.1	E876	E952.9	E982
Gastric enzymes	963.5	E852.4	E950.3	E980.3
Gaultheria procumbens	988.2	E868	E950.9	E980.9
Gee's linctus	965.0	E853.0	E950.3	E980.3
Gelatin				
absorbable (sponge)	964.4	E852.8	E950.3	E980.3
intravenous	964.9	E852.9	E950.3	E980.3
Gelsemine	965.9	E853.9	E950.3	E980.3
Gelsemium (sempervirens)	988.2	E868	E950.9	E980.9
Gemonil	967.0	E854.0	E950.0	E980.0
Gentamicin	960.9	E850.4	E950.3	E980.3
Gentian violet	961.9	E850.9	E950.3	E980.3
Ginger, Jamaica	989.9	E869	E950.9	E980.9
Gitalin	973.1	E857.1	E950.3	E980.3
Glandular extract (medicinal) NEC	977.9	E859.9	E950.3	E980.3
Glaucarubin	961.9	E850.9	E950.3	E980.3

Substance	Nature of Injury	External Cause (E-Code)		
		Accident	Suicide (attempt)	Undeter- mined
Globin zinc insulin	962.3	E851.3	E950.3	E980.3
Glucagon	962.3	E851.3	E950.3	E980.3
Glucochloral	967.1	E854.1	E950.3	E980.3
Glutamic acid (hydrochloride)	974.9	E858.9	E950.3	E980.3
Glutaraldehyde	977.8	E859.8	E950.3	E980.3
Glutathione	963.9	E852.4	E950.3	E980.3
Glutethimide	967.9	E854.9	E950.3	E980.3
Glycerin (lotion)	977.0	E859.7	E950.3	E980.3
Glyceryl trinitrate	973.4	E857.4	E950.3	E980.3
Glycobiarsol	961.1	E850.6	E950.3	E980.3
Glycols (ether)	982.9	E864	E950.9	E980.9
Glycopyrrolate	972.1	E855.4	E950.3	E980.3
Glymidine	962.3	E851.3	E950.3	E980.3
Gold (compounds) (salts)	976.2	E859.4	E950.3	E980.3
Golden sulfide of antimony	985.9	E866	E950.9	E980.9
Goldylocks	988.2	E868	E950.9	E980.9
Gonadal tissue extract	962.9	E851.9	E950.3	E980.3
female	962.2	E851.2	E950.3	E980.3
male	962.1	E851.1	E950.3	E980.3
Grain alcohol	980.0	E860	E950.9	E980.9
Gramicidin	960.9	E850.4	E950.3	E980.3
Gratiola officinalis	988.2	E868	E950.9	E980.9
Gray oil	985.0	E850.9	E950.3	E980.3
Grease	989.9	E869	E950.9	E980.9
Green hellebore	988.2	E868	E950.9	E980.9
Grifulvin	960.1	E850.1	E950.3	E980.3
Griseofulvin	960.1	E850.1	E950.3	E980.3
Guaiacol	977.8	E859.8	E950.3	E980.3
Guaiphenesin	977.8	E859.8	E950.3	E980.3
Guanatol	961.9	E850.9	E950.3	E980.3
Guanethidine	973.5	E857.5	E950.3	E980.3
Guano	989.9	E865	E950.9	E980.9
Guanoclor	973.5	E857.5	E950.3	E980.3
Guanoctine	973.5	E857.5	E950.3	E980.3
Guanoxan	973.5	E857.5	E950.3	E980.3
Haemostatics	964.4	E852.8	E950.3	E980.3
Halethazole	961.9	E850.9	E950.3	E980.3
Hallucinogenics	970.9	E855.2	E950.2	E980.2
Haloperidol	970.1	E855.1	E950.2	E980.2
Halothane	968.1	E856.2	E952.9	E982
Halquinols	961.3	E850.8	E950.3	E980.3
Hashish	967.9	E854.9	E950.3	E980.3
Headache cures, drugs, powders NEC	977.9	E859.9	E950.3	E980.3
Heavy metal antagonists	963.9	E852.4	E950.3	E980.3

Substance	Nature of Injury	External Cause (E-Code)		
		Accident	Suicide (attempt)	Undeter- mined
Hedaquinium...	961.9	E850.9	E950.3	E980.3
Hedge hyssop...	988.2	E868	E950.9	E980.9
Hedonal..	967.9	E854.9	E950.3	E980.3
Helenin..	961.9	E850.9	E950.3	E980.3
Hellebore (black) (green) (white)................	988.2	E868	E950.9	E980.9
Hemlock...	988.2	E868	E950.9	E980.9
Hemostatics..	964.4	E852.8	E950.3	E980.3
Henbane...	988.2	E868	E950.9	E980.9
Heparin (sodium)......................................	964.2	E852.6	E950.3	E980.3
Heptabarbital, heptabarbitone....................	967.0	E854.0	E950.0	E980.0
Heptachlor..	989.2	E865	E950.9	E980.9
Heptalgen...	965.0	E853.0	E950.3	E980.3
Herbicides—see Pesticides				
Heroin..	965.0	E853.0	E950.3	E980.3
Hexadimethrine (bromide).........................	964.4	E852.8	E950.3	E980.3
Hexafluorenium..	976.9	E859.4	E950.3	E980.3
Hexahydrocresol.......................................	980.9	E860	E950.9	E980.9
Hexahydrophenol......................................	980.9	E860	E950.9	E980.9
Hexalin..	980.9	E860	E950.9	E980.9
Hexamethonium..	973.3	E857.3	E950.3	E980.3
Hexamethyleneamine.................................	961.9	E850.9	E950.3	E980.3
Hexamine...	961.9	E850.9	E950.3	E980.3
Hexanone...	982.9	E864	E950.9	E980.9
Hexapropymate...	967.9	E854.9	E950.3	E980.3
Hexestrol...	962.2	E851.2	E950.3	E980.3
Hexethal (sodium)....................................	967.0	E854.0	E950.0	E980.0
Hexetidine..	961.9	E850.9	E950.3	E980.3
Hexobarbital, hexobarbitone......................	968.9	E856.3	E950.3	E980.3
Hexocyclium...	972.1	E855.4	E950.3	E980.3
Hexoestrol...	962.2	E851.2	E950.3	E980.3
Hexone..	982.9	E864	E950.9	E980.9
Hexylcaine...	969	E859.0	E950.3	E980.3
Hexylresorcinol..	983.0	E867	E950.4	E980.4
Hinkle's pills..	974.1	E858.1	E950.3	E980.3
Histalog...	977.2	E859.8	E950.3	E980.3
Histamine (phosphate)..............................	973.4	E857.4	E950.3	E980.3
Holly berries..	988.2	E868	E950.9	E980.9
Homatropine...	972.1	E855.4	E950.3	E980.3
Hormones and synthetic substitutes NEC.....	962.9	E851.9	E950.3	E980.3
Hyaluronidase...	963.5	E852.4	E950.3	E980.3
Hycodan...	965.0	E853.0	E950.3	E980.3
Hydantoin derivatives................................	966.1	E856.0	E950.3	E980.3
Hydergin(e)..	973.5	E857.5	E950.3	E980.3
Hydrabamine penicillin..............................	960.0	E850.0	E950.3	E980.3

Substance	Nature of Injury	External Cause (E-Code)		
		Accident	Suicide (attempt)	Undetermined
Hydralazine, hydrallazine	973.5	E857.5	E950.3	E980.3
Hydrargaphen	985.0	E859.7	E950.3	E980.3
Hydrazine	983.9	E867	E950.9	E980.9
Hydrochloric acid (liquid)	983.1	E867	E950.9	E980.9
medicinal	974.9	E858.9	E950.3	E980.3
vapor	987.9	E876	E952.9	E982
Hydrochlorothiazide	975.3	E859.3	E950.3	E980.3
Hydrocodone	965.0	E853.0	E950.3	E980.3
Hydrocortisone	962.0	E851.0	E950.3	E980.3
Hydrocyanic acid — see Cyanide(s)				
Hydroflumethiazide	975.3	E859.3	E950.3	E980.3
Hydrofluoric acid (liquid)	983.1	E867	E950.8	E980.8
vapor	987.9	E876	E952.9	E982
Hydrofluthiazide	975.3	E859.3	E950.3	E980.3
Hydrogen	987.9	E876	E952.9	E982
arsenide	985.1	E866	E950.7	E980.7
arseniuretted	985.1	E866	E950.7	E980.7
cyanide	989.0	E869	E950.9	E980.9
gas	987.9	E876	E952.9	E982
fluoride (liquid)	983.1	E867	E950.8	E980.8
vapor	987.9	E876	E952.9	E982
peroxide (solution)	977.8	E859.8	E950.3	E980.3
phosphuretted	987.9	E876	E952.9	E982
sulfate	983.1	E867	E950.9	E980.9
sulfide (gas)	987.9	E876	E952.9	E982
arseniuretted	985.1	E866	E950.7	E980.7
sulfuretted	987.9	E876	E952.9	E982
Hydrolin	980.9	E860	E950.9	E980.9
Hydromorphinol	965.0	E853.0	E950.3	E980.3
Hydromorphinone	965.0	E853.0	E950.3	E980.3
Hydromorphone	965.0	E853.0	E950.3	E980.3
Hydroquinone	983.0	E867	E950.4	E980.4
vapor	987.9	E876	E952.9	E982
Hydrosulfuric acid (gas)	987.9	E876	E952.9	E982
Hydroxide, caustic	983.2	E867	E950.6	E980.6
Hydroxocobalamin	963.6	E852.3	E950.3	E980.3
Hydroxyamphetamine	972.2	E855.5	E950.3	E980.3
Hydroxychloroquine	961.3	E850.8	E950.3	E980.3
Hydroxycodeine	965.0	E853.0	E950.3	E980.3
Hydroxyphenamate	970.1	E855.1	E950.2	E980.2
Hydroxyphenylbutazone	965.5	E853.5	E950.3	E980.3
Hydroxyprogesterone	962.6	E851.6	E950.3	E980.3
Hydroxyquinoline	961.3	E850.8	E950.3	E980.3
Hydroxystilbamidine	961.9	E850.9	E950.3	E980.3

Substance	Nature of Injury	External Cause (E-Code)		
		Accident	Suicide (attempt)	Undetermined
Hydroxyurea.. 963.1		E852.1	E950.3	E980.3
Hydroxyzine.. 970.1		E855.1	E950.2	E980.2
Hyoscine (hydrobromide)......................... 972.1		E855.4	E950.3	E980.3
Hyoscyamine.. 972.1		E855.4	E950.3	E980.3
Hyoscyamus (albus) (niger)...................... 988.2		E868	E950.9	E980.9
Hypnotics.. 967.9		E854.9	E950.3	E980.3
Hypochlorites—see Sodium hypochlorite				
Hypotensive agents NEC......................... 973.5		E857.5	E950.3	E980.3
Ibufenac... 965.9		E853.9	E950.3	E980.3
Idoxuridine.. 961.9		E850.9	E950.3	E980.3
IDU.. 961.9		E850.9	E950.3	E980.3
Ilex.. 988.2		E868	E950.9	E980.9
Illuminating gas—see Gas, utility				
Ilotycin... 960.3		E850.3	E950.3	E980.3
Iminomorpholinomethylguanidine............... 961.9		E850.9	E950.3	E980.3
Imipramine.. 970.0		E855.0	E950.2	E980.2
Indandione derivatives............................ 964.2		E852.6	E950.3	E980.3
Indian				
hemp... 967.9		E854.9	E950.3	E980.3
tobacco.. 988.2		E868	E950.9	E980.9
Indocin... 965.9		E853.9	E950.3	E980.3
Indomethacin... 965.9		E853.9	E950.3	E980.3
Ingested substances NEC......................... 989.9		E869	E950.9	E980.9
INH... 961.9		E850.9	E950.3	E980.3
Inhalation, gas (noxious)—see Gas				
Inositol nicotinate.................................. 973.4		E857.4	E950.3	E980.3
Inproquone.. 963.1		E852.1	E950.3	E980.3
Insect (sting), venomous.......................... 989.4		E905	E950.9	E980.9
Insecticides—see Pesticides				
Insular tissue extract.............................. 962.3		E851.3	E950.3	E980.3
Insulin (amorphous) (globin) (isophane) (lente) (NPH) (protamine) (semilente) (ultralente) (zinc)............................ 962.3		E851.3	E950.3	E980.3
Intranarcon... 968.9		E856.3	E950.3	E980.3
Iodide (see also Iodine) NEC................... 977.0		E859.7	E950.3	E980.3
mercury (ointment)............................. 985.0		E859.6	E950.3	E980.3
methylate... 977.0		E859.7	E950.3	E980.3
potassium (expectorant) NEC................ 977.8		E859.8	E950.3	E980.3
Iodine (antiseptic, external) (tincture) NEC... 977.0		E859.7	E950.3	E980.3
for thyroid conditions (antithyroid).......... 962.8		E851.8	E950.3	E980.3
vapor.. 987.9		E876	E952.9	E982
Iodobismitol.. 961.9		E850.9	E950.3	E980.3
Iodochlorhydroxyquin.............................. 961.3		E850.8	E950.3	E980.3
Iodoform... 977.0		E859.7	E950.3	E980.3

Substance	Nature of Injury	External Cause (E-Code)		
		Accident	Suicide (attempt)	Undetermined
Iodophthalein..	977.0	E859.7	E950.3	E980.3
diagnostic agent....................................	977.2	E859.8	E950.3	E980.3
Ion exchange resin.................................	963.4	E852.2	E950.3	E980.3
Iopanoic acid..	977.2	E859.8	E850.3	E980.3
Iophendylate...	977.2	E859.8	E950.3	E980.3
Iothiouracil...	962.8	E851.8	E950.3	E980.3
Ipecac...	974.6	E858.6	E950.3	E980.3
Ipecacuanha..	974.6	E858.6	E950.3	E980.3
Ipral..	967.0	E854.0	F.950.0	E980.0
Iproniazid...	970.0	E855.0	E950.2	E980.2
Iproveratril...	973.4	E857.4	E950.3	E980.3
Iron (compounds) (medicinal)....................	964.0	E852.5	E950.3	E980.3
nonmedicinal (fumes) (dust) NEC...........	985.9	E866	F.950.9	E980.9
Irritant drug..	977.9	E859.9	E950.3	E980.3
Isoamyl nitrite...	973.4	E857.4	E950.3	E980.3
Isobutyl acetate.......................................	982.9	E864	E950.9	E980.9
Isocarboxazid..	970.0	E855.0	E950.2	E980.2
Isoetharine...	972.2	E855.5	E950.3	E980.3
Isoniazid..	961.9	E850.9	E950.3	E980.3
Isopentaquine...	961.3	E850.8	E950.3	E980.3
Isophane insulin.......................................	962.3	E851.3	E950.3	E980.3
Isoprenaline..	972.2	E855.5	E950.3	E980.3
Isopropamide...	972.1	E855.4	E950.3	E980.3
Isopropyl				
acetate..	982.9	E864	E950.9	E980.9
alcohol..	980.2	F.860	E950.9	E980.9
ether...	982.9	E864	E950.9	E980.9
Isoproterenol...	972.2	E855.5	E950.3	E980.3
Isosorbide dinitrate..................................	973.4	E857.4	E950.3	E980.3
Isothipendyl..	963.0	E852.0	E950.3	E980.3
Isoxazolyl penicillin.................................	960.0	E850.0	E950.3	E980.3
Isoxsuprine...	973.4	E857.4	E950.3	E980.3
Izal (disinfectant)....................................	983.0	E862	E950.4	E980.4
Jaborandi (pilocarpus) (extract)..................	972.0	E855.3	E950.3	E980.3
Jalap...	974.1	E858.1	E950.3	E980.3
Jamaica				
dogwood (bark).....................................	965.9	E853.9	E950.3	E980.3
ginger...	989.9	E869	E950.9	E980.9
Jatropha (curcas).....................................	988.2	E868	E950.9	E980.9
Jectofer..	964.0	E852.5	E950.3	E980.3
Jequirity (bean).......................................	988.2	E868	E950.9	E980.9
Jimson weed...	988.2	E868	E950.9	E980.9
Juniper tar (oil) (ointment).......................	977.0	E859.6	E950.3	E980.3
Kallikrein..	973.4	E857.4	E950.3	E980.3

Substance	Nature of Injury	External Cause (E-Code)		
		Accident	Suicide (attempt)	Undeter- mined
Kanamycin	960.9	E850.4	E950.3	E980.3
Kantrex	960.9	E850.4	E950.3	E980.3
Kaolin	974.0	E858.0	E950.3	E980.3
Kemithal	968.9	E856.3	E950.3	E980.3
Keratolytic agent (*see also* External medi- caments)	977.0	E859.7	E950.3	E980.3
Kerosene, kerosine (fuel) (solvent) NEC	981.0	E864	E950.9	E980.9
insecticide	981.0	E865	E950.9	E980.9
vapor	987.1	E876	E952.9	E982
Ketobemidone	965.0	E853.0	E950.3	E980.3
Ketols	982.9	E864	E950.9	E980.9
Ketone oils	982.9	E864	E950.9	E980.9
Khat	971	E856.8	E950.3	E980.3
Kiln gas or vapor (carbon monoxide)	986	E875	E952.1	E982
Kosam seed	988.2	E868	E950.9	E980.9
Kwell (insecticide)	989.2	E865	E950.9	E980.9
Kwells	972.1	E855.4	E950.3	E980.3
Laburnum (leaves) (seeds)	988.2	E868	E950.9	E980.9
Lacquers	989.9	E863	E950.9	E980.9
Lactic acid	983.1	E867	E950.9	E980.9
Lactobacillus acidophilus	974.0	E858.0	E950.3	E980.3
Lactuca (virosa) extract	967.9	E854.9	E950.3	E980.3
Lactucarium	967.9	E854.9	E950.3	E980.3
Laevulose	963.4	E852.2	E950.3	E980.3
Lanatoside	973.1	E857.1	E950.3	E980.3
Largactil	970.1	E855.1	E950.2	E980.2
Larkspur	988.2	E868	E950.9	E980.9
Laroxyl	970.0	E855.0	E950.2	E980.2
Lathyrus (seed)	988.2	E868	E950.9	E980.9
Laudanum	965.0	E853.0	E950.3	E980.3
Laudexium	976.9	E859.4	E950.3	E980.3
Laurel, black or cherry	988.2	E868	E950.9	E980.9
Laurolinium	977.0	E859.7	E950.3	E980.3
Laxatives NEC	974.5	E858.5	E950.3	E980.3
Lead (carbonate) (chromate) (dust) (fumes) (iodide) (oxide) (tetraethyl) (vapor) NEC	984	E866	E950.9	E980.9
arsenate, arsenite (dust) (herbicide) (in- secticide) (vapor)	985.1	E865	E950.7	E980.7
medicinal (external) NEC	984	E859.7	E950.3	E980.3
Leptazol	971	E856.8	E950.3	E980.3
Leritin(e)	965.0	E853.0	E950.3	E980.3
Lettuce opium	967.9	E854.9	E950.3	E980.3
Leucanthone	961.9	E850.9	E950.3	E980.3

Substance	Nature of Injury	External Cause (E-Code)		
		Accident	Suicide (attempt)	Undeter- mined
Leucovorin (factor)..................................	963.6	E852.3	E950.3	E980.3
Leukeran...	963.1	E852.1	E950.3	E980.3
Levallorphan...	971	E856.8	E950.3	E980.3
Levanil..	967.9	E854.9	E950.3	E980.3
Levarterenol...	972.2	E855.5	E950.3	E980.3
Levo-dromoran..	965.0	E853.0	E950.3	E980.3
Levo-iso-methadone................................	965.0	E853.0	E950.3	E980.3
Levopropoxyphene..................................	977.8	E859.8	E950.3	E980.3
Levorphan, levorphanol...........................	965.0	E853.0	E950.3	E980.3
Levothyroxine...	962.7	E851.7	E950.3	E980.3
Levulose...	963.4	E852.2	E950.3	E980.3
Lewisite (gas) (war)................................	985.1	....	....	....
not in war...	985.1	E866	E950.7	E980.7
Librium..	970.1	E855.1	E950.2	E980.2
Lidocaine..	969	E859.0	E950.3	E980.3
Lighter fluid..	981.2	E864	E950.9	E980.9
Lignocaine..	969	E859.0	E950.3	E980.3
Ligroin(e) (solvent)................................	981.2	E864	E950.9	E980.9
vapor..	987.1	E876	E952.9	E982
Ligustrum vulgare....................................	988.2	E868	E950.9	E980.9
Lily-of-the-valley....................................	988.2	E868	E950.9	E980.9
Lime (chloride)..	983.2	E867	E950.6	E980.6
Limonene..	982.9	E864	E950.9	E980.9
Lincomycin...	960.9	E850.4	E950.3	E980.3
Lindane (insecticide) (vapor)....................	989.2	E865	E950.9	E980.9
Liniments NEC..	977.0	E859.5	E950.3	E980.3
Linoleic acid...	973.2	E857.2	E950.3	E980.3
Liothyronine...	962.7	E851.7	E950.3	E980.3
Liquid substance NEC..............................	989.9	E869	E950.9	E980.9
Liquor creosolis compositus.....................	983.0	E862	E950.4	E980.4
Lithium...	985.9	E869	E950.9	E980.9
Liver (extract) (injection).........................	964.1	E852.9	E950.3	E980.3
Lobelia...	988.2	E868	E950.9	E980.9
Lobeline..	971	E856.8	E950.3	E980.3
Lolium temulentum..................................	988.2	E868	E950.9	E980.9
Lomotil...	974.0	E858.0	E950.3	E980.3
Lophophora williamsii..............................	970.9	E855.2	E950.2	E980.2
Lotions..	977.0	E859.7	E950.3	E980.3
Lotusate...	967.0	E854.0	E950.0	E980.0
LSD (25)...	970.9	E855.2	E950.2	E980.2
Lubricating oil NEC.................................	981.9	E864	E950.9	E980.9
Lucanthone...	961.9	E850.9	E950.3	E980.3
Luminal...	967.0	E854.0	E950.0	E980.0
Lung irritant (gas) NEC............................	987.9	E876	E952.9	E982

Substance	Nature of Injury	External Cause (E-Code)		
		Accident	Suicide (attempt)	Undeter- mined
Lututrin	962.9	E851.9	E950.3	E980.3
Lye (concentrated)	983.2	E867	E950.6	E980.6
Lymecycline	960.5	E850.3	E950.3	E980.3
Lynestrenol	962.6	E851.6	E950.3	E980.3
Lypressin	962.5	E851.5	E950.3	E980.3
Lysergic acid (amide) (diethylamide)	970.9	E855.2	E950.2	E980.2
Lysine vasopressin	962.5	E851.5	E950.3	E980.3
Lysol	983.0	E862	E950.4	E980.4
Lytta (vitatta)	977.0	E859.7	E950.3	E980.3
Magnamycin	960.9	E850.4	E950.3	E980.3
Magnesium NEC	985.9	E869	E950.9	E980.9
antacid	974.0	E858.0	E950.3	E980.3
cathartic	974.3	E858.3	E950.3	E980.3
citrate	974.3	E858.3	E950.3	E980.3
fumes	987.9	E876	E952.9	E982
sulfate	974.3	E858.3	E950.3	E980.3
trisilicate	974.0	E858.0	E950.3	E980.3
Maize silk extract	975.9	E859.3	E950.3	E980.3
Malathion (insecticide)	989.3	E865	E950.9	E980.9
Male fern	961.9	E850.9	E950.3	E980.3
Mandelic acid	961.9	E850.9	E950.3	E980.3
Manganese (dioxide)	985.2	E866	E950.9	E980.9
Mannitol (medicinal) (diuretic) NEC	975.9	E859.3	E950.3	E980.3
hexanitrate	973.4	E857.4	E950.3	E980.3
mustard	963.1	E852.1	E950.3	E980.3
Mannomustine	963.1	E852.1	E950.3	E980.3
Mapharsen	961.1	E850.6	E950.3	E980.3
Marezine	963.0	E852.0	E950.3	E980.3
Marihuana	967.9	E854.9	E950.3	E980.3
Marplan	970.0	E855.0	E950.2	E980.2
Marsalid	970.0	E855.0	E950.2	E980.2
Marsh gas	987.1	E876	E952.9	E982
Marsilid	970.0	E855.0	E950.2	E980.2
Meadow saffron	988.2	E868	E950.9	E980.9
Mebanazine	970.0	E855.0	E950.2	E980.2
Mebaral	967.0	E854.0	E950.0	E980.0
Mebeverine	976.1	E859.4	E950.3	E980.3
Mebhydrolin	963.0	E852.0	E950.3	E980.3
Mebrophenhydramine	963.0	E852.0	E950.3	E980.3
Mebutamate	970.1	E855.1	E950.2	E980.2
Mecamylamine (chloride)	973.3	E857.3	E950.3	E980.3
Mechlorethamine	963.1	E852.1	E950.3	E980.3
Meclizene (hydrochloride)	963.0	E852.0	E950.3	E980.3
Meclofenoxate	971	E856.8	E950.3	E980.3

Substance	Nature of Injury	External Cause (E-Code)		
		Accident	Suicide (attempt)	Undeter- mined
Meclozine (hydrochloride)	963.0	E852.0	E950.3	E980.3
Medication NEC	977.9	E859.9	E950.3	E980.3
Medinal	967.0	E854.0	E950.0	E980.0
Medomin	967.0	E854.0	E950.0	E980.0
Medroxyprogesterone	962.6	E851.6	E950.3	E980.3
Mefenamic acid	965.9	E853.9	E950.3	E980.3
Megestrol	962.6	E851.6	E950.3	E980.3
MEK	982.9	E864	E950.9	E980.9
Meladinin	977.0	E859.7	E950.3	E980.3
Melarsoprol	961.1	E850.6	E950.3	E980.3
Melia azadirachta	988.2	E868	E950.9	E980.9
Mellaril, melleril	970.1	E855.1	E950.2	E980.2
Melphalan	963.1	E852.1	E950.3	E980.3
Menadiol sodium diphosphate	964.3	E852.7	E950.3	E980.3
Menadione (sodium bisulfite)	964.3	E852.7	E950.3	E980.3
Menthol NEC	969	E859.0	E950.3	E980.3
Mepacrine	961.3	E850.8	E950.3	E980.3
Mepazine	970.1	E855.1	E950.2	E980.2
Mepenzolate	972.1	E855.4	E950.3	E980.3
Meperidine	965.0	E853.0	E950.3	E980.3
Mephenamine	972.1	E855.4	E950.3	E980.3
Mephenesin	968.0	E856.1	E950.3	E980.3
Mephenoxalone	970.1	E855.1	E950.2	E980.2
Mephentermine	972.2	E855.5	E950.3	E980.3
Mephenytoin	966.1	E856.0	E950.3	E980.3
Mephobarbital	967.0	E854.0	E950.0	E980.0
Mepiperphenidol	972.1	E855.4	E950.3	E980.3
Mepivacaine	969	E859.0	E950.3	E980.3
Meprobamate	970.1	E855.1	E950.2	E980.2
Mepyramine (maleate)	963.0	E852.0	E950.3	E980.3
Meralluride	975.0	E859.1	E950.3	E980.3
Merbaphen	975.0	E859.1	E950.3	E980.3
Merbromin	985.0	E859.7	E950.3	E980.3
Mercaptomerin	975.0	E859.1	E950.3	E980.3
Mercaptopurine	963.1	E852.1	E950.3	E980.3
Mercumatilin	975.0	E859.1	E950.3	E980.3
Mercuramide	975.0	E859.1	E950.3	E980.3
Mercurochrome	985.0	E859.7	E950.3	E980.3
Mercurophylline	975.0	E859.1	E950.3	E980.3
Mercurosalyl	975.0	E859.1	E950.3	E980.3
Mercury, mercurial, mercuric, mercurous (compounds) (cyanide) (fumes) (nonmedicinal) (vapor) NEC	985.0	E866	E950.9	E980.9
antiseptic (external)	985.0	E859.7	E950.3	E980.3

Substance	Nature of Injury	External Cause (E-Code)		
		Accident	Suicide (attempt)	Undetermined
Mercury, mercurial, mercuric—*continued*				
chloride (antiseptic) NEC	985.0	E859.7	E950.3	E980.3
diuretic compounds	975.0	E859.1	E950.3	E980.3
insecticide (vapor)	989.3	E865	E950.9	E980.9
Merethoxylline	975.0	E859.1	E950.3	E980.3
Mersalyl	975.0	E859.1	E950.3	E980.3
Mescal buttons	970.9	E855.2	E950.2	E980.2
Mescaline (salts)	970.9	E855.2	E950.2	E980.2
Mestanolone	962.1	E851.1	E950.3	E980.3
Mestranol	962.2	E651.2	E950.3	E980.3
Metacresylacetate	961.9	E850.9	E950.3	E980.3
Metaldehyde (snail killer) NEC	989.3	E865	E950.9	E980.9
Metals (heavy) (nonmedicinal) NEC	985.9	E866	E950.9	E980.9
dust, fumes, or vapor NEC	985.9	E866	E950.9	E980.9
light NEC	985.9	E869	E950.9	E980.9
dust, fumes or vapor NEC	987.9	E876	E952.9	E982
pesticides (dust) (vapor)	989.3	E865	E950.9	E980.9
Metaphen	985.0	E859.7	E950.3	E980.3
Metaraminol	972.2	E855.5	E950.3	E980.3
Metaxalone, metaxolone	968.0	E856.1	E950.3	E980.3
Metformin	962.3	E851.3	E950.3	E980.3
Methacycline	960.5	E850.3	E950.3	E980.3
Methadone	965.0	E853.0	E950.3	E980.3
Methallenestril	962.2	E851.2	E950.3	E980.3
Methamphetamine	971	E856.4	E950.3	E980.3
Methandienone	962.1	E851.1	E950.3	E980.3
Methandriol	962.1	E851.1	E950.3	E980.3
Methandrostenolone	962.1	E851.1	E950.3	E980.3
Methane	987.1	E876	E952.9	E982
Methanol	980.1	E860	E950.9	E980.9
vapor	987.9	E876	E952.9	E982
Methantheline	972.1	E855.4	E950.3	E980.3
Methaphenilene	963.0	E852.0	E950.3	E980.3
Methapyrilene	963.0	E852.0	E950.3	E980.3
Methaqualone	967.9	E854.9	E950.3	E980.3
Metharbital, metharbitone	967.0	E854.0	E950.0	E980.0
Methdilazine	963.0	E852.0	E950.3	E980.3
Methedrine	971	E856.4	E950.3	E980.3
Methenolone	962.1	E851.1	E950.3	E980.3
Methicillin (sodium)	960.0	E850.0	E950.3	E980.3
Methimazole	962.8	E851.8	E950.3	E980.3
Methionine	974.9	E858.9	E950.3	E980.3
Methisazone	961.9	E850.9	E950.3	E980.3
Methitural	968.9	E856.3	E950.3	E980.3

Substance	Nature of Injury	External Cause (E-Code)		
		Accident	Suicide (attempt)	Undeter- mined
Methixene	972.1	E855.4	E950.3	E980.3
Methobarbital, methobarbitone	967.0	E854.0	E950.0	E980.0
Methocarbamol	968.0	E856.1	E950.3	E980.3
Methohexital, methohexitone (sodium)	968.9	E856.3	E950.3	E980.3
Methoin	966.1	E856.0	E950.3	E980.3
Methopholine	965.9	E853.9	E950.3	E980.3
Methoserpidine	970.1	E855.1	E950.2	E980.2
Methotrexate	963.1	E852.1	E950.3	E980.3
Methotrimeprazine	967.9	E854.9	E950.3	E980.3
Methoxamine	972.2	E855.5	E950.3	E980.3
Methoxsalen	977.0	E859.7	E950.3	E980.3
Methoxybenzyl penicillin	960.0	E850.0	E950.3	E980.3
Methoxychlor	989.2	E865	E950.9	E980.9
Methoxyflurane	968.1	E856.2	E952.9	E982
Methoxyphenamine	972.2	E855.5	E950.3	E980.3
Methoxypromazine	970.1	E855.1	E950.2	E980.2
Methscopolamine (bromide)	972.1	E855.4	E950.3	E980.3
Methsuximide	966.9	E856.0	E950.3	E980.3
Methyclothiazide	975.3	E859.3	E950.3	E980.3
Methyl				
acetate	982.9	E864	E950.9	E980.9
acetone	982.9	E864	E950.9	E980.9
alcohol	980.1	E860	E950.9	E980.9
amphetamine	971	E856.4	E950.3	E980.3
androstanolone	962.1	E851.1	E950.3	E980.3
atropine	972.1	E855.4	E950.3	E980.3
benzene	982.0	E864	E950.9	E980.9
benzoate	982.9	E864	E950.9	E980.9
benzol	982.0	E864	E950.9	E980.9
bromide (gas)	987.9	E876	E952.9	E982
butanol	980.9	E860	E950.9	E980.9
carbinol	980.0	E860	E950.9	E980.9
cellosolve	982.9	E864	E950.9	E980.9
cellulose	974.5	E858.5	E950.3	E980.3
chloride (gas)	987.9	E876	E952.9	E982
choline	972.0	E855.3	E950.3	E980.3
cyclohexane	982.9	E864	E950.9	E980.9
cyclohexanol	980.9	E860	E950.9	E980.9
cyclohexanone	982.9	E864	E950.9	E980.9
cyclohexyl acetate	982.9	E864	E950.9	E980.9
dihydromorphinone	965.0	E853.0	E950.3	E980.3
ergometrine	976.0	E859.4	E950.3	E980.3
ergonovine	976.0	E859.4	E950.3	E980.3
ethyl ketone	982.9	E864	E950.9	E980.9

Substance	Nature of Injury	External Cause (E-Code)		
		Accident	Suicide (attempt)	Undeter-mined
Methyl—*continued*				
glyoxal	963.1	E852.1	E950.3	E980.3
hydrazine	983.9	E867	E950.9	E980.9
isobutyl ketone	982.9	E864	E950.9	E980.9
meprobamate	970.1	E855.1	E950.2	E980.2
morphine NEC	965.0	E853.0	E950.3	E980.3
parafynol	967.9	E854.9	E950.3	E980.3
pentynol NEC	967.9	E854.9	E950.3	E980.3
peridol	970.1	E855.1	E950.2	E980.2
phenidate	971	E856.8	E950.3	E980.3
prednisolone	962.0	E851.0	E950.3	E980.3
propylcarbinol	980.9	E860	E950.9	E980.9
rosaniline NEC	961.9	E850.9	E950.3	E980.3
salicylate NEC	977.0	E859.7	E950.3	E980.3
sulfate (fumes)	987.9	E876	E952.9	E982
liquid	983.9	E867	E950.9	E980.9
sulfonal	967.9	E854.9	E950.3	E980.3
testosterone	962.1	E851.1	E950.3	E980.3
thiouracil	962.8	E851.8	E950.3	E980.3
Methylated spirit	980.1	E860	E950.9	E980.9
Methyldopa	973.5	E857.5	E950.3	E980.3
Methylene				
blue	961.9	E850.9	E950.3	E980.3
chloride or dichloride (solvent) NEC	982.9	E864	E950.9	E980.9
vapor NEC	987.9	E876	E952.9	E982
Methyprylone	967.9	E854.9	E950.3	E980.3
Methysergide	973.5	E857.5	E950.3	E980.3
Metoclopramide	963.0	E852.0	E950.3	E980.3
Metofurone	961.9	E850.9	E950.3	E980.3
Metopon	965.0	E853.0	E950.3	E980.3
Metronidazole	961.9	E850.9	E950.3	E980.3
Metyrapone	977.2	E859.8	E950.3	E980.3
Mezereon (berries)	988.2	E868	E950.9	E980.9
Migril	973.5	E857.5	E950.3	E980.3
Milk of magnesia	974.0	E858.0	E950.3	E980.3
Miltown	970.1	E855.1	E950.2	E980.2
Mineral				
oil (medicinal)	974.2	E858.2	E950.3	E980.3
nonmedicinal	981.9	E864	E950.9	E980.9
spirits	981.2	E864	E950.9	E980.9
Mithramycin (antineoplastic)	963.1	E852.1	E950.3	E980.3
Mitomycin (antineoplastic)	963.1	E852.1	E950.3	E980.3
Monkshood	988.2	E868	E950.9	E980.9
Monoamine oxidase inhibitors	970.0	E855.0	E950.2	E980.2

Substance	Nature of Injury	External Cause (E-Code)		
		Accident	Suicide (attempt)	Undetermined
Monochlorobenzene	982.0	E864	E950.9	E980.9
Monoxide, carbon—*see* Carbon monoxide				
Moroxydine (hydrochloride)	961.9	E850.9	E950.3	E980.3
Morphazinamide	961.9	E850.9	E950.3	E980.3
Morphinans	965.0	E853.0	E950.3	E980.3
Morphine NEC	965.0	E853.0	E950.3	E980.3
antagonists	971	E856.8	E950.3	E980.3
Morphinols	965.0	E853.0	E950.3	E980.3
Morphinon	965.0	E853.0	E950.3	E980.3
Morpholinylethylmorphine	965.0	E853.0	E950.3	E980.3
Moth balls (*see also* Pesticides)	989.3	E863	E950.9	E980.9
naphthalene	983.0	E865	E950.4	E980.4
Motor exhaust gas—*see* Carbon monoxide, exhaust gas				
Mucomyst	977.8	E859.8	E950.3	E980.3
Muriatic acid—*see* Hydrochloric acid				
Muscarine	972.0	E855.3	E950.3	E980.3
Mushroom, noxious	988.1	E868	E950.9	E980.9
Mussel, noxious	988.0	E868	E950.9	E980.9
Mustard (emetic)	974.6	E858.6	E950.3	E980.3
gas (war)	987.9	....	....	....
not in war	987.9	E876	E952.9	E982
nitrogen	963.1	E852.1	E950.3	E980.3
Mustine	963.1	E852.1	E950.3	E980.3
Myelobromal	963.1	E852.1	E950.3	E980.3
Myleran	963.1	E852.1	E950.3	E980.3
Mylomide	967.0	E854.0	E950.0	E980.0
Myochrysine, myocrisin	976.2	E859.4	E950.3	E980.3
Myristica fragrans	988.2	E868	E950.9	E980.9
Mysoline	966.0	E856.0	E950.3	E980.3
Nafcillin (sodium)	960.0	E850.0	E950.3	E980.3
Nalidixic acid	961.9	E850.9	E950.3	E980.3
Nalorphine	971	E856.8	E950.3	E980.3
Nandrolone (phenproprioate) (decanoate)	962.1	E851.1	E950.3	E980.3
Naphazoline	972.2	E855.5	E950.3	E980.3
Naphtha (painters') (petroleum)	981.2	E864	E950.9	E980.9
solvent	982.0	E864	E950.9	E980.9
vapor	987.1	E876	E952.9	E982
Naphthalene (chlorinated)	983.0	E867	E950.4	E980.4
insecticide or moth repellant	983.0	E865	E950.4	E980.4
vapor	987.9	E876	E952.9	E982
Naphthol	983.0	E867	E950.4	E980.4
Naphthoquinone NEC	964.3	E852.7	E950.3	E980.3
Naphthylamine	983.0	E867	E950.4	E980.4

Substance	Nature of Injury	External Cause (E-Code)		
		Accident	Suicide (attempt)	Undetermined
Narcotic (drug) NEC...............................	967.9	E854.9	E950.3	E980.3
Nardil.......................................	970.0	E855.0	E950.2	E980.2
Natrium cyanide—*see* Cyanide(s)				
Natural gas....................................	987.1	E870	E951	E981
incomplete combustion..........................	986	E870	E951	E981
Nealbarbital, nealbarbitone........................	967.0	E854.0	E950.0	E980.0
Nembutal.....................................	967.0	E854.0	E950.0	E980.0
Neoarsphenamine................................	961.1	E850.6	E950.3	E980.3
Neocinchophen.................................	965.2	E853.2	E950.3	E980.3
Neomycin.....................................	960.9	E850.4	E950.3	E980.3
Neonal.......................................	967.0	E854.0	E950.0	E980.0
Neoprontosil..................................	961.0	E850.5	E950.3	E980.3
Neosalvarsan..................................	961.1	E850.6	E950.3	E980.3
Neosilver salvarsan.............................	961.1	E850.6	E950.3	E980.3
Neostigmine...................................	972.0	E855.3	E950.3	E980.3
Neraval......................................	968.9	E856.3	E950.3	E980.3
Neravan......................................	967.0	E854.0	E950.0	E980.0
Nerium oleander................................	988.2	E868	E950.9	E980.9
Nerve gases (war)...............................	987.9	....	....	....
Neurobarb....................................	967.0	E854.0	E950.0	E980.0
Neutral spirits.................................	980.0	E860	E950.9	E980.9
Nialamide....................................	970.0	E855.0	E950.2	E980.2
Nickel (carbonyl) (tetracarbonyl) (fumes)				
(vapor)....................................	985.9	E866	E950.9	E980.9
Niclosamide...................................	961.9	E850.9	E950.3	E980.3
Nicodicodine..................................	965.0	E853.0	E950.3	E980.3
Nicotinamide..................................	963.6	E852.3	E950.3	E980.3
Nicotine (insecticide) (spray) (sulfate) NEC...	989.3	E865	E950.9	E980.9
not insecticide..............................	989.9	E869	E950.9	E980.9
Nicotinic acid.................................	963.6	E852.3	E950.3	E980.3
Nicotinyl alcohol...............................	973.4	E857.4	E950.3	E980.3
Nicoumalone..................................	964.2	E852.6	E950.3	E980.3
Nifenazone...................................	965.5	E853.5	E950.3	E980.3
Nifuraldezone.................................	961.9	E850.9	E950.3	E980.3
Nightshade, deadly..............................	988.2	E868	E950.9	E980.9
Nikethamide..................................	971	E856.8	E950.3	E980.3
Niridazole....................................	961.9	E850.9	E950.3	E980.3
Nisentil.....................................	965.0	E853.0	E950.3	E980.3
Nitrazepam...................................	970.1	E855.1	E950.2	E980.2
Nitric				
acid (liquid)	983.1	E867	E950.9	E980.9
vapor................................	987.9	E876	E952.9	E982
oxide (gas).................................	987.9	E876	E952.9	E982
Nitrite, amyl (medicinal) (vapor)	973.4	E857.4	E950.3	E980.3

Substance	Nature of Injury	External Cause (E-Code)		
		Accident	Suicide (attempt)	Undetermined
Nitroaniline	983.0	E867	E950.4	E980.4
vapor	987.9	E876	E952.9	E982
Nitrobenzene, nitrobenzol	983.0	E867	E950.4	E980.4
vapor	987.9	E876	E952.9	E982
Nitrocellulose	989.9	E869	E950.9	E980.9
Nitrofurantoin	961.9	E850.9	E950.3	E980.3
Nitrofurazone	961.9	E850.9	E950.3	E980.3
Nitrogen (dioxide) (oxide) (gas)	987.2	E876	E952.9	E982
mustard (antineoplastic)	963.1	E852.1	E950.3	E980.3
Nitroglycerin, nitroglycerol (medicinal)	973.4	E857.4	E950.3	E980.3
nonmedicinal	989.9	E869	E950.9	E980.9
fumes	987.9	E876	E952.9	E982
Nitrohydrochloric acid	983.1	E867	E950.9	E980.9
Nitromersol	985.0	E859.7	E950.3	E980.3
Nitronaphthalene	983.0	E867	E950.4	E980.4
Nitrophenol	983.0	E867	E950.4	E980.4
Nitrothiazol	961.9	E850.9	E950.3	E980.3
Nitrotoluene, nitrotoluol	983.0	E867	E950.4	E980.4
vapor	987.9	E876	E952.9	E982
Nitrous				
acid (liquid)	983.1	E867	E950.9	E980.9
fumes	987.9	E876	E952.9	E982
oxide (anesthetic) NEC	968.1	E856.2	E952.9	E982
Noctec	967.1	E854.1	E950.3	E980.3
Noludar	967.9	E854.9	E950.3	E980.3
Noptil	967.0	E854.0	E950.0	E980.0
Noradrenalin(e)	972.2	E855.5	E950.3	E980.3
Noramidopyrine	965.5	E853.5	E950.3	E980.3
Norepinephrine	972.2	E855.5	E950.3	E980.3
Norethandrolone	962.1	E851.1	E950.3	E980.3
Norethindrone	962.6	E851.6	E950.3	E980.3
Norethisterone	962.6	E851.6	E950.3	E980.3
Norethynodrel	962.6	E851.6	E950.3	E980.3
Normorphine	965.0	E853.0	E950.3	E980.3
Nortriptyline	970.0	E855.0	E950.2	E980.2
Noscapine	965.0	E853.0	E950.3	E980.3
Novobiocin	960.9	E850.4	E950.3	E980.3
Novocaine	969	E859.0	E950.3	E980.3
Noxythiolin	961.9	E850.9	E950.3	E980.3
Numorphan	965.0	E853.0	E950.3	E980.3
Nunol	967.0	E854.0	E950.0	E980.0
Nupercaine	969	E859.0	E950.3	E980.3
Nutmeg oil (liniment)	977.0	E859.5	E950.3	E980.3
Nux vomica	989.1	E859.8	E950.5	E980.5

Substance	Nature of Injury	External Cause (E-Code)		
		Accident	Suicide (attempt)	Undetermined
Nydrazid	961.9	E850.9	E950.3	E980.3
Nylidrin	972.2	E855.5	E950.3	E980.3
Nystatin	960.1	E850.1	E950.3	E980.3
Oblivon	967.9	E854.9	E950.3	E980.3
Octafonium	961.9	E850.9	E950.3	E980.3
Octaphonium	961.9	E850.9	E950.3	E980.3
Octyl nitrite	973.4	E857.4	E950.3	E980.3
Oestradiol (cypionate) (dipropionate) (valerate)	962.2	E851.2	E950.3	E980.3
Oestriol	962.2	E851.2	E950.3	E980.3
Oestrogens	962.2	E851.2	E950.3	E980.3
Oestrone	962.2	E851.2	E950.3	E980.3
Oil (of) NEC	989.9	E869	E950.9	E980.9
bitter almond	989.0	E869	E950.9	E980.9
colors	989.9	E863	E950.9	E980.9
fumes	987.9	E876	E952.9	E982
lubricating	981.9	E864	E950.9	E980.9
niobe	982.9	E864	E950.9	E980.9
specified source, other—see substance specified				
vitriol (liquid)	983.1	E867	E950.9	E980.9
fumes	987.9	E876	E952.9	E982
wintergreen (bitter) NEC	977.0	E859.7	E950.3	E980.3
Ointments NEC	977.0	E859.6	E950.3	E980.3
Oleander	988.2	E868	E950.9	E980.9
Oleandomycin	960.9	E850.4	E950.3	E980.3
Oleovitamin A	963.6	E852.3	E950.3	E980.3
Oleum ricini	974.1	E858.1	E950.3	E980.3
Olive oil (medicinal) NEC	974.2	E858.2	E950.3	E980.3
OMPA	989.3	E865	E950.9	E980.9
Opiates, opioids, opium NEC	965.0	E853.0	E950.3	E980.3
Optochin	961.9	E850.9	E950.3	E980.3
Orciprenaline	972.2	E855.5	E950.3	E980.3
Organophosphates	989.3	E865	E950.9	E980.9
Orinase	962.3	E851.3	E950.3	E980.3
Orphenadrine	972.1	E855.4	E950.3	E980.3
Ortal	967.0	E854.0	E950.0	E980.0
Orthocaine	969	E859.0	E950.3	E980.3
Orthodichloro-ethane	982.9	E864	E950.9	E980.9
Osmic acid (liquid)	983.1	E867	E950.9	E980.9
fumes	987.9	E876	E952.9	E982
Oxacillin	960.0	E850.0	E950.3	E980.3
Oxalic acid	983.1	E867	E950.9	E980.9
Oxanamide	970.1	E855.1	E950.2	E980.2

Substance	Nature of Injury	External Cause (E-Code)		
		Accident	Suicide (attempt)	Undetermined
Oxandrolone	962.1	E851.1	E950.3	E980.3
Oxazepam	970.1	E855.1	E950.2	E980.2
Oxedrine	972.2	E855.5	E950.3	E980.3
Oxeladin	977.8	E859.8	E950.3	E980.3
Oxethazaine NEC	969	E859.0	E950.3	E980.3
Oxidizing agents NEC	983.9	E867	E950.9	E980.9
Oxophenarsine	961.1	E850.6	E950.3	E980.3
Oxtriphylline	975.1	E859.2	E950.3	E980.3
Oxybuprocaine	969	E859.0	E950.3	E980.3
Oxycodone	965.0	E853.0	E950.3	E980.3
Oxygen	987.9	E876	E952.9	E982
Oxymesterone	962.1	E851.1	E950.3	E980.3
Oxymetazoline	972.2	E855.5	E950.3	E980.3
Oxymethalone	962.1	E851.1	E950.3	E980.3
Oxymorphone	965.0	E853.0	E950.3	E980.3
Oxypertine	970.1	E855.1	E950.2	E980.2
Oxyphenbutazone	965.5	E853.5	E950.3	E980.3
Oxyphencyclimine	972.1	E855.4	E950.3	E980.3
Oxyphenisatin	974.1	E858.1	E950.3	E980.3
Oxyphenonium	972.1	E855.4	E950.3	E980.3
Oxyquinoline	961.3	E850.8	E950.3	E980.3
Oxytetracycline	960.5	E850.3	E950.3	E980.3
Oxytocics NEC	976.0	E859.4	E950.3	E980.3
Oxytocin	962.5	E851.5	E950.3	E980.3
Ozone	987.9	E876	E952.9	E982
Paint NEC	989.9	E863	E950.9	E980.9
cleaner	982.9	E864	E950.9	E980.9
fumes NEC	987.9	E876	E952.9	E982
lead (fumes)	984	E866	E950.9	E980.9
solvent NEC	982.9	E864	E950.9	E980.9
stripper	982.9	E864	E950.9	E980.9
Palfium	965.0	E853.0	E950.3	E980.3
Paludrine	961.9	E850.9	E950.3	E980.3
PAM	977.8	E859.8	E950.3	E980.3
Pamaquin(e)	961.3	E850.8	E950.3	E980.3
Panadol	965.4	E853.4	E950.3	E980.3
Pancreatic dornase	963.5	E852.4	E950.3	E980.3
Pancreatin	974.9	E858.9	E950.3	E980.3
Pangamic acid	963.6	E852.3	E950.3	E980.3
Pantopium	965.0	E853.0	E950.3	E980.3
Pantopon	965.0	E853.0	E950.3	E980.3
Pantothenol	963.6	E852.3	E950.3	E980.3
Papain	963.5	E852.4	E950.3	E980.3
Papaverine	976.1	E859.4	E950.3	E980.3

Substance	Nature of Injury	External Cause (E-Code)		
		Accident	Suicide (attempt)	Undeter- mined
Para-aminosalicylic acid	961.9	E850.9	E950.3	E980.3
Paracetaldehyde (medicinal)	967.2	E854.2	E950.3	E980.3
Paracetamol	965.4	E853.4	E950.3	E980.3
Paracodin	965.0	E853.0	E950.3	E980.3
Paraffin(s) (wax)	981.9	E864	E950.9	E980.9
liquid (medicinal)	974.2	E858.2	E950.3	E980.3
nonmedicinal	981.9	E864	E950.9	E980.9
Paraldehyde (medicinal)	967.2	E854.2	E950.3	E980.3
Paramethadione	966.0	E856.0	E950.3	E980.3
Paramethasone	962.0	E851.0	E950.3	E980.3
Paraquat	989.3	E865	E950.9	E980.9
Parasympatholytics	972.1	E855.4	E950.3	E980.3
Parasympathomimetics	972.0	E855.3	E950.3	E980.3
Parathion	989.3	E865	E950.9	E980.9
Parathyroid extract	962.9	E851.9	E950.3	E980.3
Paregoric	965.0	E853.0	E950.3	E980.3
Pargyline	973.3	E857.3	E950.3	E980.3
Paris green	985.1	E866	E950.7	E980.7
insecticide	985.1	E865	E950.7	E980.7
Parnate	970.0	E855.0	E950.2	E980.2
Paromomycin	960.9	E850.4	E950.3	E980.3
Paroxypropione	963.1	E852.1	E950.3	E980.3
Parstelin	970.9	E855.2	E950.2	E980.2
Parzone	965.0	E853.0	E950.3	E980.3
PAS	961.9	E850.9	E950.3	E980.3
PCP	989.3	E865	E950.9	E980.9
Peach kernel oil (emulsion)	974.2	E858.2	E950.3	E980.3
Peanut oil (emulsion) NEC	974.2	E858.2	E950.3	E980.3
Pecazine	970.1	E855.1	E950.2	E980.2
Pecilocin	961.9	E850.9	E950.3	E980.3
Pectin (with kaolin) NEC	974.0	E858.0	E950.3	E980.3
Pelletierine tannate	961.9	E850.9	E950.3	E980.3
Pemoline	971	E856.8	E950.3	E980.3
Pempidine	973.3	E857.3	E950.3	E980.3
Penamecillin	960.0	E850.0	E950.3	E980.3
Penethamate hydriodide	960.0	E850.0	E950.3	E980.3
Penicillamine	963.9	E852.4	E950.3	E980.3
Penicillinase	963.5	E852.4	E950.3	E980.3
Penicillins	960.0	E850.0	E950.3	E980.3
Pentachlorophenol (pesticide)	989.3	E865	E950.9	E980.9
Pentaerythritol				
chloral	967.1	E854.1	E950.3	E980.3
tetranitrate NEC	973.4	E857.4	E950.3	E980.3
Pentalin	982.9	E864	E950.9	E980.9

Substance	Nature of Injury	External Cause (E-Code)		
		Accident	Suicide (attempt)	Undetermined
Pentamethonium	973.3	E857.3	E950.3	E980.3
Pentamidine	961.9	E850.9	E950.3	E980.3
Pentanol	980.9	E860	E950.9	E980.9
Pentaquin(e)	961.3	E850.8	E950.3	E980.3
Pentazocine	965.0	E853.0	E950.3	E980.3
Penthienate	972.1	E855.4	E950.3	E980.3
Pentobarbital, pentobarbitone (sodium)	967.0	E854.0	E950.0	E980.0
Pentolinium (tartrate)	973.3	E857.3	E950.3	E980.3
Pentothal	968.9	E856.3	E950.3	E980.3
Pentylenetetrazol	971	E856.8	E950.3	E980.3
Pentylsalicylamide	961.9	E850.9	E950.3	E980.3
Pepsin	963.5	E852.4	E950.3	E980.3
Percaine	969	E859.0	E950.3	E980.3
Perchloroethylene	982.9	E864	E950.9	E980.9
medicinal	961.9	E850.9	E950.3	E980.3
vapor	987.9	E876	E952.9	E982
Percodan	965.0	E853.0	E950.3	E980.3
Perhexiline	973.4	E857.4	E950.3	E980.3
Perichlor	967.1	E854.1	E950.3	E980.3
Pericyazine	970.1	E855.1	E950.2	E980.2
Peritrate	973.4	E857.4	E950.3	E980.3
Permanganates	983.9	E867	E950.9	E980.9
Pernocton	967.0	E854.0	E950.0	E980.0
Pernoston	967.0	E854.0	E950.0	E980.0
Peronin	965.0	E853.0	E950.3	E980.3
Perphenazine	970.1	E855.1	E950.2	E980.2
Pertofran(e)	970.0	E855.0	E950.2	E980.2
Pesticides (dust) (fumes) (vapor)	989.3	E865	E950.9	E980.9
arsenic	985.1	E865	E950.7	E980.7
chlorinated	989.2	E865	E950.9	E980.9
cyanide	989.0	E865	E950.9	E980.9
kerosene	981.0	E865	E950.9	E980.9
naphthalene	983.0	E865	E950.4	E980.4
petroleum (distillate) (products) NEC	981.9	E865	E950.9	E980.9
specified ingredient NEC	989.3	E865	E950.9	E980.9
strychnine	989.1	E865	E950.5	E980.5
thallium	985.9	E865	E950.9	E980.9
Pethidine (hydrochloride)	965.0	E853.0	E950.3	E980.3
Petrichloral	967.1	E854.1	E950.3	E980.3
Petrol	981.1	E864	E950.9	E980.9
vapor	987.1	E876	E952.9	E982
Petrolatum (jelly) (ointment)	977.0	E859.6	E950.3	E980.3
liquid	974.2	E858.2	E950.3	E980.3
nonmedicinal	981.9	E864	E950.9	E980.9

Substance	Nature of Injury	External Cause (E-Code)		
		Accident	Suicide (attempt)	Undetermined
Petroleum (products) NEC.........................	981.9	E864	E950.9	E980.9
benzin(e) — *see* Ligroin				
ether — *see* Ligroin				
jelly — *see* Petrolatum				
naphtha — *see* Ligroin				
pesticide — *see* Pesticides				
vapor...	987.1	E876	E952.9	E982
Peyote..	970.9	E855.2	E950.2	E980.2
Phanodorm, phanodorn............................	967.0	E854.0	E950.0	E980.0
Phanquinone, phanquone..........................	961.9	E850.9	E950.3	E980.3
Phenacemide...	966.9	E856.0	E950.3	E980.3
Phenacetin...	965.4	E853.4	E950.3	E980.3
Phenadoxone..	965.0	E853.0	E950.3	E980.3
Phenaglycodol.......................................	970.1	E855.1	E950.2	E980.2
Phenanthroline......................................	961.9	E850.9	E950.3	E980.3
Phenantoin...	966.1	E856.0	E950.3	E980.3
Phenazocine...	965.0	E853.0	E950.3	E980.3
Phenazone...	965.5	E853.5	E950.3	E980.3
Phenazopyridine.....................................	961.9	E850.9	E950.3	E980.3
Phenbenicillin..	960.0	E850.0	E950.3	E980.3
Phenbutrazate.......................................	971	E856.4	E950.3	E980.3
Phencyclidine..	970.1	E855.1	E950.2	E980.2
Phendimetrazine.....................................	971	E856.4	E950.3	E980.3
Phenelzine...	970.0	E855.0	E950.2	E980.2
Phenergan..	967.9	E854.9	E950.3	E980.3
Phenethicillin (potassium).........................	960.0	E850.0	E950.3	E980.3
Pheneturide..	966.9	E856.0	E950.3	E980.3
Phenformin...	962.3	E851.3	E950.3	E980.3
Phenglutarimide.....................................	972.1	E855.4	E950.3	E980.3
Phenindamine..	963.0	E852.0	E950.3	E980.3
Phenindione...	964.2	E852.6	E950.3	E980.3
Pheniprazine...	970.0	E855.0	E950.2	E980.2
Pheniramine..	963.0	E852.0	E950.3	E980.3
Phenmetrazine.......................................	971	E856.4	E950.3	E980.3
Phenobal...	967.0	E854.0	E950.0	E980.0
Phenobarbital, phenobarbitone...................	967.0	E854.0	E950.0	E980.0
Phenoctide...	961.9	E850.9	E950.3	E980.3
Phenol NEC..	983.0	E867	E950.4	E980.4
disinfectant.......................................	983.0	E862	E950.4	E980.4
pesticide..	989.3	E865	E950.4	E980.4
Phenolphthalein (laxative)........................	974.1	E858.1	E950.3	E980.3
Phenomorphan......................................	965.0	E853.0	E950.3	E980.3
Phenonyl...	967.0	E854.0	E950.0	E980.0
Phenoperidine.......................................	965.0	E853.0	E950.3	E980.3

Substance	Nature of Injury	External Cause (E-Code)		
		Accident	Suicide (attempt)	Undeter-mined
Phenoquin	965.2	E853.2	E950.3	E980.3
Phenothiazines (tranquilizers) NEC	970.1	E855.1	E950.2	E980.2
insecticide	989.3	E865	E950.9	E980.9
Phenoxybenzamine	973.5	E857.5	E950.3	E980.3
Phenoxymethyl penicillin	960.0	E850.0	E950.3	E980.3
Phenprocoumon	964.2	E852.6	E950.3	E980.3
Phensuximide	966.9	E856.0	E950.3	E980.3
Phentermine	971	E856.4	E950.3	E980.3
Phentolamine	973.5	E857.5	E950.3	E980.3
Phenyl				
butazone	965.5	E853.5	E950.3	E980.3
enediamine	983.0	E867	E950.4	E980.4
ephrine	972.2	E855.5	E950.3	E980.3
hydrazine	983.0	E867	E950.4	E980.4
antineoplastic	963.1	E852.1	E950.3	E980.3
mercuric compounds — see Mercury				
propanolamine	972.2	E855.5	E950.3	E980.3
salicylate	977.0	E859.7	E950.3	E980.3
Phenyramidol, phenyramidon	965.9	E853.9	E950.3	E980.3
Phenytoin	966.1	E856.0	E950.3	E980.3
Pholcodine	965.0	E853.0	E950.3	E980.3
Phorate	989.3	E865	E950.9	E980.9
Phosgene (gas)	987.9	E876	E952.9	E982
Phosphate, tricresyl	982.9	E864	E950.9	E980.9
Phosphine	987.9	E876	E952.9	E982
Phosphoric acid	983.1	E867	E950.9	E980.9
Phosphorus (compounds) NEC	983.9	E867	E950.9	E980.9
pesticides	989.3	E865	E950.9	E980.9
Phthalimidoglutarimide	967.9	E854.9	E950.3	E980.3
Phthalylsulfathiazole	961.0	E850.5	E950.3	E980.3
Physeptone	965.0	E853.0	E950.3	E980.3
Physostigma venenosum	988.2	E868	E950.9	E980.9
Physostigmine	972.0	E855.3	E950.3	E980.3
Phytolacca decandra	988.2	E868	E950.9	E980.9
Phytomenadione	964.3	E852.7	E950.3	E980.3
Phytonadione	964.3	E852.7	E950.3	E980.3
Picric (acid)	983.0	E867	E950.4	E980.4
Picrotoxin	971	E856.8	E950.3	E980.3
Pilocarpine	972.0	E855.3	E950.3	E980.3
Pilocarpus (jaborandi) extract	972.0	E855.3	E950.3	E980.3
Pimaricin	960.1	E850.1	E950.3	E980.3
Piminodine	965.0	E853.0	E950.3	E980.3
Pine oil, pinesol (disinfectant)	983.9	E862	E950.9	E980.9
Pinkroot	961.9	E850.9	E950.3	E980.3

Substance	Nature of Injury	External Cause (E-Code)		
		Accident	Suicide (attempt)	Undetermined
Pipadone..............................	965.0	E853.0	E950.3	E980.3
Pipamazine...........................	963.0	E852.0	E950.3	E980.3
Pipazethate..........................	977.8	E859.8	E950.3	E980.3
Pipenzolate..........................	972.1	E855.4	E950.3	E980.3
Piper cubeba.........................	988.2	E868	E950.9	E980.9
Piperazine NEC......................	961.9	E850.9	E950.3	E980.3
estrone sulfate...................	962.2	E851.2	E950.3	E980.3
Piperidione..........................	977.8	E859.8	E950.3	E980.3
Piperidolate.........................	972.1	E855.4	E950.3	E980.3
Piperocaine..........................	969	E859.0	E950.3	E980.3
Pipradol.............................	971	E856.8	E950.3	E980.3
Piscidia (erythrina) (bark).........	965.9	E853.9	E950.3	E980.3
Pitch................................	983.0	E867	E950.4	E980.4
Pitkin's solution....................	969	E859.0	E950.3	E980.3
Pitocin..............................	962.5	E851.5	E950.3	E980.3
Pitressin (tannate)..................	962.5	E851.5	E950.3	E980.3
Pituitary extract (posterior)........	962.5	E851.5	E950.3	E980.3
anterior..........................	962.4	E851.4	E950.3	E980.3
Pituitrin............................	962.5	E851.5	E950.3	E980.3
Placental extract....................	962.9	E851.9	E950.3	E980.3
Placidyl.............................	967.9	E854.9	E950.3	E980.3
Plant foods or fertilizers NEC......	989.9	E865	E950.9	E980.9
Plants, noxious, used as food.......	988.2	E868	E950.9	E980.9
Plasma expanders...................	964.9	E852.9	E950.3	E980.3
Plegecil.............................	970.1	E855.1	E950.2	E980.2
Podophyllum (resin) (ointment) NEC........	977.0	E859.6	E950.3	E980.3
Poison NEC..........................	989.9	E869	E950.9	E980.9
Pokeweed (any part).................	988.2	E868	E950.9	E980.9
Poldine..............................	972.1	E855.4	E950.3	E980.3
Polish (car) (floor) (furniture) (metal) (porcelain) (silver)........	989.9	E861	E950.9	E980.9
Poloxalkol...........................	974.4	E858.4	E950.3	E980.3
Polyaminostyrene resins.............	963.4	E852.2	E950.3	E980.3
Polycycline..........................	960.5	E850.3	E950.3	E980.3
Polyestradiol (phosphate)...........	962.2	E851.2	E950.3	E980.3
Polyferose...........................	964.0	E852.5	E950.3	E980.3
Polygala root........................	977.8	E859.8	E950.3	E980.3
Polymethylsiloxane..................	974.9	E858.9	E950.3	E980.3
Polymyxin...........................	960.9	E850.4	E950.3	E980.3
Polynoxylin..........................	961.9	E850.9	E950.3	E980.3
Polyoxymethyleneurea...............	961.9	E850.9	E950.3	E980.3
Polytetrafluoroethylene (inhaled)...	987.9	E876	E952.9	E982
Polythiazide.........................	975.3	E859.3	E950.3	E980.3
Polyvinylpyrrolidone................	964.9	E852.9	E950.3	E980.3

Substance	Nature of Injury	External Cause (E-Code)		
		Accident	Suicide (attempt)	Undetermined
Pontocaine (hydrochloride)........................	969	E859.0	E950.3	E980.3
Potash (caustic).......................................	983.2	E867	E950.6	E980.6
Potassic saline injection (lactated)..............	963.4	E852.2	E950.3	E980.3
Potassium (salts) NEC.............................	963.4	E852.2	E950.3	E980.3
aminosalicylate....................................	961.9	E850.9	E950.3	E980.3
arsenite (solution)................................	985.1	E859.8	E950.3	E980.3
bichromate..	983.9	E867	E950.9	E980.9
bisulfate...	983.9	E867	E950.9	E980.9
bromide (medicinal) NEC......................	967.3	E854.3	E950.3	E980.3
carbonate...	983.2	E867	E950.6	E980.6
chlorate NEC.......................................	983.9	E867	E950.9	E980.9
chloride NEC.......................................	963.4	E852.2	E950.3	E980.3
cyanide (see also Cyanide).....................	989.0	E869	E950.9	E980.9
gluconate...	963.4	E852.2	E950.3	E980.3
hydroxide...	983.2	E867	E950.6	E980.6
iodide (expectorant) NEC......................	977.8	E859.8	E950.3	E980.3
nitrate...	989.9	E869	E950.9	E980.9
oxalate..	983.9	E867	E950.9	E980.9
perchlorate NEC..................................	983.9	E867	E950.9	E980.9
antithyroid......................................	962.8	E851.8	E950.3	E980.3
permanganate......................................	983.9	E867	E950.9	E980.9
Povidone-iodine (antiseptic, external) NEC...	977.0	E859.7	E950.3	E980.3
Pralidoxime (chloride).............................	977.8	E859.8	E950.3	E980.3
Pramoxine..	969	E859.0	E950.3	E980.3
Prednisolone...	962.0	E851.0	E950.3	E980.3
Prednisone..	962.0	E851.0	E950.3	E980.3
Pregnanediol...	962.6	E851.6	E950.3	E980.3
Preludin...	971	E856.4	E950.3	E980.3
Prenylamine..	973.4	E857.4	E950.3	E980.3
Preservatives...	989.9	E869	E950.9	E980.9
Pride of China...	988.2	E868	E950.9	E980.9
Prilocaine...	969	E859.0	E950.3	E980.3
Primaquin(e)..	961.3	E850.8	E950.3	E980.3
Primidone...	966.0	E856.0	E950.3	E980.3
Primula (veris)...	988.2	E868	E950.9	E980.9
Prinadol...	965.0	E853.0	E950.3	E980.3
Priscol, priscoline....................................	973.5	E857.5	E950.3	E980.3
Privet..	988.2	E868	E950.9	E980.9
Probanthine..	972.1	E855.4	E950.3	E980.3
Probarbital...	967.0	E854.0	E950.0	E980.0
Probenecid...	963.4	E852.2	E950.3	E980.3
Procainamide (hydrochloride).....................	973.0	E857.0	E950.3	E980.3
Procaine (hydrochloride)...........................	969	E859.0	E950.3	E980.3
penicillin..	960.0	E850.0	E950.3	E980.3

Substance	Nature of Injury	External Cause (E-Code)		
		Accident	Suicide (attempt)	Undetermined
Procarbazine	963.1	E852.1	E950.3	E980.3
Prochlorperazine	970.1	E855.1	E950.2	E980.2
Procyclidine	972.1	E855.4	E950.3	E980.3
Prodilin	965.0	E853.0	E950.3	E980.3
Producer gas	986	E875	E952.1	E982
Progesterone	962.6	E851.6	E950.3	E980.3
Progestogens	962.6	E851.6	E950.3	E980.3
Progestone	962.6	E851.6	E950.3	E980.3
Proguanil	961.9	E850.9	E950.3	E980.3
Promacetin	961.9	E850.9	E950.3	E980.3
Promazine	970.1	E855.1	E950.2	E980.2
Promethazine	967.9	E854.9	E950.3	E980.3
Promin	961.9	E850.9	E950.3	E980.3
Pronestyl (hydrochloride)	973.0	E857.0	E950.3	E980.3
Pronetalol, pronethalol	973.0	E857.0	E950.3	E980.3
Prontosil	961.0	E850.5	E950.3	E980.3
Propamidine	961.9	E850.9	E950.3	E980.3
Propanal (medicinal)	967.9	E854.9	E950.3	E980.3
Propane (distributed in mobile container)	987.0	E871	E951	E981
distributed through pipes	987.0	E870	E951	E981
incomplete combustion — see Carbon monoxide, propane				
Propanidid	968.9	E856.3	E950.3	E980.3
Propanol	980.2	E860	E950.9	E980.9
Propanolol	973.0	E857.0	E950.3	E980.3
Propantheline	972.1	E855.4	E950.3	E980.3
Proparacaine	969	E859.0	E950.3	E980.3
Propatylnitrate	973.4	E857.4	E950.3	E980.3
Propicillin	960.0	E850.0	E950.3	E980.3
Propiolactone (vapor)	987.9	E876	E952.9	E982
Propiomazine	967.9	E854.9	E950.3	E980.3
Propionaldehyde (medicinal)	967.9	E854.9	E950.3	E980.3
Propoxycaine	969	E859.0	E950.3	E980.3
Propoxyphene (hydrochloride)	965.9	E853.9	E950.3	E980.3
Propyl				
alcohol	980.2	E860	E950.9	E980.9
carbinol	980.9	E860	E950.9	E980.9
hexadrine	972.2	E855.5	E950.3	E980.3
iodone	977.2	E859.8	E950.3	E980.3
thiouracil	962.8	E851.8	E950.3	E980.3
Propylene	987.1	E876	E952.9	E982
Proscillaridin	973.1	E857.1	E950.3	E980.3
Prostigmine	972.0	E855.3	E950.3	E980.3

Substance	Nature of Injury	External Cause (E-Code)		
		Accident	Suicide (attempt)	Undetermined
Protamine (sulfate)	964.4	E852.8	E950.3	E980.3
zinc insulin	962.3	E851.3	E950.3	E980.3
Protein hydrolysate	963.4	E852.2	E950.3	E980.3
Prothionamide	961.9	E850.9	E950.3	E980.3
Prothipendyl	970.1	E855.1	E950.2	E980.2
Protokylol	972.2	E855.5	E950.3	E980.3
Protoveratrine(s) (A) (B)	973.5	E857.5	E950.3	E980.3
Protriptyline	970.0	E855.0	E950.2	E980.2
Proxymetacaine	969	E859.0	E950.3	E980.3
Proxyphylline	976.1	E859.4	E950.3	E980.3
Prunus				
laurocerasus	988.2	E868	E950.9	E980.9
virginiana	988.2	E868	E950.9	E980.9
Prussic acid	989.0	E869	E950.9	E980.9
vapor	987.9	E876	E952.9	E982
Pseudoephedrine	972.2	E855.5	E950.3	E980.3
Psilocibin	970.9	E855.2	E950.2	E980.2
Psilocin	970.9	E855.2	E950.2	E980.2
Psilocybin(e)	970.9	E855.2	E950.2	E980.2
Psychostimulant NEC	971	E856.8	E950.3	E980.3
Psychotherapeutic agents NEC	970.9	E855.2	E950.2	E980.2
Psyllium	974.5	E858.5	E950.3	E980.3
Pteroylglutamic acid	963.6	E852.3	E950.3	E980.3
Pteroyltriglutamate	963.1	E852.1	E950.3	E980.3
PTFE	987.9	E876	E952.9	E982
Pulsatilla	988.2	E868	E950.9	E980.9
Purinethol	963.1	E852.1	E950.3	E980.3
PVP	964.9	E852.9	E950.3	E980.3
Pyrahexyl	967.9	E854.9	E950.3	E980.3
Pyramidon	965.5	E853.5	E950.3	E980.3
Pyrathiazine	963.0	E852.0	E950.3	E980.3
Pyrazinamide	961.9	E850.9	E950.3	E980.3
Pyrazinoic acid	961.9	E850.9	E950.3	E980.3
Pyrazolone analgesics	965.5	E853.5	E950.3	E980.3
Pyrethrins, pyrethrum	989.3	E865	E950.9	E980.9
Pyribenzamine	963.0	E852.0	E950.3	E980.3
Pyridine (liquid)	982.0	E864	E950.9	E980.9
aldoxime methiodide	977.8	E859.8	E950.3	E980.3
vapor	987.9	E876	E952.9	E982
Pyridium	961.9	E850.9	E950.3	E980.3
Pyridostigmine	972.0	E855.3	E950.3	E980.3
Pyridoxine	963.6	E852.3	E950.3	E980.3
Pyrilamine	963.0	E852.0	E950.3	E980.3

Substance	Nature of Injury	External Cause (E-Code)		
		Accident	Suicide (attempt)	Undetermined
Pyrimethamine	961.9	E850.9	E950.3	E980.3
Pyrogallic acid	983.0	E867	E950.4	E980.4
Pyrrobutamine	963.0	E852.0	E950.3	E980.3
Pyrvinium (pamoate)	961.9	E850.9	E950.3	E980.3
Quicklime	983.2	E867	E950.6	E980.6
Quinacrine	961.3	E850.8	E950.3	E980.3
Quinalbarbitone	967.0	E854.0	E950.0	E980.0
Quinestradol	962.2	E851.2	E950.3	E980.3
Quinethazone	975.3	E859.3	E950.3	E980.3
Quinidine (salts)	973.0	E857.0	E950.3	E980.3
Quinine	961.3	E850.8	E950.3	E980.3
Quiniobine	961.3	E850.8	E950.3	E980.3
Quinolines	961.3	E850.8	E950.3	E980.3
Racemoramide	965.0	E853.0	E950.3	E980.3
Racemorphan	965.0	E853.0	E950.3	E980.3
Radiator alcohol	980.1	E860	E950.9	E980.9
Radio-opaque (drugs) (materials)	977.2	E859.8	E950.3	E980.3
Ranunculus	988.2	E868	E950.9	E980.9
Rat poison	989.3	E865	E950.9	E980.9
Rauwolfia (alkaloids)	970.1	E855.1	E950.2	E980.2
Realgar	985.1	E866	E950.7	E980.7
Reducing agents, industrial NEC	983.9	E867	E950.9	E980.9
Refrigerant gas (freon)	987.4	E876	E952.9	E982
not freon	987.9	E876	E952.9	E982
Rela	968.0	E856.1	E950.3	E980.3
Relaxants, muscle				
autonomic nervous system	972.3	E855.6	E950.3	E980.3
central nervous system	968.0	E856.1	E950.3	E980.3
Replacement solutions	963.4	E852.2	E950.3	E980.3
Rescinnamine	970.1	E855.1	E950.2	E980.2
Reserpine	970.1	E855.1	E950.2	E980.2
Resorcin, resorcinol	983.0	E867	E950.4	E980.4
Rhodine	965.1	E853.1	E950.1	E980.1
Riboflavine	963.6	E852.3	E950.3	E980.3
Ricin	989.9	E869	E950.9	E980.9
Ricinus communis	988.2	E868	E950.9	E980.9
Rimifon	961.9	E850.9	E950.3	E980.3
Ringer's injection (lactated)	963.4	E852.2	E950.3	E980.3
Ristocetin	960.9	E850.4	E950.3	E980.3
Ritalin	971	E856.8	E950.3	E980.3
Roach killers — see Pesticides				
Roburite	989.9	E869	E950.9	E980.9
Rodenticides — see Pesticides				
Rodina	965.1	E853.1	E950.1	E980.1

Substance	Nature of Injury	External Cause (E-Code)		
		Accident	Suicide (attempt)	Undetermined
Rolitetracycline	960.5	E850.3	E950.3	E980.3
Rotenone	989.3	E865	E950.9	E980.9
Rotoxamine	963.0	E852.0	E950.3	E980.3
Rough-on-rats (arsenic)	985.1	E865	E950.7	E980.7
Rubbing alcohol	980.2	E860	E950.9	E980.9
Rue	988.2	E868	E950.9	E980.9
Ruta	988.2	E868	E950.9	E980.9
Sabadilla (medicinal)	961.9	E850.9	E950.3	E980.3
pesticide	989.3	E865	E950.9	E980.9
Saccharated iron oxide	964.0	E852.5	E950.3	E980.3
Safflower oil	973.2	E857.2	E950.3	E980.3
Salicylamide	965.1	E853.1	E950.1	E980.1
Salicylate(s) NEC	965.1	E853.1	E950.1	E980.1
methyl	977.0	E859.7	E950.3	E980.3
theobromine calcium	975.1	E859.2	E950.3	E980.3
Salicylazosulfapyridine	961.0	E850.5	E950.3	E980.3
Salicylhydroxamic acid	961.9	E850.9	E950.3	E980.3
Salicylic acid (keratolytic) NEC	977.0	E859.7	E950.3	E980.3
Salinazid	961.9	E850.9	E950.3	E980.3
Salol	977.0	E859.7	E950.3	E980.3
Salt NEC	963.4	E852.7	E950.3	E980.3
Saluretics	975.3	E859.3	E950.3	E980.3
Saluron	975.3	E859.3	E950.3	E980.3
Salvarsan 606 (neosilver) (silver)	961.1	E850.6	E950.3	E980.3
Sambucus canadensis	988.2	E868	E950.9	E980.9
Sanguinaria canadensis	988.2	E868	E950.9	E980.9
Saniflush (cleaner)	983.9	E861	E950.9	E980.9
Santonin	961.9	E850.9	E950.3	E980.3
Sarkomycin	963.1	E852.1	E950.3	E980.3
Saroten	970.0	E855.0	E950.2	E980.2
Saturnine—see Lead				
Savin (oil)	977.8	E859.8	E950.3	E980.3
Scammony	974.1	E858.1	E950.3	E980.3
Scheele's green	985.1	E866	E950.7	E980.7
insecticide	985.1	E865	E950.7	E980.7
Schradan	989.3	E865	E950.9	E980.9
Schweinfurth green	985.1	E866	E950.7	E980.7
insecticide	985.1	E865	E950.7	E980.7
Scilla—see Squill				
Sclerosing agents	973.6	E857.6	E950.3	E980.3
Scopolamine	972.1	E855.4	E950.3	E980.3
Secbutabarbital, secbutabarbitone	967.0	E854.0	E950.0	E980.0
Secobarbital	967.0	E854.0	E950.0	E980.0
Seconal	967.0	E854.0	E950.0	E980.0

Substance	Nature of Injury	External Cause (E-Code)		
		Accident	Suicide (attempt)	Undetermined
Secretin	977.2	E859.8	E950.3	E980.3
Sedative (drug) NEC	967.9	E854.9	E950.3	E980.3
Sedormid	967.9	E854.9	E950.3	E980.3
Sedum	988.2	E868	E950.9	E980.9
Seed disinfectant or dressing	989.9	E865	E950.9	E980.9
Selenium NEC	989.9	E869	E950.9	E980.9
disulfide or sulfide	977.0	E859.7	E950.3	E980.3
fumes	987.9	E876	E952.9	E982
Senna	974.1	E858.1	E950.3	E980.3
Serenesil	967.9	E854.9	E950.3	E980.3
Serenium (hydrochloride)	961.9	E850.9	E950.3	E980.3
Sernyl	970.1	E855.1	E950.2	E980.2
Serotonin	977.8	E859.8	E950.3	E980.3
Sewer gas	987.9	E876	E952.9	E982
Sextol	980.9	E860	E950.9	E980.9
Sextone	982.9	E864	E950.9	E980.9
Shampoo	989.9	E861	E950.9	E980.9
Shellfish, nonbacterial or noxious	988.0	E868	E950.9	E980.9
Silicones NEC	989.9	E869	E950.9	E980.9
Silver (medicinal) (nitrate) (protein) NEC	961.2	E850.7	E950.3	E980.3
anti-infective NEC	961.2	E850.7	E950.3	E980.3
arsphenamine	961.1	E850.6	E950.3	E980.3
nonmedicinal (dust)	985.9	E866	E950.9	E980.9
salvarsan	961.1	E850.6	E950.3	E980.3
Sintrom	964.2	E852.6	E950.3	E980.3
Sleeping draught, drug, pill, tablet	967.9	E854.9	E950.3	E980.3
Slippery elm (bark)	974.0	E858.0	E950.3	E980.3
Smelter fumes NEC	985.9	E866	E950.9	E980.9
Smog	987.3	E876	E952.9	E982
Smoke NEC	987.9	E876	E952.9	E982
Snail killer	989.3	E865	E950.9	E980.9
Snake (venom) (bite)	989.4	E905	E950.9	E980.9
Snuff	989.9	E869	E950.9	E980.9
Soap (powder) (product)	989.5	E861	E950.9	E980.9
Soda (caustic)	983.2	E867	E950.6	E980.6
bicarb	963.3	E852.2	E950.3	E980.3
chlorinated — see Sodium hypochlorite				
Sodium				
acetosulfone	961.9	E850.9	E950.3	E980.3
acetrizoate	977.2	E859.8	E950.3	E980.3
amytal	967.0	E854.0	E950.0	E980.0
arsenate — see Arsenic				
bicarbonate	963.3	E852.2	E950.3	E980.3

Substance	Nature of Injury	External Cause (E-Code)		
		Accident	Suicide (attempt)	Undetermined
Sodium — *continued*				
bichromate	983.9	E867	E950.9	E980.9
biphosphate	963.2'	E852.2	E950.3	E980.3
bisulfate	983.9	E867	E950.9	E980.9
borate (cleanser)	989.9	E861	E950.9	E980.9
bromide NEC	967.3	E854.3	E950.3	E980.3
cacodylate (medicinal) NEC	985.1	E859.8	E950.3	E980.3
anti-infective	961.1	E850.6	E950.3	E980.3
calcium edetate	963.9	E852.4	E950.3	E980.3
carbonate NEC	983.2	E867	E950.6	E980.6
chlorate NEC	983.9	E867	E950.9	E980.9
chloride NEC	963.4	E852.2	E950.3	E980.3
chromate	983.9	E867	E950.9	E980.9
citrate	963.3	E852.2	E950.3	E980.3
cyanide — *see* Cyanide(s)				
cyclamate	963.4	E852.2	E950.3	E980.3
diatrizoate	977.2	E859.8	E950.3	E980.3
dibunate	977.8	E859.8	E950.3	E980.3
dioctyl sulfosuccinate	974.4	E858.4	E950.3	E980.3
fluoride — *see* Fluoride(s)				
fluoroacetate (dust) (pesticide)	989.3	E865	E950.8	E980.8
glucaldrate	974.0	E858.0	E950.3	E980.3
glucosulfone	961.9	E850.9	E950.3	E980.3
glutamate	963.4	E852.2	E950.3	E980.3
hydroxide	983.2	E867	E950.6	E980.6
hypochlorite (bleach) NEC	983.9	E869	E950.9	E980.9
medicinal (antiseptic) (external)	977.0	E859.7	E950.3	E980.3
vapor	987.9	E876	E952.9	E982
iothalamate	977.2	E859.8	E950.3	E980.3
ironedetate	964.0	E852.5	E950.3	E980.3
lactate	963.3	E852.2	E950.3	E980.3
metrizoate	977.2	E859.8	E950.3	E980.3
monofluoroacetate (dust) (pesticide)	989.3	E865	E950.8	E980.8
morrhuate	973.6	E857.6	E950.3	E980.3
nafcillin	960.0	E850.0	E950.3	E980.3
nitrate (oxidizing agent)	983.9	E867	E950.9	E980.9
nitrite (medicinal)	973.4	E857.4	E950.3	E980.3
perborate (nonmedicinal) NEC	989.9	E869	E950.9	E980.9
medicinal	977.8	E859.8	E950.3	E980.3
percarbonate — *see* Sodium, perborate				
phosphate	974.3	E858.3	E950.3	E980.3
polystyrene sulfonate	963.4	E852.2	E950.3	E980.3
propionate	961.9	E850.9	E950.3	E980.3
psylliate	973.6	E857.6	E950.3	E980.3

Substance	Nature of Injury	External Cause (E-Code)		
		Accident	Suicide (attempt)	Undeter-mined
Sodium — *continued*				
removing resins	963.4	E852.2	E950.3	E980.3
salicylate	965.1	E853.1	E950.1	E980.1
soporific	967.9	E854.9	E950.3	E980.3
sulfate	974.3	E858.3	E950.3	E980.3
sulfoxone	961.9	E850.9	E950.3	E980.3
tetradecyl sulfate	973.6	E857.6	E950.3	E980.3
Solactol	982.9	E864	E950.9	E980.9
Solanine	977.8	E859.8	E950.3	E980.3
Solanum dulcamara	988.2	E868	E950.9	E980.9
Solapsone	961.9	E850.9	E950.3	E980.3
Soldering fluid	983.1	E867	E950.9	E980.9
Solid substance NEC	989.9	E869	E950.9	E980.9
Solvents, industrial NEC	982.9	E864	E950.9	E980.9
Solvulose	982.9	E864	E950.9	E980 9
Soma	968.0	E856.1	E950.3	E980.3
Somnifaine	967.0	E854.0	E950.0	E980.0
Somnos	967.1	E854.1	E950.3	E980.3
Somonal	967.0	E854.0	E950.0	E980.0
Sonalgin	967.0	E854.0	E950.0	E980.0
Soneryl	967.0	E854.0	E950.0	E980.0
Soothing syrup	977.9	E859.9	E950.3	E980.3
Soporific drug NEC	967.9	E854.9	E950.3	E980.3
Sorbide nitrate	973.4	E857.4	E950.3	E980.3
Sorbitol NEC	963.4	E852.2	E950.3	E980.3
Spanish fly	977.0	E859.7	E950.3	E980.3
Sparine	970.1	E855.1	E950.2	E980.2
Sparteine	976.0	E859.4	E950.3	E980.3
Spasmolytics	976.1	E859.4	E950.3	E980.3
Spigelia (root)	961.9	E850.9	E950.3	E980.3
Spinocaine	969	E859.0	E950.3	E980.3
Spiramycin	960.9	E850.4	E950.3	E980.3
Spirilene	970.1	E855.1	E950.2	E980.2
Spirit(s) (neutral) NEC	980.0	E860	E950.9	E980.9
industrial	980.9	E860	E950.9	E980.9
mineral	981.2	E864	E950.9	E980.9
of salt — *see* Hydrochloric acid				
surgical	980.9	E860	E950.9	E980.9
Spironolactone	975.9	E859.3	E950.3	E980.3
Sprays (aerosol)	989.9	E869	E950.9	E980.9
cosmetic	989.9	E869	E950.9	E980.9
medicinal NEC	977.9	E859.9	E950.3	E980.3
pesticides — *see* Pesticides				
specified content — *see* substance specified				

Substance	Nature of Injury	External Cause (E-Code)		
		Accident	Suicide (attempt)	Undetermined
Spurge flax	988.2	E868	E950.9	E980.9
Spurges	988.2	E868	E950.9	E980.9
Squill (expectorant) NEC	977.8	E859.8	E950.3	E980.3
rat poison	989.3	E865	E950.9	E980.9
Squirting cucumber (cathartic)	974.1	E858.1	E950.3	E980.3
Stains	989.9	E869	E950.9	E980.9
Stannous oxide—see Tin (oxide)				
Stanolone	962.1	E851.1	E950.3	E980.3
Stanozolol	962.1	E851.1	E950.3	E980.3
Staphisagria or stavesacre (pediculicide)	961.9	E850.9	E950.3	E980.3
Stelazine	970.1	E855.1	E950.2	E980.2
Stemetil	970.1	E855.1	E950.2	E980.2
Sterculia (gum) (cathartic)	974.5	E858.5	E950.3	E980.3
Sternutator gas	987.9	E876	E952.9	E982
Steroids NEC	962.0	E851.0	E950.3	E980.3
Stibine	985.9	E866	E950.9	E980.9
Stibophen	961.9	E850.9	E950.3	E980.3
Stilbamide, stilbamidine	961.9	E850.9	E950.3	E980.3
Stilbestrol	962.2	E851.2	E950.3	E980.3
Stimulants	989.9	E869	E950.9	E980.9
central nervous system NEC	971	E856.8	E950.3	E980.3
psychotherapeutic NEC	970.9	E855.2	E950.2	E980.2
Storage batteries (cells) (acid)	983.1	E867	E950.9	E980.9
Stovaine	968.9	E856.3	E950.3	E980.3
Stovarsol	961.1	E850.6	E950.3	E980.3
Stove gas—see Gas, utility				
Stramonium (medicinal) NEC	972.1	E855.4	E950.3	E980.3
natural state	988.2	E868	E950.9	E980.9
Streptodornase	963.5	E852.4	E950.3	E980.3
Streptoduocin	960.4	E850.3	E950.3	E980.3
Streptokinase	963.5	E852.4	E950.3	E980.3
Streptomycins	960.4	E850.3	E950.3	E980.3
Stripper (paint) (solvent)	982.9	E864	E950.9	E980.9
Strobane	989.2	E865	E950.9	E980.9
Strophanthin	973.1	E857.1	E950.3	E980.3
Strophanthus hispidus or kombe	988.2	E868	E950.9	E980.9
Strychnine (salts) (pesticide)	989.1	E865	E950.5	E980.5
medicinal NEC	989.1	E859.8	E950.5	E980.5
Strychnos (ignatii)—see Strychnine				
Styramate	968.0	E856.1	E950.3	E980.3
Styrene	983.0	E867	E950.4	E980.4
Succinimide, mercuric—see Mercury				
Succinylcholine	976.9	E859.4	E950.3	E980.3
Succinylsulfathiazole	961.0	E850.5	E950.3	E980.3
Sucrose	963.4	E852.2	E950.3	E980.3

Substance	Nature of Injury	External Cause (E-Code)		
		Accident	Suicide (attempt)	Undeter- mined
Sulfacetamide	961.0	E850.5	E950.3	E980.3
Sulfachlorpyridazine	961.0	E850.5	E950.3	E980.3
Sulfadiazine	961.0	E850.5	E950.3	E980.3
Sulfadimethoxine	961.0	E850.5	E950.3	E980.3
Sulfadimidine	961.0	E850.5	E950.3	E980.3
Sulfafurazole	961.0	E850.5	E950.3	E980.3
Sulfaguanidine	961.0	E850.5	E950.3	E980.3
Sulfamerazine	961.0	E850.5	E950.3	E980.3
Sulfamethizole	961.0	E850.5	E950.3	E980.3
Sulfamethoxazole	961.0	E850.5	E950.3	E980.3
Sulfamethoxydiazine	961.0	E850.5	E950.3	E980.3
Sulfamethoxypyridazine	961.0	E850.5	E950.3	E980.3
Sulfamethylthiazole	961.0	E850.5	E950.3	E980.3
Sulfan blue (diagnostic dye)	977.2	E859.8	E950.3	E980.3
Sulfanilamide	961.0	E850.5	E950.3	E980.3
Sulfanilylguanidine	961.0	E850.5	E950.3	E980.3
Sulfaphenazole	961.0	E850.5	E950.3	E980.3
Sulfaphenylthiazole	961.0	E850.5	E950.3	E980.3
Sulfaproxyline	961.0	E850.5	E950.3	E980.3
Sulfapyridine	961.0	E850.5	E950.3	E980.3
Sulfapyrimidine	961.0	E850.5	E950.3	E980.3
Sulfarsphenamine	961.1	E850.6	E950.3	E980.3
Sulfasalazine	961.0	E850.5	E950.3	E980.3
Sulfasomidine	961.0	E850.5	E950.3	E980.3
Sulfasuxidine	961.0	E850.5	E950.3	E980.3
Sulfinpyrazone	963.4	E852.2	E950.3	E980.3
Sulfisoxazole	961.0	E850.5	E950.3	E980.3
Sulfomyxin	960.9	E850.4	E950.3	E980.3
Sulfonal	967.9	E854.9	E950.3	E980.3
Sulfonamides	961.0	E850.5	E950.3	E980.3
Sulfones	961.9	E850.9	E950.3	E980.3
Sulfonethylmethane	967.9	E854.9	E950.3	E980.3
Sulfonmethane	967.9	E854.9	E950.3	E980.3
Sulfonphthal, sulfonphthol	977.2	E859.8	E950.3	E980.3
Sulfonylureas	962.3	E851.3	E950.3	E980.3
Sulfur, sulfuretted, sulfuric, sulfurous, sulfuryl (compounds) NEC	989.9	E869	E950.9	E980.9
acid	983.1	E867	E950.9	E980.9
dioxide (gas)	987.3	E876	E952.9	E982
ether—see Ether(s)				
hydrogen	987.9	E876	E952.9	E982
medicinal (keratolytic) (ointment) NEC	977.0	E859.6	E950.3	E980.3
pesticide (vapor)	989.3	E865	E950.9	E980.9
vapor NEC	987.9	E876	E952.9	E982

Substance	Nature of Injury	External Cause (E-Code)		
		Accident	Suicide (attempt)	Undetermined
Sulph—*see* Sulf-				
Sulthiame, sultiame	966.9	E856.0	E950.3	E980.3
Superinone	977.8	E859.8	E950.3	E980.3
Suramin	961.9	E850.9	E950.3	E980.3
Surital	968.9	E856.3	E950.3	E980.3
Suxamethonium (bromide)	976.9	E859.4	E950.3	E980.3
Suxethonium	976.9	E859.4	E950.3	E980.3
Sym-dichloroethyl ether	982.9	E864	E950.9	E980.9
Sympatholytics	973.5	E857.5	E950.3	E980.3
Sympathomimetics	972.2	E855.5	E950.3	E980.3
Syrosingopine	970.1	E855.1	E950.2	E980.2
Systemic agents NEC	963.9	E852.4	E950.3	E980.3
Tablets	977.9	E859.9	E950.3	E980.3
Talbutal	967.0	E854.0	E950.0	E980.0
Tandearil, tanderil	965.5	E853.5	E950.3	E980.3
Tannic acid	983.0	E867	E950.4	E980.4
medicinal (astringent)	977.0	E859.7	E950.3	E980.3
Tansy (ragwort)	988.2	E868	E950.9	E980.9
TAO	960.9	E850.4	E950.3	E980.3
Tar NEC	983.0	E867	E950.4	E980.4
camphor—*see* Naphthalene				
fumes	987.9	E876	E952.9	E982
Taractan	970.1	E855.1	E950.2	E980.2
Tartar emetic	974.6	E858.6	E950.3	E980.3
Tartaric acid	983.1	E867	E950.9	E980.9
Tartrated antimony	974.6	E858.6	E950.3	E980.3
TCA—*see* Trichloroacetic acid				
TDI	983.0	E867	E950.4	E980.4
vapor	987.9	E876	E952.9	E982
Tear gas	987.9	E876	E952.9	E982
Teclothiazide	975.3	E859.3	E950.3	E980.3
Tellurium	989.9	E869	E950.9	E980.9
fumes	987.9	E876	E952.9	E982
TEM	963.1	E852.1	E950.3	E980.3
Tepa	963.1	E852.1	E950.3	E980.3
TEPP	989.3	E865	E950.9	E980.9
Teroxalene	961.9	E850.9	E950.3	E980.3
Terramycin	960.5	E850.3	E950.3	E980.3
Testosterone	962.1	E851.1	E950.3	E980.3
Tetrabenazine	970.1	E855.1	E950.2	E980.2
Tetracaine	969	E859.0	E950.3	E980.3
Tetrachlorethylene—*see* Tetrachloroethylene				

Substance	Nature of Injury	External Cause (E-Code)		
		Accident	Suicide (attempt)	Undetermined
Tetrachloroethane	982.9	E864	E950.9	E980.9
vapor	987.9	E876	E952.9	E982
Tetrachloroethylene (liquid)	982.9	E864	E950.9	E980.9
medicinal	961.9	E850.9	E950.3	E980.3
vapor	987.9	E876	E952.9	E982
Tetrachloromethane — *see* Carbon tetrachloride				
Tetracyclines	960.5	E850.3	E950.3	E980.3
Tetraethyl lead	984	E866	E950.9	E980.9
Tetraethyl pyrophosphate	989.3	E865	E950.9	E980.9
Tetraethylammonium chloride	973.3	E857.3	E950.3	E980.3
Tetraethylphosphate	989.3	E865	E950.9	E980.9
Tetrahydroaminacrine	971	E856.8	E950.3	E980.3
Tetrahydrocannabinol	967.9	E854.9	E950.3	E980.3
Tetrahydronaphthalene	982.0	E864	E950.9	E980.9
Tetrahydrozoline	972.2	E855.5	E950.3	E980.3
Tetralin(e)	982.0	E864	E950.9	E980.9
Tetramethylthiuram (disulfide) NEC	989.3	E865	E950.9	E980.9
medicinal	961.9	E850.9	E950.3	E980.3
Tetranitromethylaniline	983.0	E867	E950.4	E980.4
Tetronal	967.9	E854.9	E950.3	E980.3
Tetryl	983.0	E867	E950.4	E980.4
Thalidomide	967.9	E854.9	E950.3	E980.3
Thallium (compounds) (dust) NEC	985.9	E866	E950.9	E980.9
pesticide	985.9	E865	E950.9	E980.9
Thebacon	965.0	E853.0	E950.3	E980.3
Thebaine	965.0	E853.0	E950.3	E980.3
Theobromine (calcium salicylate)	975.1	E859.2	E950.3	E980.3
Theophylline	975.1	E859.2	E950.3	E980.3
Thiabendazole	961.9	E850.9	E950.3	E980.3
Thialbarbital, thialbarbitone	968.9	E856.3	E950.3	E980.3
Thiambutosine	961.9	E850.9	E950.3	E980.3
Thiamil	968.9	E856.3	E950.3	E980.3
Thiamine (hydrochloride)	963.6	E852.3	E950.3	E980.3
Thiamylal (sodium)	968.9	E856.3	E950.3	E980.3
Thiazesim	970.0	E855.0	E950.2	E980.2
Thiazides	975.3	E859.3	E950.3	E980.3
Thiethylperazine	963.0	E852.0	E950.3	E980.3
Thioacetazone	961.9	E850.9	E950.3	E980.3
Thiobismol	961.9	E850.9	E950.3	E980.3
Thiocarbamide	962.8	E851.8	E950.3	E980.3
Thiocarbarsone	961.1	E850.6	E950.3	E980.3
Thiocarlide	961.9	E850.9	E950.3	E980.3
Thioguanine	963.1	E852.1	E950.3	E980.3

Substance	Nature of Injury	External Cause (E-Code)		
		Accident	Suicide (attempt)	Undeter-mined
Thiomercaptomerin	975.0	E859.1	E950.3	E980.3
Thiomersal	985.0	E859.7	E950.3	E980.3
Thiopental, thiopentone (sodium)	968.9	E856.3	E950.3	E980.3
Thiopropazate	970.1	E855.1	E950.2	E980.2
Thioproperazine	970.1	E855.1	E950.2	E980.2
Thioridazine	970.1	E855.1	E950.2	E980.2
Thio-tepa, thiotepa	963.1	E852.1	E950.3	E980.3
Thiouracil	962.8	E851.8	E950.3	E980.3
Thiourea	962.8	E851.8	E950.3	E980.3
Thiphenamil	972.1	E855.4	E950.3	E980.3
Thiram NEC	989.3	E865	E950.9	E980.9
medicinal	961.9	E850.9	E950.3	E980.3
Thonzylamine	963.0	E852.0	E950.3	E980.3
Thorazine	970.1	E855.1	E950.2	E980.2
Thornapple	988.2	E868	E950.9	E980.9
Thrombin	964.4	E852.8	E950.3	E980.3
Thymol	983.0	E867	E950.4	E980.4
Thymus extract	962.9	E851.9	E950.3	E980.3
Thyroid (derivatives) (extract)	962.7	E851.7	E950.3	E980.3
Thyrotrophin, thyrotropin	977.2	E859.8	E950.3	E980.3
Thyroxin(e)	962.7	E851.7	E950.3	E980.3
Tigloidine	968.0	E856.1	E950.3	E980.3
Tin (chloride) (dust) (oxide) NEC	989.5	E866	E950.9	E980.9
anti-infective	961.9	E850.9	E950.3	E980.3
Tincture, iodine — see Iodine				
Tindal	970.1	E855.1	E950.2	E980.2
Titanium (compounds) (vapor)	985.9	E866	E950.9	E980.9
ointment	985.9	E859.6	E950.3	E980.3
TMTD — see Tetramethylthiuram (disulfide)				
TNT	989.9	E869	E950.9	E980.9
fumes	987.9	E876	E952.9	E982
Toadstool	988.1	E868	E950.9	E980.9
Tobacco NEC	989.9	E869	E950.9	E980.9
Indian	988.2	E868	E950.9	E980.9
Tocopherol	963.6	E852.3	E950.3	E980.3
Tofranil	970.0	E855.0	E950.2	E980.2
Toilet deodorizer	989.9	E869	E950.9	E980.9
Tolazamide	962.3	E851.3	E950.3	E980.3
Tolazoline	973.5	E857.5	E950.3	E980.3
Tolbutamide	962.3	E851.3	E950.3	E980.3
Tolnaftate	961.9	E850.9	E950.3	E980.3
Tolpropamine	963.0	E852.0	E950.3	E980.3
Tolserol	968.0	E856.1	E950.3	E980.3
Toluene (liquid)	982.0	E864	E950.9	E980.9

Substance	Nature of Injury	External Cause (E-Code)		
		Accident	Suicide (attempt)	Undetermined
Toluene (liquid) – *continued*				
diisocyanate	983.0	E867	E950.4	E980.4
vapor	987.9	E876	E952.9	E982
Toluidine	983.0	E867	E950.4	E980.4
vapor	987.9	E876	E952.9	E982
Toluol (liquid)	982.0	E864	E950.9	E980.9
vapor	987.9	E876	E952.9	E982
Toluylenediamine	983.9	E867	E950.9	E980.9
Tolylene-2,4-diisocyanate	983.0	E867	E950.4	E980.4
Tonics, cardiac	973.1	E857.1	E950.3	E980.3
Toxaphene (dust) (spray)	989.2	E865	E950.9	E980.9
Tractor fuel NEC	981.1	E864	E950.9	E980.9
Tramazoline	972.2	E855.5	E950.3	E980.3
Tranquilizers	970.1	E855.1	E950.2	E980.2
Tranylcypromine	970.0	E855.0	E950.2	E980.2
Trecator	961.9	E850.9	E950.3	E980.3
Triacetin	961.9	E850.9	E950.3	E980.3
Triacetyloleandomycin	960.9	E850.4	E950.3	E980.3
Triamcinolone	962.0	E851.0	E950.3	E980.3
Triamterene	975.9	E859.3	E950.3	E980.3
Triaziquone	963.1	E852.1	E950.3	E980.3
Tribromacetaldehyde	967.3	E854.3	E950.3	E980.3
Tribromethanol	968.9	E856.3	E950.3	E980.3
Tribromide	967.3	E854.3	E950.3	E980.3
Tribromoethanol	968.9	E856.3	E950.3	E980.3
Tribromomethane	967.3	E854.3	E950.3	E980.3
Trichlormethiazide	975.3	E859.3	E950.3	E980.3
Trichloroacetic acid	983.1	E867	E950.9	E980.9
medicinal (keratolytic)	977.0	E859.7	E950.3	E980.3
Trichloroethanol	967.9	E854.9	E950.3	E980.3
Trichloroethyl phosphate	967.9	E854.9	E950.3	E980.3
Trichloroethylamine	963.1	E852.1	E950.3	E980.3
Trichloroethylene	982.9	E864	E950.9	E980.9
anesthetic (gas)	968.1	E856.2	E952.9	E982
vapor NEC	987.9	E876	E952.9	E982
Trichlorofluoromethane NEC	987.4	E876	E952.9	E982
local anesthetic	969	E859.0	E950.3	E980.3
Triclofos	967.9	E854.9	E950.3	E980.3
Tricresyl phosphate	989.9	E869	E950.9	E980.9
Tricyclamol	972.1	E855.4	E950.3	E980.3
Tridihexethyl	972.1	E855.4	E950.3	E980.3
Triethanolamine NEC	983.2	E867	E950.6	E980.6
detergent	983.2	E861	E950.6	E980.6
trinitrate	973.4	E857.4	E950.3	E980.3

Substance	Nature of Injury	External Cause (E-Code)		
		Accident	Suicide (attempt)	Undetermined
Triethanomelamine	963.1	E852.1	E950.3	E980.3
Triethylene melamine	963.1	E852.1	E950.3	E980.3
Triethylenephosphoramide	963.1	E852.1	E950.3	E980.3
Triethylenethiophosphoramide	963.1	E852.1	E950.3	E980.3
Trifluoperazine	970.1	E855.1	E950.2	E980.2
Triflupromazine	970.1	E855.1	E950.2	E980.2
Trihexyphenidyl	972.1	E855.4	E950.3	E980.3
Trilene — *see* Trichloroethylene				
Trimeprazine	963.0	E852.0	E950.3	E980.3
Trimetazidine	973.4	E857.4	E950.3	E980.3
Trimethadione	966.0	E856.0	E950.3	E980.3
Trimethaphan	973.3	E857.3	E950.3	E980.3
Trimethidinium	973.3	E857.3	E950.3	E980.3
Trimethobenzamide	963.0	E852.0	E950.3	E980.3
Trimethylcarbinol	980.9	E860	E950.9	E980.9
Trimeton	963.0	E852.0	E950.3	E980.3
Trimipramine	970.0	E855.0	E950.2	E980.2
Trimustine	963.1	E852.1	E950.3	E980.3
Trinitrin	973.4	E857.4	E950.3	E980.3
Trinitrobenzol	983.0	E867	E950.4	E980.4
Trinitrophenol	983.0	E867	E950.4	E980.4
Trinitrotoluene	989.9	E869	E950.9	E980.9
fumes	987.9	E876	E952.9	E982
Trional	967.9	E854.9	E950.3	E980.3
Triorthocresyl phosphate	989.0	E869	E950.9	E980.9
Trioxide of arsenic — *see* Arsenic				
Tripelennamine	963.0	E852.0	E950.3	E980.3
Triperidol	970.1	E855.1	E950.2	E980.2
Triphenylphosphate	989.9	E869	E950.9	E980.9
Triprolidine	963.0	E852.0	E950.3	E980.3
Trolnitrate (phosphate)	973.4	E857.4	E950.3	E980.3
Trometamol	963.3	E852.2	E950.3	E980.3
Tromethamine	963.3	E852.2	E950.3	E980.3
Troxidone	966.0	E856.0	E950.3	E980.3
Tryparsamide	961.1	E850.6	E950.3	E980.3
Trypsin	963.5	E852.4	E950.3	E980.3
Tryptizol	970.0	E855.0	E950.2	E980.2
Tuaminoheptane	972.2	E855.5	E950.3	E980.3
Tubocurare, tubocurarine	976.9	E859.4	E950.3	E980.3
Tuinal	967.0	E854.0	E950.0	E980.0
Turpentine (spirits of)	982.9	E864	E950.9	E980.9
vapor	987.9	E876	E952.9	E982
Tybamate	970.1	E855.1	E950.2	E980.2
Tymazoline	972.2	E855.5	E950.3	E980.3

Substance	Nature of Injury	External Cause (E-Code)		
		Accident	Suicide (attempt)	Undetermined
Tyrothricin	960.9	E850.4	E950.3	E980.3
Ulmus fulva (bark)	974.0	E858.0	E950.3	E980.3
Undecenoic acid	961.9	E850.9	E950.3	E980.3
Undecylenic acid	961.9	E850.9	E950.3	E980.3
Upas	989.9	E869	E950.9	E980.9
Uracil mustard	963.1	E852.1	E950.3	E980.3
Uramustine	963.1	E852.1	E950.3	E980.3
Urari	976.9	E859.4	E950.3	E980.3
Urea	975.9	E859.3	E950.3	E980.3
Urethan(e) (antineoplastic)	963.1	E852.1	E950.3	E980.3
Urginea (maritima) (scilla) — see Squill				
Urotropin(e).	961.9	E850.9	E950.3	E980.3
Urtica	988.2	E868	E950.9	E980.9
Utility gas — see Gas, utility				
Valethamate	972.1	E855.4	E950.3	E980.3
Valium	970.1	E855.1	E950.2	E980.2
Valmid	967.9	E854.9	E950.3	E980.3
Vam	968.1	E856.2	E952.9	E982
Vanadium	985.9	E866	E950.9	E980.9
Vancomycin	960.9	E850.4	E950.3	E980.3
Vapor (see also Gas)	987.9	E877	E952.9	E982
kiln (carbon monoxide)	986	E875	E952.1	E982
lead — see Lead				
specified source, other (see also substance				
specified)	987.9	E876	E952.9	E982
Varnish	989.9	E863	E950.9	E980.9
cleaner	982.9	E864	E950.9	E980.9
Vasodilators NEC	973.4	E857.4	E950.3	E980.3
Vasopressin	962.5	E851.5	E950.3	E980.3
Vasopressor drugs	962.5	E851.5	E950.3	E980.3
Veganin	965.0	E853.0	E950.3	E980.3
Venom (centipede) (insect) (reptile) (snake)				
(spider)	989.4	E905	E950.9	E980.9
Veramon	967.0	E854.0	E950.0	E980.0
Veratrine	973.5	E857.5	E950.3	E980.3
Veratrum (album) (viride)	988.2	E868	E950.9	E980.9
Verdigris (see also Copper)	985.9	E866	E950.9	E980.9
Veronal	967.0	E854.0	E950.0	E980.0
Veroxil	961.9	E850.9	E950.3	E980.3
Versidyne	965.9	E853.9	E950.3	E980.3
Vienna				
green	985.1	E866	E950.7	E980.7
insecticide	985.1	E865	E950.7	E980.7

Substance	Nature of Injury	External Cause (E-Code)		
		Accident	Suicide (attempt)	Undeter-mined
Vienna—*continued*				
red	989.9	E869	E950.9	E980.9
pharmaceutical dye	977.1	E859.8	E950.3	E980.3
Vinbarbital, vinbarbitone	967.0	E854.0	E950.0	E980.0
Vinblastine	963.1	E852.1	E950.3	E980.3
Vincristine	963.1	E852.1	E950.3	E980.3
Vinesthene, vinethene	968.1	E856.2	E952.9	E982
Vinyl				
bitone	967.0	E854.0	E950.0	E980.0
ether	968.1	E856.2	E952.9	E982
Vioform	961.3	E850.8	E950.3	E980.3
Viomycin	960.9	E850.4	E950.3	E980.3
Viprynium (embonate)	961.9	E850.9	E950.3	E980.3
Virugon	961.9	E850.9	E950.3	E980.3
Vitamins NEC	963.6	E852.3	E950.3	E980.3
K	964.3	E852.7	E950.3	E980.3
Warfarin	964.2	E852.6	E950.3	E980.3
rodenticide	989.3	E865	E950.9	E980.9
Water				
balance agents NEC	963.4	E852.2	E950.3	E980.3
gas	986	E872	E951	E981
hemlock	988.2	E868	E950.9	E980.9
supply lead	984	E866	E950.9	E980.9
Wax (paraffin) (petroleum)	981.9	E864	E950.9	E980.9
automobile	989.9	E861	E950.9	E980.9
Weedkillers—*see* Pesticides				
Welldorm	967.9	E854.9	E950.3	E980.3
White				
arsenic—*see* Arsenic				
hellebore	988.2	E868	E950.9	E980.9
spirit	981.2	E864	E950.9	E980.9
Whitewashes	989.9	E863	E950.9	E980.9
Wild				
black cherry	988.2	E868	E950.9	E980.9
parsnip	988.2	E868	E950.9	E980.9
poisonous plants NEC	988.2	E868	E950.9	E980.9
Window cleaning fluid	989.9	E861	E950.9	E980.9
Wintergreen (oil)	977.0	E859.7	E950.3	E980.3
Witch hazel	977.0	E859.7	E950.3	E980.3
Wood				
alcohol	980.1	E860	E950.9	E980.9
spirit	980.1	E860	E950.9	E980.9
Woorali	976.9	E859.4	E950.3	E980.3

Substance	Nature of Injury	External Cause (E-Code)		
		Accident	Suicide (attempt)	Undetermined
Wormseed, American................................	961.9	E850.9	E950.3	E980.3
Xanthine diuretics......................................	975.1	E859.2	E950.3	E980.3
Xanthocillin..	960.0	E850.0	E950.3	E980.3
Xenysalate...	977.0	E859.7	E950.3	E980.3
Xylene..	982.0	E864	E950.9	E980.9
vapor..	987.9	E876	E952.9	E982
Xylocaine..	969	E859.0	E950.3	E980.3
Xylol...	982.0	E864	E950.9	E980.9
vapor..	987.9	E876	E952.9	E982
Xylometazoline...	972.2	E855.5	E950.3	E980.3
Yellow jasmine...	988.2	E868	E950.9	E980.9
Yew..	988.2	E868	E950.9	E980.9
Zactane...	965.9	E853.9	E950.3	E980.3
Zerone...	980.1	E860	E950.9	E980.9
Zinc (compounds) (fumes) (vapor) NEC........	985.9	E866	E950.9	E980.9
anti-infectives.......................................	961.9	E850.9	E950.3	E980.3
pesticides...	989.3	E865	E950.9	E980.9
undecylenate..	961.9	E850.9	E950.3	E980.3
Zoxazolamine...	968.0	E856.1	E950.3	E980.3
Zygadenus (venenosus).............................	988.2	E868	E950.9	E980.9
14-hydroxydihydromorphinone	965.0	E853.0	E950.3	E980.3
2, 4-D...	989.3	E865	E950.9	E980.9
2, 4-toluene diisocyanate...........................	983.0	E867	E950.4	E980.4

SECTION IV

ALPHABETICAL INDEX TO SURGICAL OPERATIONS, DIAGNOSTIC AND OTHER THERAPEUTIC PROCEDURES

Section IV

SURGICAL OPERATIONS,
DIAGNOSTIC AND OTHER THERAPEUTIC PROCEDURES

A

Abbe operation
  construction of vagina 71.5
  division, esophageal stricture 35.1
  intestine - see Anastomosis
  reconstruction of lip 93.1
  repair of defect in upper lip 93.1
  repair of vermilion border 93.1
Ablation, inner ear (ultrasound)
    (cryosurgery) 18.0
Abortion (therapeutic) (induced)
  by
    dilation and curettage 74.7
    hysterectomy 74.6
    hysterotomy 74.6
    intra-amniotic injection 74.8
Abrasion
  epicardial 29.8
Acetabuloplasty - see categories 87.0-87.1
Acromionectomy 80.4
Acromioplasty 81.9
Adams operation
  advancement of round ligament 70.7
  crushing nasal septum 19.3
  excision palmar fascia 89.2
Adelmann operation (finger amputation)
    85.0
Adenoidectomy 21.3
  with tonsillectomy 21.2
Adipectomy 94.5
Adrenalectomy (complete) (partial) 23.1
Adrenalotomy 23.1
Advancement
  ocular muscle (oblique) (rectus) 10.6
    with resection of same muscle 10.5
  tendon 88.5
    hand 89.4
AGG - see Asymmetrogammagram
Albee operation
  bone peg, femoral neck 81.1
  graft for slipping patella 81.1
  sliding inlay graft, tibia 81.1

Albert operation (arthrodesis, knee) 87.6
Alexander operation
  ligation of vertebral artery 26.8
  prostatectomy, suprapubic 58.1
    perineal 58.3
  shortening of round ligaments 70.7
Alveolectomy 99.7
Alveoloplasty 99.7
Alveolotomy, dental 99.0
Ammon operation
  dacryocystotomy 06.0
Amniocentesis (transuterine) 74.0
Amniotomy to induce labor 75.0
  transuterine, antepartum 74.0
Amputation
  abdominopelvic 85.9
  above-elbow 85.3
  above-knee 85.8
  ankle through malleoli, tibia, and fibula
    85.7
  arm through humerus 85.3
  below-knee 85.7
  cervix 70.4
  clitoris 72.3
  ear, external 16.1
  elbow 85.3
  finger except thumb 85.0
    thumb 85.1
  foot (transmetatarsal) 85.6
  forearm through radius and ulna 85.2
  hand 85.2
  hindquarter 85.9
  hip disarticulation 85.9
  interthoracoscapular 85.4
  knee disarticulation 85.8
  leg through tibia and fibula 85.7
  penis 61.3
  ramus (jaw) 97.5
  shoulder 85.4
  supracondylar, above-knee 85.8
  supramalleolar, foot 85.6
  thigh through femur 85.8
  thumb 85.1

Anastomosis—*continued*
ureter - *see* categories 55.1-55.5
ureterocolic   55.3
ureterovesical   55.5
vas deferens   60.9
veins
   base of brain   26.7
   intra-abdominal   27.7
   intracranial   26.7
   intrathoracic   28.8
    vein to artery   28.8
   neck   26.7
   peripheral   24.8
   portal to inferior vena cava   27.7
   pulmonary to
    azygos vein   28.8
    right atrium   28.8
   splenic and renal   27.7
   vena cava, inferior   27.7
   vena cava, inferior, and pulmonary
    vein to atrium 27.7 and 28.8
   vena cava, superior, to pulmonary
    artery   28.8
  vena cava, superior, to pulmonary
    artery   28.8
  ventricular   02.2
  ventriculoatrial   02.2
  ventriculopleural   02.2
Anderson operation (lengthening, tendon)
  88.7
Andrews bottle operation
  (hydrocelectomy)   59.1
Andrews operation - *see* Repair, hernia
Andrews Wyllys operation - *see* Repair,
  hernia
Anel operation - *see also* Repair,
  aneurysm
dilation of lacrimal duct   06.4
Anesthesia, spinal - omit coding
Aneurysmectomy
  arteriovenous (fistula)
   base of brain   26.4
   intra-abdominal   27.4
   intracranial   26.4
   intrathoracic   28.2
   neck   26.4
   pelvic   27.4
   peripheral vessels   24.6
  base of brain   26.3
  intra-abdominal, except aorta   27.4
   aorta   27.3
  intracranial   26.3
  intrathoracic vessels (aorta)   28.2
  neck   26.3
  peripheral vessel   24.5
Aneurysmoplasty - *see* Aneurysmectomy

Aneurysmorrhaphy - *see*
  Aneurysmectomy
Aneurysmotomy - *see* Aneurysmectomy
Angiectomy, peripheral   24.2
Angiography   A8.6
  carotid   A8.3
  cerebral   A8.3
  coronary   A8.6
  extremities   A8.5
  head   A8.3
  heart   A8.6
  intracranial   A8.3
  neck   A8.3
  pulmonary   A8.6
  renal   A8.6
Angioplasty (patch graft)
  intra-abdominal   27.6
  peripheral   24.8
Angiorrhaphy, peripheral   24.8
Angiotomy
  base of brain   26.0
  intra-abdominal   27.0
  intracranial   26.0
  intrathoracic   28.0
  neck   26.0
  peripheral vessels   24.0
Angiotripsy, peripheral   24.9
Ankylosis, production of - *see*
  Arthrodesis
Annuloplasty (posteromedial)   29.2
Anoplasty   51.6
Anoscopy - *see* category A4.5
Antrectomy (pyloric) (gastric)   46.2
Antrotomy
  Caldwell-Luc (sinusotomy) (bilateral)
   (unilateral)   19.6
  exploratory
   maxillary   19.6
   other sinus   19.7
  intranasal   19.7
  mastoid   17.3
  maxillary, radical   19.6
  maxillary, simple   19.7
Antrum window operation - *see* Window
  operation
Aortic window operation   28.4
Aortography   A8.4
Aortotomy
  abdominal   27.0
  intrathoracic   28.0
A-P repair, cystocele-rectocele   71.4
Apicectomy (apicoectomy)   99.5
  petrous pyramid   17.3
Apicolysis   34.5
Apicostomy, alveolar   99.0
Aponeurorrhaphy   88.4
  hand   89.3

Aspiration—*continued*
  hernia   40.9
  hyphema   13.1
  joint   86.2
    jaw   97.9
  kidney by incision (cyst)   54.0
    percutaneous   54.9
  liver abscess (percutaneous)   42.6
  lung (by incision) (puncture)   34.0
  nasal sinus   19.7
  ovary   67.0
  pericardium (wound)   29.0
  pituitary gland   01.2
  pleural cavity   32.1
  Rathke's pouch   01.2
  skin or subcutaneous tissue   92.0
  spermatocele   60.9
  spinal (puncture)   R9.5
  subarachnoid space   01.2
  subdural space   01.2
  tunica vaginalis (hydrocele)   59.0
  vitreous (and replacement)   14.9
    for retinal reattachment   13.5
Astragalectomy   80.6
Asymmetrogammagram   A9.8
Atrioseptopexy   29.5
Atrioseptoplasty   29.5
  with prosthetic device   29.6
Attachment
  eye muscle
    orbicularis to eyebrow   07.4
    rectus to frontalis   10.9
  pedicle graft or flap   93.6
    hand   93.5
Atticoantrotomy (ear)   17.3
Atticotomy   17.1
Austin-Moore prosthesis, hip arthroplasty   87.1
Avulsion
  nerve
    peripheral   04.3
    phrenic   34.5
Azygography   A8.6

B

Baffes operation (venous shunts to atrium)
    28.8 and 27.7
  with outflow patch prosthesis - code
    also 29.6
Baffle, atrial   29.6
Balanoplasty   61.4
Baldy-Webster operation (uterine
    suspension)   70.7
Banding, pulmonary artery   28.4

Bankart's operation (capsulorrhaphy,
    shoulder)   87.3
Bardenheurer operation (ligation
    innominate artery)   28.7
Barwell operation - *see* Osteotomy
Basiotripsy   76.8
Bassini operation - *see* Repair, hernia
Battery change, pacemaker   30.5
Beck I (myocardial revascularization)
    29.8
Bicuspidization of valves   29.2
Biesenberger operation (size reduction,
    breast)   94.5
Bigelow operation (litholapaxy)   56.8
Billroth operation (gastric resection)
  type I   46.2
  type II 46.2 and 46.5
Biopsy (endoscopic) (punch) (needle)
  abdominal wall   A1.7
  adenoids   A1.3
    adenoids and tonsils   A1.4
  adrenal gland   A2.0
  anus   A1.8
  aorta, thoracic   A1.6
    abdominal   A2.6
  appendix   A1.8
  artery   A2.6
    thoracic   A1.6
  Bartholin's gland   A2.4
  bile duct   A1.9
  biliary (hepatic) tract   A1.9
  bladder (cystotomy) (endoscopy)   A2.1
  bone (periosteum)   A2.7
  bone marrow   A2.7
  brain tissue   A1.0
  breast   A2.3
  bronchus   A1.6
  buccal cavity   A1.4
  bursa   A2.8
  carotid body   A1.0
  cartilage   A2.8
  cerebral meninges   A1.0
  cervix except by curettage   A2.5
    with curettage   70.3
  chest wall   A1.6
    associated with breast conditions
      A2.3
  choroid   A1.2
  ciliary body   A1.2
  clitoris   A2.4
  colon (endoscopic)   A1.8
  conjunctiva   A1.2
  cornea   A1.2
  cul-de-sac (Douglas')   A2.5
  diaphragm   A1.7
  ear, external   A1.3

Biopsy, etc. —*continued*
  endometrium except by curettage
      A2.5
    with curettage   70.3
  epididymis   A2.2
  esophagus   A1.6
  eyebrow   A1.2
  eyelid (skin)   A1.2
  fallopian tube   A2.5
  fascia   A2.8
  gallbladder   A1.9
  gingiva   A1.4
  gum   A1.4
  heart   A1.6
  hepatic duct   A1.9
  intestine   A1.8
  intracranial tissue   A1.0
  iris   A1.2
  joint structure (capsule)   A2.8
  kidney (capsule) (pelvis)   A2.0
  labia (majora) (minora)   A2.4
  lacrimal apparatus   A1.2
  larynx   A1.4
  lens (eye)   A1.2
  ligament   A2.8
  lip   A1.4
  liver   A1.9
  lung   A1.6
  lymph nodes   A2.6
  lymphatic channels   A2.6
  mammary duct   A2.3
  mediastinum   A1.6
  meninges, spinal   A1.1
    cerebral   A1.0
  mesentery   A1.7
  muscle   A2.8
  nasopharynx   A1.4
  neoplasm - *code to* biopsy of site
  nerve, peripheral   A1.1
  nipple (areola)   A2.3
  nose   A1.3
  omentum   A1.7
  orbit   A1.2
  ovary   A2.5
  palate   A1.4
  pancreas   A1.9
  parathyroid gland   A1.5
  pelvirectal tissue   A1.8
  penis   A2.2
  perianal tissue   A1.8
  pericardium   A1.6
  perineum   A2.4
    male   A2.2
  periosteum   A2.7
  peripheral vessels   A2.6
  perirectal tissue   A1.8

Biopsy, etc. —*continued*
  perirenal tissue   A2.0
  peritoneum   A1.7
    pelvic, female   A2.5
  periurethral tissue   A2.1
  perivesical tissue   A2.1
  pharynx   A1.4
  pineal body   A1.0
  pituitary   A1.0
  placenta   74.5
  pleura   A1.6
  premammary tissue   A2.3
  prostate   A2.2
  rectum   A1.8
  retromammary tissue   A2.3
  salivary gland or duct   A1.4
  sclera   A1.2
  scrotum (skin)   A2.2
  sigmoid colon   A1.8
  sinus, nasal   A1.3
    accessory   A1.3
  skin (subcutaneous tissue)   A2.9
  skull (bone)   A2.7
  spermatic cord   A2.2
  spinal cord   A1.1
  spinal meninges   A1.1
  spleen   A1.9
  sternal, sternum   A2.7
  stomach   A1.8
  synovial tissue (fluid)   A2.8
  tendon (sheath)   A2.8
  testis   A2.2
  thymus   A1.6
  thyroglossal duct   A1.5
  thyroid   A1.5
  tongue   A1.4
  tonsils   A1.4
  trachea   A1.6
  tunica vaginalis   A2.2
  ureter   A2.1
  urethra   A2.1
  uterus except by curettage   A2.5
    with curettage   70.3
  uvula   A1.4
  vagina   A2.4
  vas deferens   A2.2
  vein   A2.6
    thoracic   A1.6
  vocal cords   A1.4
  vulva   A2.4
Bischoff operation (ureteroneocystostomy)
    55.5
Blalock-Hanlon operation (creation of
    atrial septal defect)   29.5
Blalock-Taussig operation (subclavian-
    pulmonary)   28.4

Blaskovics' lateral canthoplasty 07.6
Blepharoplasty 07.4
Blepharorrhaphy 07.3
Blepharotomy 07.0
Block
   celiac ganglion 46.8
   celiac plexus 46.8
   gasserian ganglion 04.8
   paravertebral stellate ganglion 05.2
   peripheral nerve 04.8
   stellate 05.2
   sympathetic nerve 05.2
   trigeminal nerve 04.8
Blount operation
   osteotomy, femur 80.1
   stapling, epiphyseal plate 81.2
Boari operation (bladder flap) 55.5
Bobb operation (cholelithotomy) 43.4
Bone age studies A9.9
Bone block for stabilization - see
   Arthrodesis
Bonney (abdominal hysterectomy) 69.2
Boyd below-knee amputation 85.7
Brauer operation (cardiolysis) 29.0
Breech extraction - see categories 76.0-
   76.1
Brewer operation - see Arterioplasty
Bricker's operation (urinary diversion)
   55.2 and 47.4
Brisement force, jaw 97.8
Brock valvulotomy 29.2
Bronchography A0.7
Bronchoplasty 33.5
Bronchorrhaphy 33.5
Bronchoscopy - see category A4.3
Bronchostomy 33.5
Bronchotomy 33.0
Browne (Denis) operation
   repair of hypospad 4
Buckling, scleral (with implant) 13.5
Bunionectomy (radical) 87.2
Bunnell operation, hand
   arthrodesis, wrist 87.6
   reconstruction of thumb 89.6
   tendon transference or transplant 89.4
Burr holes (for decompression) (bilateral)
   (unilateral) 01.0
Bursectomy 88.3
Bursotomy 88.0
Bypass
   aortic-femoral 27.5
   aortic-iliac 27.5
   aortic-iliac to popliteal 27.5
   aortic-renal 27.5
   aortopopliteal 27.5
   arterial - see Graft, artery

Bypass—continued
   cardiac revascularization - see category
     29.8
   cardiopulmonary in open heart surgery
     30.7
     other surgery R9.4
   femoropopliteal 24.7
   iliofemoral 24.7
   peripheral artery 24.7
   renal artery 27.5
   right heart (Glenn operation) 28.8
   stomach without gastric resection 46.5
   Y graft to renal arteries 27.5

C

Caldwell-Luc operation (sinusotomy)
   (bilateral) (unilateral) 19.6
Callander above-knee amputation 85.8
Calycectomy, renal 54.4
Campbell operation
   bone block, ankle 87.5
   knee stabilization 87.6
Canaliculodacryocystorhinostomy 06.3
Canaliculoplasty 06.4
Canaliculorhinostomy 06.3
Canaloplasty, external acoustic meatus
   16.2
Cannulation, sinus 19.7
Cannulization
   lacrimal apparatus (postoperative) 06.9
Canthectomy 07.6
Canthocystostomy 06.2
Canthoplasty 07.6
Canthorrhaphy 07.6
Canthotomy 07.6
Capsulectomy
   joint 86.9
     jaw 97.4
   kidney 54.9
   lens (eye) 14.3
     with lens extraction 14.4
   ovary 67.1
Capsulo-iridectomy 14.3
Capsuloplasty - see Repair, joint
Capsulorrhaphy - see Repair, joint
Capsulotomy
   joint 86.1
     temporomandibular 97.4
   lens 14.1
Carbolization, pterygium 08.6
Cardiac massage, open 30.0
   closed 30.1
Cardiectomy 46.2
Cardiocentesis 29.0

Cholecystogastrostomy 43.6
Cholecystography, intravenous
(percutaneous) A8.8
Cholecystoileostomy 43.6
Cholecystojejunostomy (Roux-Y) 43.6
Cholecystopancreostomy 43.6
Cholecystopexy 43.9
Cholecystorrhaphy 43.9
Cholecystostomy (removal of calculus)
43.4
Choledochectomy 43.1
Choledochoduodenostomy 43.2
Choledochoenterostomy 43.2
Choledochojejunostomy 43.2
Choledocholithotomy 43.0
Choledocholithotripsy 43.0
Choledochoplasty 43.3
Choledochorrhaphy 43.3
Choledochostomy 43.0
Choledochotomy (removal of calculus)
43.0
Cholelithotomy 43.4
Chondrectomy 86.9
intervertebral cartilage 86.4
knee 86.5
nasal 19.1
temporomandibular 97.4
Chondroplasty 87.3
foot and toes 87.2
hip 87.0
with mechanical device 87.1
jaw 97.5
with inert substitutes 97.6
Chondrotomy 86.1
jaw 97.4
nasal 19.1
Chordotomy (anterolateral) 03.2
percutaneous 03.2
spinothalamic 03.2
Ciliarotomy 12.6
Cinch, cinching
for retinal reattachment 13.5
ocular muscle (oblique) (rectus) 10.8
Cineplasty - see Amputation
Cineradiography, NEC A9.9
Circumcision, male 61.2
female 72.3
Clamping
carotid artery 26.8
Clavicotomy 80.3
fetal (to assist delivery) 76.8
Cleft lip operation 93.1
Cleft palate operation 96.5
Cleidotomy 80.3
fetal (to assist delivery) 76.8

Clipping
aneurysm
base of brain vessel 26.3
carotid artery 26.3
cerebral artery 26.3
intracranial 26.3
neck 26.3
frenum linguae (frenulum) 96.1
tip of uvula 96.4
Clitoridectomy 72.3
Clitoridotomy 72.3
Closed reduction - see Reduction
Closure
anastomosis
stomach 46.7
appendicostomy 41.3
artificial opening
bile duct 43.3
bladder, urinary 56.6
gallbladder 43.9
hepatic duct 43.3
intestine 48.5
larynx 20.4
bronchostomy 33.5
cecostomy 48.5
colostomy 48.5
cystostomy, urinary 56.6
delayed granulating wound of
abdominal wall 40.1
duodenostomy 48.5
enterostomy 48.5
esophagostomy 35.6
fenestration
aortic-pulmonary (valve) 29.2
septal, heart 29.5
fistula
anus 51.7
appendix 41.3
biliary tract 43.9
bladder, urinary 56.6
branchial cleft 21.7
bronchocutaneous 33.5
bronchopleural 33.5
cervicovesical 56.6
cholecystojejunal 43.9
cornea 11.2
with lamellar graft 11.4
ear, middle 17.3
esophagus 35.6
fecal 48.5
gastrocolic 46.6
gastrojejunocolic 46.6
in ano 51.7
jejunum 48.5
kidney 54.6
larynx 20.4
lymph 25.5

Closure—*continued*
  fistula—*continued*
    mouth, external   96.9
    oro-nasal   19.9
    perineal   72.5
    pharynx   21.7
    rectovaginal   71.3
    salivary gland   95.5
    stomach, external   46.6
      gastrostomy   46.7
    thoracic duct   25.5
    trachea   20.8
    tracheoesophageal   35.6
    ureter   55.6
    ureterovaginal   71.3
      with ureterovesical anastomosis -
        code also 55.5
    urethra   57.4
    urethrorectal   57.4
    urethrovaginal   71.3
    uterovesical   56.6
    vaginal   71.3
    valve, heart   29.2
    vesicocolic   56.6
    vesicoenteric   56.6
    vesicorectal   56.6
    vesicouterine   56.6
    vesicovaginal   71.3
  gastroduodenostomy   46.7
  gastrojejunostomy   46.7
  gastrostomy   46.7
  ileostomy   48.5
  jejunostomy   48.5
  myelomeningocele   03.4
  nephrostomy   54.6
  peptic ulcer, perforated   46.6
  perforation, septum   19.3
  proctostomy   50.5
  punctum   06.4
  pyelostomy   54.6
  rectostomy   50.5
  septal defect (heart)   29.5
    with prosthetic device   29.6
  sigmoidostomy   48.5
  stoma, artificial, intestines   48.5
  tracheostomy   20.8
  urethrostomy   57.4
Coagulation - *see also* Electrocoagulation
  cervix   70.2
  pharynx (by diathermy)   21.6
  post T and A (with suture)   21.4
  rectal polyp   50.2
Coccygectomy   80.6
Coccygotomy   80.3
Cocked-hat procedure thumb   89.6
Coffey operation (uterine suspension)
    70.7

Colectomy
  anterior resection for malignancy   47.5
  complete (abdominoperineal)   47.6
  hemicolectomy   47.5
  left (radical)   47.5
  partial (subtotal)   47.5
  partial, in 2 stages - *see* categories 47.1,
    47.3
  right (radical)   47.5
  segmental   47.5
Collapse, surgical, lung (extrapleural)
    (intrapleural)   34.5
Colocentesis   48.9
Colocolostomy   48.2
  proximal to distal segment   47.5
Colocystoplasty 56.5 and 47.5
Coloileotomy   47.0
Colonoscopy - *see* category A4.5
  transabdominal approach - *see* category
    A5.2
Colopexy   48.6
Coloplication   40.2
Coloproctostomy   48.2
Colorectostomy   48.2
Colorrhaphy   48.4
Colosigmoidostomy   48.2
Colostomy (iliac) (perineal) (transverse)
    47.8
Colotomy   47.0
Colpectomy   71.2
Colpocentesis   71.9
Colpocleisis   71.2
Colpomicroscopy - *see* category A4.7
Colpoperineoplasty   71.5
  with repair of urethrocele   71.4
Colpoperineorrhaphy   71.3
  following delivery   78.3
Colpopexy   71.5
Colpoplasty   71.5
Colporrhaphy   71.3
  for cystocele and rectocele   71.4
  for urethrocele   71.4
Colposcopy - *see* category A4.7
Colpotomy   71.0
  for pelvic peritoneal drainage   71.8
Combined operation (revised) (vagotomy
    and hemigastrectomy) 46.2 and
    46.8
Commando procedure
  glossectomy   96.2
  hemimandibulectomy   97.3
  radical neck procedure   25.2
Commissurotomy   29.2
Conduit, ileal - *see* categories 55.2-55.5
Condylectomy   86.9
  jaw   97.4
Condylotomy   80.3

Condylotomy—*continued*
femur 80.1
mandible 97.1
Conization, cervix 70.4
Conjunctivodacryocystostomy 06.2
Conjunctivoplasty 08.5
Conjunctivorhinostomy (tear drainage)
06.3
Constriction of globe for reattachment of
retina 13.5
Construction - *see also* Reconstruction
esophagus, artificial - *see* categories
35.4-35.5
venous valves, peripheral 24.8
Control
hemorrhage
adenoids 21.4
intrapleural 32.0
laparotomy site, recent 39.1
prostate 58.9
thorax 32.0
thyroid, postoperative 22.0
tonsils 21.4
Cordectomy, vocal 20.2
Cordopexy, vocal 20.4
Cordotomy - *see also* Chordotomy
spinal 03.2
vocal 20.0
Corelysis 12.5
Coreoplasty 12.3
Corneo-conjunctivoplasty 08.5
Correction
atresia, nasopharynx 21.7
cleft palate 96.5
coarctation of aorta 28.4
hammertoe 87.2
overlapping toes 87.2
palate, except cleft 96.6
tetralogy of Fallot - *see* Repair,
tetralogy
Cosmetic operation - *see* categories 93.0-
94.9
Costectomy, except incidental to thoracic
operation 80.6
Costochondrectomy 32.9
Costotomy 80.3
Cotte operation (presacral neurectomy)
05.1
Cotting operation (repair of ingrowing
toenail) 92.4
Countershock, cardiac 30.8
Craniectomy 01.0
strip, for premature closure of cranial
suture 02.0
Cranioclasis 76.8
Cranioplasty 02.0

Cranioplasty—*continued*
with
bone graft 02.0
metal or plastic plate 02.0
for skull defect 02.0
Craniotomy 01.0
with removal of blood clot NEC 01.3
extradural hematoma 01.0
fetal (to assist delivery) 76.8
Craterization, bones 80.4
jawbones 97.3
Creation - *see* Formation
Cricoidectomy 20.2
Cricothyreotomy 20.0
Cricothyroidectomy 20.2
Cricotomy 20.0
Cricotracheotomy 20.0
Crushing
bone, except jawbones 81.9
calculus (stone)
bile (hepatic) passage 43.0
bladder, urinary 56.8
ganglion, sympathetic 05.0
nasal septum 19.3
nerve
peripheral 04.1
phrenic 34.5
sympathetic 05.0
Cryocyclotherapy 12.7
Cryoextraction, intracapsular 14.5
extracapsular 14.4
Cryohypophysectomy 01.7
Cryopexy, retinal 13.5
Cryoretinopexy 13.5
Cryosurgery (freezing) - *see also*
Destruction
biopsy, eye A1.2
brain lesion 01.6
ear, inner 18.0
eye enucleation 10.1
tonsil 21.1
Cryothalamotomy 01.5
Cryotherapy
ciliary body 12.7
Coats' disease 13.9
corneal lesion (ulcer) 11.2
to reshape cornea 11.4
Eales' disease 13.9
iris 12.1
pterygium 08.6
retina, except for reattachment 13.9
Cryptectomy (anus) 51.2
Cryptorchidectomy, bilateral 59.5
unilateral 59.4
Culdocentesis 71.9
Culdoscopy - *see* Category A5.4

Culp-DeWeerd operation (pyeloplasty)
54.6
Curettage - *see also* Dilation and
curettage
anus 51.2
bladder, except for biopsy 56.9
bone 80.4
jawbones 97.2
bursa 88.3
cartilage 86.3
chalazion 07.1
conjunctiva 08.2
eyelids, except chalazion 07.2
joint 86.3
jaw 97.4
kidney 54.9
for biopsy A2.0
muscle 88.2
sclera 11.8
tendon 88.2
Curette evacuation, lens 14.2
Cushing operation
ureterorrhaphy 55.6
Cutting
ganglion, sympathetic 05.0
nerve
peripheral 04.1
sympathetic 05.0
nerve root, spinal 03.1
pedicle (tube) graft 93.4
pylorus (pyloromyotomy) 46.1
ureterovesical orifice 55.9
urethral sphincter 57.9
Cyclectomy (partial) 12.9
Cyclicotomy 12.6
Cycloanemization 12.6
Cyclocryotherapy 12.7
Cyclodialysis 12.6
Cyclodiathermy 12.6
Cycloelectrolysis 12.1
Cystectomy, urinary (complete) (partial)
(simple) (total) (subtotal) 56.3
with reference to a cyst - *see* Excision,
cyst
resection of lesion only - *see* categories
56.1-56.2
Cystocolostomy 56.4
Cystography A9.3
Cystolithotomy 56.0
Cystopexy 56.6
Cystoplasty - *see* categories 56.5-56.6
Cystoproctostomy 56.4
Cystoprostatectomy, radical 56.3
Cystorrhaphy 56.6
Cystoscopy - *see* category A4.6
Cystosigmoidostomy 56.4
Cystostomy (urinary bladder) 56.0

Cystotomy 56.0
Cystourethrography A9.3
Cystourethroscopy - *see* category A4.6
Czerny operation - *see* Repair, hernia

D

Dacryoadenectomy 06.1
Dacryoadenotomy 06.0
Dacryocystectomy 06.1
Dacryocystography A8.2
Dacryocystorhinostomy 06.3
Dacryocystostomy 06.2
Dacryocystosyringotomy 06.0
Dacryocystotomy 06.0
Dana operation (spinal nerve root section)
03.1
Davis operation (ureterotomy for
pyeloplasty) 54.6
Debridement
abdominal wall 39.5
compound fracture 80.7
skin 92.1
skull 02.0
teeth 99.9
valve, heart 29.2
Decapitation (fetal) 76.8
Decapsulation, kidney 54.9
Decompression
anus, for imperforate 50.0
cranial 01.0
heart 29.0
median nerve 04.0
nerve
auditory (VII) 17.9
peripheral 04.0
orbit 09.0
intracranial approach - code also 01.0
pericardium 29.0
rectum 50.0
spinal cord 03.0
suboccipital 01.0
subtemporal 01.0
trigeminal nerve root 04.0
Decortication
cerebral 01.6
heart 29.1
kidney 54.9
lung 32.4
nose 19.3
periarterial 05.9
pericardium 29.1
ventricle, heart 29.5
De-epicardialization 29.1
with revascularization - code also 29.8

Defibrillation, electric, heart   30.8
Delaying of pedicle graft   93.4
Delimiting, cornea   11.0
Delivery procedure (to induce) (to assist)
   75.0-76.9
   breech extraction, partial   76.0
      spontaneous delivery - omit operative
         code
      total   76.1
   cesarean section - see Cesarean section
   destruction of fetus   76.8
   dilation of cervix   76.9
   episiotomy without forceps   75.9
   forceps
      with episiotomy
         high 75.8 and 75.9
         low   75.6
         mild 75.7 and 75.9
         outlet   75.4
      aftercoming head - see category 76.0
      breech extraction, partial   76.0
         ~total   76.1
      for rotation of fetal head   76.2
      Piper - see category 76.0
      without episiotomy
         high   75.8
         low   75.5
         mid   75.7
         outlet   75.3
   incision of cervix   76.9
   insertion of bag, pack or bougie   76.9
   puerperal (abortion) - see categories
      78.0-78.9
   rupture of membranes, artificial   75.0
   Scanzoni operation   76.2
   surgical induction of labor   75.0
      missed abortion   74.8
   vacuum extraction   76.3
   version, external   75.1
      internal   75.2
Delorme 1 operation (thoracoplasty)   34.5
Delorme operation
   pericardiectomy   29.1
   repair of prolapsed rectum   50.5
Delpech operation (axillary artery)   24.2
Denonvillier operation (plastic, ala nasi)
   (see also category 94.2)   19.3
Dermabrasion   93.7
Dermatoplasty - see categories 93.0-93.7
Desmotomy   86.1
Destruction - see also Electrocoagulation
   fetal   76.8
   lesion - see Excision of lesion
Detorsion of testis (digital) (incision)
   59.9
   with orchiopexy   59.7

Dialysis
   kidney   R9.3
   peritoneum   R9.3
   recirculation   R9.3
Diaphysectomy   80.4
Diathermy - see also Excision, lesion
   chalazion (marginal)   07.1
   choroid   13.0
      for reattachment of retina   13.5
   ciliary body (artery)   12.6
   conjunctival lesion   08.2
   esophagus   35.1
   labyrinth   18.0
   rectum   50.2
   retina   13.9
      for other lesions   13.9
      for reattachment   13.5
   sclera   11.9
      for reattachment of retina   13.5
   sinus, nasal   19.7
   transcleral for retinal reattachment
      13.5
   vestibule of ear   18.0
Dickson operation (muscle transplant)
   88.5
Dieffenbach hip amputation   85.9
Dilatation - see Dilation
Dilation
   artificial opening, intestine   48.9
   bladder (neck)   57.5
   bronchus   33.9
   cervix, nonobstetrical   70.9
      for examination only - omit coding
      to assist delivery   76.9
   duct of Wirsung   44.9
   endoscopic - code to dilation of site
   esophagus   35.7
   lacrimal duct (nasolacrimal)   06.4
   larynx (endoscopic)   20.9
   nasal duct, frontal   19.5
   pharynx   21.9
   punctum (with syringing)   06.4
   rectum (instrumental) (manual)   50.8
   salivary duct   95.5
   sphincter
      anal   51.8
      cardiac   35.7
   stoma, artificial, intestines   48.9
   trachea   20.9
   ureter (by catheter)   55.7
   ureterovesical orifice   55.7
   urethra   57.5
   urethrovesical junction   57.5
   vagina   71.6
Dilation and curettage (uterus) (cervix)
   diagnostic   70.3
   following abortion   78.1

D'Ombrain operation - *see* Pterygium operation
Douglas operation (suture, lip to tongue) 96.3
Drainage - *see also* Incision and drainage
abdomen 39.4
abdominal wall 39.0
abscess
  abdominal wall 39.0
  appendix 41.0
  auditory canal, external 16.0
  auditory meatus, external 16.0
  auricle 16.0
  Bartholin's gland 72.0
  breast 65.0
  buccal space 96.0
  cornea 11.0
  ear 16.0
  external site, NEC 92.0
  extraperitoneal 39.0
  facial region 96.0
  groin 39.3
  iliac fossa 39.3
  infratemporal space 96.0
  intestine (diverticulum) 47.0
  intrahepatic 42.0
  intranasal 19.5
  ischiorectal 51.1
  kidney 54.0
  lacrimal sac 06.0
  larynx 20.0
  lip 96.0
  lymph node 25.0
  nose 19.5
  omental 39.3
  orbit - *see* category 09.0
  ovary 67.0
  parotid gland 95.5
  pelvic, nos 71.8
  pelvirectal 50.1
  perianal 51.1
  perigastric 39.3
  perineum, female 72.0
    male 92.0
  perirectal 50.1
  perirenal tissue 54.2
  perisplenic 39.3
  peritoneum, pelvic 71.8
  prostate 58.0
  pulmonary - *see* category 34.0
  rectum, submucous (supralevator) 50.1
  retroperitoneal 39.3
  retropharyngeal 21.5
  salivary gland 95.5
  sclera 11.6
  scrotum 59.0

Drainage — *continued*
abscess — *continued*
  Skene's gland 72.0
  skin or subcutaneous tissue 92.0
  subdiaphragmatic 39.0
  subhepatic 39.3
  sublingual 96.0
  subphrenic 39.0
  teeth, supporting structures of 99.0
  thyroid 22.0
  urethra 57.0
  vulva 72.0
appendix 41.0
bile (hepatic) ducts 43.0
bladder (urinary)
  with incision (cystostomy) 56.0
  without incision 56.8
bone (marrow) 80.0
  jawbones 97.0
breast 65.0
bulbourethral gland 57.9
bursa 88.0
by anastomosis
  kidney (renal pelvis) 54.6
  ureter - *see* categories 55.1-55.5
by catheter to kidney 55.7
by myringotomy 17.0
by ureteroenterostomy 55.3
by ureterostomy - *see* category 55.2
cellulitis
  teeth, supporting structures of 99.0
chalazion 07.0
conjunctiva 08.0
cranial sinus (lateral) (sigmoid) 01.3
craniobuccal pouch by incision 01.3
craniopharyngioma 01.3
cyst
  dentigerous 99.0
  ovary 67.0
  thyroglossal 22.0
  thyroid 22.0
duodenal 47.9
ear, inner 18.0
epididymis 60.9
epidural space, cerebral 01.3
  spinal 03.0
esophagus (endoscopic) 35.0
eyelid 07.0
fascia 88.0
fistula, anus 51.0
gallbladder 43.4
hematoma
  nasal sinus 19.7
hordeolum 07.0
joint structures 86.0
  jaw 97.0
kidney 54.0

Drainage — *continued*
  kidney — *continued*
    by catheter to kidney   55.7
      renal pelvis   54.1
    lacrimal gland or sac   06.0
    larynx (for perichondritis)   20.0
    liver   42.0
    lung, by incision (closed) (open)   34.0
    lymph node (lymphadenitis)   25.0
    mediastinum (cervical) (transthoracic)
      32.2
    meibomian gland (cyst)   07.0
    Moll's gland   07.0
    mouth NEC   96.9
    mucocele, frontal sinus (nasal)   19.7
    muscle   88.0
    orbit - *see* category 09.0
    ovary   67.0
    pancreas (cyst)   44.0
    penis   61.9
    pericardium   29.0
    perineum, female   72.0
      male   92.0
    periprostatic tissue only   58.9
    perirectal   50.1
    periurethral tissue   57.9
    perivesical tissue   56.9
    petrous pyramid   17.1
    pharynx   21.5
    pilonidal cyst (sinus)   52.0
    pleura   32.0
    prostate   58.0
    pulp canal, teeth   99.0
    Rathke's pouch by incision   01.3
    retina   13.9
      with retinal reattachment - *see*
        categories 13.4 and 13.5
    salivary gland   95.5
    seminal vesicles   58.5
    sinus, nasal (accessory)   19.7
    skull (bone)   01.0
    spermatic cord   59.0
    spinal cord   03.0
    spleen   45.0
    sty   07.0
    subarachnoid space, cranial   01.3
      spinal   03.0
    subdural space cerebral   01.3
    tendon   88.0
    testis   59.0
    thorax (open) (closed)   32.0
    tunica vaginalis   59.0
    urethra (urethrostomy)   57.0
    vagina   71.0
    ventricular - *see* Shunt, ventricle
    vulva   72.0
    Zeis' gland   07.0

Drilling, bone   80.0
  jawbones   97.0
Dunn operation (arthrodesis foot)   87.5
Duodenectomy   47.4
Duodenocholedochotomy   43.0
Duodenoduodenostomy   48.0
  proximal to distal segment   47.4
Duodenoileostomy   48.0
Duodenojejunostomy   48.0
Duodenorrhaphy   48.4
Duodenostomy   47.9
Duodenotomy   47.0
Dupuytren operation (shoulder
    disarticulation)   85.4
Duraplasty   02.1
Durham operation (division of muscle)
    88.1

E

Echo-encephalography (ultrasonic)   A9.9
Eggers operation (transplantation
    hamstring, knee)   88.5
Electrocoagulation - *see also* Coagulation
    and Fulguration
  aneurysm, peripheral vessels   24.5
  brain tissue, not dura   01.4
  ear, external (fistula)   16.1
    inner   18.0
  nose, for epistaxis   19.5
  prostate   58.9
  retina   13.5
  semicircular canals   18.0
  urethrovesical junction, transurethral
    56.1
Electroconvulsive therapy - *see* category
    R9.0
Electrodesiccation
  skin and subcutaneous tissue   92.1
    wide or radical   92.2
Electrolysis   93.8
  cilia (eyelashes)   07.5
  ciliary body   12.1
  retina   13.9
Electroresection - *see also* Resection
  bladder neck, transurethral   56.1
  prostate - *see* Prostatectomy
Electroshock therapy   R9.0
Elevation
  bone fragments
    cranial   02.0
    spinal   03.4
  bone, fractured
    sinus (frontal) (maxillary)   19.9
  pedicle graft   93.4

Elliot's operation (corneoscleral trephining with excision) 11.7
Eloesser operation (thoracoplasty) 34.5
Embolectomy - *see also* Removal, embolus
    peripheral vessels 24.0
    pulmonary 28.0
Embryectomy NEC 77.8
Embryotomy 76.8
Emmet operation
    bladder fistulization 56.0
    trachelorrhaphy 70.6
Encephalography A8.0
    isotopic A9.8
Encephalopuncture 01.2
Encirclement, cervical os 70.5
Encircling, sclera (fascia lata) (tubing) 13.5
Endarterectomy (gas) (with patch graft)
    abdominal aorta 27.1
    aorto-iliac 27.1
    base of brain 26.1
    carotid 26.1
    common iliac 27.1
    coronary (with patch graft) 29.8
    intra-abdominal vessels 27.1
    intracranial 26.1
    intrathoracic 28.1
    mesenteric artery 27.1
    neck 26.1
    peripheral vessels 24.1
    subclavian, thoracic 28.1
    thoracic aorta 28.1
Endoaneurysmorrhaphy - *see* Repair, fistula arteriovenous
Endometrectomy, interna (uterine) 70.2
    excision of external implants only
        bladder, urinary 56.2
        cervix 70.2
        cul-de-sac 71.1
        ligaments, uterosacral 70.2
        vagina 71.1
Endoscopy, NEC - *see* category A4.9
    with
        surgical approach, NEC - *see* category A5.9
Enlargement
    aortic lumen, intrathoracic 28.4
    introitus 72.0
    orbit (eye) (mechanical) (mould) 09.3
    palpebral fissure 07.6
    punctum 06.4
Enterectomy NEC 47.4
Enteroanastomosis - *see* categories 48.0-48.2
Enterocelectomy 38.9
    female - *see also* category 71.5

Enterocentesis 47.0
    colocentesis 48.9
Enterocolectomy NEC 47.4
Enterocolostomy 48.1
Enteroenterostomy NEC 48.0
Enterolithotomy 47.0
Enterolysis 40.3
Enterorrhaphy 48.4
Enterostomy NEC 47.9
Enterotomy 47.0
Enucleation
    cyst
        broad ligament 70.2
        dental 99.2
        ovary 67.1
        salivary gland 95.1
    eyeball (bulb) (globe) 10.1
    lesion, jaw 97.2
    myoma - *see* Myomectomy
    prostate - *see* Prostatectomy
Epididymectomy except with orchiectomy 60.5
Epididymisoplasty 60.9
Epididymoplasty 60.9
Epididymotomy 60.9
Epididymovasostomy 60.9
Epiglottidectomy (endoral) (external) 20.2
Epilation, eyelid (cilia) 07.5
Epiphysiodesis 81.2
Epiploectomy 39.7
Epiplopexy 40.2
Epiplorrhaphy 40.2
Episioperineoplasty 72.5
Episioperineorrhaphy 72.5
    during postpartum 78.3
Episioplasty 72.5
Episiorrhaphy 72.5
    during postpartum 78.3
Episiotomy 75.9
    with high forceps 75.9 and 75.8
    with low forceps 75.6
    with mid forceps 75.9 and 75.7
    with outlet forceps 75.4
Equalization, leg
    bone fusion 81.2
    epiphyseal arrest 81.2
    ostectomy, partial 80.4
    osteotomy - *see* categories 80.1, 80.3
Esophagectomy (partial) (subtotal) (total) 35.2
Esophagocolostomy, antethorax 35.5
    intrathorax 35.4
Esophagoduodenostomy, intrathorax 35.4
    with complete gastrectomy 46.3
Esophagoenterostomy, antethorax 35.5

Excision—*continued*
  chalazion 07.1
  choroid 13.0
  choroid plexus 02.1
  cicatrix 92.1
  cilia base 07.2
  ciliary body, prolapsed 12.9
  coarctation of aorta 28.4
  condyle 86.9
    jawbone 97.4
  cornea (epithelium) 11.2
  cusp, heart valve 29.2
  cyst - *see also* Excision, lesion
    apical, tooth 99.2
    bile duct 43.1
    breast 65.2
    broad ligament 70.2
    conjunctiva 08.2
    dentigerous 99.2
    ear 16.1
    epididymis 60.4
    eyebrow 07.2
    eyelid 07.2
    Gartner's duct 71.1
    knee, lateral meniscus 86.5
      popliteal (Baker's) 88.2
      semilunar cartilage 86.5
    labia 72.1
    lymph 25.1
    Moll's gland 07.2
    Morgagni, female 68.9
    nabothian 70.2
    odontogenic 99.2
    orbit 09.1
    ovary 67.1
    parovarian 70.2
    pericardial 29.1
    periodontal 99.2
    popliteal artery 24.9
    scrotum 59.3
    skin and subcutaneous tissue 92.1
    thyroglossal 22.4
    thyroid 22.1
    tooth, involving 99.2
    urachal 39.5
    vagina 71.1
  cystic hygroma 25.1
  dentinoma 99.2
  diaphragm 38.1
  disk
    articular, jaw 97.4
    intervertebral, prolapsed 86.4
  dissecting hematoma, intrathoracic, with
    graft implantation 28.4
  diverticulum
    bladder 56.2
      transurethral 56.1

Excision—*continued*
  diverticulum—*continued*
    duodenum 47.2
    esophagus 35.1
    Meckel's 47.4
    pharyngoesophageal 21.6
    stomach 46.2
    ventricle, heart 29.5
  duct, thyroglossal 22.4
  ear, external 16.1
  endoscopic - *code to* excision of the site
  epulis (gum) 99.2
  eye (with implant) 10.1
  eyelid (redundant skin) 07.2
  fascia, for graft 88.3
    hand 89.2
  fibroadenoma, breast 65.2
  fissure, anus 51.2
  fistula - *see also* Fistulectomy
    arteriovenous
      base of brain 26.4
      intra-abdominal 27.4
      intracranial 26.4
      intrathoracic 28.2
      neck 26.4
      pelvic 27.4
      peripheral 24.6
    lacrimal gland and sac 06.1
    vesico-vaginal 71.1
  frenum, labial (lip) 96.9
    lingual (tongue) 96.1
  gallbladder 43.5
  ganglion
    sympathetic nerve 05.1
    tendon sheath (wrist) 88.2
  gingiva 99.1
  goiter, intrathoracic, by mediastinotomy
    22.3
  hematocele
    spermatic cord 59.1
    tunica vaginalis 59.1
  hematoma - *see* Incision, hematoma
  hemorrhoidal tags 51.3
  hydatid cyst, liver 42.1
  hydatid of Morgagni, male 59.9
  hydrocele
    canal of Nuck (female) 72.1
    round ligament 70.2
    spermatic cord 59.1
    tunica vaginalis 59.1
  intervertebral disc 86.4
  keloid (scar) 92.1
  lacrimal gland or sac 06.1
  lesion
    abdominal wall 39.5
    adenoid 21.4
    alveolus 99.7

Excision—*continued*
  lymph node, simple 25.1
    radical 25.2
  lymphangioma 25.1
  lymphatic channel 25.2
    pedicle graft - code also 93.6
  median bar, transurethral approach
      56.1
  meibomian gland (granuloma) 07.1
  meniscus 86.9
    knee 86.5
    temporomandibular 97.4
  mucous membrane of sinus 19.9
  myositis ossificans 88.2
  nail (nailbed) (nailfold) 92.4
  neoplasm - *see* Excision, lesion of the
      site
  nerve, sympathetic 05.1
  neuroma 04.2
  nipple 65.1
  ocular muscle segment 10.5
  odontogenic tumor 99.2
  orbital contents 09.2
  osteochondritis dissecans 86.3
  ovary - *see* categories 67.1-67.5
  parathymus 22.5
  parathyroid (ectopic) 22.5
  parotid gland (duct) 95.1
  patella, complete 80.6
  perianal skin tabs 51.1
  perianal tissue 51.1
  periprostatic tissue 58.9
  perirectal tissue 50.1
  perirenal tissue 54.2
  periurethral tissue 57.9
  pilonidal cyst (sinus) 52.1
  pleura 32.4
  polyp - *see* Excision, lesion of the site
  prostate - *see* Prostatectomy
  pterygium - *see* Pterygium operation
  rectal mucosa 50.2
  redundant mucosa of colostomy 47.2
  ring of conjunctiva around cornea 08.3
  salivary gland 95.1
  scar - *see also* Excision, lesion of the
      site
  septum, vagina 71.2
  sinus
    spinal (dermal sinus) 03.3
    thyroglossal 22.4
    urachal 39.5
  skin and subcutaneous tissue
    donor site, graft - omit coding
    local 92.1
    radical 92.2
    wide 92.2
  spermatocele 60.4

Excision—*continued*
  spinal 03.3
  stricture
    urethra 57.2
  subdural membranous sac 01.6
  submaxillary gland 95.1
  tarsal plate 07.2
  tattoo (accidental) 92.1
    by dermabrasion 93.7
  tendon sheath 88.3
    hand 89.2
  tendon, for graft 88.3
    hand 89.2
  thymus 23.0
  thyroid gland, aberrant, by transsternal
      route 22.3
  tonsil tag 21.1
  tooth 99.4
    from nasal sinus 19.9
    residual root 99.4
    root apex 99.5
  torus, mandible 97.2
  tract, thyroglossal 22.4
  ulcer
    duodenum 46.2
    peptic 46.2
    stomach 46.2
  ureteral stricture 55.1
  ureterocele 55.6
  urethral valves (endoscopic) 57.9
  uvula 96.4
  varicocele, spermatic cord 59.2
  vein
    intra-abdominal 27.2
    intracranial 26.2
    intrathoracic 28.9
    neck 26.2
    peripheral, except varicose 24.3
    varicose 24.4
  vitreous opacity (transcleral) 14.9
Exenteration
  ethmoid sinus 19.8
  orbit (with graft) 09.2
  pelvic (organs), female 69.7
    male 56.3
  petrous pyramid 17.3
Exodontia - *see* categories 99.3 and 99.4
Exploration - *see also* Incision
  abdomen 39.1
  abdominal wall 39.0
  adrenal gland 23.1
  axilla 92.0
  bile (hepatic) ducts 43.0
  bladder, by incision 56.0
    endoscopic A4.6
  blood vessels
    base of brain 26.0

Exploration — *continued*
  blood vessels — *continued*
    intra-abdominal   27.0
    intracranial   26.0
    intrathoracic   28.0
    neck   26.0
    peripheral   24.0
  bone   80.0
  breast   65.0
  bronchus   33.0
    endoscopic   A4.3
  bursa   88.0
  ciliary body   12.9
  colon (sigmoid)   47.0
  cranial   01.0
  esophagus, by incision   35.0
    endoscopic   A4.4
  fascia   88.0
  fossa - *see* category 92.0
  frontonasal duct   19.5
  gallbladder   43.4
  groin   92.0
  inguinal ring (groin)   39.0
  intestine, by incision   47.0
  intra-abdominal vessels   27.0
  intrathoracic   32.0
  jawbones   97.0
  joint structures   86.0
    jaw   97.0
  kidney   54.0
    renal pelvis   54.1
  lacrimal gland or sac   06.0
  larynx, by incision   20.0
    by endoscopy   A4.2
  liver   42.0
  lung, by incision   34.0
  maxillary sinus   19.6
  mediastinum   32.2
    endoscopic   A5.1
  muscle   88.0
  nerve, peripheral   04.0
    auditory   04.0
    root, spinal   03.0
  orbit   09.0
    intracranial approach - code also 01.0
  pancreas   44.0
  parotid gland   95.5
  pelvic laparotomy   39.1
  pericardium   29.0
  perineum, by incision, female   72.0
    male   92.0
  peripheral vessels   24.0
  perirenal tissue   54.2
  perivesical tissue   56.9
  petrous pyramid cells   17.1
  pilonidal sinus   52.0
  pleura   32.0

Exploration — *continued*
  popliteal space   92.0
  rectum, by incision   50.0
    endoscopic   A4.5
  salivary gland   95.5
  sclera   11.6
  sinus except maxillary, by incision
       19.7
  skin (sinus tract)   92.0
  spinal cord   03.0
  spleen   45.0
  stomach, by incision   46.0
    endoscopic   A4.4
  subcutaneous tissue   92.0
  subdiaphragmatic space   39.0
  tendon   88.0
  thyroid   22.0
  trachea, by incision   20.0
    by endoscopy   A4.2
  tympanum by transtympanic route
       17.1
  ureter   55.0
    endoscopic   A4.6
  urethra, by incision   57.0
    endoscopic   A4.6
  vagina, by incision   71.0
    by endoscopy   A4.7
  vulva, by incision   72.0
Expression, trachoma follicles   08.2
Extension - *see* Traction or Lengthening
Exteriorization
  intestine   47.1
Extirpation
  aneurysm
    arteriovenous (fistula)
      base of brain   26.4
      intra-abdominal   27.4
      intracranial   26.4
      intrathoracic   28.2
      neck   26.4
      pelvic   27.4
      peripheral   24.6
    base of brain   26.3
    intra-abdominal, except aorta   27.4
      aorta   27.3
    intracranial   26.3
    intrathoracic vessels (aorta)   28.2
    neck   26.3
    peripheral vessels   24.5
  larynx   20.2
  nerve of tooth - *see* category 99.5
  varicose veins   24.4
Extracorporeal circulation   R9.4
  in open heart surgery   30.7
Extraction
  breech - *see* categories 76.0-76.1

Fistulectomy—*continued*
    skin and subcutaneous tissue   92.1
    stomach   46.2
    thorax   32.4
    ureter   55.1
    urethra   57.2
    vagina   71.1
    vocal cords   20.1
Fistulization
    appendix   41.2
    esophagus, external   35.3
    lacrimal sac into nasal cavity   06.3
    larynx   20.6
    orbit   09.0
    salivary gland   95.5
    subarachnoid space   02.1
    thoracic duct   25.3
    trachea   20.6
    ventricle, cerebral   02.2
Fistulotomy, anal   51.0
Fixation
    bone without fracture reduction - *see*
        categories 81.5-81.6
    breast, pendulous   65.7
        size-reduction   94.5
    device (cast) (nail) (plate) (Note - *see*
        Includes and Excludes notes in
        Volume 1, page 632)
        external without manipulation for
            reduction   81.6
        internal without fracture reduction
            81.5
            for fracture or dislocation - *see*
                Reduction
    fracture, bone - *see* categories 82-84
        and 98
    intestine to abdominal wall   48.6
    iris (bombe)   12.3
    joint - *see* Repair, joint
    kidney - *see* Nephropexy
    ligament
        palpebrae   07.7
    ligament, cardinal   70.7
    parametrial   70.7
    rectum (with fascia graft)   50.5
    spine with fusion   87.4
    stapes   17.5
    tendon   88.7
        hand   89.8
    testis in scrotum (trans-septal)   59.7
    urethrovaginal to Cooper's ligament
        71.5
    uterus   70.7
    vagina   71.5
Flap
    bone, cranial   02.0

Flap—*continued*
    conjunctival (hood)   08.5
    skin - *see* Graft, grafting
Flap-splitting operation for vesicovaginal
        fistula   71.3
Fluoroscopy, without injection of
        radiopaque substance - omit coding
Folding, ocular muscle (oblique) (rectus)
        10.8
Foley V-Y plasty (pyeloplasty)   54.6
Foraminotomy (spinal)   03.0
Forceps (application) - *see* Delivery
        procedure
Formation
    adhesions, pericardium and myocardium
        29.8
    anus, artificial   47.8
    pupil   12.3
        by iridectomy   12.1
Fothergill operation (A-P colporrhaphy)
        71.4
    parametrial fixation only   70.7
Fowler operation (thoracoplasty)   34.5
Fracture, surgical   81.3
Franco operation (suprapubic cystotomy)
        56.0
Frank operation (gastrostomy)   46.4
Frazier operation (chordotomy)   03.2
Frazier-Spiller operation (trigeminal
        sensory root division)   04.1
Fredet-Ramstedt operation
        (pyloromyotomy)   46.1
Freeing adhesions
    abdominal   40.3
    artery-vein-nerve bundle tissue   24.9
    biliary tract (gallbladder)   43.9
    bladder (neck)   56.9
    bone   81.9
        jawbones   97.8
    cartilage of joint   87.9
    conjunctiva   08.9
    cornea   12.5
    cortical, brain   01.4
    ear, middle   17.1
    fallopian tube   68.9
    fascia   88.9
        hand   89.9
    heart   29.0
    intestines   40.3
    iris   12.5
    joint   87.9
        jaw   97.8
    kidney   54.9
    larynx   20.9
    lung   34.5
    meninges, spinal   03.5

Freeing adhesions—*continued*
  muscle 88.9
    hand 89.9
  nerve roots, spinal 03.5
  nerve, peripheral 04.6
  nose 19.5
  orbit (eye socket) 09.3
  ovary 67.9
  pelvic, female 71.8
    male 40.3
  penis 61.9
  pericardium 29.0
  peripheral vessels 24.9
  peritoneum 40.3
  pharynx 21.9
  pleura 32.0
  rectum 50.0
  spinal cord 03.5
  spleen 45.9
  stomach 46.9
  tendon 88.9
    hand 89.9
  thorax 32.0
  tongue 96.3
  trachea 20.9
  ureter (fibrous tissue bands) 55.8
  uterus 70.8
  vulva (labia) 72.9
Freeze, gastric R9.9
Frenotomy 96.1
Frenulumectomy see Frenumectomy
Frenumectomy
  lip (labial) 96.9
  maxilla (midline) 96.9
  tongue 96.2
Fulguration - *see also* Excision, lesion of
    site
  anus 51.2
  bladder, transurethral 56.1
    by cystotomy 56.2
  eyelids 07.2
  penis 61.1
  perineum, female 72.1
  prostate, transurethral 58.2
  rectum 50.2
  retina 13.9
  scrotum 59.3
  skin and subcutaneous tissue 92.1
  urethra 57.2
  vulva 72.1
Fundectomy, uterine - *see* categories 69.1
    and 69.4
Fundusectomy, gastric 46.2
Fusion
  bone 81.2
  epiphyseal-diaphyseal 81.2

Fusion—*continued*
  epiphysiodesis 81.2
  joint (with bone graft) 87.6
    ankle 87.5
    dorsal spine 87.4
    foot 87.5
    hip 87.6
    interphalangeal, finger 87.6
    ischiofemoral 87.6
    jaw - *see* category 97.4
    lumbosacral 87.4
    pantalar 87.5
    spinal 87.4
    subtalar 87.5
    tarsal joints 87.5
    toe 87.5
  lip to tongue 96.3

G

Gait training R4.1
Ganglionectomy
  gasserian 04.3
  nerve, peripheral 04.3
  sphenopalatine (Meckel's) 05.1
  sympathetic 05.1
  tendon sheath (wrist) 88.2
Gangliorrhaphy, sympathetic 05.9
Gant operation (division femur) 80.1
Gastrectomy
  complete (total) 46.3
  partial (subtotal) (wedge) 46.2
  radical 46.3
Gastroduodenectomy
  complete (total) 46.3
  partial (subtotal) 46.2
Gastroduodenostomy 46.5
  with partial gastrectomy 46.2
Gastroduodenotomy 46.0 and 47.0
Gastroenterostomy 46.5
Gastrogastrostomy 46.5
  with partial gastrectomy 46.2
Gastrojejunostomy 46.5
Gastrojejunotomy 46.0 and 47.0
Gastrolysis 46.9
Gastroplasty 46.6
Gastroplication 46.6
Gastrorrhaphy 46.6
Gastroscopy - *see* category A4.4
Gastrostomy 46.4
Gastrotomy 46.0
Genioplasty - *see* categories 97.5-97.6
Gifford operation
  delimiting keratotomy 11.0
  destruction of lacrimal sac 06.1

Graft, grafting—*continued*
  ovary 67.6
  palate, cleft 96.5
    other 96.6
  penis 61.4
  saphenous vein - *code to* graft site
  sclera 11.8
  scrotum 59.6
  septum, heart, prosthetic 29.6
    tissue 29.5
  skin except breast, ear, eyelid, lip,
      mouth, nose, palate, penis and
      scrotum
    dermal fat 93.3
      breast augmentation 94.4
    free skin 93.3
      hand 93.2
      thumb 93.2 and 89.6
    mucous membrane 93.3
    pedicle (flap) (tube)
      attachment to site 93.6
        hand 93.5
        thumb 93.5 and 89.6
      defatting 93.4
      delayed 93.4
      elevation 93.4
      preparation of (cutting) 93.4
      revision 93.4
    vagina 71.5
  tarsal cartilage 07.4
  temporalis muscle to orbit 09.3
  tendon 88.7
    for joint repair - *see* Repair, joint
    hand 89.8
    testicle 59.6
  thumb 89.6
  tongue 96.3
  trachea 20.7
  ureter - *see* Replacement, ureter
  valve (aortic) (mitral) (pulmonary)
    aortic wall tissue 29.3
    artificial foraminal valve 29.4
    ball-valve, prosthetic 29.4
    inert material (synthetic) 29.4
    prosthetic patch graft 29.4
    tissue replacement (graft) 29.3
  ventricle, prosthetic 29.6
    tissue 29.5
  vermilion border 93.1
Grantham lobotomy (modified) 01.4
Grattage, conjunctiva 08.2
Grice operation (arthrodesis foot) 87.5
Gritti-Stokes above-knee amputation
    85.8
Guttering, bone 80.4
  jawbones 97.2
Guyon below-knee amputation 85.7

H

Hagedorn operation (cleft lip repair) 93.1
Hagner operation (epididymotomy) 60.9
Hanley operation (cavernotomy) 54.3
Harelip operation 93.1
Haultain operation (replacement, inverted
    uterus) 70.6
  puerperal (postpartum) 78.4
Hegar operation (perineorrhaphy) 72.5
Heine operation (cyclodialysis) 12.6
Heinke-Mikulicz pyloroplasty 46.1
Heller procedure (transthoracic
    cardiomyotomy) 35.0
Hemicolectomy 47.5
Hemicystectomy 56.3
Hemiglossectomy 96.2
Hemilaminectomy 03.0
Hemilaryngectomy 20.2
Hemimandibulectomy 97.3
Heminephrectomy 54.4
Hemipelvectomy 85.9
Hemispherectomy, cerebral 01.6
Hemithyroidectomy 22.1
Hemodialysis (acute) (episodic) (chronic),
    extracorporeal R9.3
Hemorrhage, control - *see* Control,
    hemorrhage
Hemorrhoidectomy 51.3
Hemostasis - *see* Control, hemorrhage
Henry operation (femoral herniorrhaphy)
    38.4
Henry-Swan operation - *see* Anastomosis,
    bile duct
Hepatectomy NEC 42.2
Hepaticodochotomy 43.0
Hepaticojejunostomy 43.2
Hepaticolithotomy 43.0
Hepaticostomy 43.0
Hepaticotomy 43.0
Hepatocholangiocystoduodenostomy
    43.6
Hepatography A8.6
  with cholangiography A8.8
Hepatopexy 42.3
Hepatorrhaphy 42.3
Hepatostomy 42.3
Hepatotomy 42.0
Hernioplasty - *see* Repair of hernia
Herniorrhaphy - *see* Repair of hernia
Herniotomy - *see* Repair of hernia
Hey foot amputation 85.6
Hibbs' operation (spinal fusion) 87.4
Hinging
  valve, mitral 29.2
Hirschel operation (resection of
    duodenum and pancreas) 44.1

Hofmeister retrocolic anastomosis 46.2 and 46.5
Hoke operation (triple arthrodesis) 87.5
Holmes operation (ostectomy, os calcis) 80.4
Holter (Spitz-Holter) valve insertion 02.2
Homograft - *see* Graft, grafting
Homotransplantation - *see* Transplantation
Hormone therapy for cancer (neoplasm) R1.8
Hufnagel operation (aortic valve replacement) 29.4
Hummelscheim operation (transplantation, rectus muscle) 10.7
Hunter operation - *see* Repair, aneurysm
Hutch operation (ureteroneocystostomy) 55.5
Hymenectomy 71.2
Hymenorrhaphy 71.3
Hymenotomy 71.0
Hynes-Anderson operation (ureteropyelostomy) 54.6 and 55.1
Hypophysectomy (complete) (partial) 01.7
Hypothermia - *see* categories 30.6-30.7
Hypotympanotomy 17.1
Hysterectomy
  abdominal approach
    with cesarean - code also C-section for termination of pregnancy 74.6
    radical (Wertheim) 69.3
    subtotal (partial) 69.1
    total (complete) 69.2
  vaginal approach
    radical (Schauta) 69.5
    subtotal (partial) 69.4
    total (complete) 69.4
Hysterocolpectomy, radical, paravaginal section 69.5
Hysterography A9.4
Hysterolysis 70.8
Hysteromyomectomy 70.1
Hysteropexy 70.7
Hysteroplasty 70.6
Hysterorrhaphy 70.6
  following delivery or abortion 78.2
Hysterosalpingography A9.4
Hysterosalpingostomy 68.3
Hysterotomy 70.0
  with removal of hydatidiform mole 70.0
  for intrauterine transfusion 74.1
  for termination of pregnancy 74.6
  vaginal, under 28 weeks' gestation 74.6
Hysterotrachelectomy 70.4

Hysterotracheloplasty 70.6
Hysterotrachelorrhaphy 70.6
  following delivery or abortion 78.2
Hysterotrachelotomy 70.0

I

Ileal bladder formation, ureterostomy 55.2 and 47.4
  closed (bladder replacement) 56.5 and 47.4
Ileal loop operation - *see* Ureteroileostomy
Ileectomy 47.4
Ileocecostomy 48.1
Ileocolectomy 47.5
Ileocolostomy 48.1
Ileocolotomy 47.0
Ileocystoplasty 56.5 and 47.4
Ileoduodenotomy 47.0
Ileoileostomy 48.0
  proximal to distal segment 47.4
Ileoproctostomy 48.1
Ileorrhaphy 48.4
Ileosigmoidostomy 48.1
Ileostomy (Brooke) (Crile-Turnbull) (Dragstedt) (end-loop) 47.7
  with plication of ileum 47.7
  closure 48.5
  reduction of prolapse 48.9
  repair of 48.3
  revision of 48.3
  transplantation to new site 47.7
Ileotomy 47.0
Ileotransversostomy 48.1
Implant, implantation
  acrylic, nasal septum (*see also* category 94.2) 19.3
  artery
    aortic branches to heart muscle 29.8
    mammary to ventricular wall 29.8
  blood vessels to myocardium 29.8
  cornea 11.5
  dentures 99.8
  electronic stimulator
    bladder 56.0
    carotid-sinus nerve 05.9 and 30.4
    heart muscle 30.4
    ureter 55.0
  fallopian tube into uterus 68.3
  heart (artificial) (homograft) 29.9
    valves only - *see* categories 29.3-29.4
  inert materials
    breast 65.7
      for augmentation 94.4
    heart, within - *see* categories 29.4 and 29.6

Implant, implantation—*continued*
  inert materials—*continued*
    hip 87.1
    jaw 97.6
    nose - *see* categories 19.3 and 94.2
    orbital (eye socket) 09.4
      re-insertion 09.4
    scleral shell (cup) with evisceration
        10.1
      secondary implantation 10.3
    Tenon's capsule, with enucleation
        10.1
      postenucleation 10.3
      secondary implantation 10.3
    ureter for repair 55.6
  nerve, peripheral 04.5
  patella to tibia 81.9
  radioactive isotope therapy R1.5
  radium (radon) R1.4
  retinal reattachment, for 13.5
  tooth 99.6
  ureters into
    "bladder 55.5
    intestine 55.3
      external diversion 55.2
    rectum 55.3
    skin 55.2
  vitreous (silicone) 14.9
    for retinal reattachment 13.5

Imre lateral canthoplasty 07.6

Incision (and drainage)
  with
    drainage - *see also* Drainage
    exploration - *see* Exploration
    removal of foreign body - *see*
            Removal, foreign body
  abdominal wall 39.0
  abscess
    alveolar 99.0
    appendix 41.0
    brain 01.3
    cerebral 01.3
    cornea 11.0
    epidural 01.3
    eyelid 07.0
    gum 99.0
    intracranial 01.3
    meningeal 01.3
    nerve root 03.0
    omental 39.3
    perigastric 39.3
    perisplenic 39.3
    peritoneal NEC 39.3
      pelvic, female 71.8
    peritonsillar 21.0
    retroperitoneal 39.3

Incision (and drainage)—*continued*
  abscess—*continued*
    skin or subcutaneous tissue 92.0
    spinal cord 03.0
    spinal meninges 03.0
    subdiaphragmatic 39.0
    subhepatic 39.3
    subphrenic 39.0
  alveolus, dental 99.0
  appendix 41.0
  auditory canal, external 16.0
  auricle 16.0
  Bartholin's gland or cyst 72.0
  bile duct 43.0
  bladder 56.0
  bone 80.0
    jawbones 97.0
  breast 65.0
  bursa 88.0
  carotid gland (body) 01.9
  cervix 70.0
    to assist delivery 76.9
    to replace inverted uterus,
            postpartum 78.4
  chalazion 07.0
    with removal of capsule 07.1
  conjunctiva 08.0
  cornea 11.0
  ear, external 16.0
  endolymphatic sac 17.9
  epididymis 60.9
  esophageal web (endoscopic) 35.0
  esophagus (cervical) (endoscopic)
          (transthoracic) 35.0
  exploratory - *see* Exploration
  external site, NEC 92.0
  eyelid 07.0
  fascia 88.0
  fistula, anus 51.0
  furuncle - *see* Incision of site
  gallbladder 43.4
  glands of skin (steatoma) 92.0
  hair follicles 92.0
  hematoma (removal)
    aorta, thoracic (with graft
            implantation) 28.4
    cerebral 01.3
    ear 16.0
    epidural 01.3
    extradural 01.0
    intracranial 01.3
    laparotomy site 39.1
    ligament, broad 70.2
    meningeal 01.3
    nerve root 03.0
    pericardium 29.0
    skin or subcutaneous tissue 92.0

Incision (and drainage)—*continued*
  hematoma, etc.—*continued*
    spinal cord 03.0
    spinal meninges 03.0
    subdural 01.3
    thyroid 22.0
  hepatic duct 43.0
  hygroma
    cerebral 01.3
    epidural 01.3
    intracranial 01.3
    meningeal 01.3
    nerve root 03.0
    spinal cord 03.0
    spinal meninges 03.0
  ingrown nail 92.0
  joint structures 86.0
    jaw 97.0
  kidney 54.0
    renal pelvis 54.1
  lacrimal gland or sac 06.0
  larynx 20.0
    emergency tracheotomy 20.5
  liver 42.0
  lymph nodes 25.0
  lymphatic channels 25.0
  meibomian gland (cyst) 07.0
  mouth, floor NEC 96.9
  muscle 88.0
  nailbed or nailfold 92.0
  nerve, peripheral 04.0
  nose 19.5
  orbit - *see* category 09.0
  palate 96.6
  pancreas 44.0
  paronychia 92.0
  parotid gland 95.5
  penis 61.9
  perianal skin 51.1
  perineum, nonobstetrical 72.0
    male 92.0
  peripheral vessels 24.0
  perirectal tissue 50.1
  perirenal tissue 54.2
  peritonitis, localized 39.3
    pelvic, female 71.8
  pilonidal sinus (cyst) 52.0
  pituitary 01.3
  salivary gland 95.5
  scrotum 59.0
  Skene's duct or gland 72.0
  skin of ear 16.0
  skin or subcutaneous tissue 92.0
  spermatic cord 59.0
  sphincter or Oddi 43.0
  tendon 88.0
  tendon sheath 88.0

Incision (and drainage)—*continued*
  testis 59.0
  trachea 20.0
    emergency tracheotomy 20.5
  tunica vaginalis 59.0
  umbilicus 39.0
  ureter 55.0
  urethra 57.0
  vagina (septum) (stenosis) 71.0
    for pelvic abscess 71.8
  valve, heart 29.2
  vulva, nonobstetrical 72.0
Incudectomy 17.4
Indentation, sclera, for retinal
    reattachment 13.5
Indian operation (plastic, nose) (*see also*
    category 94.2) 19.3
Induction, surgical, labor 75.0
Inflation
  eustachian tube 17.8
Infolding, sclera, for retinal reattachment
  13.5
Infraction, turbinate 19.2
Infundibulectomy, hypophyseal 01.7
  aortic or pulmonary valves 29.2
Infusion
  intra-arterial, chemotherapy for
    neoplasm R1.6
Injection
  air, peritoneum 39.0
    anterior chamber, NEC 13.2
  breast for augmentation (silicone) 94.4
  bursa 88.9
  ganglion, sympathetic 05.2
    ciliary 12.9
  hemorrhoids 51.9
  intra-amniotic to terminate pregnancy
    74.8
  jaw structure 97.9
  lung for surgical collapse 34.5
  nerve
    peripheral 04.8
    superior laryngeal 20.9
    sympathetic 05.2
  radiopaque substance
    uvula 96.4
  renal pelvis (cyst) 54.9
  saline, intrauterine 74.8
  varices, esophagus 35.8
Insertion
  bougie
    cervix 70.9
      to assist delivery 76.9
  breast implant 65.7
    for augmentation 94.4
  cannula, nasal sinus 19.7

Insertion—*continued*
  catheter (tube)
    anterior chamber for permanent
      drainage (glaucoma)   13.2
    bile (hepatic) ducts   43.0
    bladder, indwelling   56.8
    bronchus   A4.3
    chest   32.0
    esophagus, permanent tube (silicone)
      35.6
    for intrauterine transfusion   74.1
  electronic stimulator - *see* Implant,
    implantation
  fixation device - *see* Fixation
  globe into eye socket (implant)   09.4
  Holter (Spitz-Holter) valve   02.2
  intrauterine contraceptive device   70.9
  lens, artificial, into eye, post cataract
    extraction (plastic lens)   14.7
  orbital implant   09.4
  orthodontic appliance   99.9
  pacemaker, heart   30.4
    replacement   30.5
  pack or bag
    cervix (intrauterine)   70.9
      following delivery or abortion
        78.5
      to assist delivery   76.9
    vagina   71.9
      following delivery or abortion
        78.5
  pessary
    cervix   70.9
      after delivery   78.9
      to assist delivery   76.9
Instillation
  therapeutic agent by endoscopy - *see*
    categories A4.0-A5.9
Insufflation
  fallopian tube   68.6
Intercricothyroidotomy   20.0
Interposition operation
  esophageal reconstruction (colon)
    (jejunal)
    antethorax   35.5
    intrathorax   35.4
    retrosternal   35.4
  jaw   97.6
    with bone transplant   97.5
Intimectomy - *see* Endarterectomy
Introduction - *see also* Application
  therapeutic fluid or substance, bursa
    88.9
Intubation - *see also* Catheterization and
  Insertion
  bile (hepatic) ducts   43.0

Intubation—*continued*
  eustachian tube   17.8
  lacrimal for
    dilation   06.4
    tear drainage, nose   06.3
  nasolacrimal   06.3
  small intestine   48.9
Invagination, diverticulum
  pharynx   21.7
  stomach   46.6
Inversion, intestinal diverticulum   47.2
Iridectomy   12.1
  with
    capsulectomy   14.3
    cataract extraction - *see* categories
      14.4-14.5
Iridencleisis   12.3
Iridesis   12.3
Iridocapsulectomy   14.3
Iridocyclectomy   12.1
Iridocystectomy   12.1
Iridodesis   12.3
Iridodialysis   12.2
Iridoplasty   12.3
Iridosclerectomy   12.1
Iridosclerotomy   12.0
Iridotasis   12.4
Iridotomy   12.0
Irradiation therapy - *see* categories R1.2
  and R1.3
Irrigation, endoscopic - *see* categories
  A4.0-A5.9
Irwin's muscle section   88.1
Ischiopubiotomy   80.3
Isthmectomy, thyroid   22.1
Italian operation (plastic, nose) (*see also*
  category 94.2)   19.3
Iverson operation (dermabrasion)   93.7

J

Jaboulay abdominopelvic amputation
  85.9
Jejunectomy   47.4
Jejunocecostomy   48.1
Jejunocolostomy   48.1
Jejunoileostomy   48.0
Jejunojejunostomy   48.0
  proximal to distal   47.4
Jejunorrhaphy   48.4
Jejunostomy (feeding)   47.9
Jejunotomy   47.0
Johanson operation (urethral
  reconstruction)   57.4

Jones procedure (transplant of muscle and
     tendon, foot)   88.5
  with capsulotomy - code also   86.1
Jonnesco operation (sympathectomy)
     05.1

K

Kader operation (Stamm-Kader)
     (gastrostomy)   46.4
Keegan operation (plastic, nose) (*see also*
     category 94.2)   19.3
Keen operation (omphalectomy)   39.5
Kehrer operation (mammilliplasty)   65.7
Keller (bunionectomy)   87.2
Kelly operation
  arytenoidopexy   20.4
  fixation of uterus   70.7
  plication, urethra (sphincter)   57.4
  urethroplasty   57.4
Kelly-Kennedy operation (urethroplasty)
     57.4
  with cystocele repair - code also   71.4
Keratectomy (complete) (partial)
     (superficial)   11.2
Keratocentesis for hyphema   13.1
Keratomileusis   11.4
Keratoplasty (lamellar) (penetrating)
     (nonpenetrating) (tectonic)   11.4
Keratotomy (delimiting) (posterior)   11.0
Kidner operation (excision of bone and
     fixation tendon, foot) 80.6 and 88.7
Kineplasty - *see* Amputation
King operation (arytenoidopexy)   20.4
Kirk supracondylar amputation   85.8
Kocher operation
  excision of thyroid - *see* Thyroidectomy
  excision of tongue   96.2
  gastric resection   46.2
Koerte-Ballance operation (anastomosis
     of facial nerves)   04.5
Kraske procedure (proctectomy and
     coccygectomy) 50.3 and 80.6
Krimer operation (palatoplasty) - *see*
     categories 96.5-96.6
Krukenberg below-elbow amputation
     85.2
Kuester operation (drainage, mastoid)
     17.1
Kuhnt operation (excision mucous
     membrane, sinus)   19.9
Kuhnt-Szymanowski operation (ectropion
     repair)   07.4
Kustner operation (replacement, inverted
     uterus)   70.6
  puerperal (postpartum)   78.4

L

Labbe operation (gastrotomy)   46.0
Labiectomy   72.3
Labyrinthectomy   18.0
Labyrinthotomy (transtympanic)   18.0
Lagrange operation
  sclerectomy and iridectomy 11.7 and
     12.1
  sclerectomy and iridenclesis 11.7 and
     12.3
Lambrinudi operation (arthrodesis foot)
     87.5
Laminectomy (decompression)   03.0
  with excision of herniated intervertebral
     disc   86.4
Laminography   A8.1
Laminotomy   03.0
Lane-Lannelongue operation (cranial
     decompression)   01.0
Laparorrhaphy   40.0
Laparotomy
  exploratory (pelvic)   39.1
  reopening of recent operative site
     (control of bleeding) (exploration)
     (removal of hematoma)   39.1
Laparotrachelotomy - *see* category 77.1
Laryngectomy
  complete or total   20.2
  partial   20.2
  radical   20.3
  wide field   20.3
Laryngocentesis   20.0
Laryngofissure   20.0
Laryngography   A8.7
Laryngopharyngectomy NEC   20.2
Laryngoplasty   20.4
Laryngorrhaphy   20.4
Laryngoscopy - *see* category A4.2
Laryngostomy   20.6
Laryngotomy   20.0
Laryngotracheoscopy - *see* category A4.2
Laryngotracheostomy - *see* categories
     20.5-20.6
Laryngotracheotomy   20.0
  emergency   20.5
  permanent opening   20.6
Laser beam - *see* Photocoagulation
Lash operation (repair of cervical os)
     70.5
Latzko cesarean section   77.2
Lavage
  endoscopic - *see* cagegories A4.0-A5.9
  gastric, by stomach tube - omit coding
  intestinal for renal failure   R9.3
  peritoneal   R9.3

Le Fort operation (vaginal cleisis) 71.2
Lengthening
  bone, NEC 81.9
  fascia 88.7
    hand 89.8
  heel cord 88.7
  levator palpebrae muscle 07.7
  muscle 88.6
    hand 89.7
  palate 96.5
  tendon 88.7
    hand 89.8
Leriche operation (periarterial
    sympathectomy) 05.9
Leucotomy (leukotomy) 01.4
Ligation
  adenoid 21.4
  aneurysm - see Repair, aneurysm
  artery
    carotid (cervical) (external) 26.8
      for aneurysm 26.3
    common hepatic 27.8
    for aneurysm - see Repair, aneurysm
    gastric 27.8
    hypogastric 27.8
    innominate 28.7
    intrathoracic 28.7
    middle meningeal 02.1
    peripheral 24.2
    profunda femoris 24.2
    splenic 27.8
    vertebral 26.8
  auricle, heart 29.5
  blood vessel
    esophagus 35.8
  coronary sinus 29.8
  ductus arteriosus, patent 28.4
  fallopian tube, bilateral 68.5
    remaining tube 68.5
    unilateral 68.9
  fistula, arteriovenous - see Repair,
      fistula arteriovenous
  hemorrhoids 51.3
  intra-abdominal vessels 27.8
  lymphatics (iliac) (thoracic duct) 25.5
  meningeal vessels 02.1
  spermatic cord 59.9
    varicocele 59.2
  splenic vessels 27.8
  superior longitudinal sinus 02.1
  supernumerary fingers 85.0
  thoracic duct 25.5
  tonsil 21.4
  ureter 55.9
  varices, esophageal 35.8
  vas deferens 60.2

Ligation—continued
  vein
    intrathoracic 28.9
    peripheral, except varicose 24.3
    varicose 24.4
      scrotum 59.2
    vena cava, inferior 27.8
Light coagulation - see Photocoagulation
Lipectomy, subcutaneous tissue 94.5
Lisfranc shoulder disarticulation 85.4
Litholapaxy, bladder 56.8
Lithotomy
  bile passage 43.0
  bladder (urinary) 56.0
  gallbladder 43.4
  hepatic duct 43.0
Lithotripsy, bladder 56.8
Lobectomy
  brain 01.6
  liver 42.2
  lung
    with segmental resection of adjacent
        lobes 34.3
    complete 34.3
    partial 34.2
  thyroid 22.1
Lobotomy, brain (frontal) (prefrontal)
    01.4
Longmire hepaticojejunostomy 43.2
Lorenz bifurcation, femur 80.1
Lowman operation (fascia transplant,
    abdomen) 88.7
Ludloff operation (osteotomy, foot) 80.2
Lund operation (astragalectomy) 80.6
Lymphadenotomy 25.0
Lymphangiectomy 25.2
Lymphangiography A8.6
Lymphangioplasty 25.3
Lymphangiorrhaphy 25.3
Lymphangiotomy 25.0
Lymphaticostomy 25.3
Lymphedema of limb, operation for
    excision with graft - see category 25.2
    obliteration of lymphatics 25.5
    transplantation of autogenous
        lymphatics 25.3
Lysis of adhesions - see Freeing of
    adhesions

M

Magnet extraction - see Extraction,
    foreign body by magnet
Mammectomy - see Mastectomy
Mammilliplasty 65.7

Myectomy—*continued*
  ocular (oblique) (rectus)   10.5
  levator palpebrae   07.7
Myelography (by cisternal puncture)
  A8.1
Myomectomy, uterine (cervical)   70.1
  broad ligament   70.2
Myoplasty   88.6
  hand   89.7
Myorrhaphy   88.4
  hand   89.3
Myosuture   88.4
  hand   89.3
Myotasis   88.8
  hand   89.9
Myotenoplasty   88.7
  hand   89.8
Myotenotomy   88.1
  hand   89.1
Myotomy   88.0
  for division   88.1
  hand   89.1
  ocular (rectus) (oblique)   10.4
    levator palpebrae   07.7
Myringectomy   17.3
Myringodectomy   17.3
Myringo-malleo-labyrinthopexy   18.1
Myringoplasty   17.6
Myringostapediopexy   17.5
Myringotomy   17.0

N

Narrowing, palpebral fissure   07.6
Nasolacrimal duct radiography (sinuses)
  A8.2
Needling, lens (eye)   14.0
Nephrectomy, partial (wedge)   54.4
  complete   54.5
Nephrocolopexy   54.8
Nephrocystanastomosis   54.6
Nephrolithotomy   54.0
Nephrolysis   54.9
Nephropexy (solo procedure)   54.8
  with partial nephrectomy   54.4
Nephroplasty   54.6
Nephropyeloplasty   54.6
Nephropyeloureterostomy   54.6
Nephrorrhaphy   54.6
Nephrostomy (drainage tube)   54.0
  closure   54.6
Nephrotomography   A9.2
Nephrotomy   54.0
Nephroureterectomy   54.5
Nephroureterocystectomy 54.5 and 56.3
Neurectasis, peripheral   04.7

Neurectomy
  cranial nerves   04.3
  infraorbital   04.3
  opticociliary   12.9
  peripheral   04.3
  presacral   05.1
  spinal nerves   04.3
Neurexeresis   04.3
Neuroanastomosis
  hypoglossal facial   04.5
  peripheral   04.5
  spinal
    accessory facial   04.5
    accessory hypoglossal   04.5
Neurolysis, peripheral   04.6
Neuropaxy, peripheral   04.1
Neuroplasty, peripheral   04.5
Neurorrhaphy, peripheral   04.4
Neurotomy
  acoustic   04.1
  cranial, peripheral   04.1
  glossopharyngeal   21.9
  lacrimal branch (parasympathetic)   05.0
  peripheral   04.1
  retrogasserian   04.1
  spinal, peripheral   04.1
Neurotripsy, peripheral   04.1
Nicola operation (capsulorrhaphy,
    shoulder)   87.3
Noble operation (jejunal plication)   40.2
Notched lip operation   93.1

O

Ober operations
  capsulotomy   86.1
  division of ligaments   88.1
  muscle transplant   88.5
Obliteration
  canaliculi (electrocauterization)   06.1
  cavity, bone   81.9
    jawbones   97.5
  cul-de-sac   71.7
  lymphatics   25.5
  pleura   32.5
  Skene's gland   72.3
  vagina   71.2
Obstetrical procedure
  after delivery or abortion - *see*
      categories 78.0-78.9
  antepartum - *see* categories 74.0-74.9
  assisting delivery - *see* Delivery
      procedure
  cesarean section -'*see* Cesarean section
  inducing delivery - *see* Delivery
      procedure

Pancreatectomy (total) (subtotal) (distal) 44.1
  radical   44.2
Pancreaticoduodenectomy NEC   44.1
  Cattell   44.2
  Childs   44.2
  radical   44.2
  Whipple   44.2
Pancreaticoduodenostomy   44.3
Pancreaticoenterostomy   44.3
Pancreaticogastrostomy   44.3
Pancreaticoileostomy   44.3
Pancreaticojejunostomy   44.3
Pancreatotomy (removal of calculus) 44.0
Pancreolithotomy   44.0
Panendoscopy, bladder - see category A4.6
Panhysterectomy - see Hysterectomy, total
Paquin operation (ureteroneocystostomy) 55.5
Paracentesis
  abdominal   39.4
  anterior chamber, eye   13.1
  cornea   13.1
  eye (anterior chamber)   13.1
  thoracic   32.1
  tympanum   17.0
Parathyroidectomy (complete) (partial) 22.5
  with complete thyroidectomy   22.2
Parotidectomy   95.1
Partsch operation (marsupialization, cyst) 99.2
Passot operation (size reduction, breast) 94.5
Patellapexy   81.9
Patellaplasty, NEC   81.9
Patellectomy   80.6
PCG - see Positrocephalogram
Pean operation
  hip joint amputation   85.9
  hysterectomy - see Hysterectomy
Peet operation (splanchnic resection) 05.1
Pelvic pneumography   A9.5
Pelviolithotomy   54.1
Pelvioplasty, kidney   54.6
Pelviotomy   80.3
Pelvi-ureteroplasty   54.6
Pemberton operation (acetabuloplasty) 87.0
Pereyra operation (periurethral suspension)   57.4
Perforation
  stapes footplate   17.5

Perfusion
  radioactive isotope therapy   R1.5
Pericardiectomy   29.1
Pericardiocentesis   29.0
Pericardiolysis   29.0
Pericardioplasty   29.7
Pericardiorrhaphy   29.7
Pericardiotomy   29.0
Perinectomy   72.3
  to assist delivery   76.9
Perineoplasty   72.5
Perineorrhaphy   72.5
  during postpartum   78.3
Perineotomy, nonobstetrical   72.0
  to assist delivery - see Episiotomy
Periosteotomy   80.0
  jawbones   97.0
Peritectomy   08.3
Peritomy   08.3
Peritoneocentesis   39.4
Peritoneoscopy - see category A5.3
Peritoneotomy   39.9
Peritotomy - see Peritomy
Pettit's bow back operation   97.3
Phalangectomy, partial (distal)   80.4
Pharyngectomy   21.6
Pharyngoplasty   21.7
  for cleft palate   96.5
Pharyngorrhaphy   21.7
  for cleft palate   96.5
Pharyngotomy   21.5
Phemister operation (subperiosteal onlay graft)   81.0
Phlebectomy
  intra-abdominal   27.2
  neck   26.2
  peripheral   24.3
  varicose   24.4
Phleborrhaphy
  peripheral - see categories 24.8-24.9
Phlebotomy
  base of brain   26.0
  intra-abdominal vessel   27.0
  intracranial   26.0
  intrathoracic   28.0
  neck   26.0
  peripheral vessels   24.0
Photocoagulation
  intra-ocular foreign body, for   13.6
  iris - see categories 12.1 and 12.3
  macular hole   13.6
    for retinal reattachment   13.4
  orbital lesion   09.1
  retina for reattachment   13.4
    with diathermy - code also 13.5
    for other lesions   13.6
  periphlebitis   13.6

Photocoagulation—*continued*
  retina for reattachment—*continued*
    prophylactic 13.6
Phrenemphraxis 34.5
Phrenicectomy 34.5
Phrenicoexeresis 34.5
Phrenicotomy 34.5
Phrenicotripsy 34.5
Physical medicine - *see* categories R4.0-R4.9
Physical therapy R4.1
Pinealectomy (complete) (partial) 01.8
Pinning, ear 94.0
Pirogoff below-knee amputation 85.7
Pituitectomy (complete) (partial) 01.7
Placentogram A9.4
Planing, skin (surgical) (chemical) 93.7
Plastic repair - *see also* Repair, Graft and Reconstruction of site
  auricle of ear 94.1
  breast - *see* Mammoplasty
  ear pinning 94.0
  nose by plastic surgeon 94.2
  skin - *see* categories 93.0-93.6
Plasty, bladder neck (V-Y) 56.6
Pleating
  sclera for retinal reattachment 13.5
  superior oblique tendon (eye) 10.8
Pleuracentesis 32.1
Pleurectomy 32.4
Pleurolysis (extraperiosteal) (extrapleural) (intrapleural) 34.5
Pleuropexy 32.9
Pleurotomy 32.0
Plexectomy
  choroid 02.1
  hypogastric 05.1
Plication
  diaphragm 38.1
  fascia 88.7
    hand 89.8
  intestine (jejunum) 40.2
  ligament - *see also* Repair, joint
    broad 70.7
    sacrouterine 70.7
  ocular muscle (oblique) (rectus) 10.8
  sphincter, urinary (bladder) 56.6
  tendon 88.7
    hand 89.8
  ureter 55.6
  urethra 57.4
Plombage 34.5
Pneumocentesis 34.0
Pneumoencephalography (lumbar) A8.0
Pneumography, pelvic A9.5
Pneumonectomy
  complete 34.4

Pneumonectomy—*continued*
  left - *see* categories 34.2-34.3
  partial - *see* categories 34.2-34.3
  radical 34.4
  standard 34.4
Pneumonolysis (extraperiosteal) (extrapleural) (intrapleural) 34.5
Pneumonotomy 34.0
Pneumoperitoneum 39.0
Pneumothorax, artificial (extrapleural) (intrapleural) (peritoneal) 34.5
Pollicization, thumb 89.6 and 85.0 or 85.5
Pollock disarticulation of knee 85.8
Polya operation (gastrojejunostomy) 46.2 and 46.5
Polypectomy - *see* Excision, lesion of site
Pomeroy operation (sterilization) 68.5
Poncet operation
  lengthening of Achilles tendon 88.7
  urethrostomy, perineal 57.0
Porro cesarean section - code cesarean section and hysterectomy
Positrocephalogram A9.8
Potts-Smith anastomosis (pulmonary-aortic) 28.4
Poudrage, pleura 32.5
  intrapericardial 29.8
Preparation of pedicle (tube) graft 93.4
Preputiotomy 61.0
Probing
  canaliculus, lacrimal 06.5
  lacrimal duct or sac 06.5
  lacrimonasal duct 06.5
Proctectasis 50.8
Proctectomy (abdominoperineal) (complete) (partial) (pull-through) 50.3
Proctolysis 50.0
Proctopexy 50.5
Proctoplasty 50.5
Proctorrhaphy 50.5
Proctoscopy - *see* category A4.5
Proctosigmoidectomy 50.3
Proctosigmoidopexy 50.5
Proctosigmoidoscopy - *see* category A4.5
Proctostomy 50.4
Proctotomy (with drainage) (decompression) 50.0
  for pelvic peritoneal drainage 71.8
Proctovalvotomy 50.0
Prostatectomy
  with
    bladder neck plasty - code also 56.6
    vasectomy - code also 60.1
    vesiculectomy - code also 58.5
  perineal 58.3

Prostatectomy—*continued*
  radical NEC 58.3
  retropubic 58.3
  suprapubic (transvesical) 58.1
  transurethral 58.2
Prostatocystotomy 58.0
Prostatolithotomy 58.0
Prostatotomy 58.0
Prostatovesiculectomy - *see*
  ° Prostatectomy
Provis insufflation 68.6
Psychotherapy R9.1
Pterygium operation 08.6
  with lamellar keratoplasty 08.6 and 11.4
    conjunctival graft 08.6 and 08.5
  carbolization 08.6
  dissection with reposition 08.6
  simple excision 08.2
  subepithelial excision 08.6
Ptyalectasis 95.5
Pubiotomy 80.3
  assisting delivery 76.9
Pull-through, abdomino-anal 50.3
Pulpectomy 99.5
Punch operation - *see also* Biopsy
  bladder neck, transurethral 56.1
  prostate, except biopsy - *see*
    Prostatectomy
Puncture
  antrum (bilateral) (unilateral) 19.7
  bursa 88.0
  cisternal 01.2
  cranial (exploratory) 01.2
  fontanel, anterior 01.2
  heart 29.0
  intrathoracic vessels 28.0
  iris 12.0
  joint for aspiration 86.2
    jaw 97.9
  larynx 20.0
  lumbar· R9.5
  lung 34.0
  pericardium 29.0
  peripheral vessels 24.0
  pleural cavity 32.1
  polycystic kidney 54.0
    percutaneous (needle) 54.9
  sinus, nasal 19.7
  spinal R9.5
  spleen for biopsy A1.9
  sternal, for bone marrow biopsy A2.7
Pupillotomy by light coagulation 12.3
Putti-Platt operation (capsulorrhaphy,
  shoulder) 87.3
Puusepp operation (spinal cordotomy)
  03.2

Pyelography, intravenous A9.0
  retrograde A9.1
Pyelolithotomy 54.1
Pyeloplasty 54.6
Pyeloscopy - *see* category A4.6
Pyelostomy 54.1
  closure 54.6
Pyelotomy 54.1
  with removal of tumor 54.3
Pylorectomy 46.2
Pyloromyotomy 46.1
Pyloroplasty 46.1
Pylorostomy 46.1

R

Rachicentesis R9.5
  cranial (cisternal) 01.2
Rachitomy 03.0
Radical neck dissection - *see* Dissection,
  neck, radical
Radicotomy 03.1
Radiculectomy 03.1
Radiculotomy 03.1
Radiography, contrast - *see* categories
  A8.0-A9.9
Radioisotope examination A9.8
  therapy R1.5
Radiotherapy
  deep x-radiation (high voltage) R1.1
  implantation of radium or radon R1.4
  isotope, radioactive R1.5
  megavoltage irradiation R1.2
  particle irradiation (electron) (neutron)
    (proton) R1.3
  superficial x-radiation (low voltage)
    R1.0
  supervoltage irradiation R1.2
  teleradiotherapy - *see* categories R1.1
    and R1.2
Ramisection
  jawbones 97.1
    with excision 97.3
  other bones 80.3
  sympathetic 05.0
Ramstedt operation (Fredet-Ramstedt)
  (pyloromyotomy) 46.1
Rankin operation (partial colectomy)
  47.5
Ranschoff operation (pleurotomy) 32.0
Readjustment
  pacemaker 30.5
Reamputation, stump 81.4
Reanastomosis, intestines - *see* categories
  48.0-48.2

Reattachment
  choroid and retina   13.5
    by photocoagulation   13.4
  choroid only   13.0
  extremities
    arm (above elbow)   90.3
    finger except thumb   90.0
    foot   90.4
    hand   90.2
    leg   90.5
    thumb   90.1
  ligament - *see also* Repair, joint
    uterosacral   70.7
  muscle   88.5
    hand   89.4
  retina (and choroid)   13.5
    by photocoagulation   13.4
  tendon   88.5
    hand   89.4
  tooth   99.6
Recession
  ocular muscle (oblique) (rectus)   10.6
    with resection of same muscle   10.5
  tendon   88.5
    hand   89.4
Reconstruction - *see also* Repair and
      Graft of site
  artery - *see* Graft, artery
  bladder   56.5
    with
      ileum - code also 47.4
      sigmoid - code also 47.5
  bone, NEC   81.9
  diaphragm   38.1
  ear pinning   94.0
  ear, auricle   94.1
    external auditory meatus   16.2
  eyebrow   07.4
  eyelid   07.4
  foot and toes   87.2
  hip - *see* categories 87.0-87.1
  jawbones - *see* categories 97.5-97.6
  joints - *see* categories 87.0-87.3
  lip   93.1
  lymphatic by transplantation   25.3
  mouth   93.1
  nose (*see also* category 94.2)   19.3
  operations, NEC   94.9
  ossicles (graft) (prosthesis)   17.4
  pelvic floor   71.5
  penis (skin graft)   61.4
  thumb   89.6
  trachea   20.7
  urethra (stage 1 and 2)   57.4
  vagina, artificial   71.5
  vas deferens, divided   60.9

Rectopexy   50.5
Rectoplasty   50.5
Rectosigmoidectomy
    (abdominoendorectal)   50.3
Rectostomy   50.4
Reduction
  dislocation of joint
    closed (manipulation)   87.7
      jaw   97.7
    open (with internal fixation)   87.8
      with bone grafting - *see*
          Arthroplasty
    jaw with bone block   97.5
  epistaxis   19.5
  fracture - *see also* categories 84.4-84.7
    acetabulum - *see* categories 82.6-82.9
    alveolus, jaw (socket) - *see* category
        98.6
    ankle - *see* categories 83.0-83.2
    attempted - code the subsequent
        procedure performed
    Barton's - *see* categories 83.3-83.5
    blow-out - *see* categories 98.0-98.3
        and 09.3
    clavicle - *see* categories 84.4-84.7
    Colles' - *see* categories 83.3-83.5
    elbow - *see* categories 84.0-84.3
    epiphysis, upper femur - *see*
        categories 82.0-82.1
    femur
      lower end (condyle) (knee) - *see*
          categories 84.0-84.3
      lower epiphysis (knee) - *see*
          categories 84.0-84.3
      shaft - *see* categories 84.4-84.7
      upper end (head) (hip) (neck)
          (trochanter) - *see* categories
          82.0-82.9
      upper epiphysis (hip) - *see*
          categories 82.0-82.1
    fibula
      lower end (ankle) - *see* categories
          83.0-83.2
      lower epiphysis (ankle) - *see*
          categories 83.0-83.2
      malleolus - *see* categories 83.0-83.2
      shaft - *see* categories 84.4-84.7
      upper end of fibula (knee) - *see*
          categories 84.0-84.3
      upper epiphysis (knee) - *see*
          categories 84.0-84.3
    finger - *see* categories 84.4-84.7
    foot except ankle - *see* categories
        84.4-84.7
    hip - *see* categories 82.0-82.9

Reduction—*continued*
fracture—*continued*
humerus
epiphysis (lower) (upper) - *see*
categories 84.0-84.3
lower end (articular process)
(condyle) - *see* categories
84.0-84.3
shaft - *see* categories 84.4-84.7
upper end (neck) (tuberosity) (head)
- *see* categories 84.0-84.3
intertrochanteric - *see* categories
82.2-82.5
jaw - *see* categories 98.0-98.6
wiring without reduction 97.9
knee - *see* categories 84.0-84.3
Le Fort I, II or III - *see* Reduction,
fracture, site of facial bone
malar (jaw) - *see* categories 98.0-98.1
mandible (condyle) (gonial angle) - *see*
categories 98.4-98.5
wiring without reduction 97.9
maxilla - *see* categories 98.2-98.3
nasal (closed) (open) 19.4
orbit (infra) (supra) - *see* categories
98.0-98.3 and 19.9
Pott's - *see* categories 83.0-83.2
pyramidal, jaw - *see* category 98.6
radio-ulnar - *see* categories 83.3-83.5
radius
lower end (wrist) - *see* categories
83.3-83.5
lower epiphysis (wrist) - *see*
categories 83.3-83.5
radiocarpal - *see* categories 83.3-
83.5
shaft - *see* categories 84.4-84.7
styloid process - *see* categories
83.3-83.5
upper end (elbow) (head) (neck) -
see categories 84.0-84.3
upper epiphysis (elbow) - *see*
categories 84.0-84.3
shaft of long bones - *see* categories
84.4-84.7
shoulder - *see* categories 84.0-84.3
skull - *see* categories 02.0 and 19.9
Smith's - *see* categories 83.3-83.5
spine (coccyx) (sacrum) - *see*
categories 84.4-84.7
talus except ankle - *see* categories
84.4-84.7
tibia
lower end (ankle) - *see* categories
83.0-83.2
shaft - *see* categories 84.4-84.7

Reduction—*continued*
fracture—*continued*
tibia—*continued*
upper end (knee) - *see* categories
84.0-84.3
tibiofibular - *see* categories 83.0-83.2
ulna
lower end (wrist) - *see* categories
83.3-83.5
lower epiphysis (wrist) - *see*
categories 83.3-83.5
shaft - *see* categories 84.4-84.7
upper end (coronoid) (elbow)
(olecranon) - *see* categories
84.0-84.3
upper epiphysis (elbow) - *see*
categories 84.0-84.3
vertebra - *see* categories 84.4-84.7
wrist - *see* categories 83.3-83.5
zygoma (arch) - *see* categories 98.0-
98.1
fracture-dislocation - *see* Reduction,
fracture
hemorrhoids 51.9
hernia - *see* Repair, hernia
incarcerated bowel in hernia - *see*
Repair, hernia
intussusception 48.8
malrotation
intestine 48.8
prolapse
artificial opening, intestine 48.9
colostomy 48.9
enterostomy 48.9
ileostomy 48.9
rectum (manipulation) 50.8
uterus - *see* categories 70.6, 70.7, and
70.9
separation, epiphysis (slipped) - *see*
Reduction, fracture
torsion
kidney pedicle 54.6
omentum 40.2
spermatic cord 59.9
testis (digital) (incision) 59.9
with orchiopexy 59.7
volvulus
intestine 48.8
stomach 46.9
Reefing
joint capsule 87.3
jaw 97.5
Re-entry operation, thoracic aorta 28.2
Refracture
bone for nonunion (malunion) 81.3
bone with wrench 81.3

Removal—*continued*
  foreign body—*continued*
    larynx—*continued*
      endoscopic A4.2
    liver 42.0
    lung, by incision 34.0
    mediastinum 32.2
    muscle 88.0
    nerve
      peripheral 04.0
      root 03.0
    nose 19.5
    pericardium 29.0
    perineum 72.0
    perirenal tissue 54.2
    pharynx 21.9
    pleura 32.0
      endoscopic A5.1
    rectum, by incision 50.0
      endoscopic A4.5
    scrotum 59.9
    sinus, nasal 19.7
    skin, by incision 92.0
    skull, except plate 01.0
    spermatic cord 59.9
    spinal cord 03.0
    spinal meninges 03.0
    stomach, by incision 46.0
      endoscopic A4.4
    subcutaneous tissue, by incision
      92.0
    tendon 88.0
    testis 59.9
    thorax 32.0
      endoscopic A5.1
    tonsil 21.4
    trachea, by emergency incision 20.5
      endoscopic A4.2
    tunica vaginalis 59.9
    ureter 55.0
      endoscopic A4.6
    vulva 72.0
  gallstones outside gallbladder 43.0
  granulation tissue
    cranial 02.0
    spinal process 03.4
  hair follicle 92.0
  hematoma - *see* Incision, hematoma
  hydatidiform mole 70.2
    by
      hysterectomy - code only
        hysterectomy
      hysterotomy 70.0
  impacted feces, rectum 50.9
  intrauterine contraceptive device 70.9
  lesion - *see* Excision, lesion
  mucous membranous labyrinth 18.0

Removal—*continued*
  nail 92.4
  nasal polyp 19.0
  odontoma, tooth 99.2
  osteocartilagenous loose body, joint
      structures 86.0
    jaw 97.0
  patella 80.6
    partial 80.4
  phlebolith - *see* Removal, embolus
  plate
    skull 02.0
  pterygium - *see* Pterygium operation
  redundant skin, eyelids 07.2
  remaining ovary 67.4
    tube 68.2
    tube and ovary 67.5
  remaining testis 59.5
  retained placenta, manual 78.0
    with curettage 78.1
  rhinolith 19.0
  rice bodies, tendon sheaths 88.0
  secundines, manual 78.0
    with curettage 78.1
  sequestrum 80.0
    jawbones 97.0
    nose 19.0
    skull 01.0
  suture
    cervix 70.9
  symblepharon 08.9
  thrombus - *see* Removal, embolus
  tissue, endoscopic - *code to* excision of
      the site
  tooth (multiple)
    forceps extraction 99.3
    surgical 99.4
  tube, encircling, eye 13.9
  ventricular shunt 02.4
  vitreous, opaque flake of 14.9
Renipuncture 54.0
Re-opening
  craniotomy site
    for examination 01.0
    for ventriculostomy 02.2
  laminectomy site for examination 03.0
  osteotomy site 80.0
    jawbones 97.0
  recent laparotomy site 39.1
  recent operation site, liver 42.0
  wound
    thyroid 22.0
Repair - *see also* Graft, grafting
  alveolus 99.7
  anal sphincter 51.6
    postpartum 78.3

Repair—*continued*
  hernia—*continued*
    esophageal hiatus—*continued*
      thoracic route   38.1
    femoral (extraperitoneal)   38.4
      recurrent   38.5
    incisional   38.6
    inguinal   38.2
      recurrent   38.3
    internal   38.9
    ischiatic   38.9
    ischiorectal   38.9
    lumbar   38.9
    obturator   38.9
    paraesophageal   38.0
    parahiatal   38.0
    parasternal   38.1
    perineal (enterocele)   38.9
      for rectal prolapse   50.5
    sciatic   38.9
    spigelian   38.7
    umbilical   38.8
    ventral   38.6
  hydrocele
    spermatic cord   59.1
    tunica vaginalis   59.1
  hypospadias   61.4
  ileostomy   48.3
  ingrown toenail   92.4
  joint (capsule)   87.3
    foot (metatarsals)   87.2
    hallux valgus   87.2
    hip - *see* categories 87.0-87.1
    jaw - *see* categories 97.5-97.6
    toe(s)   87.2
  kidney   54.6
  laceration
    skin   92.5
  laceration, obstetrical, during
      postpartum
    cervix   78.2
    perineal (1st, 2nd, 3rd degree)   78.3
    uterus   78.2
    vagina   78.3
  lacrimal apparatus   06.4
  larynx   20.4
  ligament - *see also* Repair, joint
    broad   70.6
  lip - *see* categories 92.5 and 93.1
  liver   42.3
  meninges
    cerebral   02.1
    spinal   03.4
  meningocele
    cranial   02.1
    spinal   03.4
  mouth - *see* categories 93.1 and 96.0-
      96.9

Repair—*continued*
  musculotendinous cuff, shoulder   88.4
  nasopharynx atresia   21.7
  nose   19.3
  orbit   09.3
  ovary   67.6
  pacemaker, heart   30.5
  palate, except cleft   96.6
  pelvic floor   72.5
    during postpartum   78.3
  penis   61.4
  pericardium   29.7
  perineum   72.5
  peritoneum   40.2
  pharynx   21.7
  plastic - *see* Repair of site
    open wound without skin graft   92.5
  prolapsed rectal mucosa   50.5
  ptosis, eyelid   07.7
  rectocele   71.4
  rectum   50.5
  retina (and choroid)   13.5
  salivary gland or duct   95.5
  sclera   11.8
  scrotum   59.6
  sinus, nasal   19.9
  spermatic cord   59.6
  spina bifida   03.4
  spinal cord   03.4
  spleen   45.2
  stoma, artificial, intestines   48.3
  stomach   46.6
  synovial membrane, joint - *see* Repair,
      joint
  testis   59.6
  tetralogy of Fallot
    anastomosis (shunt)
      aortopulmonary   28.4
      subclavian-pulmonary   28.4
    correction of septal defect - *see*
      categories 29.5-29.6
    valvulotomy, pulmonary   29.2
  thymus gland   23.0
  tooth - *see* categories 99.6-99.9
  trachea   20.8
  tunica vaginalis   59.6
  tympanum - *see* categories 17.6-17.7
  ureter   55.6
  urethra   57.4
  urethrocele   71.4
  uterus   70.6
    following delivery or abortion   78.2
  uvula   96.4
  vagina - *see* categories 71.3-71.5
    during postpartum   78.3
  vaginal wall   71.3

Repair—*continued*
  vaginal wall—*continued*
    for
      cystocele 71.4
      hernia 71.4
      rectocele 71.4
      urethrocele 71.4
    varicocele 59.2
    vas deferens 60.9
    ventricular septal defect 29.5
      with prosthetic device 29.6
    vertebral arch defect (spina bifida)
        03.4
    vulva 72.5
    wound without skin graft 92.5
Replacement
  bladder with ileal loop 56.5 and 47.4
    with sigmoid (colonic loop) 56.5 and
        47.5
  femoral head by prosthesis 87.1
  graft - *see* Graft, grafting
  heart - *see* category 29.9
  heart valve - *see* categories 29.3-29.4
  inverted uterus, postpartum (puerperal)
        78.4
    hydrostatic, postpartum 78.4
    manual, postpartum 78.4
    nonobstetrical (chronic) 70.6
  iris 12.3
  pacemaker, heart 30.5
  testis in scrotum (Note - error in
        Tabular List of inclusions) 59.7
    abdomen 59.6
  umbilical cord 76.9
  ureter
    with bladder flap 55.5 and 55.1
    with ileal segment, implanted into
        bladder 55.5 and 55.1 and 47.4
  valve, heart - *see* categories 29.3-29.4
  vitreous 14.9
    for retinal reattachment 13.5
Replantation - *see* Reimplantation
Reposition, cilia base 07.4
Resection - *see also* Excision of site
  aneurysm - *see* Aneurysmectomy
  artery, intrathoracic 28.7
    aorta, thoracic 28.4
    pulmonary 28.4
  bladder neck - *see* categories 56.1-56.2
  bladder, urinary (complete) (partial)
        56.3
    endoscopic 56.1
    local resection of lesion - *see*
        categories 56.1-56.2
    wedge resection 56.1
  bone 80.4
    jawbones 97.3

Resection—*continued*
  bronchus (en bloc) (wide sleeve) 33.4
  bursa 88.3
  cecum 47.5
  chest wall 32.9
  colon, partial 47.5
    anterior for neoplasm 47.5
      for prolapsed rectum 50.3
    complete 47.6
    sigmoid 47.5
  conjunctiva for pterygium - *see*
        Pterygium operation
  esophagus 35.2
  exteriorized intestine 47.3
  fascia 88.3
    hand 89.2
  gallbladder 43.5
  infundibular 29.2
  intestine, small 47.4
  joint structure NEC 86.9
    jaw 97.4
  kidney (wedge) 54.4
  levator palpebrae muscle (with
        advancement)   07.7
  ligament 86.9
  lip (wedge) 92.1
  liver 42.2
  lung, segmental (basilar) (superior)
        (wedge) 34.2
  Meckel's diverticulum 47.4
  mesentery 39.9
  muscle 88.3
    hand 89.2
  nasal septum 19.1
  nerve
    lacrimal branch 05.1
    peripheral 04.3
    phrenic 34.5
    sympathetic 05.1
  nose, for removal of lesion 19.0
  ocular muscle 10.5
    levator palpebrae 07.7
    oblique (inferior) (superior) 10.5
    orbicularis 07.2
    rectus (lateral) (medial) (superior)
        (inferior) 10.5
  ovary, partial (wedge) 67.1
  palate except cleft 96.6
  pancreas 44.1
    radical 44.2
  pelvic viscera, en masse, female 69.7
    male 56.3
  penis 61.3
  pharynx 21.6
  prostate, transurethral 58.2
    other - *see* Prostatectomy
  rectosigmoid (pull-through) 50.3

Suture—*continued*
  artery—*continued*
    peripheral NEC 24.9
      division and end-to-end suture
        24.8
  bile duct 43.3
  bladder 56.6
  breast (skin) 65.7
  bronchus 33.5
  canaliculus 06.4
  cervix 70.6
    during postpartum 78.2
  cleft palate 96.5
  conjunctiva 08.4
  cornea (with air injection) 11.3
  cul-de-sac 71.7
  ear, external 16.3
  esophagus 35.6
  eyeball 10.2
  eyebrow 07.3
  eyelid 07.3
  face 92.5
  fascia 88.4
    hand 89.3
    to skeletal attachment 88.7
      hand 89.8
  ganglion
    sympathetic 05.9
  gum 99.1
  heart 29.7
  hepatic duct 43.3
  intestine (injury) (perforation) (rupture) 48.4
  kidney 54.6
  larynx 20.4
  ligament 87.3
    broad 70.6
    Cooper's 71.5
    foot and toes 87.2
    jaw 97.5
    knee 87.3
    other - *see* Repair, joint
    sacrouterine 71.5
  lip 92.5
  liver 42.3
  mesentery 40.2
  mouth 96.9
  muscle 88.4
    hand 89.3
  nerve
    peripheral 04.4
    sympathetic 05.9
  nose
    external 19.3
    internal (for epistaxis) 19.5
  ovary 67.6
  palate, except cleft 96.6

Suture—*continued*
  palpebral fissure 07.6
  pancreas 44.9
  peptic ulcer, perforated 46.6
  pericardium 29.7
  perineum, female 72.5
    during postpartum 78.3
    male 92.5
  peritoneum 40.0
  pharynx 21.7
    that for cleft palate 96.5
  rectum 50.5
  retina for reattachment 13.5
  salivary gland 95.5
  sclera 11.8
  scrotum (skin) 59.6
  secondary
    abdominal wall 40.1
    peritoneum 40.1
  skin (mucous membrane) 92.5
    breast 65.7
    ear 16.2
    eyebrow 07.4
    eyelid 07.4
    nose 19.3
    penis 61.4
    scrotum 59.6
    vulva 72.5
  spermatic cord 59.6
  spleen 45.2
  stomach 46.6
  tendon (end-to end) 88.4
    hand 89.3
    to skeletal attachment 88.7
      hand 89.8
  testis 59.6
  tongue 96.3
  trachea 20.8
  tunica vaginalis 59.6
  ulcer, perforated duodenal 48.4
  ureter 55.6
  urethra 57.4
  uterus 70.6
    during postpartum 78.2
  uvula 96.4
  vagina 71.3
    during postpartum 78.3
  vas deferens 60.9
  vein
    intra-abdominal 27.8
    intrathoracic 28.9
    peripheral 24.9
  venous injuries
    iliac 27.8
    peripheral - *see* categories 24.8-24.9
    vena cava, inferior 27.8

Suture — *continued*
 vulva 72.5
  during postpartum 78.3
Sweep, anterior iris 12.5
Sweet pyloroplasty 46.1
Swenson operation
 bladder reconstruction 56.5
 proctectomy 50.3
Swinney operation (urethral
   reconstruction) 57.4
 with cystostomy - code also 56.0
Syme operation
 amputation at ankle 85.6
Sympathectomy
 cervical 05.1
 lumbar 05.1
 periarterial 05.9
 renal 05.1
 tympanum 17.9
Sympatheticotripsy 05.0
Symphysiotomy 76.9
 kidney 54.6
Symphysis, pleural 32.5
Synchondrotomy 86.1
 temporomandibular 97.4
Syndesis - *see* Arthrodesis
Synechiotomy 12.5
Synovectomy, joint 86.6
 jaw 97.4
Syringing
 lacrimal sac 06.9
 lacrimonasal duct 06.9
  with dilation 06.5

T

Taarnhoj operation (trigeminal nerve root
   decompression) 04.0
Take-down - *see* Removal and Revision
Talma-Morison operation (omentopexy)
   40.2
Tamponade
 intrauterine (intracervical) 70.9
  following delivery or abortion 78.5
  to assist delivery 76.9
 vaginal 71.9
  following delivery or abortion 78.5
Tap
 abdomen 39.4
 chest 32.1
 cisternal 01.2
 joint 86.2
  jaw 97.9
 spinal R9.5
 subdural 01.2
Tarsal rotation operation, eyelid 07.4

Tarsectomy 07.2
Tarsoplasty 07.4
Tarsorrhaphy 07.3
Tattooing
 cornea (chemical) (lamellar) (mechanical)
   11.5
Tautening eyelid for entropion 07.4
Tendon loop operation, hand 89.4
Tenectomy 88.3
 hand 89.2
 ocular 10.5
  levator palpebrae 07.7
Tennison (repair of cleft lip) 93.1
Tenodesis 88.7
 hand 89.8
Tenolysis 88.9
 hand 89.9
Tenoplasty 88.7
 hand 89.8
Tenorrhaphy - *see* Suture, tendon
Tenosuture - *see* Suture, tendon
Tenosynovectomy 88.3
 hand 89.2
Tenotomy 88.1
 hand 89.1
 levator palpebrae 07.7
 ocular (bridled) (controlled) (free) 10.4
  levator palpebrae 07.7
 scalenus muscle 88.1
Tensing, orbicularis oculi 07.4
Termination of pregnancy
 by
  dilation and curettage 74.7
  hysterectomy 74.6
  hysterotomy 74.6
  intra-amniotic injection 74.8
  other 74.9
Thalamectomy (cryosurgery) 01.5
Thalamotomy 01.5
Theleplasty 65.7
Therapy
 blind rehabilitation R4.8
 cancer, NEC R1.9
 chemotherapy for cancer R1.6
 educational R4.5
 electroconvulsive R9.0
 hormone for cancer R1.8
 insulin shock R9.0
 isotope, radioactive R1.5
 manual arts R4.4
 occupational R4.3
 physical R4.1
 psychotherapy R9.1
 radiation - *see* catègories R1.0-R1.3
 radium (radon) R1.4
 recreation R4.7
 rehabilitation, NEC R4.9

Tuffier operation—*continued*
   vaginal hysterectomy 69.4
Tunnel, subcutaneous, antethorax - *see*
   categories 35.5-35.6
Turbinectomy (complete) (partial) 19.2
Tympanectomy 17.1
Tympanoplasty - *see* categories 17.6-17.7
   type I 17.6
   type II, III, IV, V 17.7
Tympanosympathectomy 17.9
Tympanotomy 17.0

U

Ultrafiltration - *see* Hemodialysis
Umbilectomy 39.5
Undercutting of hair follicle 92.0
Uptake of radioactive iodine examination
   (with scan) A9.8
Uranoplasty - *see* categories 96.5-96.6
Uranorrhaphy - *see* categories 96.5-96.6
Urban operation (extended radical
   mastectomy) 65.6
Ureterectomy 55.1
Ureterocecostomy 55.3
Ureterocolostomy 55.3
Ureterocystostomy 55.5
Ureteroenterostomy 55.3
Ureteroileostomy
   external diversion (ileostomy) 55.2 and
      47.4
   internal diversion only 55.3
Ureterolithotomy 55.0
Ureterolysis 55.8
Ureteroneocystostomy 55.5
Ureteropexy 55.6
Ureteroplasty 55.6
Ureteroplication 55.6
Ureteroproctostomy 55.3
Ureteropyelography, intravenous A9.0
   retrograde A9.1
Ureteropyelostomy 54.6
Ureterorrhaphy 55.6
Ureteroscopy - *see* category A4.6
Ureterosigmoidostomy 55.3
Ureterostomy (cutaneous) (external) (ileal)
   (tube) 55.2
Ureterostomy-in-situ, tube drainage 55.2
Ureterotomy 55.0
Ureteroureterostomy 55.5
   division with end-to-end anastomosis
      55.5
   excision with end-to-end anastomosis
      55.1
Urethrocystography, retrograde A9.3

Urethrocystopexy (Note - cancel category
   56.7 in Tabular List) 57.4
Urethrolithotomy 57.0
Urethrolysis 57.9
Urethropexy 57.4
Urethroplasty 57.4
Urethrorrhaphy 57.4
Urethroscopy - *see* category A4.6
   for control of hemorrhage of prostate
      58.9
Urethrostomy 57.0
Urethrotomy, external 57.0
   internal (endoscopic) 57.9
Urography (antegrade) (intravenous)
   (retrograde) A9.2
Uteropexy 70.7
Uvulectomy 96.4
Uvulotomy 96.4

V

Vacuum extraction 76.3
Vagectomy, subdiaphragmatic 46.8
Vaginectomy 71.2
Vaginofixation 71.5
Vaginoperineotomy 71.0
Vaginoplasty 71.5
Vaginorrhaphy 71.3
Vaginoscopy - *see* category A4.7
Vaginotomy 71.0
   for pelvic abscess 71.8
Vagotomy (gastric) 46.8
Valvotomy (aortic) (mitral) (pulmonary)
   29.2
Valvulectomy - *see* categories 29.2-29.4
Valvuloplasty - *see* categories 29.2-29.4
Valvulotomy 29.2
Varicocelectomy, spermatic cord 59.2
Varicotomy, peripheral vessels 24.0
Vasectomy 60.1
Vasoligation 60.2
   gastric 27.8
Vasotomy 60.2
Vasovasotomy 60.9
Veau operation
   repair of cleft lip 93.1
   repair of cleft palate 96.5
Venectomy
   intra-abdominal 27.2
   neck 26.2
   peripheral 24.3
   varicose 24.4
Venipuncture
   base of brain 26.0
   intracranial 26.0
   neck 26.0

Venipuncture—*continued*
peripheral vessels   24.0
Venisection, peripheral vessels   24.0
Venography   A8.6
dural sinus   A8.3
extremity   A8.5
intraosseous   A8.6
mesenteric   A8.6
Venotomy, peripheral   24.0
intra-abdominal   27.0
intrathoracic   28.0
Venovenostomy
base of brain   26.7
intra-abdominal   27.7
intracranial   26.7
intrathoracic   28.8
neck   26.7
peripheral   24.8
Ventriculocisternostomy (by tube)   02.2
Ventriculocordectomy   20.2
Ventriculography   A8.0
Ventriculopuncture   01.2
Ventriculoseptopexy   29.5
Ventriculoseptoplasty   29.5
with prosthetic device   29.6
Ventriculostomy   02.2
Ventrofixation   70.7
Ventrosuspension   70.7
Verneuil operation (iliac colostomy)   47.8
Version, obstetrical
combined (internal and external)   75.2
external   75.1
internal (combined) (cephalic) (podalic)   75.2
Vesicolithotomy (suprapubic)   56.0
Vesicourethroplasty   56.6
Vesiculectomy   58.5
Vesiculotomy   58.5
Vestibuloplasty, dental   99.8
Vestibulotomy   18.0
Vicq d'Azyr operation (laryngotomy)   20.0
Vidal operation (ligation for varicocele)   59.2
Vidianectomy   05.1
Villusectomy   86.3
Vineberg (mammary artery implantation)   29.8
Voice training   R4.6
Vulvectomy   72.3
V-Y operation
eyelid   07.3

W

Wagner operation (cranioplasty)   02.0

Ward-Mayo operation (hysterectomy and pelvic floor repair)   69.4
Wardrop operation - *see* Repair, aneurysm
Waters cesarean section   77.2
Webster (Baldy) suspension   70.7
Weir operation (appendicostomy)   41.2
Weir operation (correction of nostrils)   94.2
Wertheim's operation   69.3
Wharton-Jones operation (cicatricial eyelid repair)   07.3
Wheeler operation (entropion repair)   07.4
Whipple operation (resection) (modified) (pancreas)   44.2
Whitehead operation
excision of hemorrhoids   51.3
Wieting operation (femoral vein to artery anastomosis)   24.8
Wilms operation (thoracoplasty)   34.5
Window operation
antrum   19.7
maxillary   19.6
aortic   28.4
bone cortex   80.0
jawbones   97.9
Winiwarter operation (cholecystoenterostomy)   43.6
Wiring
aneurysm - *see also* Suture, aneurysm
hypogastric   27.4
subclavian, thoracic   28.2
dental - *see* categories 98.0-98.6
mandible fracture without reduction   97.9
Witzel operation (gastrostomy)   46.4
Wood operation
cystoplasty   56.6
herniorrhaphy - *see* Repair, hernia
Wullstein operation (tympanoplasty)   17.7
Wyeth hip joint amputation   85.9

X

X-radiation therapy, superficial   R1.0
deep   R1.1
X-ray
contrast - *see* Radiography, contrast
diagnostic without injection of radiopaque substance - omit coding
therapeutic - *see* Therapy

Y

Young operation
  repair of epispadias   61.4
Yount procedure (division of iliotibial
        band)   88.1

Z

Ziegler operation (pupil formation by
        iridectomy)   12.1
Zonolysis - *see* category   14.5
Z-plasty
  eyelid   07.3
    epicanthus   07.6
  other relaxing - *see* category   93.0

THE STORY OF

ARCHAEOLOGY

on
below